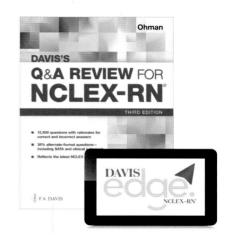
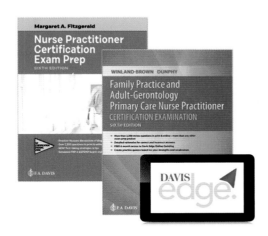

SEVENTH EDITION

Family Health Care Nursing

Theory, Practice, and Research

Melissa Robinson, PhD, RN
Professor and Division Chair
University of Providence
Great Falls, Montana

Deborah Padgett Coehlo, PhD, C-PNP, PMHS, CFLE
Developmental and Behavioral Specialist/Certified Pediatric
  Nurse Practitioner and Pediatric Mental Health Specialist
Juniper Ridge Developmental and Behavioral Pediatrics
Faculty
Oregon State University–Cascades
Bend, Oregon

Paul S. Smith, PhD, RN, CNE
Associate Dean of Nursing and Associate Professor
Linfield University–Good Samaritan School of Nursing
Portland, Oregon

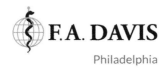

F.A. DAVIS

Philadelphia

F. A. Davis Company
1915 Arch Street
Philadelphia, PA 19103
www.fadavis.com

Printed in the United States of America

Last digit indicates print number: 10 9 8 7 6 5 4 3 2 1

Acquisitions Editor: Jacalyn Sharp
Manager of Project and eProject Management: Catherine H. Carroll
Senior Content Project Manager: Christine M. Abshire
Art and Design Manager: Carolyn O'Brien

As new scientific information becomes available through basic and clinical research, recommended treatments and drug therapies undergo changes. The author(s) and publisher have done everything possible to make this book accurate, up to date, and in accord with accepted standards at the time of publication. The author(s), editors, and publisher are not responsible for errors or omissions or for consequences from application of the book, and make no warranty, expressed or implied, in regard to the contents of the book. Any practice described in this book should be applied by the reader in accordance with professional standards of care used in regard to the unique circumstances that may apply in each situation. The reader is advised always to check product information (package inserts) for changes and new information regarding dose and contraindications before administering any drug. Caution is especially urged when using new or infrequently ordered drugs.

Library of Congress Cataloging-in-Publication Data

Names: Robinson, Melissa, author. | Coehlo, Deborah Padgett, author. |
    Smith, Paul S. (Associate professor of nursing), author.
Title: Family health care nursing: theory, practice, and research /
    Melissa Robinson, Deborah Padgett Coehlo, Paul S. Smith.
Description: Seventh edition. | Philadelphia: F.A. Davis, [2022] |
    Includes bibliographical references and index.
Identifiers: LCCN 2021030479 (print) | LCCN 2021030480 (ebook) | ISBN
    9781719642965 (paperback) | ISBN 9781719646697 (ebook)
Subjects: MESH: Family Nursing | Family Health | Family
Classification: LCC RT120.F34 (print) | LCC RT120.F34 (ebook) | NLM WY
    159.5 | DDC 610.73--dc23
    LC record available at https://lccn.loc.gov/2021030479
    LC ebook record available at https://lccn.loc.gov/2021030480

Dedication

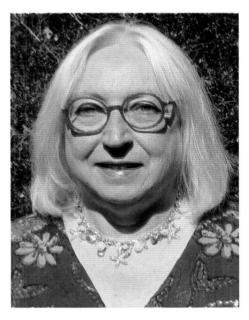

Dr. Joanna Rowe Kaakinen, PhD, RN, recently retired from a stellar career in nursing after many years specializing in nursing education. Dr. Kaakinen assumed the role of lead editor for the fourth, fifth, and sixth editions of Family Health Care Nursing: Theory, Practice, and Research, *from Dr. Shirley May Harmon Hanson, a pioneer in family nursing. Dr. Kaakinen carried on the work with renewed energy and tireless dedication until her retirement.*

Countless family nursing scholars, faculty members, nursing students, and families, both nationally and internationally, have been positively affected by the contributions of Dr. Hanson and Dr. Kaakinen. Their commitment and passion for family nursing is reflected in the work of this textbook to advance family nursing science, knowledge, and theory.

In the late 1980s, Dr. Hanson was teaching at Oregon Health and Science University when she recognized the need for a comprehensive nursing text that specifically focused student learning on the health needs of the whole family in all specialty aspects of nursing practice. Thus, the first edition of Family Health Care Nursing: Theory, Practice, and Research *was published in 1991. The book received the* American Journal of Nursing Book of the Year Award *in its category for both the 2005 and 2015 editions, and for the Community and Public Health category in 2018.*

We are grateful for the work Dr. Kaakinen did throughout her career in nursing and nursing education. It is our honor to carry on the legacy of family nursing knowledge, research, and nursing care that Dr. Hanson and Dr. Kaakinen have left.

—With fondness and gratitude, Melissa, Debbie, and Paul

Overview of The Seventh Edition

Individuals often share a variety of emotions and details when they describe significant experiences that affected one of their family members, their own lives, or their entire families. Every person in the family is influenced by her or his own individual experience and by the structure, function, and processes within the family. People who have little interaction with their families of origin may still be influenced by their family experiences. The value of relationships within families and the impact they have on individual and family function over the course of their lives have been studied extensively in a variety of disciplines, including nursing.

Working in partnership with families to identify what they need to support their health and how they navigate the health care system has become more important than ever. It has also become critical to understand the unique circumstances of individuals and families in their communities. The social determinants of health have a significant influence on every person and family and on their health, no matter where they live or what their background. When families access the health care system, they may be experiencing stress and/or trauma or they may be in crisis, and they need nurses' understanding, knowledge, and guidance.

The purpose of this book is to provide nursing students as well as practicing nurses with the understanding, knowledge, and guidance to practice family nursing in any setting and across the life span. Since the last edition, there have been changes in families, family health, health policy, and the environment, all of which affect the health of families. Each chapter reflects those changes with current, evidence-based information.

Use of the Book

Family Health Care Nursing: Theory, Practice, and Research, Seventh Edition, is organized so that it can be used on its own to structure a course in family nursing. An alternative approach for the use of this text is for students to purchase the book at the beginning of their program of study so that specific chapters can be assigned for specialty courses throughout the curriculum. For example, Chapter 7, "Family Health Promotion," and Chapter 19, "Families and Population Health," could be used for teaching courses in public health nursing; Chapter 16, "Family Nursing in Acute-Care Adult Settings," could be studied during a pediatric course or in conjunction with a concept-based curriculum for chronic illness and acute-care courses. In graduate programs, specific chapters such as Chapter 4, "Families and Health Policy," or Chapter 9, "Genomics and Family Nursing Across the Life Span," may be relevant for a specific course. The textbook could be integrated throughout the undergraduate or graduate nursing curriculum.

While it is true that the United States and Canada have different health care systems, families in North America are very similar based on what they need to promote their health and achieve healthy outcomes. Each of the chapters in this edition includes information on trends, statistical data, research findings, evidence-based interventions, and programs and resources in the community that are family-centered for both Canada and the United States.

New in the Seventh Edition

Chapter 6, "Environmental Health and Families," is a new chapter that applies the Ecological Systems Theory of population health to human health, with human health at the center of multiple intersecting influences including behavior, social, family, community, living and working conditions, and the broader influences of national or global factors. Environmental justice and environmental literacy are examined as key issues affecting family health. Chapter 13, "Relational Nursing and Family Nursing in Canada," was moved from the online resources in the sixth edition to the print textbook for this edition due to the importance of developing strong relationships as nurses work directly with families to identify their needs and support their health. Practice and reflection questions have been added to every case study in this edition. The questions are designed to help nursing students develop their ability to reflect on their practice of working with families and to challenge their own assumptions, beliefs, and biases.

Structure of This Book

The book is divided into three units. Unit 1, "Foundations in Family Health Care Nursing," which includes Chapters 1 to 6; Unit 2, "Families Across the Health Continuum," which includes Chapters 7 to 13; and Unit 3, "Nursing Care of Families in Clinical Areas," which includes Chapters 14 to 19. Each chapter begins with the critical concepts to be addressed within that chapter. The purpose of placing the critical concepts at the beginning of the chapter is to focus the reader's thinking and learning and offer a preview and outline of what is to come. Another organizing framework for the book is presented in Chapter 2, "Theoretical Foundations for the Nursing of Families." This chapter covers the importance of using theory to guide the nursing of families and presents five theoretical perspectives; it also includes a case study demonstrating how to apply these five theoretical approaches in practice. These three family nursing theories—Family Systems Theory, Developmental and Family Life Cycle Theory, and Bioecological Theory—are threaded throughout the book and are applied in many of the chapter case studies. Most of the chapters include two case studies, and many of the case studies contain family genograms and ecomaps.

Resources

The *Family Health Care Nursing Active Classroom Instructor's Guide* is an online faculty guide that provides assistance to faculty members teaching family nursing or the nursing care of families in a variety of settings. Instructors will also find PowerPoint presentations, test bank questions for each chapter, and suggested answers for the practice and reflection questions in the case studies.

The references, answers to the NCLEX®-style questions in the appendix, and the Friedman Family Assessment Model are available to students and instructors on fadavis.com.

UNIT 1

"Foundations in Family Health Care Nursing"

Chapter 1, "Family Health Care Nursing: An Introduction," provides foundational information that is essential to understanding families and family nursing. The chapter introduces dimensions of family nursing and defines the terms *family*, *family health*, and *healthy families*. The chapter follows with an explanation of family health care nursing and the nature of interventions in the nursing care of families, along with the four approaches to family nursing: context, client, system, and component of society. The chapter presents the concepts or variables that influence family nursing, family nursing roles, and obstacles to family nursing practice, and offers an introduction to understanding family structure, family functions, and family processes.

Chapter 2, "Theoretical Foundations for the Nursing of Families," lays the theoretical groundwork needed to practice family nursing. A background for why nurses should understand the interactive relationships among theory, practice, and research is provided. It also makes the point that no single theory adequately describes the complex relationships of family structures, functions, and processes. The chapter introduces three theoretical/conceptual models specific to family nursing: Family Systems Theory, Developmental and Family Life Cycle Theory, and Bioecological Theory. Using a family case study, the chapter explores how each of the three theories could be used to assess and plan interventions for a family. This approach enables learners to see how different interventions are derived from different theoretical perspectives.

Chapter 3, "Family Demography," provides nurses with a basic contextual orientation to the demographics of families and health. This chapter examines changes and variations in North American families in order to understand what these changes portend for family health care nursing. The subject matter of the chapter is structured to provide family nurses with background on changes in the North American family so that they can understand their patient populations. The chapter provides some trends on demographic patterns that influence family nursing.

Chapter 4, "Families and Health Policy," explores the complex factors influencing health policy and family health. The roles that nurses play in providing care within a framework of family nursing and in multiple sociopolitical contexts are integrated throughout the chapter. Specifically, key theoretical models guide family policies that intersect with social, economic, political, cultural, and environmental factors. Health outcomes are examined in the context of social health determinants, family policy, and the educational and advocacy role of nurses that enhance development and positive health outcomes. A case study is used to demonstrate the role of the nurse in advocating for family-centered policies. At the completion of this chapter, nurses will have developed a broad understanding of family policy and how it can contribute to or mitigate poor health outcomes.

Chapter 5, "Family Nursing Assessment and Intervention," presents a systematic approach for developing a plan of action for the family, *with* the family, to address its most pressing needs. This chapter is built on the traditional nursing process model to create a dynamic, systematic family nursing assessment approach. Assessment strategies include selecting assessment instruments, determining the need for interpreters, assessing for health literacy, building on family strengths, and learning how to diagram family genograms and ecomaps. The chapter also explores ways to involve families in shared decision making and explores analysis, a critical step in the family nursing process that helps focus the nurse and the family on identification of the family's primary concern(s). The chapter uses a family case study as an exemplar to demonstrate the family nursing assessment and intervention.

Chapter 6, "Environmental Health and Families," addresses various aspects of environmental health and their impact on family health. Environmental health topics are presented within the scope of public health nursing, although the concepts discussed in this chapter provide background information to any area of nursing practice, with interventions designed to address a family's health being affected at the individual family level or at the community/population level. Topics include various types of environmental pollution and climate change; the impact of natural disasters; chemical, physical, and biological hazards; food safety; and more. Environmental justice issues are identified, and the role of the nurse as a family health advocate and the importance of advancing environmental health literacy are explored.

UNIT 2

"Families Across the Health Continuum"

Chapter 7, "Family Health Promotion," examines family health and family health promotion from the perspective of health equity. The chapter authors contextualize the definition of family through an equity lens and discuss the application of theoretical frameworks in nursing care for diverse families with attention to social determinants of health. Strategies for promoting family health are discussed with a focus on family assessment and promoting health through empowerment. The chapter applies the Bioecological Systems Model to promote health equity at multiple levels and to promote understanding of the determinants of health using the Integrated Life Course and Social Determinants Model of Aboriginal Health.

Chapter 8, "Nursing Care of LGBTQ+ Families," focuses on families with LGBTQ+ members who are working to achieve the same socially prescribed functions of all families and to rear responsible and independent children, provide emotional and instrumental support to one another, and provide family member health care across the life span. Nurses care for families with members with unique gender identities, sexual orientations, and family structures in a variety of settings and circumstances with increasing visibility and frequency. The purpose of this chapter is to provide nurses with an evidence-based foundation and to facilitate the delivery of culturally competent family nursing care, thus decreasing health risks and disparities among this vulnerable population. In this chapter, historical, political, sociocultural, religious, and economic contexts that influence the meaning of gender, gender identities, and gender expressions are explored. Language and social ideas about gender are always evolving. Therefore, information regarding terms and pronouns is presented to assist nurses in using correct terminology to create safe and respectful dialogue from the position of learner when caring for LGBTQ+ individuals and their families. The chapter presents

LGBTQ+ family structures and family processes that are unique to LGBTQ+ families and explores them across the life span. Health challenges and disparities in LGBTQ+ families are also presented using a life span approach. A case study demonstrates evidence-based family nursing practice. The acronym LGBTQ+ has been used throughout this textbook to represent individuals who identify as lesbian, gay, bisexual, transgender, questioning, and "plus," which represents other sexual identities that don't identify as straight or cisgender.

Chapter 9, "Genomics and Family Nursing Across the Life Span," describes nursing responsibilities for families of persons who have or who are at risk for having genetic conditions. The ability to apply an understanding of genetics in the care of families is a priority for nurses and for all health care providers. As a result of genomic research and the rapidly changing body of knowledge regarding genetic influences on health and illness, more emphasis has been placed on involving all health care providers, including family nurses, in this field. Genetic conditions are lifelong, so families living with genetic conditions need ongoing care and support. These responsibilities are described for nurses working with individuals and families across the life span. The goal of the chapter is to describe the relevance of genetic information within families when there is a question about genetic aspects of health or disease for family members. The chapter begins with a brief introduction to genomics and genetics and then goes on to explain how families react to finding out they are at risk for genetic conditions and how they decide and with whom to disclose genetic information. The critical aspect of confidentiality is then discussed. The chapter outlines the components of conducting a genetic assessment and history and offers interventions that include education and resources. Several specific case examples and a detailed case study illustrate nurses working with families that have a member(s) with a genetic condition.

Chapter 10, "Families Living With Chronic Illness," describes ways for nurses to think about the impact of chronic illness on families and to consider strategies for helping families manage chronic illness. The chapter begins with the importance of integrating ethnoculture in family health care and the impact of chronic illness on family life. Four theoretical approaches are introduced for assisting nurses to think about the best way to assist the family living with chronic illness. The rest of the chapter captures a variety of possible nursing actions to assist these families. Two case studies are presented in this chapter: one family who has a member living with type 1 diabetes and another family helping an older parent and grandparent managing Parkinson's disease. Although every family and illness experience is completely individual, many of the trials that these two families demonstrate are universal to other families supporting members living with different chronic illnesses.

Chapter 11, "Families in Palliative and End-of-Life Care," details the key components to consider in providing palliative and end-of-life care, as well as families' most important concerns and needs when a family member experiences a life-threatening illness or is dying. The chapter also presents some concrete strategies to assist nurses in providing optimal palliative and end-of-life care to all family members. More specifically, the chapter begins with a brief definition of palliative and end-of-life care, including its focus on improving quality of life for patients and their families. The chapter then outlines principles of palliative care and ways to apply these principles across all settings, regardless of whether death results from chronic illness or a sudden or traumatic event. Three evidence-based, palliative-care and end-of-life case studies conclude the chapter.

Chapter 12, "Trauma and Family Nursing," helps nurses develop knowledge about trauma and family nurses' key role in the field of trauma. It emphasizes the importance of prevention, early treatment, encouraging family resilience, and helping the family to make meaning out of negative events. This chapter also stresses an understanding of secondary trauma, or the negative effects of witnessing the trauma of others. This discussion is particularly salient for family nurses because they are some of the health care providers who are most likely to encounter traumatized victims in their everyday practice. Two case studies demonstrate family nursing when working with families who are experiencing the effects of traumatic life events.

Chapter 13, "Relational Nursing and Family Nursing in Canada," offers a unique and intentional focus on attending to the diversity of families when providing nursing care. The chapter offers a specific approach to care that emerged from family nursing in Canada and that considers the contextual nature of family health and illness experiences and how family members' lives are shaped by their circumstances. The chapter authors recommend that nurses orient their care through an understanding of the family's unique experience, structure, risks, and strengths. They offer strategies for developing relationships with families that allow nurses to address the well-being of the family as a whole. Perspectives on understanding risks for families related to health inequities, socioeconomic barriers, and challenges in rural communities are shared. A case study provides an experience attending to context of one family's unique circumstances.

UNIT 3

"Nursing Care of Families in Clinical Areas"

Chapter 14, "Family Nursing With Childbearing Families," focuses on family relationships and the health of all family members in childbearing families. Nurses working with childbearing families use family concepts and theories as part of developing the plan of nursing care. A review of the literature provides current evidence about the processes that families experience when deciding on and adapting to childbearing, including theory and clinical application of nursing care for families planning pregnancy, experiencing pregnancy, adopting and fostering children, struggling with infertility, and coping with illness during the early postpartum period. The chapter covers specific issues that childbearing families may experience, including postpartum depression, attachment concerns, and postpartum illness. Nursing interventions are integrated throughout this chapter to demonstrate how family nurses can help childbearing families prevent complications; increase coping strategies; and adapt to their expanded family structure, development, and function. Two case studies explore family adaptations to stressors and changing roles related to childbearing.

Chapter 15, "Family Child Health Nursing," builds on the major task of families to nurture children to become healthy, responsible, creative adults who can develop meaningful relationships across the life span. Families experience the stress

of normative transitions with the addition of each child and situational transitions when children experience illness. Knowledge of the family life cycle, child development, and illness trajectory provides a foundation for offering anticipatory guidance and coaching at stressful times. Family life influences the promotion of health and the experience of illness in children and is influenced in turn by children's health and illness. This chapter provides a brief history of family-centered care of children and then presents foundational concepts that guide nursing practice with families with children. Case studies illustrate the application of family-centered care across settings.

Chapter 16, "Family Nursing in Acute-Care Adult Settings," discusses how the hospitalization of an adult family member for an acute illness, injury, or exacerbation of a chronic illness is stressful for patients and their families. Adults who are experiencing illness are often in a physiological crisis when they enter the hospital, and the family that accompanies them may also be in an emotional crisis. Families with members who are acutely or critically ill are seen in adult medical-surgical units, intensive-care or cardiac-care units, or emergency departments. The purpose of this chapter is to describe family nursing in acute-care settings, including families in the critical-care units and medical-surgical units. The chapter begins with a review of the literature that captures the major stressors families face during hospitalization of an adult family member: the transfer from one unit to another, being discharged home, participation in cardiopulmonary resuscitation, withdrawing life support therapy, and organ donation. A case study highlights the issues that families experience and adapt to when an adult member is ill. The case study applies the Family Systems Theory in order to demonstrate one theoretical approach for working with families.

Chapter 17, "Families and Aging," examines families using a variety of different theoretical approaches, including Family Systems Theory, Family Life Cycle Theory, and Bioecological Systems Theory. The chapter presents evidence-based practice for working with adults in mid- and later life, including a review of living choices for older adults with chronic illness, and the importance of peer relationships and intergenerational relationships for quality of life. This chapter includes extensive information about family caregiving for and by older adults, including spouses, adult children, and grandparents. A case study demonstrates the generational challenges facing older adults, particularly during transitions in care, and a second case study illustrates the experiences of an older parent who is the legal guardian for her son, who suffers from developmental and physical disabilities and is also aging.

Chapter 18, "Family Mental Health Nursing," begins with a brief demographic overview of the pervasiveness of mental health conditions in both Canada and the United States. The remainder of the chapter focuses on the impact that a specific mental health condition can have on the individual with the condition, individual family members, and the family as a unit. Although the chapter does not go into specific diagnostic criteria for various conditions, it does offer nursing interventions to assist families. One case study explores the impact

and treatment of substance abuse. The second presents how a family nurse can work with a family to improve the health of all family members when one of them lives with paranoid schizophrenia.

Chapter 19, "Families and Population Health," provides a description of population health, public health nursing interventions, and community health nursing in promoting the health of families in communities. It discusses the concepts and principles that guide the work of these nurses, the roles they enact in working with families and communities, and the various settings in which they work. This discussion is organized around a visual representation of community health nursing. The chapter ends with a discussion of current trends in community and public health nursing. A case study depicts working with a family member experiencing homelessness.

Contributors

Ridwaanah Ali, MSN, RN
Research Assistant, Lawrence S. Bloomberg School of Nursing
University of Toronto and Hospital for Sick Children
Toronto, Ontario, Canada

Jennifer M. Babitzke, MS
Graduate Student, Department of Sociology
University of Kansas
Lawrence, Kansas

Annette Bailey, PhD, RN
Associate Professor
Ryerson University
Toronto, Ontario, Canada

Henny Breen, PhD, RN, CNE, COI
Professor of Nursing
Linfield University, Good Samaritan School of Nursing
Portland, Oregon

Helen Brown, PhD, RN
Associate Professor of Nursing
The University of British Columbia
Vancouver, British Columbia, Canada

Liz Cave, RN, MA
Graduate Student, The University of British Columbia
Vancouver, British Columbia, Canada

Deborah Padgett Coehlo, PhD, C-PNP, PMHS, CFLE
Developmental and Behavioral Specialist
Juniper Pediatrics
Faculty Member
Oregon State University–Cascades
Bend, Oregon

Laura Fairley, MN, RN, CHPCN(C)
Assistant Professor
University of Toronto, Bloomberg School of Nursing
Toronto, Ontario, Canada

Jordan Ferris, MSN, RN
Assistant Professor
Linfield University, Good Samaritan School of Nursing
Portland, Oregon

Julie S. Fitzwater, PhD, RN, CNRN, CNE
Assistant Professor, Director of Clinical Education
Linfield University, Good Samaritan School of Nursing
Portland, Oregon

Louise Fleming, PhD, MSN-ED, RN
Associate Dean of Undergraduate Programs and Division
UNC School of Nursing
Chapel Hill, North Carolina

Kiki Fornero, MSN, RN
Assistant Professor
Linfield University, Good Samaritan School of Nursing
Portland, Oregon

Tammy L. Henderson, PhD, CFLE
Professor, Family and Consumer Sciences
Lamar University
Beaumont, Texas

Kimberly Dupree Jones, PhD, FNP, FAAN
Professor and Dean of Nursing
Linfield University, Good Samaritan School of Nursing
Portland, Oregon

Shahin Kassam, MN, RN, PhD(c)
University of Victoria
Victoria, British Columbia, Canada

Kimberly E. Kintz, DNP, ANP-BC, RN
Associate Professor
Linfield University, Good Samaritan School of Nursing
Portland, Oregon

TRACEY A. LAPIERRE, PhD, MSc
Associate Professor, Department of Sociology
University of Kansas
Lawrence, Kansas

GARY LAUSTSEN, PhD, FNP, RN, FAANP,
  FAAN
Professor of Nursing
MSN Program Coordinator
Linfield University, Good Samaritan School of
  Nursing
Portland, Oregon

CHUCK LESTER, MPH
Grant Coordinator
Oklahoma State University
Stillwater, Oklahoma

SHAN MOHAMMED, RN, MN, PhD
Assistant Professor
University of Toronto, Bloomberg School of
  Nursing
Toronto, Ontario, Canada

JOYCE M. O'MAHONY, PhD, RN
Associate Professor
Thompson Rivers University, School of Nursing
Kamloops, British Columbia, Canada

MICHÈLE PARENT-BERGERON, PhD, RN
Principal, Indigenous Health Scholar and
  Consulting
Adjunct Faculty, Arthur Labatt Family School of
  Nursing
Adjunct Faculty, Western University and Laurentian
  University School of Nursing
Toronto, Ontario, Canada

MELISSA ROBINSON, PhD, RN
Professor and Division Chair
University of Providence
Great Falls, Montana

PATRICK ROBINSON, PhD, RN, ACRN, CNE,
  ANEF, FAAN
Provost and Senior Vice President of Academic
  Affairs
Arizona College
Phoenix, Arizona

LYNETTE SAVAGE, PhD, RN
Associate Professor of Nursing
MSN Program Director
University of Providence
Great Falls, Montana

PAUL S. SMITH, PhD, RN, CNE
Associate Dean of Nursing and Associate
  Professor
Linfield University, Good Samaritan School
  of Nursing
Portland, Oregon

ELIZABETH STRAUS, MN, RN, COI, PhD(c)
Assistant Professor of Nursing
Linfield University, Good Samaritan School of
  Nursing
Portland, Oregon

MORGAN TORRIS-HEDLUND, PhD, MPA,
  MS, CEN, PHNA-BC, NHDP-BC,
  FAWM
Assistant Professor of Nursing
Linfield University, Good Samaritan School
  of Nursing
Portland, Oregon

MANDANA VAHABI, PhD, RN
Professor
Ryerson University, Daphne Cockwell School
  of Nursing
Toronto, Ontario, Canada

MARCIA VAN RIPER, PhD, RN, FAAN
Professor and Chair of Family Health
  Division
University of North Carolina at Chapel Hill
Chapel Hill, North Carolina

COLLEEN VARCOE, PhD, RN
Professor of Nursing
The University of British Columbia
Vancouver, British Columbia, Canada

DELENE VOLKERT, PhD, RN, CNE
Associate Professor
Galen College of Nursing
Louisville, Kentucky

JACQUELINE F. WEBB, DNP, FNP-BC, RN
Associate Professor, School of Nursing
Director, Family Nurse Practitioner Program
Oregon Health and Sciences University
Portland, Oregon

KIMBERLEY A. WIDGER, PhD, RN, CHPCN(C)
Associate Professor
Lawrence S. Bloomberg School of Nursing
University of Toronto
Toronto, Ontario, Canada

Karline Wilson-Mitchell, DNP, MSN, CNM, RN, RM, FACNM
Director and Associate Professor, Midwifery Education Program
Ryerson University
Toronto, Ontario, Canada

Josephine Pui-Hing Wong, PhD, RN
Professor and Research Chair in Urban Health
Ryerson University, Daphne Cockwell School of Nursing
Toronto, Ontario, Canada

Mindy B. Zeitzer, PhD, MBE, RN
Assistant Professor of Nursing
Linfield University, Good Samaritan School of Nursing
Portland, Oregon

Reviewers

Stephanie M. Chalupka, EdD, RN,
  PHCNS-BC, FAAOHN, FNAP
Professor and Director, Master of Science in
  Nursing Program
Worcester State University
Worcester, Massachusetts

Sally Doshier, EdD, MS, RN
Associate Professor
Northern Arizona University, School of Nursing
Flagstaff, Arizona

Patricia Ellen Freed, MSN, EdD, RN, CNE
Associate Professor
Saint Louis University, Trudy Bush Valentine
  School of Nursing
St. Louis, Missouri

Susan Goebel, MS, RN, WHNP
Associate Professor of Nursing
Colorado Mesa University
Grand Junction, Colorado

Contents

Available online at fadavis.com: References

Foundations in Family Health Care Nursing

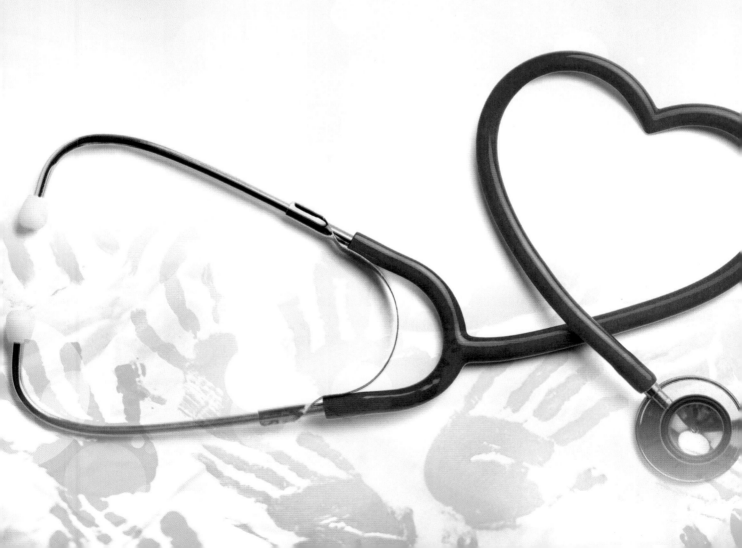

chapter 1

Family Health Care Nursing
An Introduction

Melissa Robinson, PhD, RN

Critical Concepts

- Family health care nursing is an art and a science that has evolved as a way of thinking about and working with families.
- The term *family* is defined in many ways, but the most salient definition is: *the family is who the members say it is.*
- Health and illness are family events.
- Health and illness affect all members of families.
- Families influence the process and outcome of health care.
- Understanding families enables nurses to assess the family health status, ascertain the effects of the family on individual family members' health status, predict the influence of alterations in the health status of the family system, and work with families as they plan and implement actions to improve the health of family members and the family as a whole.
- Knowledge about each family's structure, function, and process informs the nurse about how to optimize nursing care in families and provide individualized nursing care, tailored to the uniqueness of every family system.

Family health care nursing is an art and a science, a philosophy, and a way of interacting with families about health care. It has evolved in recent decades as a way of thinking about family health promotion and working with families when an individual within the family experiences a health problem. The philosophy and practice of family health care nursing encompasses the following assumptions:

- Health and illness affect all members of families.
- Health and illness are family events.
- Families influence the process and outcome of health care.

All health care practices, attitudes, beliefs, behaviors, and decisions are made within the context of larger family and societal systems. Families are diverse in structure, function, and processes. The structure, functions, and processes of the family influence and are influenced by each individual family member's health status and the overall health status of the whole family. Families vary within given cultures because every family has its own unique culture. People who come from the same family of origin create different families over time. Knowledge of the theories of families, as well as the structure, function, and processes of families, can assist nurses when supporting families in achieving or maintaining a state of health.

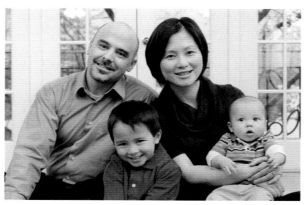

© iStock.com/YinYang

When families are considered the unit of care—as opposed to individuals—nurses have much broader perspectives for approaching the health care needs of both individual family members and the family unit as a whole (Kaakinen, 2018). Understanding families enables nurses to assess the health status of the family, ascertain the effects of the family on individual family members' health status, predict the influence of alterations in the health status of the family system, and work with family members to develop action plans aimed at improving the health of each individual family member and the family as a whole.

Constant changes within the health care system, which include advances in technology, increasingly complex care of chronic conditions, persistent socioeconomic disparities, changes in health care policy, and the need to provide more health care in the home and community, have required a shift in the delivery of nursing care from an individual-centered focus to a family-centered approach that cares for the family as a whole. The family-centered approach has affected the development and application of family theory, practice, research, social policy, and education. It is critical for nurses to be knowledgeable of the importance of family-centered care within the health care system. The American Nurses Association (ANA) defines the expectations and obligations of nursing in the *Guide to Nursing's Social Policy Statement* as "the protection, promotion, and optimization of health and abilities, prevention of illness and injury, alleviation of suffering through the diagnosis and treatment of human response, and advocacy in the care of individuals, families, communities, and populations" (Fowler, 2015, p. 23). The ANA *Scope and Standards of Practice* mandates that nurses provide family care (Fowler, 2015). In addition, the *Nursing Alliance for Quality Care* (American Nurses Association, 2021), the *Agency for Healthcare Research and Quality* (2017), and *QSEN – Quality and Safety Education for Nurses* (2020), all prioritize patient and family-centered care that engages each person and family as partners in their health care, ensures optimal patient and family experiences, improves health outcomes, and contributes to safety within the health care system.

The goal of this textbook is to enhance nurses' knowledge and skills in the theory, practice, research, and social policy surrounding nursing care of families. This chapter provides a broad overview of family health care nursing. It begins with an exploration of the definitions of family and family health care nursing, as well as the concept of healthy families. Four approaches to working with families are described: family as context, family as client, family as system, and family as a component of society. The chapter presents diverse family structures and explores family functions relative to reproduction, socialization, affective function, economic issues, and health care. Finally, the chapter discusses family processes so that nurses know how their practice makes a difference when families experience stress because of the illness of individual family members.

THE FAMILY AND FAMILY HEALTH

Three foundational components of family nursing are (1) determining how family is defined, (2) understanding the concepts of family health, and (3) knowing the current evidence about the elements of a healthy family.

What Is the Family?

Family life is a universal human experience and no two individuals have the exact same experience within a family (Galvin et al., 2015). However, there is no universally agreed-upon definition of family. Now more than ever, the traditional definition of family is being challenged and is shifting. Canada enacted the Civil Marriage Act in 2005, recognizing that all couples have equal access to marriage for civil purposes (Government of Canada, 2020). Spain had legalized same-sex marriage less than a month earlier and in June 2015, the United States became the 21st country to legalize same-sex marriage nationwide (Pew Research Center, 2015). *Family* is a word that conjures up different images for each individual and group, and the word has evolved in its meaning over time. Definitions of *family* also differ by discipline, for example:

- *Legal:* relationships through blood ties, adoption, guardianship, or marriage
- *Biological:* genetic biological networks among and between people
- *Sociological:* groups of people living together with or without legal or biological ties
- *Psychological:* groups with strong emotional ties

Historically, early family social science theorists (Burgess & Locke, 1953, pp. 7–8) adopted the following traditional definition of families in their writing:

The family is a group of persons united by ties of marriage, blood, or adoption, constituting a single household; interacting and communicating with each other in their respective social roles of husband and wife, mother and father, son and daughter, brother and sister; and creating and maintaining a common culture.

More recently, the U.S. Census Bureau (2020) defined a family as a group of two or more people related by birth, marriage, or adoption and residing together; all such people (including related subfamily members) are considered members of one family. The definition of a family provides a foundation for the implementation of many social programs and policies. It is important to note that the definition excludes many diverse individuals and groups who identify as families and who perform family functions, such as economic, reproductive, social, and affective functions. Families are also represented by, and are not limited to, married or remarried couples with biological or adoptive children, cohabiting same-sex couples, single-parent families with children, extended families living together, and grandparents raising grandchildren.

The definition of *family* adopted by this textbook (Kaakinen, 2018) is as follows:

Family refers to two or more individuals who depend on one another for emotional, physical, and economic support. The members of the family are self-defined.

Nurses who work with families should ask clients who they consider to be members of their family and should include those persons in health care planning with their permission.

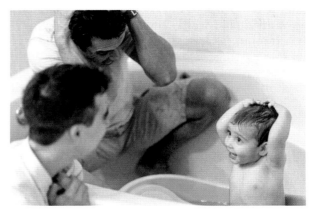

© iStock.com/Juanmonino

What Is Family Health?

According to the World Health Organization (WHO, 2020a), at least half of the world's population cannot obtain essential health services and are living in poverty due to health care costs that they must pay out of their own pockets. Currently, 800 million people spend at least 10 percent of their household budgets on health expenses for themselves, a sick child, or other family member (WHO, 2020a). In response to the need for essential services, the *Framework on Integrated People-Centered Health Services* was developed (WHO, 2020b). The framework states that care should be coordinated around the needs of the people; care should respect the preferences of individuals and families; and care should be safe, effective, timely, affordable, and of acceptable quality. The framework is not about patient-centered care, which focuses on the individual, but is about people-centered care that expands the care to individuals, families, communities, and society (WHO, 2020b). The term *family health* is often used interchangeably with *family functioning, healthy families,* or *familial health.* To some, family health is the composite of individual family members' physical health because it is impossible to make a single statement about the family's physical health as a single entity.

The definition of *family health* adopted in this textbook (Kaakinen, 2018) is as follows:

> *Family health is a dynamic, changing state of well-being, which includes the biological, psychological, spiritual, sociological, and cultural factors of individual members and the whole family system.*

This definition combines all aspects of life for individual members, as well as for the whole family. On the wellness-to-illness continuum, an individual's health affects the entire family's functioning, and in turn, the family's ability to function affects each individual member's health. Assessment of family health involves collecting data on the health and functional status of each individual as well as the whole family system (Kaakinen, 2018).

What Is a Well-Functioning Family?

Although it is possible to define family health, it is more difficult to describe characteristics of a family that is well-functioning. Characteristics used to describe healthy, well-functioning families have varied throughout time in the literature. A "healthy family" is one in which the needs of the family members are being met (Vander Wielen, 2020). Otto (1963) was the first scholar to develop psychosocial criteria for assessing family strengths and emphasized the need to focus on positive family attributes instead of the pathological approach that accentuated family problems and weaknesses. Later, Pratt (1976) introduced the idea of the "energized family" as one whose structure encourages and supports individuals to develop their capacities for full functioning and independent action, thus contributing to family health. Characteristics of healthy families were also summarized by Kaloupek (2018) based on experiences in a family-focused counseling practice working with diverse families that included foster families, blended families, single-parent families, nuclear families, extended families, and more. Characteristics of healthy families are listed in Box 1-1.

The Circumplex Model of Marital and Family Systems is used to describe three major dimensions of family function including flexibility, cohesion, and communication (Olson et al., 2019). The model has been used to describe family systems

---

BOX 1-1
Characteristics of Healthy Families

- Communicates and listens
- Fosters table time and conversation
- Affirms and supports each member
- Teaches respect for others
- Develops a sense of trust
- Has a sense of play and humor
- Has a balance of interaction among members
- Maintains appropriate boundaries
- Spends quality time together
- Exhibits a sense of shared responsibility
- Teaches a sense of right and wrong
- Engages in rituals and traditions
- Shares a religious core
- Respects the privacy of each member
- Values service to others
- Admits to problems and seeks help
- Manages conflict and crisis when they occur
- Offers forgiveness, comfort, and support

and how they change over time. Three major hypotheses form the Circumplex Model:

1. Balanced couples and families are happier and more functional than unbalanced systems;
2. Balanced couples and families demonstrate more effective communication than unbalanced systems;
3. Balanced couples and families adapt to stressors and changes over time by being flexible and becoming more cohesive, compared to unbalanced systems (Olson et al., 2019).

Balanced families will function more effectively across the life cycle, resulting in higher levels of success and happiness. Families can achieve healthier outcomes when their communication skills enable them to plan ahead and adapt to challenges and stressors. Being flexible can allow individual family members to contribute to the overall cohesion of the family, thus promoting the health and well-being of the family. Figure 1-1 (flexibility) and Figure 1-2 (cohesion) illustrate the continuum of family function and dysfunction in the Circumplex Model.

The Circumplex Model has been applied to other settings such as in the assessment of parenting, classroom styles, leadership styles, and more. Studies conducted within families have addressed how families change over time, illustrated developmental changes, or illustrated situational factors such as the assessment of how families function during times of stress and trauma (Olson et al., 2019). In a study by Tafa et al. (2016), family function was measured in families with female adolescents suffering from eating disorders. Researchers found that adolescents and their parents had very different perceptions of the way their family was functioning. The adolescents believed their family was highly disengaged, rigid, and poor in communication, while their parents described the family as more balanced, flexible, and cohesive, with positive communication patterns (Tafa et al., 2016). The model is fluid and assumes that the needs of the family will evolve. Each family member also has their own set of perspectives on how the family functions; therefore, the model requires nurses to perform individualized assessment when applying a model to family nursing.

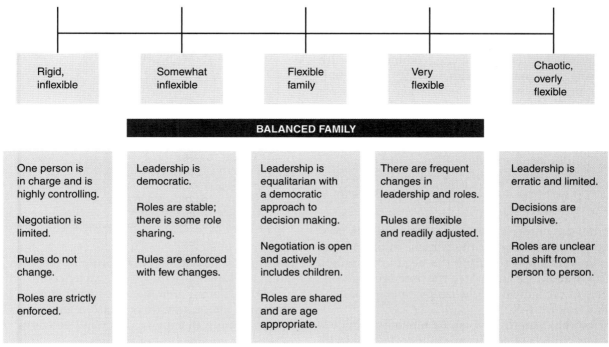

FIGURE 1-1 Family Flexibility Continuum

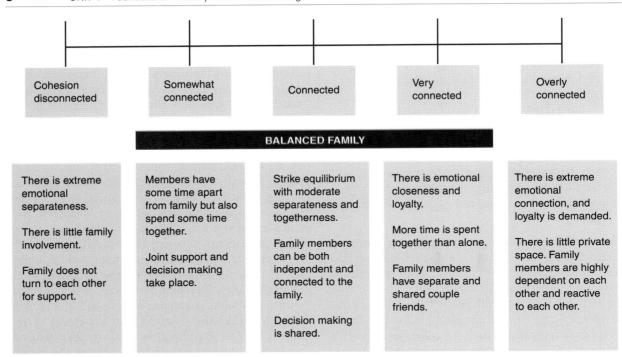

Cohesion disconnected	Somewhat connected	Connected	Very connected	Overly connected
BALANCED FAMILY				
There is extreme emotional separateness. There is little family involvement. Family does not turn to each other for support.	Members have some time apart from family but also spend some time together. Joint support and decision making take place.	Strike equilibrium with moderate separateness and togetherness. Family members can be both independent and connected to the family. Decision making is shared.	There is emotional closeness and loyalty. More time is spent together than alone. Family members have separate and shared couple friends.	There is extreme emotional connection, and loyalty is demanded. There is little private space. Family members are highly dependent on each other and reactive to each other.

FIGURE 1-2 Family Cohesion Continuum

FAMILY HEALTH CARE NURSING

The specialty area of family health care nursing has been evolving since the early 1980s. Some question how family health care nursing is distinct from other specialties that involve families, such as maternal-child health nursing, community health nursing, and mental health nursing. The definition and framework for *family health care nursing* adopted by this textbook and that applies from the previous edition (Kaakinen, 2018) is as follows:

> *The process of providing for the health care needs of families that are within the scope of nursing practice. This nursing care can be aimed toward the family as context, the family as a whole, the family as a system, or the family as a component of society.*

At the same time, it cuts across the individual, family, and community for the purpose of promoting, maintaining, and restoring the health of families. This framework illustrates the intersecting concepts of the individual, the family, nursing, and society (Figure 1-3).

Another way to view family nursing practice is conceptually, as a confluence of theories and strategies from nursing, family therapy, and family social science, as depicted in Figure 1-4. Over time,

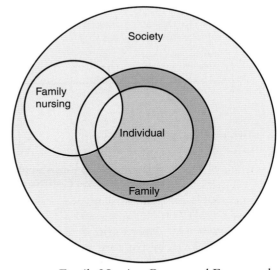

FIGURE 1-3 Family Nursing Conceptual Framework

family nursing continues to incorporate ideas from family therapy and family social science into the practice of family nursing. Chapter 2 includes a discussion about how theories from family social science, family therapy, and nursing converge to inform the nursing care of families.

The International Family Nursing Association (IFNA, 2020) represents 340 members from

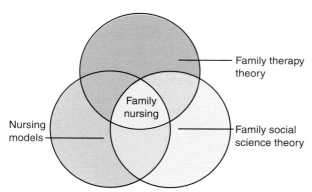

FIGURE 1-4 Family Nursing Practice

Table 1-1	**Family Nursing Competencies: Generalist**

1. Enhance and promote family health.

2. Focus nursing practice on family's strengths, the support of family and individual growth, the improvement of family self-management abilities, the facilitation of successful life transitions, the improvement and management of health, and the mobilization of family resources.

3. Demonstrate leadership and systems thinking skills to ensure the quality of nursing care with families in everyday practice and across every context.

4. Commit to self-reflective practice based on examination of nurse actions with families and family responses.

5. Practice using an evidence-based approach.

Source: International Family Nursing Association (IFNA). (2015). *IFNA Position Statement on Generalist Competencies for Family Nursing Practice.*

28 countries with the mission to transform family health by serving as a unifying force and voice for family nursing globally. IFNA (2015) developed a position statement that defines five family nursing competencies for generalist nurses practicing globally; see Table 1-1.

The following 10 interventions are used by family nurses to provide structure to working with families regardless of the theoretical underpinning of the nursing approach. These are enduring ideas that support the practice of family nursing (Kaakinen, 2018):

1. Family care is concerned with the experience of the family over time. It considers both the history and the future of the family group.

2. Family nursing considers the community and cultural context of the group. The family is encouraged to receive from, and give to, community resources.

3. Family nursing considers the relationships between and among family members and recognizes that, in some instances, all individual members and the family group will not achieve maximum health simultaneously.

4. Family nursing is directed at families with both healthy and ill members, regardless of the severity of the illness in the family member.

5. Family nursing is often offered in settings where individuals have physiological or psychological problems. Together with competency in treatment of individual health problems, family nurses must recognize the reciprocity between an individual family member's health and collective health within the family.

6. Family nursing requires the nurse to manipulate the environment to increase the likelihood of family interaction. The physical absence of family members, however, does not preclude the nurse from offering family care.

7. The family system is influenced by any change in its members. In family nursing, the focus includes the individual as well as how the family system and all family members are affected by the health event. Family nursing requires the nurse to manipulate the environment to increase the likelihood of family interaction. The physical absence of family members, however, does not preclude the nurse from offering family care.

8. The family nurse recognizes that the person in a family who is most symptomatic may change over time; this means that the focus of the nurse's attention will also change over time.

9. Family nursing focuses on the strengths of individual family members and the family group to promote their mutual support and growth.

10. Family nurses must define with the family which persons constitute the family and where they will place their therapeutic energies.

These are the distinctive intervention statements specific to family nursing that appear continuously in the care and study of families in nursing, regardless of the theoretical model in use.

APPROACHES TO FAMILY NURSING

Four different approaches to care are inherent in family nursing: (1) family as the context for individual development, (2) family as a client, (3) family as a system, and (4) family as a component of society (Kaakinen, 2018). Figure 1-5 illustrates these approaches to the nursing of families. Each approach derived its foundations from different nursing specialties: maternal-child nursing, primary care nursing, psychiatric/mental health nursing, and community health nursing, respectively. All four approaches have legitimate implications

Family as Context

Individual as foreground
Family as background

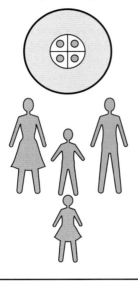

Family as Client

Family as foreground
Individual as background

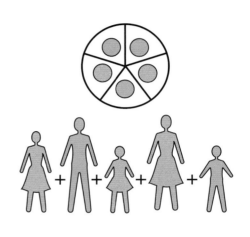

Family as System

Interactional family

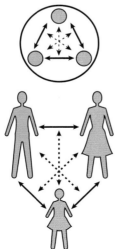

Family as Component of Society

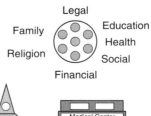

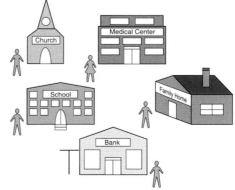

FIGURE 1-5 Approaches to Family Nursing

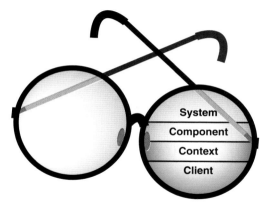

FIGURE 1-6 Four Views of Family Through a Lens

should take a family-centered approach to understanding their unique function. This approach can reveal the strengths of the family as well as areas of growth and opportunity for planning nursing care that will meet the support needs of the family.

When assessing the family, the nurse might ask individuals in the family the following types of questions: "What kinds of activities does your family enjoy doing for fun?" "When your family makes decisions about important issues, what does this include?" "Who in your family assists when someone is ill or needs medications?" or "How do your family members communicate with each other when things are stressful for your family, such as when someone is experiencing illness?"

for nursing assessment and intervention. The approach that nurses use is determined by many factors, including the health care setting, family circumstances, and nurse resources. Figure 1-6 shows how a nurse can view all four approaches to families through just one set of eyes. It is important to keep all four perspectives in mind when working with any given family.

Family as Context

The first approach to family nursing care focuses on the assessment and care of an individual client in which the family is the context. Alternate labels for this approach are *family centered* or *family focused*. This is the traditional nursing focus in which the emphasis is on the individual and the family is in the background. Most existing nursing theories or models were originally conceptualized using the individual as a focus. One example of the approach, family as context, includes understanding how the family functions when an adult family member is suffering from illness. The family can serve as a resource and source of support, or as a stressor to the individual that is experiencing illness.

In a concept analysis exploring family functioning within the context of adult illness, Zhang (2018) identified the following experiences of family function that may be affected, including: how well family members communicate with each other, how they support each other and adjust to changes in family roles, how they continue with family routines, how they adapt to family stressors, and how they relate to each other during times of stress. During assessment of family function, nurses

Family as Client

The second approach to family nursing care centers on the assessment of the family as a whole. The family nurse is focused on the way that all family members are affected by the health event or illness experience. Family-centered care in the neonatal intensive care unit (NICU) is an example of the approach to family nursing that considers the family as the client. The focus on interventions in the NICU have expanded to a focus on protection and prevention, on the vulnerability of the child in their physical and social environment, on interactions with their family, and on developmental and physical milestones (Hernandez et al., 2019). To ensure the optimal health and well-being of the child, the nurse also assesses and provides support for each person in the family. The family members may include parents, siblings, grandparents, or other significant persons identified by the family. Depending on the circumstances, care may continue for a short time or for an extended period of time. From this perspective, the nurse may focus on family-centered strategies to support the family that include demonstrating compassion and supportive communication, including family members in care routines, providing education for family members, celebrating developmental milestones, and providing access to home and community resources that support the family.

Family as System

The third approach to family nursing care views the family as a system. Family systems theory

(FST) sees the family as a complex, interconnected system within their environment. The basic tenets of FST include (1) families determine membership, (2) families strive to maintain equilibrium, (3) resources are needed to adapt and change, and (4) families have rules and routines (Pratt & Skelton, 2018). The emphasis for nursing assessment and intervention using FST is on the interactions and interconnectedness of the family members. Due to the family dynamics involved in childhood obesity, FST can assist nurses in engaging multiple family members in treatment to influence overall family functioning and long-term behavior modification (Pratt & Skelton, 2018). By addressing family routines, rules, communication patterns, and overall family function, changes can be most successful. Nurses can use FST-informed approaches when working with families to develop healthy new routines, such as:

1. Adults will provide structure for healthy eating and physical activity.
2. Rules will be established for eating and exercising at home and outside the home.
3. Communication will be focused on health rather than on weight or size.
4. Health goals will be identified, implemented, and reinforced.
5. Family members will get involved with each other to work on health goals.
6. Family will build on previous successes and healthy behaviors.
7. Adults will address household barriers in order to make health changes (Haines et al., 2016; Pratt & Skelton, 2018).

Family as Component of Society

The fourth approach to care looks at the family as a component of society, in which the family is viewed as one of many institutions in society, similar to health, educational, religious, or economic institutions. The family is a basic or primary unit of society, and it is part of the larger system of society (Figure 1-7). A family nursing approach considers that the family interacts with multiple other institutions for communication, services, and support. Community health nursing is an example of this perspective based on the interface between families and community agencies. More specifically, nurses working in correctional facilities have the opportunity to apply a family nursing approach to

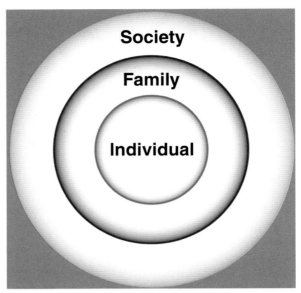

FIGURE 1-7 Family as Primary Group in Society

caring for persons with life-limiting conditions or to those persons with the need for hospice or end-of-life care. Nurses play a key role in addressing multilevel barriers to palliative and hospice care within corrections institutions, including those that are individual, relational, institutional, physical, and sociocultural (Burles, 2021). By advocating for holistic support of symptoms, ensuring greater dignity for individuals that are suffering, and improving family and peer support, outcomes for the dying can be improved (Burles, 2021).

VARIABLES THAT INFLUENCE FAMILY NURSING

Family health care nursing has been influenced by many variables that are derived from both historical, community, and current social events and the profession of nursing. Examples include changing nursing theory, practice, education, and research; new knowledge derived from family social sciences and the health sciences; national and state health care policies; changing health care behavior and attitudes; and national and international political events. Chapters 2 and 4 provide detailed discussions of theoretical foundations of family nursing and health and social policies that affect families.

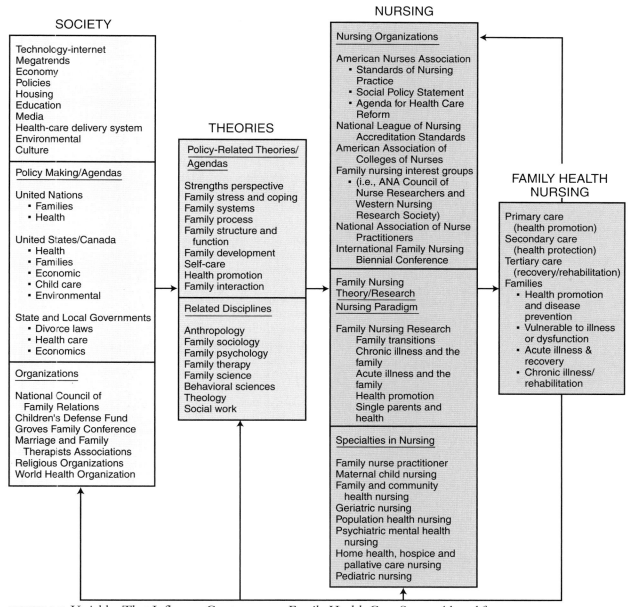

FIGURE 1-8 Variables That Influence Contemporary Family Health Care *Source: Adapted from Bomar, P. J. (Ed.). (2004). Promoting health in families: Applying family research and theory to nursing practice (3rd ed., p. 17). Philadelphia, PA: Saunders/Elsevier, with permission.*

Figure 1-8 illustrates how many variables influence contemporary family health nursing, making the point that the status of family nursing depends on what is occurring in the wider society—family as community. An example of the influence of societal issues affecting family health is access to health care. Health policy changes that result in higher health care costs and greater numbers of people that are either underinsured or uninsured have a significant impact on quality of life and health for families. To ensure that every person has access to affordable health care, a major shift in priorities, funding, and services is needed. The movement toward health promotion and family care in the community will greatly affect the evolution of family nursing.

FAMILY NURSING ROLES

Families are the basic unit of every society, but it is also true that families are complex, varied, dynamic, and adaptive, which is why it is crucial for all nurses to be knowledgeable about the scientific discipline of family nursing, and the variety of ways nurses may interact with families (Kaakinen, 2018). The roles of family health care nurses are evolving along with the specialty. Figure 1-9 lists the many roles that nurses can assume with families as the focus. This figure was constructed from some of the first examples of family nursing literature that appeared, and it is a composite of what various scholars believe to be the role of nurses when caring for families.

Educator The family nurse teaches about family wellness, illness, relations, and parenting, to name a few topics. The nurse educator function is ongoing in all settings in both formal and informal ways. Examples include teaching new parents how to care for their infant and giving instructions about diabetes to a newly diagnosed adolescent boy and his family members.

Coordinator, Collaborator, Navigator, and Liaison The family nurse coordinates the care that families receive, collaborating with the family to plan care. For example, if a family member has been in a traumatic accident, the nurse would be a key person in helping families to access resources—from inpatient care, outpatient care, home health care, and social services to rehabilitation. Nurse navigators provide a holistic approach to care delivery by working with patients and families as a care coordinator and patient advocate with the purpose of giving each patient/family under their care a consistent point of connection in a highly fragmented, complex health care industry. Nurse navigators help patients and their family access the health care system and overcome barriers to receiving care, as well as facilitate the provision of timely, quality care in a culturally sensitive manner.

Care Provider and Supervisor of Care The family nurse either provides direct care or supervises the care that families receive in various settings. To do this, the nurse must be a technical expert in terms of both knowledge and skill. For example, the nurse may be the person going into the family home on a daily basis to consult with the family and help take care of a child on a respirator.

Family Advocate The family nurse advocates for families and empowers family members to speak with their own voices, or the nurse speaks out for the family. An example is a school nurse advocating for special education services for a child with attention deficit-hyperactivity disorder.

Consultant The family nurse serves as a consultant to families when necessary. For example, a hospice and palliative care nurse may be asked to meet with a family and assess their loved one for hospice eligibility. The nurse may consult with the patient, family, and provider to develop a plan of care that supports the patient's condition and goals for care.

Counselor The family nurse has a therapeutic role in helping individuals and families solve problems or change behavior. An example from the mental health arena is a family that requires help with coping with a long-term chronic condition, such as when a family member has been diagnosed with schizophrenia. The family nurse may also make referrals to resources in the community to support the needs of the family.

Contact Tracing (Epidemiology) The family nurse may be involved in contact tracing for a family member that has been recently diagnosed with a communicable disease. The nurse would engage in investigating the sources of the transmission, notifying members of the family or community of potential exposure, and providing resources for others to seek treatment. Screening families and subsequent referral of the family members may be part of this role.

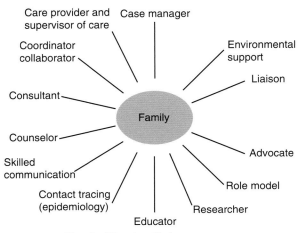

FIGURE 1-9 Family Nursing Roles

Environmental Support The family nurse consults with families and collaborates with other health care providers to modify the environment to enhance patient safety, function, and independence. For example, if a man with paraplegia is about to be discharged from the hospital to home, the nurse assists the family in modifying the home environment so that the patient can move around in a wheelchair and engage in self-care.

Skilled Communication The nurse is skilled in multiple communication strategies, clarifying and interpreting information to families in all settings. The family nurse develops rapport with the family and demonstrates compassion and care through effective communication. For example, if a child in the family has a complex disease, such as leukemia, the nurse clarifies and interprets information pertaining to the diagnosis, treatment, and prognosis of the condition to parents and extended family members.

Researcher The family nurse should identify practice problems and find the best solution for dealing with these problems through the process of scientific investigation. An example might be collaborating with a colleague to find a better intervention for helping families cope with incontinent older adults living in the home.

Role Model The family nurse is continually serving as a role model to other people. The nurse models care and compassion, safe health behaviors, professionalism, and high-quality communication.

Case Manager Nurse case managers serve important roles coordinating care and collaborating between individuals, families, and the health care system. For example, a family nurse working with seniors in the community may work with the family as an older adult experiences health changes and requires a higher level of care or support, such as transitioning from an independent living situation to a residential care facility.

FAMILY NURSING PRACTICE

There is a significant amount of literature available about families; however, some nurses may not have had exposure to family-focused nursing or family theory during their undergraduate education.

Traditional models of nursing care have focused on the individual as the patient or client rather than on the family. Families are diverse and complex; therefore, even with several family assessment models and approaches, no single assessment or treatment approach fits all family situations.

Family-centered care may be somewhat limited in certain settings. The established hours for health care facilities, such as primary care office hours, may not be conducive to family members accompanying their loved ones. Some clinics and outpatient settings offer evening and weekend hours, making it possible for family members to come in together. Some hospitals and residential care centers have limited visiting hours for family members and may not include family members in treatment meetings, even if the care has an impact on family members. When challenges affect the nurse's ability to provide family-focused nursing care, it is important that the nurse attempt to connect with family members in alternative ways as well as to advocate for changes that support caring for the family as a whole.

FAMILY STRUCTURE, FUNCTION, AND PROCESS

Knowledge about family structure, functions, and processes is essential for understanding the complex family interactions that affect health, illness, and well-being (Kaakinen, 2018). Knowledge emerging from the study of family structure, function, and process suggests concepts and a framework that nurses can use to provide effective assessment and intervention with families. Many internal and external family variables affect individual family members and the family as a whole. An important influence on how nurses provide care to all families is related to the wide range of diversity present within every family. Internal family variables include unique individual characteristics, communication, preferences, and interactions, whereas external family variables include location of family household, community factors, social policy, and economic trends. Family members may have complicated responses to these factors, particularly during crisis or when faced with health challenges that affect the family. Even when external factors may not be modifiable, nurses can assist family members with coping during conflict or as the needs of the family are changing. For example, economic or employment changes within the family can affect the function of the family significantly. Understanding the unique circumstances of patients and families can help the nurse plan more effective interventions, such as connecting them to the resources in the community that will support their needs. Nurses can assist individuals and families with coping skills, communication patterns, location of needed resources, effective use of information, or creation of family rituals or routines (Kaakinen, 2018).

Nurses who understand the concepts of family structure, function, and process can use this knowledge to educate, counsel, and implement changes that enable families to cope with illness, family crisis, chronic health conditions, and mental illness. Nurses serve an important role assisting families with life transitions that occur across the life span (Kaakinen, 2018). For example, when a family member experiences a chronic condition such as diabetes, family roles, routines, and power dynamics within the family may be challenged. Nurses must be prepared to address the complex challenges that result from illness and the circumstances that families experience as well as to care for the individual's health care needs.

Family Structure

Family structure is the ordered set of relationships within the family, without respect to roles and function. The family form or structure does not indicate how healthy the family is or how it functions. In terms of family nursing, it is logical to begin with "who" makes up the family and how they define their relationships. Identifying the family structure is an important component of caring for families and includes the following:

- The individuals who comprise the family
- The relationships between them
- The interactions between the family members
- The interactions with other social systems

Family relationships are unique and consequential for the well-being of the family across the life course (Thomas et al., 2017). Family relationships also reflect the diversity of the family structure, including marital relationship, multigenerational

relationships, blended with a mix of sibling ties, single-parent families, and domestic partnerships, all of which also have an impact on family function. The variation in family and household structures range from traditional in form and pattern, to diverse and nontraditional (Table 1-2).

Individuals often experience multiple family forms during their lifetime. Figure 1-10 depicts the variety of familial forms that individuals may live through. Nurses encounter families structured differently from their own families of origin, which may conflict with their personal or professional value systems. For nurses to work effectively with families, they must maintain openness and compassion. Nurses experience variation not only in their personal lives but also with individuals and families they work with in health care settings (Kaakinen & Webb, 2015). Understanding family structure enables nurses assisting families to identify effective coping strategies for daily challenges, health promotion activities, and disease prevention (Ferrara et al., 2016; Kaakinen, 2018). In addition, nurses have an essential role advocating for social and economic policies that address

Table 1-2	Variations of Family and Household Structures	
FAMILY TYPE	**COMPOSITION**
Single family	Living alone, never married
Nuclear dyad/childless	Married couple, no children
Nuclear	Two generations of family, parents, and biological or adopted children residing in the same household
Binuclear	Two postdivorce families with children as members of both
Extended/multigenerational	Two or more adult generations and one that includes grandparents and grandchildren living in the same household
Blended/reconstituted	One or more of the parents have been married previously and they bring with them children from their previous marriage
Single-parent family	One parent and child(ren) residing in one household
Commune	Group of men, women, and children
Cohabitation (domestic partners)	Unmarried couple sharing a household who are involved in an emotional and/or sexually intimate relationship

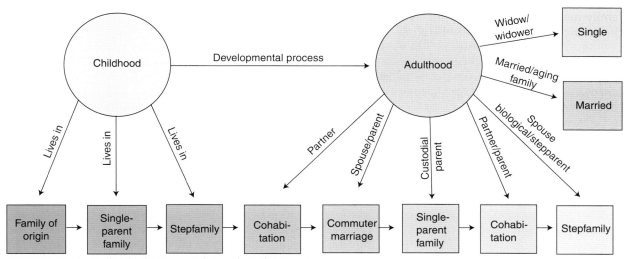

FIGURE 1-10 An Individual's Potential Family Life Experiences

the needs of families, for example, taking political action to increase the availability of affordable and high-quality child care for single-parent families, or collaborating with community organizations to meet the caregiving and respite needs of families caring for chronically or terminally ill loved ones. Nurses that are well informed about different family structures can identify specific needs of unique families, provide appropriate clinical care to enhance family resilience, and act as change agents to enact social policies that reduce family burdens. Chapter 4 includes a deeper discussion on how families are affected by health and social policies and the role of nurses.

Family Functions

A functional perspective has to do with the ways that families serve and support their members. One way to describe the functional aspect of family is to see the unit as made up of intimate, interactive, and interdependent persons who share some values, goals, resources, responsibilities, decisions, and commitment over time. The literature on family functioning suggests that effective families result when family members play their respective roles, successfully perform practical tasks, and maintain relationships within and beyond the family context (Cuhadar et al., 2015; Zhang, 2018).

It is important to be clear that there is a distinction between the concepts of family function (social and cultural norms about the roles of family

in society) and family functioning (the processes of family life). Family function includes the ways that family members care for each other, the way they have children and interact to socialize younger members of the family, the way they work cooperatively to meet their economic needs, and how they function within the community and society.

Nurses should ask about specific characteristics that factor into achieving the unique goals of the family. Certain functional processes such as socialization, reproduction, economics, and issues affecting health care are areas that nurses can assess and support during health care interactions. Nursing interventions can enhance the family's protective health function when teaching and counseling are tailored to the unique learning needs of the family. The cultural context and individual health literacy of the family members are closely related to the functional needs of the family. Nursing interventions that assist families to identify social support and community resources during times of family transitions and health crisis have a significant impact on family health. Five specific functions of the family are explored in the following sections: reproduction, socialization, affective, economic, and health care.

Reproductive Functions of the Family

Traditionally, the family has been organized around the biological function of reproduction. Reproduction was viewed as a major concern for thousands of years during which efforts to populate the world were continually threatened by famine, disease, war, and other life uncertainties. In recent years, the fertility rate has declined for a variety of reasons, including personal and family choices. According to a recent study conducted at the University of Washington on fertility, mortality, migration, and population scenarios, Vollset et al. (2020) found that continued trends in female educational attainment and access to contraception hasten declines in fertility and slow population growth. Nurses working with families are involved in various care scenarios related to family planning and health promotion, including abortion, various contraception and fertility options, and assistive reproductive technologies. Family planning also includes discussions with families about adoption, surrogacy, and fostering children. Nurses encounter a variety of ethical, legal, moral, and technological scenarios when caring for the reproductive functions of families.

Socialization Functions of the Family

The family is the first and one of the most influential settings for socialization. Parents and caregivers are the primary source of individual development for children and where they are prepared with the skills, resources, beliefs, cultural values, and behaviors that they need to succeed as adults (American Psychological Association, 2021). A major function for families is to teach children to be well-integrated and participating members of society. Socialization also includes how children acquire culture and ethnic identity through language and the modeling of others in the family, particularly from parental figures (Kim et al., 2018). Individuals learn and adopt cultural norms through the socialization process.

Families have great variability in the ways they address the physical and emotional needs, moral values, and economic needs of children, and these patterns are influenced specifically by the role of parenting and somewhat by the larger society (Pérez-Fuentes et al., 2019). Children are born into families without knowledge of the values, language, norms, morals, communication, or roles of the society in which they live. A major function of the family continues to be to socialize them about family life and ground them in the societal identity of which they are part. Although the family is not the only institution of society that participates in socialization of children, it is generally viewed as having primary responsibility for this function. As children are socialized and grow older, they gain independence and the dynamic of the family changes over time.

Socialization is the primary way children acquire the social and psychological skills needed to take their place in the adult world. Parents combine social support and social control as they prepare children to meet future life tasks. Parental figures interact in multiple roles such as friends, lovers, child-care providers, housekeepers, financial providers, recreation specialists, and counselors. Children growing up within families learn the values and norms of their parents and extended families.

Another role of families in the socialization process is to guide children through various rites of passage. Rites of passage are ceremonies that announce a change in status in the ways members are viewed. Examples include events such as a baptism, communion, circumcision, puberty ritual, graduation, wedding, and death. These occasions signal to others changes in role relationships and new expectations. Understandings about families' traditions can assist nurses working with diverse health care needs.

Affective Functions of the Family

Affective function is one of the basic functions of the family. Fulfilling this function and providing positive emotional relationships among family members are essential for creating a harmonious and stable environment that is optimal for healthy child development and for the satisfaction of all family members. Affective function has to do with the way family members relate to one another and those outside the immediate family boundaries. Well-functioning families are able to maintain a consistent level of involvement with one another yet at the same time not become too involved in each other's lives (Peterson & Green, 2009). Well-functioning families have empathetic interaction where family members care deeply about each other's feelings and activities and are emotionally invested in each other. Families with a strong affective function are the most effective type of families (Peterson & Green, 2009). All families have boundaries that help to buffer stresses and the pressure of systems outside the family on its members. Well-functioning families protect their boundaries but at the same time give members room to negotiate their independence. Achieving this balance is often difficult in our fast-paced culture. It is also particularly difficult in families with adolescents (Pérez-Fuentes et al., 2019). Emotional involvement is a key to successful family functioning. Researchers have identified several characteristics of strong families. Among these are expressions of appreciation, spending time together, strong commitment to the family, good communication, and positive conflict resolution (Vander Wielen, 2020). When family members feel that they are supported and encouraged and that their personal interests are valued, family interaction becomes more effective.

Families provide a sense of belonging and identity to their members. This identity often proves to be vitally important throughout the entire life cycle. Within the confines of families, members learn dependent roles that later serve to launch them into independent ones. Families serve as places to learn about intimate relationships and establish the foundation for future personal interactions. Families provide the initial experience of self-awareness, which includes a sense of knowing one's own gender, ethnicity, race, religion, and personal characteristics. Families help members become acquainted with who they are and experience themselves in relationships with others. Families provide the substance for self-identity, as well as a foundation for other-identity. Within the confines of families, individual members learn about love, care, nurturance, dependence, and support of the dying.

Resilience implies an ability to rebound from stress and crisis and the capacity to be optimistic, solve problems, be resourceful, and develop caring support systems. Although unique traits alter potential for emotional and psychological health, individuals exposed to resilient family environments tend to have greater potential to achieve normative developmental patterns and positive sibling and parental relationships (Walsh, 2016a).

Variables such as the quality of couples' relationships, the ways families' conflicts are handled, whether abuse or violence has previously occurred in the households or members' lives, frequency of children's contact with nonresidential parents, shared custody arrangements, and emotional relationships between parents and children appear to be important predictors of family affective functions.

Affective functions can best be understood by gathering information from *all* the members involved within a household. When families are managing illness, family functioning is the outcome of the efforts of the family members to maintain balance, harmony, and coherence, despite stress and differing views (Zhang, 2018).

Economic Functions of the Family

Families are the means whereby children are supplied with necessities such as food, shelter, and clothing. Families have an important function in keeping both local and national economies viable. Economic conditions significantly affect families. Turbulent economies affect families' structures, functions, and processes. People make decisions about when to enter the labor force, when to marry, when to have children, and when to retire or come out of retirement based on economic factors.

Family income provides a substantial part of family economics, but an equally important aspect has to do with economic interactions and consumerism related to household consumption and finance. Money management, housing decisions, consumer spending, insurance choices, retirement planning, and savings are some of the issues that affect the family economically. These values and skills are passed down to children within the family structure.

In order to meet their own economic needs and maintain family life and health, family members take upon themselves several contributory roles for obtaining and utilizing the wages. Family nurses should explore the types of resources available or lacking as families engage in providing health care functions to their members.

Health Care Functions of the Family

The family is the primary place where individuals learn how to maintain health, protect health, and restore health. Families are expected to provide care for sick family members. Families influence well-being, prevention, illness care, maintenance care associated with chronic illness, and rehabilitative care. Individuals regularly seek services from a variety of health care providers, but the family is the primary social context in which health issues are addressed. Within the family, decisions are made about health care, such as when to seek professional treatment and whether to follow or ignore treatment options. Families can become particularly vulnerable when they encounter health threats, and family-focused nurses are in a position to provide education, counseling, and assistance with locating resources. Family-focused care implies that when a single individual is the target of care, the entire family is still viewed as the unit of care.

Health care functions of the family include many aspects of family life. Family members have different ideas about health and illness, and often these ideas are not discussed within families until problems arise. Availability and cost of health care insurance is a concern for many families, but many families lack clarity about what is and is not covered until they encounter a problem. Lifestyle behaviors, such as healthy diet, regular exercise, and alcohol and tobacco use, are areas that family members may not associate with health and illness outcomes. Risk reduction, health promotion and maintenance, rehabilitation, and caregiving are areas where families often need information and assistance. Family members spend far more time taking care of health issues of family members than professionals do.

Family Processes

Family process refers to the interactions among members of a family, including their relationships, communication patterns, time spent together, and satisfaction with family life. In part, family process makes every family unique within its own particular culture. Families with similar structures and functions may interact differently. Family process, at least in the short term, appears to have a greater effect on the family's health status than family structure because it influences how a family functions. In any illness situation, processes within families are affected by alterations in health status. Families mobilize and organize their resources, buffer stresses, and at times reorganize who does what in the family to fit the changing conditions (Walsh, 2016b). During times of change, family nurses can assist family members to restabilize by helping the family determine how to accomplish daily routines (family roles), facilitate communication, locate needed resources, and use a shared decision-making approach to foster family resilience and coping.

Family Coping

In any kind of crisis, families function best when the whole family can come together in offering support, resources, and nurturance (Walsh, 2015, 2016b). "Informal kin and chosen family members can be lifelines for resilience, especially for under-resourced single parents, immigrants, refugees, and migrant workers" (Walsh, 2016b, p. 77).

Every family has its own set of coping strategies that may or may not be adequate in times of stress, such as when a family member experiences an altered health event. Even families who function at optimal levels with well-established coping strategies may experience difficulties when stressful events pile up (Walsh, 2015, 2016b). Families with support can withstand and rebound from difficult stressors or crises (Walsh, 2016b), which is referred to as *family resilience*. "Family resilience refers to the capacity of the family system to withstand and rebound from adversity, strengthened and more resourceful. More than coping with or surviving an ordeal, resilience involves positive adaptation, (re)gaining the ability to thrive, with personal and relational transformation and positive growth forged through the experience" (Walsh, 2016a, p. 616).

For many reasons, not all families have the same ability to cope. There is no universal list of key effective factors that contribute to family resilience, but a review of research and literature by Black and Lobo (2008) found the following similarities across studies for those families that cope well: a positive outlook, spirituality, family member accord, flexibility, communication, financial management, time together, mutual recreational interests, routines and rituals, and social support. According to Walsh (2016a, 2016b), some key processes in family resilience include belief system, organizational patterns, and family communication. The family's belief system involves making meaning of adversity, maintaining a positive outlook, and being able to transcend adversity through a spiritual/faith system (Walsh, 2016a, 2016b). The families' organization patterns, which speak to their flexibility, connectedness, and social and economic resources, help the family maintain resilience. Finally, families who communicate with clarity, allow open emotional expression, and have a collaborative problem-solving approach facilitate family resilience (Walsh, 2016a, 2016b).

Nurses have the ability to support families in times of stress and crisis through empowering processes that work well and are familiar to the family. Using a strengths-based approach, family nurses help families to adjust and adapt to stressors (Walsh, 2015, 2016b).

Family Roles

All families have a variety of different roles and responsibilities for the individuals in the family. A role is an expected pattern or set of behaviors associated with a particular position within the family. Roles are defined as formal when they are associated with position and structure. Roles can be defined according to the job that a role performs to help the family function on a daily basis. Other roles are informal and may be related to the family member's personality.

Within the family, regardless of structure, each family position has several attached roles, and each role is accompanied by expectations. The following formal roles defined by family structure are typically present in all families in some fashion: parent, child, brother, sister, spouse/partner, grandparent, aunt/uncle, and grandchild. The *family genogram* is a basic fundamental tool used to illustrate a detailed record of family history and information (Cuartas, 2017). Genograms include basic details about the family members and the family structure, as well as provide information about the medical and social history of the family. The tool can be used during assessment of strengths and risks within the family, and may help the nurse identify any complexities or opportunities for support and intervention. Family genograms are utilized throughout the book to illustrate the unique and complex nature of families.

Functional roles help the family accomplish tasks that keep the family organized in getting the work of the family done. Some of these roles include the tasks of provider, caregiver, organizer and planner, and decision maker. Some of the duties of the family are done by specific family members as a matter of routine, such as chores and housework, child care, grocery shopping, cooking, home repairs, driving, managing the finances, and so on. These duties and roles can change when a new family member is added, such as with the birth or adoption of a child, or due to a marriage or a change in the relationships in the family. When a family member becomes ill due to a short-term illness, the family may need to adapt to the change. When the disruption is caused by chronic illness, the changes may require more creativity and teamwork to reduce the stress on the family. When a family experiences the loss of a family member due to death or divorce, roles are shifted more significantly, which may cause a family crisis. When death is caused by a long-term chronic situation, the family must still adjust to the permanent change in structure and roles.

Health-Promoting Behaviors

Typically, individuals learn health-promoting behaviors in their immediate families or from close caregivers and role models. The family unit is an "unparalleled player" for maintaining, promoting, and supporting health while also preventing disease and conditions because members support and nurture each other throughout the life span (Barnes et al., 2020, p. 1). The family also contributes to the health of the public and community by promoting the family system. Throughout the discipline of public health, there is an emphasis on empowering the public to ensure that everyone can be healthy, which includes engaging with families for strategic partnerships and health promotion programming (South et al., 2018). When engaged as full partners in the promotion of health within the family, families may facilitate improved outcomes for individuals and communities (Dinkel et al., 2017). The following perspectives are important to supporting family engagement, family diversity, family stability, and family responsibility when it comes to health promotion for the family:

1. Consider the larger context of the family (all members) when planning and implementing health promotion activities.
2. Advocate for family health in policy decisions.
3. Partner with families to demonstrate optimism or belief in their capacity to improve health outcomes.
4. Focus on strengthening family mentors in the community.
5. Strengthen family capacity to model memorable and positive health practices.
6. Empower families to assess their own needs, abilities, and possible solutions to their problems (South et al., 2019).

Each of these perspectives supports the nurse's role as clinician, caregiver, advocate, educator, and researcher to partner with families to promote the overall health of the family and each member.

Family Communication

Communication is an ongoing, complex social interaction within families. Family communication affects family health and the function of the family. During health care interactions, effective communication establishes the joint agreement between health care providers and individuals and families to engage in a two-way process (expressive and receptive) in which messages are negotiated and understood by both parties (Joint Commission, 2021). Successful communication is achieved when providers understand and integrate information shared by individuals and families and, in turn, when individuals and families demonstrate that they comprehend accurate, timely, and complete messages from providers in a way that enables them to participate fully in their care (The Joint Commission, 2021). Nurses have a unique and important role related to communication with individuals and when working with families.

The role of the nurse is to facilitate family communication. Nurses model communication skills through listening, reflection, and summarizing communication in order to enhance understanding among family members. Nurses also support family members through communication that occurs during times of stress such as during a health crisis experienced by a member of the family, when supporting a family during childbirth, during a mental health crisis affecting a family or community, or at the time of loss or grief experienced when a family member is lost due to death.

The goals of nurse-family communication include (1) establishing a trusting relationship; (2) providing emotional support to families; (3) helping families to understand diagnosis, prognosis, and treatment options; (4) developing an understanding of the patient as an individual and as part of a family; and (5) supporting an environment that supports discussion and decision making that is individual- and family-centered (Seaman et al., 2017). Ultimately, nurses support family communication to ensure the safety and comfort of the family members while helping them to achieve a successful, healthy outcome. Communication strategies that nurses use when working with families are discussed in subsequent chapters throughout this text.

Family Decision Making

Several factors influence decision making within families, including the choices and decisions that are made about health care. Family decision making is a group effort that can be complex and socially interactive (Slade, 2017), and it is also informed by the culture and history of the family. Every family has their own communication style when it comes to making decisions about health care for the family and for individual family members. Within the context of the health care system, it is rare for individuals to make decisions alone or based solely on their own perspective. In addition to input they may have from family members, caregivers, or other support persons, they also have perspectives and information shared by health care professionals. In fact, it is critical for health care professionals to educate individuals and families about their treatment options so they can make the best decisions possible (Seaman et al., 2017). Within the health care system, decision making for individuals and families relies on information that comes from providers and allows patients and families to take an informed, active role in collaborating on their treatment plan (Slade, 2017).

The Agency for Healthcare Research and Quality (2020) prioritizes shared decision making between health care providers and individuals and families so they may work together to make health care decisions that are in their best interest. The most effective decisions consider the best evidence and information that has been provided about every option available, the health care provider's knowledge and experience, and the individual's values and preferences (Agency for Healthcare Research and Quality, 2020). A family-centered approach places the family in the process of shared decision making, which is important if individuals have made the choice to include family members when making choices about health care. The SHARE Approach is a five-step process for shared decision making that engages health care providers, individuals, and families in meaningful discussion about their choices:

1. Seek your patient's participation.
2. Help your patient explore and compare treatment options.
3. Assess your patient's values and preferences.
4. Reach a decision with your patient.
5. Evaluate your patient's decision (Agency for Healthcare Research and Quality, 2020).

Shared decision making is beneficial for health care providers and for individuals and families. While there is evidence to indicate that health outcomes and patient satisfaction are improved when patients participate more fully in health care decision making (Hibbard & Green, 2013; Parchman et al., 2010), Satin et al. (2017) suggested that some outcome-based metrics used in health care can be insensitive to patient and family preferences. They proposed elements of shared decision making in family medicine that include (1) discussing relevant information about health conditions, possible treatments, and likely outcomes with patients and families; (2) clarifying and understanding patients' unique values and priorities when making treatment decisions; and (3) providing patients the choice in a care plan that fits their personal goals (Satin et al., 2017). High-quality communication between health care providers and individuals and families, which is at the center of shared decision making, has a meaningful impact on individual and family satisfaction within the health care system.

In a recent study that examined nursing staff confidence with communicating with family members of patients in the intensive care unit, family-member satisfaction with the quality of communication was rated higher than the level of patient-care satisfaction (Edward et al., 2020). Nurses that expressed confidence with patient- and family-centered approaches to communication that engaged them in shared decision making helped to reduce the anxiety and stress levels of family members (Edward et al., 2020). Researchers conducting a quality improvement study on family engagement were able to transform care in an intensive care unit from a primarily patient-focused model to a model built on family involvement, shared decision making, mutual respect, and ongoing collaboration (McAndrew et al., 2020). Themes identified by families about their overall experience included family interactions with the team, information sharing and effective communication, family navigation of the care environment, family engagement, and quality of patient care. Families consistently identify effective communication and information sharing as key to reducing their anxiety and stress during times of illness. Nurses have a crucial role in transforming family-centered care due to their ongoing presence and interactions with families (Auriemma et al., 2021; McAndrew et al., 2020).

Family Rituals and Routines

All families have unique rituals and routines that provide organization, give meaning to family life, and help families cope when in crisis. Family rituals and traditions allow families to make memories, share special moments, celebrate milestones, and develop the values of the family. Routines are patterned behaviors or interactions that provide a sense of continuity through daily or regular activities, such as bedtime procedures, mealtimes, greetings, and treatment of guests (Walsh, 2016b).

Routines keep the family on track with what needs to be done and keeping the family functioning. Families use routines to provide structure and order so that the family works together to serve the needs of the family as a whole and of each member. Family routines can create structure that build confidence in each family member, particularly when the family experiences stress or crisis. Some purposes that family routines accomplish for families are (Kiser, 2015, p. 26):

- Accomplish tasks in order to meet basic needs
- Provide structure
- Clarify roles
- Provide rules and structure
- Establish boundaries around who is part of the family
- Support family communication and cohesion
- Establish an identity by personalizing routines in the family
- Provide predictability within the family, which in turn provides comfort and confidence

Rituals involve symbolic communication among the family members that provides for a feeling of belonging (Fraser-Thill, 2020). Rituals are actions family members undertake individually and collectively as a family for a specific purpose; they provide meaning to who that family is, reveal what the members believe, and identify what is important to that family. Rituals can be created about any aspect of life, but they often are associated with formal celebrations, cultural or family traditions, and religious and spiritual observances with symbolic meaning that all provide a shared meaning for life events.

When family rituals and routines are disrupted by illness, the family system as a whole is affected; therefore, it can affect the health of each family member and the family as a whole (Walsh, 2016b). Family rituals and routines are important aspects that influence positive health outcomes during times of stress and illness that affect the family.

- Established family routines and rituals were performed less as the illness interfered with the timing or ability of members to participate.
- New routines and rituals were established to help the family adapt to changing needs.
- Routines and rituals provided opportunities for family members to support each other emotionally.
- Rituals and routines offered the family a sense of normalcy amid the challenges posed by chronic conditions.
- Rituals and routines supported positive health and adaptation outcomes for both patients and family members.

Assessing rituals and routines related to specific health or illness needs provides a basis to envision distinct family interventions and to devise specific plans for health promotion and disease management, especially when adherence to medical regimens is critical or caregiving demands are burdensome to the families (Denham, 2016). Family nurses who support families in conducting their routines help families have a sense of normalcy in the face of stress from a family member's illness.

Nurses can help families establish new routines that provide structure and meet the needs of the family (Denham, 2016). Nurses can facilitate family rituals by navigating organizational obstacles that may prevent the family from conducting or participating in an important family ritual. Nurses can assist families to establish daily routines that support the functioning of the family.

SUMMARY

This chapter provides an introduction and broad overview to family health care nursing. The following major concepts were discussed in this chapter:

- Family health care nursing is an art and a science that has evolved as a way of thinking about and working with families.
- Family nursing is a scientific discipline based in theory.
- Health and illness are family events.
- The term *family* is defined in many ways, but the most salient definition is *the family is who the members say it is.*
- An individual's health affects the entire family's functioning; in turn, the family's ability to function affects each individual member's health.
- The family is well positioned to maintain, promote, and support the health of the family while also preventing disease; family members support and nurture each other throughout the life span.
- Family health care nursing knowledge and skills are important for nurses who practice in generalized and in specialized settings.
- Knowledge about each family's structure, function, and process informs the nurse in how to optimize nursing care in families and provide individualized nursing care, tailored to the uniqueness of every family system.

chapter 2

Theoretical Foundations for the Nursing of Families

Lynette Savage, PhD, RN

Critical Concepts

- Theories inform the practice of nursing. Practice informs theory and research. Theory, practice, and research are interactive, and all three are critical to the profession of nursing and family care.

- The major purpose of theory in family nursing is to provide knowledge and understanding that improves the quality of nursing care of families.

- By understanding theories and models, nurses are prepared to think more creatively and critically about how health events affect family clients. Theories and models provide different ways of comprehending issues that may be affecting families and offer choices for action.

- The theoretical/conceptual frameworks and models that provide the foundations for nursing of families have evolved from three major traditions and disciplines: family social science, family therapy, and nursing.

- No single theory, model, or conceptual framework adequately describes the complex relationships of family structure, function, and process. Nor does one theoretical perspective give nurses a sufficiently broad base of knowledge and understanding to guide assessment and interventions with families. No one theoretical perspective is better, more comprehensive, or more correct than another. Nurses who use an integrated theoretical approach build on the strengths of families in creative ways. Nurses who use a singular theoretical approach to working with families limit the possibilities for families they serve. By integrating several theories, nurses acquire different ways to conceptualize problems, thus enhancing their thinking about interventions.

By understanding theories and models, nurses are prepared to think creatively and critically about how health events affect the family client. The reciprocal or interactive relationship between theory, practice, and research is that each aspect informs the other, thereby expanding knowledge and nursing interventions to support families. Theories and models extend thinking to higher levels of understanding problems and circumstances that may be affecting families and thereby offer more choices and options for nursing interventions.

Currently, no single theory, model, or conceptual framework adequately describes the complex relationships of family structure, function, and process. Nor does one theoretical perspective give nurses a sufficiently broad base of knowledge and understanding to guide assessment and interventions with families. No one theoretical perspective is better, more comprehensive, or more correct than another (Doane & Varcoe, 2015; Kaakinen, 2019). The goal for nurses is to have a deep understanding of the stresses that families experience when their family clients have a health event and to support and implement family interventions based on theoretical perspectives that best match the needs identified by the family.

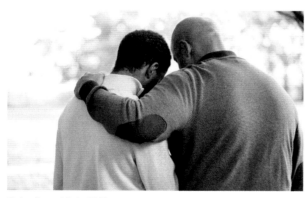

© istock.com/digitalskillet

Many theoretical approaches exist to help understand families. The purpose of this chapter is to demonstrate how families who have members experiencing a health event are conceptualized differently depending on the theoretical perspective. This chapter shows how nurses seek different data depending on which theory is being used, both to understand the family experience and to determine the interventions offered to the family to support the health and well-being of each individual and the family as a whole.

This chapter begins with a brief review of the components of the three chosen theories and how the

components contribute to the nursing care of families. Each theoretical approach is presented, ranging from a broader to a more specific perspective:

- Family Systems Theory
- Developmental and Family Life Cycle Theory
- Bioecological Theory

The chapter utilizes a case study of a family with a member who is experiencing progressive multiple sclerosis (MS) to demonstrate these three different theoretical approaches to nursing care of families.

RELATIONSHIP BETWEEN THEORY, PRACTICE, AND RESEARCH

In nursing, the relationship of theory to practice constitutes a dynamic feedback loop rather than a static linear progression. Theory, practice, and research are mutually interdependent. Theory grows out of observations made in practice and is tested by research; then tested theory informs practice; and practice, in turn, facilitates the further refinement and development of theory. Figure 2-1 depicts the dynamic relationship between theory, practice, and research.

Theories do not emerge all at once. Rather, they build slowly over time as data are gathered through practice, observation, assimilation of meaningful experiences, and analysis of evidence. Relating together the various concepts that emerge from observation and evidence occurs through a purposeful, thoughtful reasoning process. *Inductive reasoning* is a process that moves from specific pieces of information toward a general or broader idea; it is thinking about

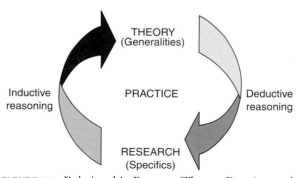

FIGURE 2-1 Relationship Between Theory, Practice, and Research *Source: Adapted from Smith, S. R., Hamon, R. R., Ingoldsby, B. B., & Miller, J. E. [2008]. Exploring family theories [2nd ed.]. New York, NY: Oxford University Press.*

how the parts create the whole. *Deductive reasoning* goes in the opposite direction from inductive reasoning. Deductive reasoning occurs when the broader ideas of a given theory generate more specific questions. These specific questions further clarify the theory and filter back into the cycle. Deductive reasoning helps refine understanding of the specific details of the theory and how to apply the theory to practice (Smith & Hamon, 2016; White et al., 2014).

Assimilating meaningful experiences is the cognitive process of making new information fit with an individual's existing understanding of the world (Cherry, 2020). This adaptation process, described by Piaget, is when an individual either assimilates or accommodates new experiences into existing individual knowledge (Bormanaki & Khoshhal, 2017). This allows the individual to expand an ever-growing knowledge base from various experiences and to make both large and small adjustments to their existing thought processes.

Theories are designed to make sense of the world by showing how one concept is related to another and how together they make a meaningful pattern that can predict the consequences of certain clusters of characteristics or events. Theories are abstract, general ideas that are subject to rules of organization. Theories provide a general framework for understanding data in an organized way, as well as showing us how to predict patterns and more accurately intervene to prevent, stabilize, or treat problems. We live in a time when tremendous amounts of information are readily available and quickly accessible in multiple forms. Therefore, theories provide ways to transform this large volume of information into organized knowledge and to integrate the information in order to help us make better sense of the world (White et al., 2014). Ideally, nursing theories represent logical and intelligible patterns that make sense of the observations that nurses make in practice and enable nurses to predict what is likely to happen to clients based on observed patterns (Polit & Beck, 2021). Theories are tools for reasoning, critical thinking, and decision making and thus lead to quality nursing practice (Alligood, 2018). The major function of theory in family nursing is to provide knowledge and understanding that improves nursing care for families.

Another important aspect of theories is that they explain what is happening; they provide answers to "how" and "why" questions, help to interpret and make sense of complex phenomena, and predict what could happen in the future based

on careful thought and study about what has happened in the past. All scientific theories use the same components: *concepts*, *relationships*, and *propositions*. Theories also construct hypotheses (i.e., what is expected to happen) and conceptual models (i.e., relationships between several concepts).

Concepts, the building blocks of theory, are words that create mental images or abstract representations of phenomena of study. Concepts, the major ideas expressed by a theory, may be abstract or concrete, and they may have different meanings in various conceptual or theoretical frameworks (Hardin, 2018). The more concrete the concept, the easier it is to figure out when it applies or does not apply (White et al., 2014). For example, one concept in Family Systems Theory is that families have boundaries. A highly abstract aspect of this concept is that the boundary reflects the energy between the environment and the system. A more concrete aspect of this concept is that families open or close their boundaries, or their willingness to let others into their lives, in times of stress.

Propositions are statements about the proposed relationship between two or more concepts or a logical deduction from a theoretical statement (Hardin, 2018). A proposition might be a statement such as the following: Families as a whole influence the health of individual family members. The word *influence* proposes a link between the two concepts of "families as a whole" and "health of individual family members." Propositions suggest a relationship between the subject and the object. Propositions may lead to hypotheses. Theories are generally made up of several propositions that suggest the relationships among the concepts in that specific theory.

A *hypothesis* is a way of stating an expected relationship between concepts or an expected proposition (Hardin, 2018). The concepts and propositions in the hypothesis are derived from and driven by the original theory. For example, using the concepts of family and health, one could hypothesize that there is an interactive relationship between how a family is coping and the eventual health outcome of family members. In other words, the family's ability to cope with stress affects the health of individual family members; in turn, the health of an individual family member influences the family's ability to cope. The proposed relationship, or hypothesis, is that the concept of coping is related to the concept of health in families. This hypothesis may be tested by a research study that measures family coping strategies and family members' health over time and that uses statistical procedures to look at the relationships between the two concepts.

A *conceptual model* is a set of general propositions that integrate concepts into an explanation of phenomena (Alligood, 2018). Conceptual models in nursing are based on the observations, insights, and deductions that combine ideas from several fields of inquiry. Conceptual models provide a frame of reference and a coherent way of thinking about nursing phenomena. A conceptual model is more abstract and more comprehensive than a theory. Similar to a conceptual model, a conceptual framework is a way of integrating concepts into a meaningful pattern; however, conceptual frameworks are often less definitive than models. They provide useful conceptual approaches or ways to look at a problem or situation rather than a definite set of propositions about relationships between concepts.

In this text, the terms *conceptual model or framework* and *theory or theoretical framework* are often used interchangeably. In part, this is because no single theoretical base exists for the nursing of families. Rather, nurses typically draw from many theoretical conceptual foundations using a more pluralistic and eclectic approach. The interchangeable use of these various terms reflects the fact that there is considerable overlap among ideas in the various theoretical perspectives and conceptual models/frameworks and that many influences and perspectives are important for family nurses to understand, consider, and incorporate into practice. As might be expected, a substantial amount of cross-fertilization among disciplines has occurred, such as between social science and nursing, and concepts originating in one theory or discipline have been translated into similar concepts for use in another discipline. Currently, no one theoretical perspective or one discipline gives nurses a sufficiently broad base of knowledge and understanding to guide assessment and interventions with families.

THEORETICAL AND CONCEPTUAL FOUNDATIONS FOR THE NURSING OF FAMILIES

Nursing is a scientific discipline; thus, nurses are concerned about the relationships between ideas and data. Nurse scholars have developed theories based on empirical observations, aspects of nursing practice, and testable practice questions that can be used as evidence in evidence-based practice (Alligood, 2018). In nursing, evidence-based

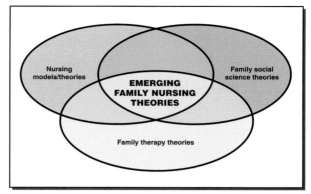

FIGURE 2-2 Theoretical Frameworks That Influence the Nursing of Families

practice is practice that is based on the best available evidence, patient preferences, and clinical judgment (Schmidt & Brown, 2019). Nurse researchers investigate and test the models and relationships. Nurses in practice use theories, models, and conceptual frameworks to decide on interventions that will help clients achieve the best outcomes (Kaakinen, 2019). In nursing, evidence, in the form of theory, is used to explain and guide practice. The theoretical foundations, theories, and conceptual models that explain and guide the practice of nursing families have evolved from three major traditions and disciplines: family social science theories, family therapy theories, and nursing models and theories. Figure 2-2 shows the theoretical frameworks that influence the nursing of families.

Family Social Science Theories

Of the three sources of theory, *family social science theories* are the best developed and informative about family phenomena. Examples of such theories include the following: family function, the environment-family interchange, interactions and dynamics within the family, changes in the family over time, and the family's reaction to health and illness. Table 2-1 summarizes the basic family social science theories and provides some classic references where these theories originate. It is challenging to use the purist form of family social science theories as a basis for nursing assessment and intervention because of the abstract nature of theory. Despite this challenge, in recent years, nursing and family scholars have made strides in extrapolating and morphing these theories for use in clinical work (Kaakinen, 2019).

Table 2-1	Family Social Science Theories Used in Family Nursing Practice
FAMILY SOCIAL SCIENCE THEORY	**SUMMARY**
Structural Functional Theory	
Friedman, Bowden, and Jones (2003) Nye and Berardo (1981)	The focus is on families as an institution and how they function to maintain the family and social network.
Symbolic Interaction Theory	
Hill and Hansen (1960)	The focus is on the interactions within families and the symbolic communication.
Nye (1976)	
Rose (1962)	
Turner (1970)	
Developmental and Family Life Cycle Theory	
Carter and McGoldrick (2005)	The focus is on the life cycle of families and representing normative stages of family development.
Duvall (1977)	
Duvall and Miller (1985)	
Pelton (2011)	Expanding the family life cycle to address the needs of voluntarily childfree couples.
Falicov (2016)	Expanding the family life cycle to address the needs of migrant families.
Family Systems Theory	
von Bertalanffy (1950, 1968)	The focus is on the circular interactions among members of family systems. These circular interactions result in functional or dysfunctional outcomes.
Family Stress Theory	
Hill (1949, 1965)	The focus is on the analysis of how families experience and cope with stressful life events.
McCubbin and McCubbin (1993)	
McCubbin and Patterson (1983)	
Theory of Comfort	
Kolcaba (2003)	Kolcaba described (a) comfort as existing in three forms: *relief, ease,* and *transcendence* and (b) four contexts in which patient comfort can occur: *physical, psychospiritual, environmental,* and *sociocultural.*
Change Theory	
Maturana (1978)	The focus is on how families remain stable or change when there is change within the family structure or from outside influences.
Maturana and Varela (1992)	
Watzlawick, Weakland, and Fisch (1974)	
Shajani & Snell (2019)	
Wright and Watson (1988)	
Transition Theory	
White (2005)	The focus is on understanding and predicting the transitions that families experience over time by combining Role Theory, Family Development Theory, and Life Course Theory.
White, Klein, and Martin (2014)	

Family Therapy Theories

Family therapy theories are newer than and not as well developed as family social science theories. Table 2-2 lists these theories and the names of some foundational scholars who first developed them. These theories emanate from a practice discipline of family therapy rather than from an academic discipline of family social science. Family therapy theories were developed to work with troubled families and therefore focus primarily on family pathology. Nevertheless, these conceptual models describe family dynamics and patterns that are found, to some extent, in all families (Tadros, 2019). Because these models are concerned with what can be done to facilitate change in dysfunctional families, they are both descriptive and prescriptive. They describe and explain observations made in practice, treatment, and intervention strategies.

Nursing Conceptual Frameworks

Finally, of the three types of theories, *nursing conceptual frameworks* are the least developed theories in relation to the nursing of families. Table 2-3 lists several of the theories and theorists from within the nursing profession. During the 1960s and 1970s, nurses placed great emphasis on the development of nursing models. Other than the Neuman Systems Model (Neuman & Fawcett, 2010) and the Behavioral Systems Model for Nursing (Johnson, 1980), both of which were based on family social science theories, the majority of the classic nursing theorists from the 1970s focused on individual patients and not on families as a unit of care/analysis. The nursing models, in large part, represent a deductive approach to the development of nursing science (general to specific). Although they embody an important part of our nursing heritage, these nursing conceptual frameworks and their

Table 2-2	Family Therapy Theories Used in Family Nursing Practice
FAMILY THERAPY THEORIES	**SUMMARY**
Structural Family Therapy Theory	
Minuchin (1974)	This systems-oriented approach views the family as an open sociocultural system that is continually faced with demands for change, both from within and from outside the family. The focus is on the whole family system; its subsystems, boundaries, and coalitions; as well as family transactional patterns and covert rules.
Minuchin and Fishman (1981)	
Minuchin, Rosman, and Baker (1978)	
Nichols (2004)	
International Family Therapy Theory	
Jackson (1965)	This approach views the family as a system of interactive or interlocking behaviors or communication processing. Emphasis is on the here and now rather than on the past. Key interventions focus on establishing clear, congruent communication and clarifying and changing family rules.
Watzlawick, Beavin, and Jackson (1967)	
Family Systems Therapy Theory	
Freeman (1992)	This approach focuses on promoting differentiation of self from family and promoting differentiation of intellect from emotion. Family members are encouraged to examine their processes to gain insight and understanding into their past and present. This therapy requires a long-term commitment.
Kerr and Bowen (1988)	
Toman (1961)	

Table 2-3	Nursing Theories and Models Used in Family Nursing Practice
NURSING THEORIES AND MODELS	**SUMMARY**
Nightingale Nightingale (1859)	Family is described as having both positive and negative influences on the outcome of family members. The family is seen as a supportive institution throughout the life span for its individual family members.
Rogers's Science of Unitary Human Beings Rogers (1970, 1986, 1990)	The family is viewed as a constant open system energy field that is ever-changing in its interactions with the environment.
Roy's Adaptation Model Roy (1976) Roy and Roberts (1981)	The family is seen as an adaptive system that has inputs, internal control, and feedback processes and output. The strength of this model is an understanding of how families adapt to health issues.
Johnson's Behavioral Systems Model for Nursing Johnson (1980)	The family is viewed as a behavioral system composed of a set of organized, interactive, interdependent, and integrated subsystems that adjust and adapt to internal and external forces.
King's Goal Attainment Theory King (1981, 1983, 1987)	The family is seen as the vehicle for transmitting values and norms of behavior across the lifespan, including behaviors during health and illness. The family is responsible for addressing the health care function of the family. Family is seen as both an interpersonal and a social system. The key component is the interaction between the nurse and the family as client.
Neuman's Systems Model Neuman (1983, 1995)	The family is viewed as a system. The family's primary goal is to maintain its stability by preserving the integrity of its structure by opening and closing its boundaries. It is a fluid model that depicts the family in motion and is not a static view of family from one perspective.
Orem's Self-Care Deficit Theory Gray (1996) Orem (1983a, 1983b, 1985)	The family is seen as the basic conditioning unit in which the individual learns culture, roles, and responsibilities. Specifically, family members learn how to act when one is ill. The family's self-care behavior evolves through interpersonal relationships, communication, and culture that is unique to each family.
Parse's Human Becoming Theory Parse (1992, 1998)	The concept of family and who makes up the family is viewed as continually becoming and evolving. The role of the nurse is to use therapeutic communication to invite family members to uncover their meaning of the experience, to learn what the meaning of the experience is for each other, and to discuss the meaning of the experience for the family as a whole.
Friedemann's Framework of Systemic Organization Friedemann (1995)	The family is described as a social system that has the expressed goal of transmitting culture to its members. The elements central to this theory are family stability, family growth, family control, and family spirituality.
Denham's Family Health Model Denham (2003)	Family health is viewed as a process over time of family member interactions and health-related behaviors. Family health is described in relation to contextual, functional, and structural domains. Dynamic family health routines are behavioral patterns that reflect self-care, safety and prevention, mental health behaviors, family care, illness care, and family caregiving.

deductive approach are viewed more critically today. As the science of nursing has evolved, more inductive approaches to nursing theory have developed (specific to general) and are now being used in everyday nursing practice.

Table 2-4 shows the differences between family social science theories, family therapy theories, and nursing models/theories as they inform the practice of nursing with families. The following case study is used to demonstrate how the three different theoretical approaches may guide a nurse's work with one family. Box 2-1 compares these three theories as they apply to the Jones family case study.

Table 2-4	Family Social Science Theories, Family Therapy Theories, and Nursing Models/Theories		
CRITERIA	FAMILY SOCIAL SCIENCE THEORIES	FAMILY THERAPY THEORIES	NURSING MODELS/THEORIES
Purpose of theory	Descriptive and explanatory (academic models); to explain family functioning and dynamics.	Descriptive and prescriptive (practice models); to explain family dysfunction and guide therapeutic actions.	Descriptive and prescriptive (practice models); to guide nursing assessment and intervention efforts.
Discipline focus	Interdisciplinary (although primarily sociological).	Marriage and family therapy; family mental health; new approaches focus on family strengths.	Nursing focus.
Target population	Primarily "normal" families (normality-oriented).	Primarily "troubled" families (pathology-oriented).	Primarily families with health and illness problems.

BOX 2-1

Comparison of Theories as They Apply to the Jones Family

Family Systems Theory

Conceptual

Family is viewed as a whole. What happens to the family as a whole affects each individual family member, and what happens to individuals affects the totality of the family unit. Focus is on the circular interactions among members of the family system, resulting in functional or dysfunctional outcomes.

Assessment

The family may be assessed together or individually. Assessment questions relate to the *interaction* between the individual and the family, and the *interaction* between the family and the community in which the family lives.

Intervention Examples

- Complete a family genogram to understand patterns and relationships over several generations over time.
- Complete a family ecomap to see how individuals/family relate to the community around them.
- Collect data about the family as a whole and about individual family members.
- Conduct care-planning sessions that include family members.

Strengths

Focus is on family as a whole, its subsystems, or both. It is a generally understood and accepted theory in society.

Weaknesses

Theory is broad and general. It does not give definitive prescriptions for interventions.

Application to the Jones Family

All members of the Jones family are affected by the mother's progressive chronic health condition and changes. Family structure, functions, and processes of the family are influenced, thus changing family roles and dynamics. Everyone in the family has his or her own concerns and needs attention from health care professionals.

Family Developmental and Life Cycle Theory

Conceptual

Family is viewed as a whole over time. All families go through similar developmental processes, starting with the birth of the first child to death of the parents. Focus is on the life cycle of families and represents normative stages of family development.

BOX 2-1

Comparison of Theories as They Apply to the Jones Family—cont'd

Assessment

The family may be assessed together or individually. Assessment questions relate to the normative predictable events that occur in family life over time. It also includes non-normative, unexpected events.

Intervention Examples

- Conduct a family interview to determine where the family is in terms of cognitive, social, emotional, spiritual, and physical development.
- Complete a family genogram and ecomap.
- Determine the normative and non-normative events that have occurred to the family as a whole or to individuals within the family.
- Analyze how an individual's growth and developmental milestones may affect the family developmental trajectory.

Strengths

Focus is on the family as a whole. The theory provides a framework for predicting what a family will experience at any given stage in the family life cycle so that nurses can offer anticipatory guidance.

Weaknesses

The traditional linear family life cycle is no longer the norm. Modern families vary widely in their structure and roles. Divorce, remarriage, gay parents, and never-married parents have changed the traditional trajectory of growth and developmental milestones. The theory does not focus on how the family adapts to the transitions from one stage to the other; rather, it simply predicts what transitions will occur.

Application to the Jones Family

The Jones family is in the stages of "families with adolescents" and "launching young adults." The non-normative health condition of the mother is changing the predictable normative course of development for the individuals and for the family as a whole. These health events will change the cognitive, social, emotional, spiritual, and physical development as the family shifts to integrate new roles into their lives as family members.

Bioecological Systems Theory

Conceptual

Bioecological systems theory combines children's biological disposition and environmental forces that come together to shape the development of human beings. This theory has a basis in both developmental theory and systems theory to understand individual and family growth. It combines the influence of both genetics and environment from the individual and family with the larger economic/political structure over time. The basic premise is that individual and family development are contextual over time. The different levels of the theory that apply to the family at any one point in time vary depending on what is happening at that time. Therefore, the interaction of the systems varies over time as the situation changes.

Assessment

Assess all levels of the larger ecological system when interviewing the family. Determine the microsystem, mesosystem, exosystem, macrosystem, and chronosystem of the individual and of the family as a whole.

Intervention Examples

- Conduct a family interview to determine the family's status in relationship to four locational/spatial contexts and one time-related context.
- Complete a family genogram and ecomap.
- Determine how individuals are doing in relationship to their entire environment, which includes immediate family, extended family, home, school, and community.
- Analyze the family in its smaller and larger contextual aspects.

Strengths

Focus is on a holistic approach to human/family development. A biological, psychological, sociological, cultural, and spiritual approach to understanding how individuals and families develop and adapt over time in their society is a more complete approach.

Weaknesses

This holistic approach is not specific enough to define contextual changes over time. Nor can the larger context in which individuals/families are embedded be predicted or controlled.

Application to the Jones Family

- *Microsystem:* The Jones family consists of school-age children living at home. The parental roles have been traditional until recent health events.
- *Mesosystem:* Family has much interaction with schools, church, and extended family.
- *Exosystem:* Family influenced by father's work at the factory and other institutions in the community.
- *Macrosystem:* Family consistent with community culture, attitudes, and beliefs. Their community is largely Caucasian, middle class, and Christian.
- *Chronosystem:* At this time in the illness story of the Jones family, with the mother's illness changing, the family situation changes and moves between stability and crisis.

Family Case Study: Jones Family

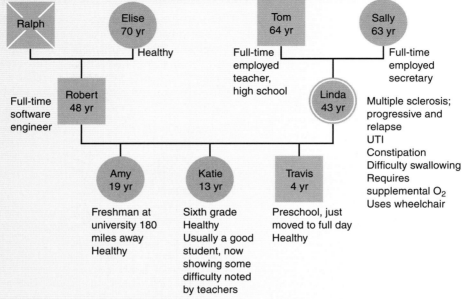

FIGURE 2-3 Jones Family Genogram

Setting: Inpatient acute care hospital.

Nursing Goal: Work with the family to assist them in preparation for discharge that is planned to occur in the next 2 days.

Family Members:
The Jones family is a nuclear family. The Jones family genogram and ecomap are illustrated in Figures 2-3 and 2-4, respectively.

- Robert: 48 years old; father, software engineer, full-time employed.
- Linda: 43 years old; mother, stay-at-home homemaker, has progressive MS, which recently has worsened significantly.
- Amy: 19 years old; oldest child, daughter, freshman at university in town 180 miles away.
- Katie: 13 years old; middle child, daughter, sixth grade, usually a good student.
- Travis: 4 years old; youngest child, son, just started attending an all-day preschool because of his mother's illness.

Jones Family Story
Linda was diagnosed with MS at age 30 when Katie was 3 months old. After her diagnosis, Linda had a well-controlled, slow progression of her illness. Travis was a surprise pregnancy for Linda at age 39; he is described as "a blessing." Linda and Robert are devout Baptists. They did discuss abortion in light of the fact that Linda's illness could progress significantly after the birth of Travis. Their faith and personal beliefs did not support abortion. They made the decision to continue with Linda's pregnancy, knowing the risk that it might exacerbate and speed up her MS. Linda had an uncomplicated pregnancy with Travis. She felt well until three months postpartum with Travis when she noted a significant relapse of her MS.

During the last four years, Linda has experienced development of progressive relapsing MS, which is a progressive disease from onset with clear, acute relapses without full recovery after each relapse. The periods between her relapses are characterized by continuing progression of the disease. She now has secondary progressive MS because of her increased weakness. Robert and Linda are having sexual issues with decreased libido and painful intercourse for Linda. Both are experiencing stress in their marital roles and relationship.

Currently, Linda has had a serious relapse of her MS. She is hospitalized for secondary pneumonia from aspiration. She has weakness in all limbs, left foot drag, and increasing ataxia. Linda will be discharged with a wheelchair (this aid is new because she has used a cane up until this admission). She has weakness of her neck muscles and cannot hold her head steady for long periods. She has difficulty swallowing, which probably caused her aspiration. She has numbness and tingling of her legs and feet.

Family Case Study: Jones Family—cont'd

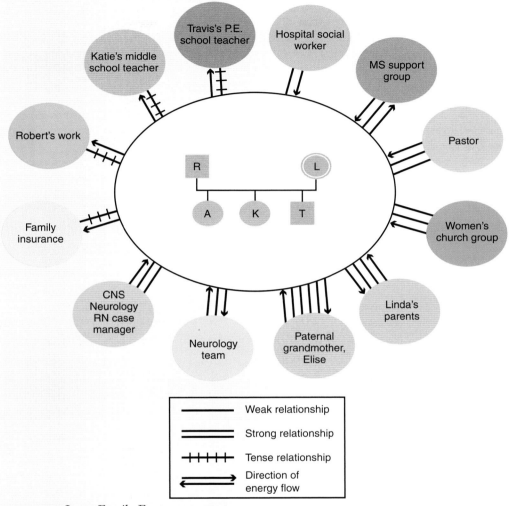

FIGURE 2-4 Jones Family Ecomap

periods. She has difficulty swallowing, which probably caused her aspiration. She has numbness and tingling of her legs and feet. She has severe pain with flexion of her neck. Her vision is blurred. She experiences vertigo at times and has periodic tinnitus. Constipation is a constant problem, together with urinary retention that causes periodic urinary tract infections.

Health Insurance
Robert receives health insurance through his work that covers the whole family. Hospitalizations are covered 80/20, so they have to pay 20 percent of their bills out of pocket. Although Robert is employed full-time, this cost adds heavily to the financial burden of the family. Robert has shared with the nurses that he does not know whether he should take his last week of vacation when his wife comes home or whether he should save it for a time when her condition worsens. Robert works for a company that offers family leave; however, it is without pay.

Family Members
Robert reports being continuously tired from caring for his wife and children as well as working full-time. He asked the doctor for medication to help him sleep and decrease his anxiety. He said that he is afraid that he may not hear Linda in the night when

(continued)

Family Case Study: Jones Family—cont'd

she needs help. He is open to his mother moving in to help care for Linda and the children. He begins counseling sessions with the pastor in their church.

Amy is a freshman at a university that is 180 miles away in a different town. Her mother is proud of Amy going to college on a full scholarship. Amy does well in her coursework; she travels home weekends to help the family and her mother. Amy is considering giving up her scholarship to transfer home to attend the local community college. She has not told her parents about this idea yet.

Katie is in the sixth grade. She is typically a good student; however, her latest report card showed that she dropped a letter grade in most of her classes. Katie is quiet. She stopped having friends over to her home about six months ago when her mother began to have more ataxia and slurring of speech. Linda used to be very involved in Katie's school; however, she is no longer involved because of her illness. Katie has been involved in Girl Scouts and the youth group at church.

Travis just started going to preschool two months ago for full days because of his mother's illness. This transition to preschool has been difficult for Travis because he had been home full-time with Linda until her disease worsened. He is healthy and developmentally on target for his age.

Linda's parents live in the same town. Her parents, Tom and Sally, both work full-time and are not able to help. Robert's widowed mother, Elise, lives by herself in her own home about 30 minutes out of town and has offered to move into the Jones's home to help care for Linda and the family.

Discharge Plans: Linda will be discharged home in two days.

Questions for reflection on the nursing care of the Jones family:

1. What strengths and challenges exist for the family as Linda prepares to discharge from the hospital?
2. What nursing interventions would you prioritize in caring for the Jones family as a whole and/or as individuals?
3. What approaches to communication would help the nurse build a relationship with the Jones family?
4. What resources in the community would you consider to support the Jones family?

THEORETICAL PERSPECTIVES AND APPLICATION TO FAMILIES

The case of the Jones family is used throughout the rest of this chapter to demonstrate how assessments, interventions, and options for care vary based on the particular theoretical perspective chosen by nurses caring for this family.

Family Systems Theory

Family Systems Theory has been the most influential of all the family social science frameworks (Kaakinen, 2019; Shajani & Snell, 2019). Much of the understanding of how a family is a system derives from physics and biology perspectives that organisms are complex, organized, and interactive systems (Bowen, 1978; von Bertalanffy, 1950, 1968). Nursing theorists who have expanded the concept of systems

theory include Etchin et al. (2020), Hanson (2001), Johnson (1980), Neuman (1995), Neuman and Fawcett (2010), Smith and Parker (2014), and Walker (2005).

The Family Systems Theory is an approach that allows nurses to understand and assess families as an organized whole and/or as individuals within family units who form an interactive and interdependent system (Kaakinen, 2019). Family Systems Theory is constructed of concepts and propositions that provide a framework for thinking about the family as a system. In family nursing, we typically look at three-generational family systems (Goldenberg et al., 2017).

One of the major assumptions of Family Systems Theory is that family system features are designed to maintain stability, although these features may be adaptive or maladaptive. At the same time, families change constantly in response to stresses and strains from both the internal and external environments. Family systems increase in complexity

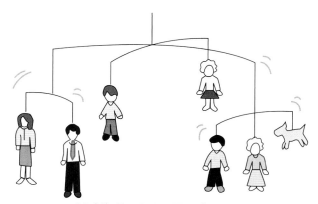

FIGURE 2-5 Mobile Depicting Family System

over time and increase their ability to adapt and to change (Smith & Hamon, 2016). The family systems theoretical perspective encourages nurses to see individual clients as participating members of a larger family system. Figure 2-5 depicts a mobile showing how family systems work. Any change in one member of the family affects all members of the family. As it applies to the Jones family, nurses who use this perspective would assess the impact of Linda's illness on the entire family as well as the effects of family functioning on Linda. The goal of nurses is to help maintain or restore the stability of the family in order to help family members achieve the highest level of functioning that they can. Therefore, emphasis should be on the whole rather than on an individual. Some of the concepts of systems theory that help nurses working with families are explained in the following sections.

Concept 1: All Parts of the System Are Interconnected

What influences one part of the system influences all parts of the system. When an individual in a family experiences a health event, all members are affected because they are connected. The effect on each family member varies in intensity and quality. In the Jones case study, all members of the Jones family are touched when Linda's health condition changes, requiring her to be hospitalized. Linda takes on the role of a sick person and must give up some of her typical at-home mother roles; she is physically ill in the hospital. She feels guilty about not being at home for her family. Robert is affected because he has to assume the care of Katie and Travis. These tasks require getting them ready for school, transporting them to school and other

events, and making lunches. Katie gives up some after-school activities to help Travis when he gets home from preschool. Travis misses the food his mother prepared for him, his afternoon alone time with his mother when they read a story, and being tucked into bed at night with songs and a back rub. Amy, who is a freshman in college, finds it difficult to concentrate while reading and studying for her college classes. The formal and informal roles of all these family members are affected by Linda's hospitalization. What affects Linda affects all the members of the Jones family in multiple ways.

Concept 2: The Whole Is More Than the Sum of Its Parts

The family as a whole is composed of more than the individual lives of family members. It goes beyond parents and children as separate entities. Families are not just relationships between the parent and child; rather, all family members are in relationships together. As we look at the Jones family, it is a nuclear family—mother, father, and three children. They are a family system that is experiencing the stress of a chronically ill mother who is deteriorating over time; each of them is individually affected; therefore, the family as a whole is affected by this unexpected (non-normative) family health event. The individuals in this family may wonder at times what will happen to them as a family (whole) when Linda dies.

One way of visualizing the family as a whole is to think of how the Jones family has built the concept of the "Jones Family Easter." Even though Linda always decorates the house and bakes several special dishes for the family for this holiday, this year she has been too ill to decorate or cook for Easter. The family as a whole feels stressed by the loss of routine and ritual as it represents a change in their family tradition and beliefs. Thus, the family loss is larger than individual loss of this tradition.

Concept 3: All Systems Have Some Form of Boundaries or Borders Between the System and Its Environment

Families control the inflow of information and people coming into its family system to protect individual family members or the family as a whole. Boundaries are physical or abstract imaginary lines that families use as barriers or filters to control the impact of stressors on the family system (Smith & Hamon, 2016; White et al., 2014). Family boundaries include levels of permeability in that they can be closed; flexible; or too open to information, people, or other forms of resources. Some families have closed boundaries as exemplified by statements such as, "We as a family pull together and don't need help from others," or "We take care of our own." For example, if the Jones family were to have a *closed boundary*, they would not want to meet with the social worker or, if they did, they would reject the idea of a home-health aide and respite care.

Some families have *flexible boundaries*, which they control and selectively open or close to gain balance or adapt to the situation. For example, the Jones family welcomes a visit from the pastor yet turns down visits from some of the women in Linda's Bible study group. Some families have *too open boundaries* in which they are not discriminating about who knows their family situation or the number of people from whom they seek help. Open boundaries can invite chaos and unbalance if the family is not selective in the quantity or quality of resources. If the Jones family were to have truly *open boundaries*, it may reach out to the larger community for resources and have different church members come stay with the children every evening. The permeability of boundaries resides on a continuum and varies from family to family.

Concept 4: Systems Can Be Further Organized Into Subsystems

In addition to conceptualizing the family as a whole, nurses can think about the subsystems of the family, which may include husband to wife, mother to child, father to child, child to child, grandparents to parents, grandparents to grandchildren, and so forth. These subsystems consider the three dimensions of families discussed in Chapter 1: structure, function (including roles), and processes (interconnection and dynamics). By understanding these three dimensions, family nurses can streamline interventions to achieve specific family outcomes. For example, the Jones family has the following subsystems: parents, siblings, parent-child, a daughter subsystem, an in-law subsystem, and a grandparent subsystem. The nurse may work to decrease family stress by focusing on the marital spouse subsystem to help Linda and Robert continue couple time, or the nurse may focus on the sibling subsystem of Katie and Travis and their after-school activities.

Application of Family Systems Theory to the Jones Family

The focus of the nurses' practice from this perspective is family as the client. Nurses work to help families maintain and regain stability. Assessment questions of family members are focused on the family as a whole. While planning for Linda's discharge that is scheduled in the next couple of days, a nurse would ask questions such as the following to explore with Linda or with Linda and Robert:

- Who are members of your family? (See Concept 1.)
- How do you see your family being involved in your care once you go home? (See Concept 1.)
- Who in your family will experience the most difficulty coping with the changes, especially now that you will be using a wheelchair? (See Concept 1.)
- How are the members of your family meeting their personal needs at this time? (See Concept 1.)
- The last time your condition worsened, what was the most help to your family? (See Concept 2.)
- The last time your condition worsened, what was the least help to your family? (See Concept 2.)
- Who outside your immediate family do you see as being a potential person to help your family during the next week when you go home? (See Concept 3.)
- How do you feel your family would react to having a home-health aide come to help you twice a week? (See Concept 3.)
- Are there some friends, church members, or neighbors who might be able to help with some of the everyday management issues, such as carpooling to school, or providing some after-school care for Travis so Katie could go to her after-school activities? (See Concepts 3 and 4.)
- What are your thoughts about how the children will react to having Grandma Elise here to help the family? (See Concept 4.)

Interventions by family nurses must address individuals, subsystems within the family, and the whole family all at the same time. Caring and open communication is a strategy that can help the nurse assess family process and functioning. Once the nurse learns more from the family about their preferences and their daily functioning, specific interventions can be offered to support the family. Some of the following questions can assist nurses to assess family functioning:

- Linda and Robert, from what you have told me, it appears that your oldest daughter, Amy, has been a significant help supporting the family by running errands, helping with transportation, and shopping for groceries. Now that Amy is off to college, have you thought about the chores that you may need help with when you get home? Is someone available to support you?

- You both shared that your family likes to go bowling on family night out. Let's talk about how this will work for you as you accommodate for Linda being in a wheelchair.

- Have you had a chance to discuss some of the legal aspects of making health care decisions? Linda, as your condition changes, there may come a time when you would rely on Robert to assist you by making health care decisions. A durable power of attorney for health care is a document that can identify your wishes and give Robert permission to carry those out on your behalf. Does this sound like something that would be beneficial? Let us discuss what those types of health care decisions might involve. Linda, please tell me how your close, personal relationships are going for you now that you have recognized more physical challenges.

The goal of using a family systems perspective is to help the family reach stability by building on their strengths as a family, using knowledge of the family as a social system, and understanding how the family is an interconnected whole that is adapting to the changes brought about by the health event of a given family member.

Strengths and Weaknesses of Family Systems Theory

The strengths of the general systems framework are that this theory covers a large array of phenomena and views the family and its subsystems within the context of its suprasystem (the larger community in which it is embedded). Moreover, it is an interactional and holistic theory that looks at processes within the family rather than at the content and relationships between the members (Tadros, 2019). The family is viewed as a whole, not as merely a sum of its parts. Another strength of this approach is that it is an excellent data-gathering method and assessment strategy, for example, using a family genogram to gather a snapshot of the family as a whole. The genogram and other family system assessment instruments are discussed in Chapter 5.

Systems theory also has its limitations (Smith & Hamon, 2016; Tadros, 2019). Because this theoretical orientation is so global and abstract, it may not be specific enough for beginners to define family nursing interventions. It is important for family nurses to be able to understand conceptually how important the family as a whole is to the practice of family nursing. As health care systems continue to emphasize the autonomy of the individual, it takes time and practice to develop ways to understand deeply how a family as a whole is greater than the members of the family.

Developmental and Family Life Cycle Theory

Developmental and Family Life Cycle Theory provides a framework for nurses to understand normal family changes and experiences over the members' lifetimes; the theory assesses and evaluates both individuals and families as a whole because individual family members and the family as a whole develop and change over time. This approach views the evolving needs and priorities of family members and the family. Developmental stages for individuals are seen as a system in that what happens at one level has powerful ramifications at other levels of the system. Families are seen as the basic social unit of society and as the optimal level of intervention.

The family developmental theories are specifically geared to understanding families and not individuals (Smith & Hamon, 2016). Families, similar to individuals, are in constant movement and change throughout time—the family life cycle. Family developmental theorists who inform the nursing of families include Duvall (1977), Duvall and Miller (1985), McGoldrick, Garcia Preto, and Carter (2016), R. Walsh (2015), and F. Walsh (2016). The original work of Duvall (1977), and later Duvall and Miller (1985), examined how families were affected or changed cognitively, socially, emotionally, spiritually, and physically when all members experienced developmental changes. The relationships among family members are affected by changes in individuals, and changes in the family as a whole affect the individuals within the family. These theorists recognized that families are stressed at common and predictable stages of transition and need to undergo adjustment to regain family stability. This early theoretical work was primarily based on the experiences of White Anglo middle-class nuclear families, with a married couple, children, and extended family.

McGoldrick et al. (2016) expanded on the original Developmental and Family Life Cycle Theory because they recognized the dramatically changing landscape of family structure, functions, and processes that was making it increasingly difficult to determine normal predictable patterns of change in families. They replaced the concept of "nuclear family" with "immediate family," which takes into consideration all family structures, such as stepfamilies, LGBTQ+ families, and divorced families. Instead of addressing the legal aspects of being a married couple, they viewed the concept of couple relationships and commitment as a focal point for family bonds. There is much value in nurses studying the normative sequential new experiences, challenges, and opportunities regardless of the type of family because all these normative stressors will be affected when a family also experiences events that are not expected, such as illness, death, or disability. R. Walsh (2015) and F. Walsh (2016) explored the life cycle perspective on family development to understand the family's ability to withstand and rebound from adversity and to increase understanding of family resilience over time. For example, an earlier experience with overcoming an adverse situation is not indicative that the family will manage the current situation with ease or resiliency.

What are thought of as normal development and family life are largely influenced by socially constructed, subjective worldviews from the historical era of the oldest family members. These normative milestones are associated with chronological ages of family members and the family (Duvall, 1977; Duvall & Miller, 1985). McGoldrick et al. (2016), R. Walsh (2015), and F. Walsh (2016) recognized that previous "normative changes" do not apply, especially related to chronological ages (i.e., a woman can have her first child at 16, and then marry, divorce, and restart a family at age 35). Many previous family phases repeat themselves with blended families and grandparents raising grandchildren.

By examining the life cycle perspective of family development, R. Walsh (2015) and F. Walsh (2016) noted how individual family members and the family as a whole manage stresses, conflict, and disruptive life changes by using short-term and long-term adaptive strategies, thereby increasing family resilience.

Concept 1: Families Develop and Change Over Time

According to Developmental and Family Life Cycle Theory, family interactions among family members change over time in relation to structure, function (roles), and processes. The stresses created by these changes in family systems are somewhat predictable for different stages of family development.

The first way to view family development is to look at predictable stresses and changes as they relate to the expected age of the family members at certain transitions (i.e., societal expectation that most couples marry before turning 30 years old) and the social norms that the individuals experience throughout their development. The classic traditional work of Duvall (1977) and Duvall and Miller (1985) identified overall family tasks that need to be accomplished for each stage of family development as related to the developmental trajectory of the individual family members. It starts with couples getting married and ends with one member of the couple dying. Refer to Table 2-5 for a detailed list of the traditional family life cycle stages and developmental tasks.

According to this theory, families have a predictable natural history. The first stage involves the couple pairing; the family group then becomes more complex over time with the addition of new members. When the younger generation leaves home to take jobs, attend college, or marry, the original family group changes in roles, expectations, and adjustment back to a smaller core within the household.

The second way to view family development is to assess the predictable stresses and changes in families based on the stage of family development and how long the family is in that stage. For example, suppose each of the following couples have made a choice to be childless: a newly married couple, a

Table 2-5 Traditional Family Life Cycle Stages and Developmental Tasks	
STAGES OF FAMILY LIFE CYCLE	**FAMILY DEVELOPMENTAL TASKS**
Married couple	Establishing relationship as a married couple.
	Blending of individual needs; developing conflict-and-resolution approaches, communication patterns, and intimacy patterns.
Childbearing families with infants	Adjusting to pregnancy and then infant.
	Adjusting to new roles as mother and father.
	Maintaining couple bond and intimacy.
Families with preschool children	Understanding normal growth and development.
	If more than one child in family, adjusting to different temperaments and styles of children.
	Coping with energy depletion.
	Maintaining couple bond and intimacy.
Families with school-age children	Working out authority and socialization roles with school.
	Supporting child in outside interests and needs.
	Determining disciplinary actions and family rules and roles.
Families with adolescents	Allowing adolescents to establish their own identities and still be part of the family.
	Thinking about the future, education, jobs, and working.
	Increasing roles of adolescents in family, cooking, repairs, and power base.
Families with young adults: launching	After family member moves out, reallocating roles, space, power, and communication.
	Maintaining supportive home base.
	Maintaining parental couple intimacy and relationship.
Middle-aged parents	Refocusing on marriage relationship.
	Ensuring security after retirement.
	Maintaining kinship ties.
Aging families	Adjusting to retirement, grandparent roles, death of spouse, and living alone.

couple who have been married for three years, and a couple who have been married for 15 years (White et al., 2014). The stresses each couple experiences from this decision would be different because of societal expectations of childbearing and child rearing.

Concept 2: Families Experience Transitions From One Stage to Another

Disequilibrium occurs in the family during the transitional periods from one stage of development to the next. When transitions occur, families experience changes in kinship structures, family roles, social roles, and interaction. Family stress is considered to be greatest at the transition points as families adapt to achieve stability, redefine their concept of family in light of the changes, and realign relationships because of the changes

(McGoldrick et al., 2016; R. Walsh, 2015; F. Walsh, 2016). For example, marriage changes the status of all family members, creates new relationships for family members such as including extended family into the married dyad, and joins two different complex family systems.

Although some family developmental needs and tasks must be performed at each stage of the family life cycle, developmental tasks are general goals rather than specific jobs that must be completed at that time. Achievement of family developmental tasks enables individuals within families to realize their own individual tasks. According to Developmental and Family Life Cycle Theory, every family is unique in its composition and in the complexity of its expectations of members at different ages and in different roles. Families, similar to individuals, are influenced by their history and traditions and by the social context in which they live. Furthermore, families change and develop in different ways because their internal/external demands and situations differ. Families may also arrive at similar developmental levels using different processes. For example, the launching phase in one family might have a child attend community college and live at home whereas another may have their college-age child live in the dorm in the same town in which they live or the college student may attend a college across the country. How the child launches is different while many of the tasks of the family are the same. Another example would be a family with a stay-at-home mother caring for an infant and another family with a working mother needing day care for their infant.

Despite their differences, however, families have enough in common to make it possible to chart family development over the life span in a way that applies to most families (Friedman et al., 2003). Families experience stress when they transition from one stage to the next. The predictable changes that are based on these family developmental steps are called *normative* changes. When changes occur in families out of sequence, "off time," or are caused by a different family event, such as illness, they are called *non-normative*. For example, it is expected to lose a parent to death during the seventh to ninth decade of life. If a parent dies during his or her forties, then that is considered an "off time" or non-normative event.

In contrast with Duvall's (1977) and later Duvall and Miller's (1985) traditional developmental approach, Carter and McGoldrick (1989) and McGoldrick et al. (2016) built on this work by approaching family development from the perspective of family life cycle stages. They explored what happens within families when family members enter or exit their family group; they focus on specific family experiences, such as disruption in family relationships, roles, processes, and family structure. Examples of a family member leaving would be divorce, illness, miscarriage, incarceration, or death of a family member. Examples of family members entering would include birth, adoption, marriage, or other formal union. Examples of family structures would include traditional, blended, LGBTQ+ cohabitation, single parent, multiple generations in one household, grandparents raising grandchildren, or living apart yet

feeling together (e.g., deployed adults causing separation from their family).

Today, the Developmental and Family Life Cycle Theory remains useful as long as it is viewed generally for use with families, despite all the current variations of families. McGoldrick et al. (2016) expanded the family life cycle to incorporate the changing family patterns and broadened the view of both development and the family. McGoldrick et al. (2016) expanded the traditional Developmental and Family Life Cycle Theory to address changes in the family that undergoes a divorce. Table 2-6 outlines the emotional process of a family undergoing a divorce and describes the developmental tasks that the family deals with at different stages.

Acquired brain injury (ABI) is caused by head trauma or a cerebrovascular event and can result in cognitive, behavioral, emotional, and affective changes, interfering with family relationships and disrupting the life cycle and normal family transitions (Larrata, 2020; Thomas et al., 2017). The impact on each family member and the family as a whole depends on the severity of the brain injury; however, stressors may include (1) disruptions in interpersonal relationships, (2) adapting to the family member's disability, and (3) supporting the family member's overall functioning (Larrata, 2020). Family members may experience burden as they take on the role of caregiver or experience financial challenges. The impact of disability on spouse caregivers and in families where the spouse of the patient with a brain injury had an adult child have been characterized by a higher level of burden (Larrata, 2020). In this situation, an acute injury can lead to long-term consequences that have an impact on the family life cycle and transitions of family members and the family as a whole.

Pelton (2011) described specific stressors and tasks relative to couples that elect to remain child-free or childless by choice. The first task is making the decision not to have children. The second task for this couple is to manage the stigma and pressure that family, friends, acquaintances, and society place on them. In fact, this stress is one the couple will face until the woman is no longer biologically able to have children. The third task for the child-free couple is defining their identity that does not include children. During this task, couples may elect to focus on their chosen career, determine how to spend their leisure time, and decide if there are projects in which they would like to volunteer

Table 2-6	**Family Life Cycle for Divorcing Families**	
PHASE	**EMOTIONAL PROCESS OF TRANSITION: PREREQUISITE ATTITUDE**	**DEVELOPMENTAL ISSUES**
Divorce		
The decision to divorce	Acceptance of inability to resolve marital tensions sufficiently to continue relationship.	Acceptance of one's own part in the failure of the marriage.
Planning the breakup of the system	Supporting viable arrangements for all parts of the system.	a. Working cooperatively on problems of custody, visitation, and finances. b. Dealing with extended family about the divorce.
Separation	a. Willingness to continue cooperative coparented relationships and joint financial support of children. b. Work on resolution of attachment to spouse.	a. Mourning loss of intact family. b. Restructuring marital and parent-child relationships and finances; adaptation to living apart. c. Realignment of relationships with extended family; staying connected with spouse's extended family.
The divorce	More work on emotional divorce: overcoming hurt, anger, and guilt, among other emotions.	a. Mourning loss of intact family. b. Retrieval of hopes, dreams, and expectations from the marriage. c. Staying connected with extended families.
Postdivorce Family		
Single parent (custodial household or primary residence)	Willingness to maintain financial responsibilities, continue parental contact with ex-spouse, and support contact of children with ex-spouse and his or her family.	a. Making flexible visitation arrangements with ex-spouse and family. b. Rebuilding own financial resources. c. Rebuilding own social network.
Single parent (noncustodial)	Willingness to maintain financial responsibilities and parental contact with ex-spouse and to support custodial parent's relationship with children.	a. Finding ways to continue effective parenting. b. Maintaining financial responsibilities to ex-spouse and children. c. Rebuilding own social network.

Source: Adapted from Carter, B., and McGoldrick, M. (2005). The divorce cycle: A major variation in the American family life cycle. In B. Carter and M. McGoldrick (Eds.), *The expanded family life cycle: Individual, family, and social perspectives* (3rd ed., 2005). New York, NY: Allyn and Bacon.

their time and expertise. The fourth major task of a childfree couple is to build a support system with other couples who do not have children. During this task, the members of the childfree couple work together to determine the legacy they will leave to future generations. Childless couples approach the developmental stage of generativity in different ways. For example, childless couples often choose careers that involve children (teachers, counselors, etc.), or they consciously seek to give to the next generation through writing or art.

Normal developmental tasks and stressors can be intensified by cultural contrasts in situations such as migration to a new country (Falicov, 2016).

For example, in the case of immigration, parents may be separated from their children. Young adults may elect not to leave the family to venture out on their own in the same time frame, which places them in a non-normative developmental progression. If the children are savvier with language acquisition, there may be a reversal of roles, with decision making and power within the family given to the children rather than the parents.

Application of Developmental and Family Life Cycle Theory to the Jones Family

When conducting family assessments using the developmental model, nurses begin by determining the family structure and where this particular family falls in the family life cycle stages. Using the developmental tasks outlined in the developmental model, the nurse has a ready guide to anticipate stresses that the family may be experiencing or to assess the developmental tasks that are not being accomplished or are being accomplished "off time."

According to Duvall and Miller (1985), the Jones family is in the *Families With Young Adults: Launching Phase* because Amy left home and is now a freshman at a college. She is living away from home for the first time. Although the Jones family is experiencing a non-normative event (unexpected, developmental stressor) because Linda, the mother, is now in the hospital, the family is also experiencing the normative or expected challenges for a family when the oldest child leaves home. This family is undergoing the Launching Phase at the same time that they are raising an adolescent and a toddler. Although Duvall (1977; Duvall & Miller, 1985) recommended focusing on the older child, later researchers noted that this does not work because transitions for each child have an impact on all family members.

This is a good example of where major individual and whole family events coincide and present challenges for families. Questions to explore with the family relative to Amy might include the following:

1. How has the family addressed the reallocation of family household physical space since Amy left for school (for example, the allocation of bedrooms or the arrangement of space within the bedroom if Katie and Amy shared the bedroom)?
2. How has Amy developed as an indirect caregiver (such as calling home to chat with Dad and see how he is doing, talking with the siblings and teasing or supporting their efforts, or sharing with parents her school life to reduce their worry about her adjustment)?
3. How have family roles changed since Amy left for school? What roles did Amy perform for the family that someone else needs to pick up now? For example, who will perform roles such as chauffeur, grocery shopper, errand runner, and babysitter now that Linda is not able and Amy is gone?
4. How has the power structure of the family shifted now that Katie is more responsible for the care of Travis?

5. How has the parents' couple time changed since Amy went to college?

Questions to explore about Travis, the 4-year-old preschool child, include:

1. Children at this age need to develop increasingly complex social relationships. Travis is struggling with suddenly being introduced to preschool, so can the transition be designed so that he attends preschool only 2 days a week for now and gradually increase as he becomes adjusted to this new experience?
2. Are there any extended family members who have children the same age as Travis that he can interact with?
3. Could it be arranged that Travis has some special time with Mom when he gets home from preschool so that he feels like he is still center stage with his mother's attention?
4. What type of ritual and routine would help provide Travis with stability and change?

Finally, questions that might be explored relative to 13-year-old Katie follow. Katie's position in the family is between the school-age child and the teenager. Katie wants to move toward more independence at the same time that she is being asked to babysit Travis. Questions for Katie might include:

1. Can the family negotiate allowing Katie to have special time when she is not responsible at home to hang out with her friends, to go to youth camp with the Girl Scouts, or to be with the youth group at church?
2. Are there activities at the church that Travis and Katie could attend at the same time? For example, are there preschool and teen youth group activities for them to attend with children their own age?
3. Are there other ways that Katie can help support the family rather than provide childcare for Travis?
4. Would it be helpful for the school counselor to reach out to Katie about her stress or explore having a child-life specialist work with Katie?

With the developmental approach, nursing interventions may include helping the family understand individual and family developmental tasks. Interventions could also include helping the family understand the normalcy of disequilibrium during these transitional periods. Another intervention is helping the family mitigate these transitions by building on the strengths of family routines and traditions. Strong family rituals are predictive of attachment security and family cohesion (Prime et al., 2020), which may decrease the anxiety caused by changes in the family dynamic. Family nurses must recognize that every family must accomplish both individual and family developmental tasks for every stage of the Developmental and Family Life Cycle. Events at one stage of the cycle have powerful effects at other stages. Helping families adjust and adapt to these transitions is an important role for family nurses. It is important for nurses to keep in mind the needs and requirements of both the family as a whole and the individuals who make up the family.

Strengths and Weaknesses of the Developmental and Family Life Cycle

A major strength of the developmental approach is that it provides a systematic framework for predicting what a family may be experiencing at any stage in the family life cycle. Family nurses can assess a family's stage of development, the extent to which the family has achieved the tasks associated with that stage of family development, and problems that may or may not exist. It is a superb theoretical approach for assisting nurses who are working with families on health promotion. Family strengths and available resources are easier to identify because they are based on assisting families achieve developmental milestones.

A primary criticism of family development theory is that it best describes the trajectory of intact, two-parent, heterosexual nuclear families. The original eight-stage model was based on a nuclear family, assumed an intact marriage throughout the life cycle of the family, and was organized around the oldest child's developmental needs. It did not consider divorce, death of a spouse, remarriage, unmarried parents, childless couples, the developmental needs of subsequent children, or cohabitating or gay and lesbian couples. It normalized one type of family and ignored others (Smith & Hamon, 2016). Today's families vary widely in their structure and related roles. The traditional view of families moving in a linear direction from getting married, tracking children from preschool to launching, middle-aged parents, and aging families is no longer the majority family structure or development, and therefore the traditional view

has become questionable. Carter (2005), Carter and McGoldrick (1989, 2005), and McGoldrick et al. (2016) expanded the family developmental model to include stresses in the remarried family. A serious shortcoming of these models is that they ignore the importance of cultural diversity and health disparities in families, and the impact on family development (Falicov, 2016). As family structures continue to change in response to cultural factors and the ecologic system, trajectories of families likely will not fit within the traditional developmental framework (White et al., 2014). Future theory development and research are needed to expand understanding of family development across time while considering changes and diversity within family development.

Bioecological Systems Theory

Urie Bronfenbrenner was one of the world's leading scholars in the field of developmental psychology (Bronfenbrenner, 1972a, 1972b, 1979, 1981, 1986, 1997; Bronfenbrenner & Morris, 1998). He contributed greatly to the ecological theory of human development, which concentrated on the interaction and interdependence of humans—as biological and social entities—within the environment. Originally this idea was called the *Human Ecology Theory*, then it was changed to *Ecological Systems Theory*, and it finally evolved into the *Bioecological Systems Theory* (Bronfenbrenner & Lerner, 2004; Rosa & Tudge, 2013). The Bioecological System is the combination of children's biological disposition and environmental forces coming together to shape the development of human beings. This theory combines both developmental theory and systems theory to understand individual and family growth.

Before Bronfenbrenner, child psychologists studied children, sociologists examined families, anthropologists analyzed society, economists scrutinized the economic framework, and political scientists focused on political structures. Through Bronfenbrenner's groundbreaking work in human ecology, environments from the individual and family to larger economic/political structures have come to be viewed as part of systems interacting across the life course, from infancy through adulthood. This bioecological approach to human development crosses over barriers among the social sciences and builds bridges among the disciplines, allowing for better understanding to emerge about key elements in the larger social structure that are vital for optimal human development (both individual and family) (Rosa & Tudge, 2013).

The human ecology framework brings together other diverse influences. From evolutionary theory and genetics comes the view that humans develop as individual biological organisms with capacities limited by genetic endowment (*ontogenetic development*) that lead to hereditary familial characteristics. From population genetics comes the perspective that populations change by means of natural selection. For the individual, this means that individuals/families demonstrate their fitness by adapting to ever-changing environments. From ecological theories comes the notion that human and family development is contextualized and "interactional" over time (Rosa & Tudge, 2013; White et al., 2014). All this leads to the ongoing debate related to the dual nature of humans as constructions of both biology and culture; hence, the argument of nature versus nurture. Although this debate has not been resolved, scientists have moved beyond debate to the realization that the development of most human traits depends on a nature/nurture interaction rather than on one influence having priority over the other (White et al., 2014). Thus, Bronfenbrenner moved his own theory and ideas from the concept and terminology of ecology (environment) to bioecology (both genetics and society) as a way of embracing two developmental origins for this theory (Rosa & Tudge, 2013). His Bioecological Systems Theory emphasizes the interaction of both the biological/genetics (ontologic/nature) and the social context (society) characteristics of development (Rosa & Tudge, 2013; Smith & Hamon, 2016; White et al., 2014).

The human bioecological perspective consists of a framework of four locational/spatial contexts and one time-related context (Rosa & Tudge, 2013; White et al., 2014). A primary feature of this theory is the premise that individual and family development is contextual over time. According to Bronfenbrenner (1986), individual development is affected by five types or levels of environmental systems (Figure 2-6). Family Bioecological Theory describes the interactions and influences on the family from systems at different levels of engagement.

Microsystems are the settings in which individuals/families experience and create day-to-day reality. They are the places people inhabit, the people with whom they live, and the things they do together. In this level, people fulfill their roles in families, with peers, in schools, and in neighborhoods where they are in the most direct interaction with agents around them.

Mesosystems are the relationships among major microsystems in which persons or families actively participate, such as families and schools, families and religion, and families with peers. For example, how does the interaction between families and schools affect families? Can the relationship between families and their religious/spiritual communities be used to help families?

Exosystems are external environments that influence individuals and families indirectly. The person may not be an active participant within these systems; however, the system has an effect on the persons/families. For example, a parent's job experience affects family life, which in turn affects the children (parent's travel requirements for a job, job stress, salary). Furthermore, governmental funding to other microsystems environments—schools, libraries, parks, health care, and day care—affects the experiences of children and families.

Macrosystems are the broad cultural attitudes, ideologies, or belief systems that influence institutional environments within a particular culture/subculture in which individuals/families live. Examples include the Judeo-Christian ethic, democracy, ethnicity, and societal values. Mesosystems and exosystems are set within macrosystems, and together they are the blueprints for the ecology of human and family development.

Chronosystems are time-related contexts where changes occur over time and have an effect on the other four levels/systems of development mentioned earlier. Chronosystems include the patterning of environmental events and transitions over the life course of individuals/families. These effects are created by time or critical periods in development and are influenced by sociohistorical conditions, such as parental divorce, unexpected death of a parent, or a war. Individuals/families have no control over the evolution of such external systems over time.

Within each one of these levels are roles, norms, and rules that shape the environment. Bronfenbrenner's model of human/family development acknowledges that people develop not in isolation but in relation to their larger environment: families, homes, schools, communities, and

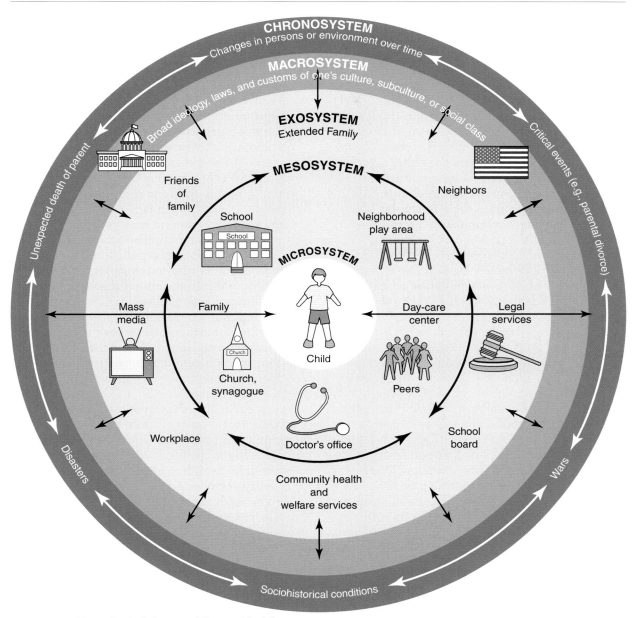

FIGURE 2-6 Bioecological Systems Theory Model

societies. All these interactive, ever-changing, and multilevel environments over time are key to understanding human/family development.

Bronfenbrenner uses the term *bidirectional* to describe the influential interactions that take place between children and their relationships with parents, teachers, and society. All relationships among humans/families and their environment are bidirectional or interactional. The environment influences individuals and families; in turn, individuals/families influence what happens in their own environments. This interaction is also basic to Family Systems Theory.

Within the bioecological framework, what happens outside family units is as important as what happens inside individual members and family units.

Developing families are on center stage as an active force shaping their social experiences for themselves. The ecological perspective views children/families and their environments as mutually shaping systems, each changing and adapting over time (again, also included in the Family Systems Theory perspective). The bioecological approach addresses both opportunities and risks. Opportunities refer to what the environment offers families, such as material, emotional, and social encouragement compatible with their needs and capacities. Risks to family development are composed of direct threats or the absence of opportunities, such as poverty, mental health challenges, or social isolation.

Application of the Bioecological Systems Theory to the Jones Family

Assessment using the *Bioecological Systems Theory* consists of looking at all levels of the system when interviewing the family in a health care setting. Assessment of the *microsystem* reveals that the Jones family consists of five members: two parents and three children. They live in a two-story home with four bedrooms in an older suburban section of town. Mother Linda had been a full-time homemaker before experiencing health problems related to her diagnosis of MS. The *mesosystem* assessment for the family consists of identifying the schools the children attend, the neighborhood, friends, extended family, and religious affiliation. The oldest daughter is a college student who travels home on weekends to help the family. The second daughter is in a local middle school and can walk back and forth to her school. The youngest child, a boy, attends an all-day preschool and is transported by his parents or other parents from the preschool. The family has attended a Protestant church in the neighborhood. The family lives in a house in an older established neighborhood and has made friends through the schools, church, and neighborhood contacts. Part of the extended family (grandparents) live nearby, and all the family members get together for the holidays; neither parent has siblings who live nearby. The *exosystem* assessment shows that father Robert works 40 hours a week for an industrial plant at the edge of town, and he drives back and forth daily. The father has some job stress because he is in a middle-management position. His salary is average for middle-class families in the United States. State and county funding to the area schools, libraries, and recreational facilities are always a struggle in this community. The town has physicians/clinics of all specialties and has one community hospital. An assessment of the *macrosystem* shows that this community is largely White, with only 10 percent of residents from other backgrounds. Most people in the community embrace a Christian ethic.

The community value system includes a family focus and a strong work ethic. Many of the people prefer the Democratic Party. In terms of the time-related contexts of the *chronosystem*, a few things are notable. These time-related events put more stress on the family than usual non-normative events. Linda's disease process with MS has sped up recently, placing additional strain on the family system. Robert's own dad died in the past year, leaving him extra responsibility for his widowed mother in addition to his responsibility for his own children and now ill wife. The economy in the country and region is going through a recession, leading people to feel some fear about their economic futures. Robert had hoped that his wife could go to work part-time when their youngest child went to school; however, that no longer seems to be a possibility. The family assessment would include how the family at each of the earlier mentioned levels is influenced by the changes brought about by Linda's progressing debilitative disease and recent hospitalization. The family is experiencing disturbance at many of these levels.

Interventions include the following possibilities. In general, nurses can also look for additional systems that the family could interact with to help support family functioning during this family illness event. Nurses could make home visits to assess the living arrangements of the family and to determine how the home could be changed to accommodate a wheelchair/walker. The nurses should talk with the parents about their relationship to the schools, church, and extended family support systems. The parents might be advised to inform the school(s), church, workplace, and grandparents of what is happening to their family. The nurses could make suggestions relative to Travis's current behavior with having to go to all-day preschool. The nurses also could explore with the family the larger external environment, including community resources (e.g., Multiple Sclerosis Society, visiting nurse service, or counseling services). The nurses should contact the medical doctor(s) and discharge planning nurse at the hospital to obtain information to interpret the diagnosis, prognosis, and treatment of MS for the family. The nurses might talk to the family members about how their faith can be of help during these tough times and what their primary concerns are as a family. The nurses should get in touch with the social workers at the hospital to coordinate care and social well-being strategies for the posthospitalization period as well as in the future. Strategies may involve application to Social Security for the disabled. A family-care planning meeting should be set up to involve as many caretakers and stakeholders as possible.

Evaluation of the interventions would consist of follow-up with the family through periodic home visits and telephone contact. The nurses would explore how the family is adapting to its situation, how the father is dealing with the extra responsibility, how the children are coping, and the physical and mental health of the mother. Because MS is a chronic progressive relapsing disorder, a plan would be put into place for periodic evaluations that might involve changing the plan of care.

Strengths and Weaknesses of the Bioecological Systems Theory

The strength of the bioecological perspective is that it represents a comprehensive and holistic view of human/family development—a biological, psychological, sociological, cultural, and spiritual approach to the understanding of how humans and families develop and adapt to the larger society. It includes both the *nature* (biological context) and *nurture* (environmental context) aspects of growth and development for both individuals and families. It directs our attention to factors that occur within as well as to the layered influences of factors that occur outside individuals and families. The bioecological perspective provides a valuable complement to other theories that may offer greater insight into how each aspect of the holistic approach affects individuals and families over time.

The strength of this theory is also part of its weakness. The different systems show nurses what factors to think about that may affect the family; however, the direction of how the family adapts is not specifically delineated in this theory. In other words, the biological, psychological, sociological, cultural, and spiritual aspects of human/family growth and development are not detailed enough to define how individuals/families can accomplish

or adapt to these contextual changes over time. Aspects of the theory—specifically, the influence of biological and cognitive processes and how they interact with the environment—require further delineation and testing.

SUMMARY

Theory is used in all aspects of nursing care and assists the practicing nurse in organizing, understanding, and analyzing information. Essentially, theory provides a systematic, consistent way of thinking about nursing care. Nurses who understand the relationship between theory and practice use multiple approaches in their practice with families and can thereby explore more options for families in providing health care. By understanding theories and models, nurses are better prepared to think creatively and critically about how health events affect the family. This chapter introduced nurses to the concept of theory-guided, evidence-based family nursing practice. It presented the relationship between theory, practice, and research, and explained crucial aspects of theory. The chapter then explored three theories for the nursing care of families and applied the theories to the case study in the chapter:

- Family Systems Theory
- Developmental and Family Life Cycle Theory
- Bioecological Systems Theory

The chapter revealed how nurses can practice family nursing differently with the Jones family according to the different theoretical perspectives.

The following points highlight critical concepts that are addressed in this chapter:

- No single theory, model, or conceptual framework adequately describes the complex relationships of family.
- No one theoretical perspective gives nurses a sufficiently broad base of knowledge and understanding to guide assessment and interventions with all families.
- No one theoretical perspective is better, more comprehensive, or more correct than another.
- Nurses who draw from multiple theories are more effective in tailoring their

nursing practice and family interventions to reach the optimal outcomes. Using multiple theories substantially increases the likelihood that the family will be able to achieve stability and health as a family unit.

■ Family nursing is guided by theory and is evidence-based.

This chapter presents approaches to providing quality family health care nursing that is theory driven and evidence based. By using different lenses to view family health issues, a variety of solutions and interventions become available. Due to the complex health events and diverse circumstances experienced by families, there is no one theoretical perspective that provides all nurses practicing in all settings a sufficiently broad base of knowledge. Rather, nurses use multiple theoretical perspectives to guide their practice with the nursing care of families.

chapter 3

Family Demography

Continuity and Change in North American Families

Tracey A. LaPierre, PhD, MSc

Jennifer M. Babitzke, MS

Critical Concepts

- Technological, economic, social, and cultural changes have increased the diversity and complexity of North American families and resulted in a growing disconnect between who we live with and who we consider family.
- Family structure and functioning typically vary according to other demographic characteristics such as gender, sexual orientation, age, race/ethnicity, nativity, and socioeconomic status.
- Marriage rates have declined, and marriage is frequently preceded or replaced by cohabitation. In addition, families are becoming smaller and nonmarital, and the rate of MPF has increased.
- Compared to older generations, young adults are pursuing higher levels of education, delaying entry into the labor market, living with their parents longer, and transitioning into marriage and parenthood at older ages.
- Family instability, MPF, ART, and changing trends in adoption are creating new family forms with ambiguous rights and responsibilities.
- Gender norms are changing to recognize more diverse gender identities, and expectations for gender roles have become more egalitarian; however, significant differences in attachment to the labor force, economic equality, and the gendered division of household labor persist.
- Demographic trends related to fertility, life expectancy, and immigration are changing the composition of the Canadian and U.S. populations, resulting in population aging and increased ethnic/racial diversity that will intensify in the coming decades if current trends continue.

As a social institution, the word *family* implies clearly defined roles with shared expectations for behavior (Seltzer, 2019). Legally and socially, members of the family are afforded certain rights and responsibilities and are viewed as more stable and permanent than relationships with unrelated individuals (Tillman & Nam, 2008). Historically, Western culture has recognized and privileged the standard nuclear family, traditionally viewed as an opposite-sex married couple and their minor biological children, as a basic social unit (Tillman & Nam, 2008). Indeed, it was not that long ago that most North American children were born into the standard nuclear family and typically lived in households with only their parents and full siblings until adulthood (Napolitano et al., 2013). However, evolving social norms, family structure, and transitions, including changing family formation and dissolution behaviors, have altered traditional family roles, responsibilities, and expectations and the long-term stability of these relationships. They have also resulted in a proliferation of new types of family structures and connections, many with ambiguous rights and responsibilities. As a result, families today are increasingly varied and complex, and they have varying levels of social and institutional support.

Family demographers seek to identify and explain family demographic trends and to uncover the implications of these trends for individual, family, and societal well-being. This knowledge can be used to develop policies and programs to support and sustain families and serve as an early warning system for potential future needs. At the core of family demography is the study of the composition of families, transitions into and out of different family structures, and the socioeconomic characteristics associated with different types of family structures. Family demographers are also interested in the factors that influence stability and change in the structure of families over time and in the implications of these family characteristics for individuals and society. As the discipline evolves, it is expanding its focus to include family functioning and roles and responsibilities within different types of families, such as the division of paid and unpaid labor, gender roles, power dynamics, communication, and exchanges of support across time among family members (Seltzer, 2019).

The purpose of this chapter is to familiarize family nursing students and professionals with key themes and trends in family demography in the United States and Canada. Whenever possible, the statistics in this chapter reflect entire populations, drawing on census data and nationally representative surveys collected at different points in time. These data provide the most accurate picture of population-level trends and allow demographers to investigate changes over time and differences within and between different cohorts. By using this data to determine key demographic characteristics of the population and projecting current population trends forward, demographers can also make educated predictions about the future. Family demography helps connect these macro-level trends to the meso and micro levels of families and individuals and back again.

In addition to utilizing the most recently available data, important material from historical records and older studies are used to illustrate population-level changes over time. Findings from seminal studies, qualitative research, and research drawing on more focused or geographically restricted populations are incorporated as needed to help interpret and explain the implications of population dynamics. In most cases, the raw data and data reports for this chapter come from government agencies such as Statistics Canada or the U.S. Census Bureau. Due to variations in the gathering and reporting of raw data, comparable data between the United States and Canada are not always available for some topics covered in this chapter. It is also important to note that, in many cases, the data used to calculate similar statistics were not collected in the same year, and differences in how a family indicator is defined or measured can change across the two countries at different times, as well as within the same country over time. Finally, different data sources use different defining groups and thus terms to delineate groups, such as race, reflect those differences.

Family composition and transitions tend to vary by other demographic variables such as age, race/ethnicity, gender, sexual orientation, nativity, education, and geographic location (rural/urban differences as well as across states, provinces, and territories). Key subgroup differences are frequently noted, but it is beyond the scope of this chapter to attend to each of these differences. Unless explicitly stated otherwise, it is likely that important differences exist that are not mentioned in this chapter, and students are encouraged to seek out additional details about these differences on their own. The list of references and suggested websites included with this chapter offer a great starting point for this exploration and can be a continued source of the most recent data going forward.

To capture fully the role of families and family transitions as a social determinant of health, one needs to consider not just current family status but also family and household history. The development and availability of longitudinal data on individuals and families have allowed family demographers to move beyond snapshots of population-level changes to consider family change as a dynamic process. While much of this research focuses on isolated transitions or a specific type of family change, a holistic approach that considers a collective set of changes is emerging, with unique insights into the role of repeated family changes on well-being (Cavanagh & Fomby, 2019). Longitudinal data are also critical for teasing out factors that increase the risk of an individual experiencing a particular family structure or transition and the impact of that family structure or transition on individual factors.

This chapter begins by providing a demographic portrait of families and change over time in the United States and Canada. The formation and dissolution of romantic unions, becoming a parent, household composition and living arrangements, and family roles and responsibilities related to work and home are described. In the second part of the chapter, demographic theories that try to account for how and why families have changed over time are discussed. These theories focus on the changing social and economic conditions of families and changing gender and family norms and attitudes. Concurrent demographic trends related to life expectancy and immigration and racial/ethnic diversity are also considered. The chapter ends with a discussion of why demography matters and its implications for nurses.

While covering a range of family indicators over time and across different countries and subgroups of the population, it is easy to become overwhelmed by all the statistics. Keep in mind that exact values are given as a reference to articulate how large or small an indicator is, to illustrate how indicators are changing over time, and to compare across groups. While the exact figures are constantly changing, the trends and patterns tell a story across time. What is more important is recognizing these overall trends and noticing when patterns change or diverge from what is expected.

A DEMOGRAPHIC PORTRAIT OF FAMILIES AND CHANGE OVER TIME

Modern family relationships can originate from biological connections, legal connections, and even social and emotional connections that transcend more limited understandings of family. Significant family connections are more likely to extend across multiple households than they did in the past. Therefore, there can be disagreement as to who are the members of the family. This broad view of family better captures the network of linked lives that represent families today but makes research on family structure more difficult due to measurement challenges. With that in mind, the demographic portrait of families presented here considers different types of connections (biological, legal, social/emotional) and co-residence as important components of family structure.

The Formation and Dissolution of Romantic Unions

The study of families starts with the first step in forming a family, which traditionally has started with marriage. This start has changed across time, however, and most notably in the last 50 years as couples have decided to share residences and often parenthood before or instead of marriage. This section will explore the different ways that families are formed and dissolved across North America.

Marriage

Historically, a marital union between a man and a woman was the foundation for a family. Demographic data indicate a reduction in marriage among family structures in both the United States and Canada. One indicator of this is a decline in marriage rates over the past 40 years. The marriage rate represents the number of marriages per 1,000 population in any one year. In the United States, since the most recent peak of 10.9 marriages (per 1,000 population) in 1972, rates fluctuated a bit before starting a steady decline from the early 1980s until 2009. These lower rates became relatively stable (between 6.8 and 7.0 per 1,000 population) until 2017, followed by an all-time low rate of 6.5 observed in 2018 (Curtin & Sutton, 2020).

The retreat from marriage is also evident when you look at the percentage of the population 15 years and older who are currently married. In Canada, 45.8% of men and 43.8% of women were married in 2019, down from 61.8% of men and 60.8% of women in 1971 (Statistics Canada, 2020c). In the United States, 53.2% of men and 50.9% of women were married in 2020, down from 66.8% of men and 61.9% of women in 1970 (see Figure 3-1).

Marriage is also strongly related to education, with the nature of this relationship reversing over time in both Canada and the United States. Historically, women with a university education were less likely than women without a university education to be married, whereas now they are more likely to be married (Martin & Hou, 2010; Torr, 2011). This is consistent with cross-national research that shows more highly educated women are less likely to be married than less educated women in societies with traditional gender roles, but they are more likely to be married than their less educated counterparts in gender-egalitarian countries (Kalmijn, 2013), which reflects the changing gender norms in Canada and the United States during this time.

A large part of the decline in the proportion of the adult population that is married can be attributed to changes in the timing of marriage. The average ages of entry into marriage dipped to an all-time low during the post–World War II

baby-boom years, when the median age at first marriage was 20 years for women and 23 years for men during 1948; it hovered at this median until the early 1960s and was followed by a steady increase. The most current data show a median age of first marriage of 30.5 years for men and 28 years for women in 2020 (U.S. Census Bureau, 2020a). Statistics Canada no longer publishes data on the average age at first marriage. The most recently available data show the average age at first marriage in 2008 was 31 years for men and 30 years for women, up from 23 years for women and 25 years for men in the early 1970s (Statistics Canada, 2017a).

These general trends obscure differences in age at first marriage by race and education. Looking at 2017 data, Payne (2019b) found the median age at first marriage in the United States to be highest among Black men (32 years) and Black women (30.4 years). For both men and women, the next highest racial category was Asians (30.4 years for men and 28.9 years for women). However, among men, this group was followed by those who identify as Hispanic, who had a slightly higher median age than their White counterparts (29.8 years versus 29.4 years); whereas among women, those who identify as Hispanic had the lowest median age (27.5 years), with the median age for White women being slightly older (28 years). The relationship between age at first marriage and education varies by gender. For men, the relationship is U-shaped, with the highest median age observed for men with a master's degree or higher (31.7 years), followed by men without a high-school degree (29.9 years), and then those with education

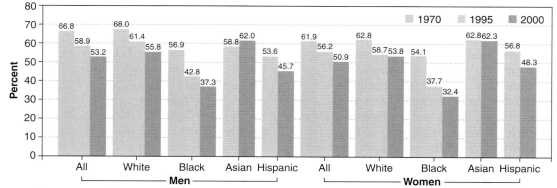

FIGURE 3-1 Percentage of the Population 15 Years Old and Over Who Are Married—by Sex, Race and Hispanic Origin: United States 1970, 1995, 2000 *Source: Data from U.S. Census Bureau, Historical Marital Status Tables, Table MS-1.*

levels in between having a slightly lower median age (approximately 29 years) (Payne, 2019a). For women, the median age at first marriage tends to increase with higher levels of education, with almost a five-year difference in the median age at first marriage between those without a high school or GED diploma (25.9 years), and those with a master's degree or higher (Payne, 2019a). Even though men and women with higher levels of education tend to get married at older ages, the overall likelihood of ever marrying increases with education (Smock & Schwartz, 2020).

Marriage under the age of 18 years, or child marriage, has been determined to be against human rights by the United Nations (United Nations, 2016). While commonly thought of as only being a problem in other parts of the world, child marriages are still occurring in the United States and Canada. Estimates using survey data suggest approximately six out of every 1,000 children in the United States have been married, with children of Native American or Chinese descent and immigrant children being at highest risk (Koski & Heymann, 2018). In Canada, approximately 1% of children are estimated to be married or in common-law unions (Zaman & Koski, 2020). As of 2020, only four U.S. states (New Jersey, Delaware, Pennsylvania, and Minnesota) and the U.S. Virgin Islands fully outlaw marriage for people under the age of 18 years without exceptions (Coffey, 2020). In Canada, the Civil Marriage Act was amended in 2015 to prohibit legal marriage before the age of 16 (Government of Canada, 2015), which still allows 16- and 17-year-old individuals to marry with parental consent (Zaman & Koski, 2020). Child marriage is associated with a younger age at first birth and associated obstetrical risks, higher number of births, higher risk of domestic violence, lower levels of educational attainment, and isolation (Morin, 2017).

Despite the decrease in adults choosing marriage in any given year and a smaller proportion of the population being married at any given moment, young men and women in the United States and Canada still see marriage as a desirable status and expect to marry someday (Anderson, 2016). Indeed, a majority of North Americans still marry eventually. In 2017, more than 90% of adults aged 50 years or older in the United States had been married at least once (U.S. Census Bureau, 2017). Comparable data from Canada in 2016 found slightly lower rates of ever being married among this age group, with 86% of men and 89% of women having been married at least once (Statistics Canada, 2017a). However, the proportion of never-married adults in the United States and Canada continues to grow, and it is projected that an increasing proportion of them will reach older adulthood without ever having married.

An exception to the retreat from marriage has been observed among same-sex couples. Many same-sex couples are embracing legal marriage, and dramatic increases in the number of married same-sex couples have been observed because of changes in the laws to allow these marriages. For example, in Canada, just over half of the country's population had access to same-sex marriage after it was legalized in Ontario and British Columbia in 2003. However, the number of same-sex married couples nearly tripled in the five years following the passage of the 2005 federal Civil Marriage Act that made same-sex marriage legal across all of Canada (Statistics Canada, 2016). The overall number of same-sex couples in Canada continues to increase and represents 0.9% of all couples, one-third of which are married (Statistics Canada, 2017e).

Massachusetts became the first state in the United States to allow same-sex marriage, in 2004, and a total of 37 states had done the same before the Supreme Court ruling in 2015 that struck down all state bans on same-sex marriage, thus making same-sex marriage legal across the country. Just prior to this change, in 2014, 43% of all same-sex households were marriages (U.S. Census Bureau, 2020j). That figure increased to 58% in 2019 but ranges from 35.7% in Wyoming to 72.5% in North Dakota (U.S. Census Bureau, 2020j). Same-sex couples live primarily in larger metropolitan areas and are more likely than opposite-sex couples to have at least one member of the couple with a bachelor's degree or higher (U.S. Census Bureau, 2019d).

Cohabitation

One of the most significant household changes in the second half of the 20th century in North America is the increase in men and women living together without being married. This trend continues, although the pace has slowed somewhat since the rapid rise in the 1970s and 1980s (LaPlante & Fostik, 2016; Smock & Schwartz, 2020). The first co-residential union for most young adults is now one of cohabitation rather than marriage (Sassler & Lichter, 2020). Approximately 60% of adults aged 18 to 44 in the United States have cohabited, more than the proportion who have ever been married (50%) (Horowitz et al., 2019). In 1987, only one in three women in this age group reported having ever cohabited (Manning, 2020). While a majority of couples getting married today live together before getting married, most cohabiting unions do not result in marriage (Eickmeyer & Manning, 2018).

Cohabiting couples in Canada are known as common-law couples. While most couples who live together are married, the proportion who are in common-law relationships continues to grow. When census data on common-law relationships was first collected in Canada in 1981, 6.3% of couples living together were not married, but this grew to 21.3% of couples by 2016 (Statistics Canada, 2017e). Considerable differences by age and regional variability are noteworthy. In 2016, 12% of Canadians aged 15 years and older were living in common-law relationships, with the highest proportion found among 25- to 29-year-old women (16.3%), and 30- to 34-year-old men (14.3%) (Statistics Canada, 2017e). Common-law relationships are most common in Nunavut (50%) and Quebec (40%).

Rates of cohabitation are increasing even among older adults. In 2017, of those 65 years and older, 6% of those are partners in cohabiting households compared to 2% in 1996 (Roberts & Ogunwole, 2018). The characteristics of older adult cohabiting relationships differ from those of younger adults (Brown et al., 2012). Researchers found that cohabitation among adults over the age of 65 years tends to last longer (8 years on average); is not a reflection of financial strain; and serves as an alternative to marriage rather than a step toward marriage, as it is with younger adults (Brown et al., 2012). Researchers have found that cohabiting older adults seem to experience the same level of relationship satisfaction, physical pleasure, and openness as their married counterparts (Brown & Kawamura, 2010).

Divorce

In 2020, not taking into account cohabiting status, divorced was the current marital status for almost 10% of the adult population aged 15 and older in the United States, whereas in 1970 it was less than 3% (U.S. Census Bureau, 2020f). Comparable statistics in Canada show approximately 7% were divorced in 2020, compared to less than 1% in 1971 (Statistics Canada, 2020c). These statistics do not capture divorced individuals who are remarried or separated individuals who are in the process of getting a divorce. These data reflect a higher risk of divorce than in the past.

In the United States, the divorce rate for women (the number of divorces per 1,000 women in the population) increased sharply between 1960 (9.2) and the peak in 1980 (22.6), and have gradually declined since then, with a slight uptick between 2000 and 2010 that has since reversed and now sits at 15.7 (Schweizer, 2020a). While the overall divorce rate has been declining, this trend differs by age. The decline in divorce rates is observed only among individuals less than 45 years of age, with divorce rates for those 45 years and older doubling since at least the 1990s (Allred, 2019). This phenomenon has been dubbed gray divorce. Approximately 16% of Canadian women aged 55 years and older, and 13% of their male counterparts, were separated or divorced from a marriage in 2017 (Statistics Canada, 2019a). In the United States, in 2016, 15.1% of American women over the age of 65 years were divorced compared to 11.9% of men (Roberts & Ogunwole, 2018).

Research shows that the risk factors for divorce among older adults are similar to those among younger couples, and they include duration factors (shorter marriages are more likely to end in divorce), remarriages, lower educational attainment, interracial marriages, financial stressors, and poor marital quality (Brown & Lin, 2012; Brown & Wright, 2017). Divorce is a significantly stressful life event regardless of the ages of the partners, but outcomes may have unique positive and negative outcomes for older North Americans. For partners who are financially secure and in good health, divorce may provide reduced stress and an increased sense of freedom. For individuals who are not financially secure or have poorer health, they have fewer years within the labor force as they reach retirement, and they may be left without caregivers to offer support during health crises (Brown & Wright, 2017).

Across age groups, highly educated individuals have a lower risk of marital dissolution than do those with less education. While the probability of divorce declines with educational attainment for both men and women, the protective effect of education is greater for men than for women. The Analysis of the National Longitudinal Survey of Youth (ANLSY) found that by age 46 years, 56.6% of the first marriages of men with less than a high school diploma had ended in divorce, whereas only 23.7% of first marriages of men with at least a bachelor's degree had ended in divorce (Aughinbaugh et al., 2013). Comparable figures for women showed that 59.9% of first marriages among those with less than a high school diploma ended in divorce by age 46, while 35.4% of those with a bachelor's degree or higher were divorced by this time (Aughinbaugh et al., 2013).

A number of researchers have looked at the relationship between premarital cohabitation and subsequent divorce. Early research on cohabitation found that marriages preceded by cohabitation were more likely to end in divorce; however, more recent research is calling this connection into question, finding that those who cohabitate with the intention of getting married are less likely to later divorce than are those that start their cohabitation without intending to marry later (Smock & Schwartz, 2020).

Trends in the dissolution of cohabiting relationships have not been adequately captured at the population level. With many cohabiting relationships ending before marriage, the result has been more young adults experiencing co-residential union dissolutions than previous cohorts, despite declining rates of marriage and divorce. This pattern changes depending on the intent with cohabitation, with those sharing residences for financial and convenience reasons more likely to dissolve compared to those sharing residences with the intent to marry later (Eickmeyer & Manning, 2018).

Widowhood

In 2020, approximately 5% of Canadians and 6% of U.S. residents aged 15 years and older identified their marital status as widowed (Statistics Canada, 2020d; U.S. Census, 2020f). The proportion of women who are currently widowed is consistently higher than the proportion of men, reflecting both the longer life expectancy of women compared to men and the lower likelihood of remarriage following the death of a spouse for women. In Canada, the rate of widowed women climbed from 1.25 million in 2000 to 1.5 million in 2020. Fewer men

were widowed during the same time period, with 260,000 widowed in 2000 compared to 444,515 widowed in 2020 (Statistics Canada, 2020d). In the United States, the trend is similar for men, with 2.6 million men being widowed in 2000 compared to 3.5 million men in 2020; women's rates have been more constant, with 11.1 million women being widowed in 2000 compared to 11.4 million women in 2020 (U.S. Census Bureau, 2020f). The larger number of widowed women across both countries indicates that widowhood is another factor increasing the risk of isolation and poverty in older women compared to other demographics.

Repartnering

Most statistics on repartnering focus on remarriage following divorce or widowhood, but information on repartnership via cohabitation and repartnership after the dissolution of a cohabiting relationship is increasingly being examined. In Canada, more than one in four adults who are in a couple relationship are in their second or subsequent marriage or common-law union (Statistics Canada, 2019g). In the United States, one in three adults aged 19 to 44 years have experienced multiple cohabiting relationships in their lifetime (Horowitz et al., 2019), and approximately one in four married individuals have been previously married (Schwiezer, 2020b).

Like first marriages, remarriage rates (the number of marriages per 1,000 divorced or widowed individuals) have also been in decline in recent decades (Schweizer, 2020a). There is considerable sociodemographic variability in who gets remarried. Remarriage rates are progressively higher among those with more education, highest among Asians, and lowest among Black women (Reynolds, 2020a). Men are consistently more likely than women to remarry and to remarry more quickly (Schwiezer, 2020b). Divorced individuals with children are less likely to intend to remarry, especially for women (Di Nallo, 2019).

Older men tend to remarry rather than cohabitate, yet older women tend to remain single or single longer (Brown et al., 2019; Carr & Utz, 2020). The disparity between gendered trends of repartnership are related to several factors, including the longer lives of women; men's preference to remarry younger women compared to women's preference to marry same-age or older men; women being more likely to have children in the home, which decreases repartnering rates; and decreasing numbers of eligible men to marry as women age. Men have been found to experience higher levels of distress and loneliness during the first year after divorce, which may motivate repartnering (Leopold, 2018). These decisions are also influenced by changing attitudes, caregiver role status, financial security, health status, age, race, and previous marital status (Brown et al., 2019).

Becoming a Parent

Pathways to parenthood have become increasingly diverse and add to the complexity of family structures observed in contemporary families. Individuals have shifted to limiting parenting options to parenting only within a heterosexual marriage, with limited access to parenting nonbiological children, to a number of diverse decisions, from not parenting at all to parenting before marriage, without a partner, with a same-sex partner, through adoption, and through technological advances such as in vitro fertilization.

Total Fertility Rate and Family Size

In the United States and Canada, fertility has exhibited a trend of long-term decline for more than a century, interrupted by the baby-boom period and other small fluctuations. Like many other developed countries, the United States and Canada are both below replacement-level fertility. *Replacement-level fertility* refers to the required number of children each woman in the population would have to bear on average to replace herself

and her partner, and it is conventionally set at 2.1 children per woman for countries with low mortality rates. This threshold is set slightly above two in order to account for a negligible rate of childhood mortality and a small proportion of individuals who do not survive to their reproductive age (Livingston, 2019).

Figure 3-2 shows the trends in the total fertility rate since the 1930s for the United States and Canada. The total fertility rate reflects the total number of children a woman would have, assuming current age-specific birth rates. As this graph shows, both countries experienced a post–World War II baby boom during the 1950s and 1960s, after which fertility began to decline again. In the mid-1970s, Canada and the United States had similar below-replacement total fertility rates, but the decline in fertility in the United States began to stabilize, and in the 1980s, it increased again, hovering around replacement level until the Great Recession of 2007–2009. Since then, the total fertility rate has continued to decline and now sits at its lowest point ever, at 1.73. In Canada, the fertility rate continued a slower decline into the 1980s, with smaller bouts of recovery and most recently a decline since the Great Recession that has fallen to around 1.5.

Fertility varies by demographic characteristics. Fertility rates decrease with increasing amounts of education (U.S. Census Bureau, 2019). In Canada and the United States, the age-specific birth rate is highest among women aged 30 to 34 (Martin et al., 2019). Immigrants tend to exhibit higher fertility rates than the native-born population. Recently,

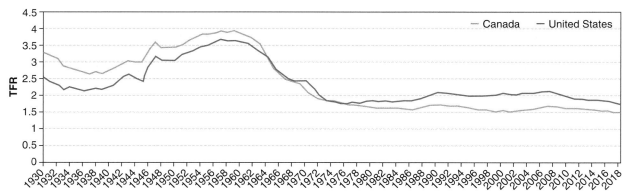

FIGURE 3-2 Total Fertility Rate for the United States and Canada: 1930–2018 *Sources: Data from Statistics Canada, Canadian Vital Statistics, Births Database, 1921 to 2016, Survey 3231 and Demography Division, Demographic Estimates Program (DEP); Trends in Fertility in the United States, Vital and Health Statistics Services 21-No. 28, Table 13 (1977); The World Bank, Fertility rate, total (births per woman), 1960–2018.*

however, there has been a dramatic decline in fertility among Hispanic immigrants that has contributed to the overall fertility decline in the United States. In 2018, native-born women aged 45 to 50 had given birth to 1.96 children on average; the comparable figure for foreign-born women was 2.21 children (U.S. Census Bureau, 2019a). Part of the decline in fertility among Hispanic immigrants has been attributed to a reduction in recent immigrants from Mexico, who tend to have high fertility rates (Cherlin et al., 2013). Fertility also varies by race/ethnicity. In 2018 in the United States, the total fertility rate was the highest among Native Hawaiian or among other Pacific Islanders (2.11), followed by Hispanic women (1.96), African Americans (1.79), and European Americans (1.64), and the lowest rate was observed among Asian women (1.53) (Martin et al., 2019).

Age at First Birth

Overall, women have delayed childbirth in both the United States and Canada. After sharp increases in the mean age at first pregnancy during the 1970s and 1980s, the pace slowed during the 1990s and 2000s but began to increase more rapidly again since the late 2000s (Guzzo & Payne, 2018). The average age at first birth in Canada in 2016 was 29.2 years, up from 23.5 years in the mid-1960s (Provencher et al., 2018; Statistics Canada, 2017g). In 2018, the average age at first birth in the United States was 26.9 years, but it varies considerably by race/ethnicity. Native American/Alaska Native women had the youngest average age at first birth, at 23.5 years, and Asian American women had the oldest, at 30.5 years; for African American and Hispanic American women, it was about 25 years, and for European American women it was 27.7 years (Martin et al., 2019).

Two trends related to age and birth rates are contributing to the increased age at first birth. First, the birth rate among teenagers declined in both Canada and the United States over the past decade, but more dramatically in the United States than in Canada. In the United States, the birth rate among 15- to 19-year-old women dropped by more than 58% between 2008 and 2018, with the largest declines among Asian, Hispanic, and Black teenagers (Martin et al., 2019). While the economic downturn associated with the Great Recession of 2007–2009 may be a factor, increasing levels of abstinence coupled with

higher rates of contraceptive use and the use of more effective contraceptive methods among sexually active women in this age group also played a role (Livingston & Thomas, 2019). Despite dramatic reductions in teenage fertility in the United States and a record low of 17.4 births per 1,000 women aged 15 to 19 in 2018, the rate is still nearly twice that of Canada.

Second, while birth rates for younger women have been decreasing, there has been a countertrend of increasing birth rates among women over the age of 30, particularly among those of so-called advanced maternal age who are over the age of 35 (Martin et al., 2019). Delayed childbirth has been shown to further shrink family size and decrease fertility rates. While delaying childbirth allows women to pursue more easily higher education and more professional opportunities, delay marriage, and pursue more personal goals, waiting for childbirth increases risks for infertility, complications with pregnancy, and chromosomal defects (e.g., Down's syndrome). Nurses can assist families in making informed decisions regarding their desire for childbearing balanced with the risk involved in delaying childbearing.

Marital Versus Nonmarital Births

A majority of births in both Canada and the United States are to married women, but the proportion of births to unmarried women has increased significantly. In 1969 in the United States and in 1970 in Canada, only 10% of births were to unmarried women. This percentage essentially quadrupled in size over the subsequent 40 years. A number of reports highlighted the alarming growth in nonmarital births during this time. Since 2009, the percentage of births to unmarried women has remained relatively stable in both countries, even decreasing slightly in recent years; in 2018, births to unmarried women accounted for 39.6% of births in the United States and 39.2% of births in Canada (Statistics Canada, 2020c; Martin et al., 2019).

There is tremendous variation in nonmarital births by age, race, and education level. In the United States, the majority of births to women ages 15 to 19 years (90%) and ages 20 to 24 years (66%) are to unmarried women, with the percentage decreasing at older age groups until ages 40 to 44 years, where it ticks up slightly before declining again (Vital Statistics Birth Data, 2018;

author calculations). However, nonmarital births for women younger than 30 years have been on the decline for more than a decade, and nonmarital birth rates for women older than 30 years have been increasing.

Figure 3-3 shows nonmarital childbearing by race-ethnicity and education level in the United States in 2018. More than 60% of births to women with less than a high school education were nonmarital, compared to 13% for women with a bachelor's degree and less than 7% for women with a graduate or professional degree. Asians have the lowest levels of nonmarital childbearing (11%), followed by non-Hispanic White women (29%). In all other racial groups, more than 50% of births in 2018 were nonmarital. Patterns by race and education show a decline in the proportion of nonmarital groups as education increases for all racial groups except Asian, where women with less than a high school degree are less likely to have a nonmarital birth than Asian women with a high school or associate's degree. The magnitude of the decline varies by race, but for most groups the greatest decreases are observed between those with an associate's degree or some college and those having a bachelor's degree. This is consistent with higher rates of marriage at higher levels of education, increasing the likelihood that a couple will be married when a pregnancy occurs.

Multiple-Partner Fertility

Multiple-partner fertility (MPF) occurs when someone has biological children with more than one partner. While the behavior itself is not new, it is increasing, and the context of MPF has changed, from primarily occurring as the result of young widows remarrying and having children with their new partner in the 19th century, to the same behavior following divorce in the late 20th century, to the current context, in which MPF increasingly involves nonmarital births (Fostik & Le Bourdais, 2020; Guzzo, 2014; Monte, 2019). Because of the diversity of patterns leading to MPF, research on exact numbers of children with different biological parents for diverse reasons living under the same household is limited.

In 2014, the Survey of Income and Program Participation (SIPP) became the first nationally representative survey to ask specifically about MPF. For U.S. adults, an estimated 10.1% of all persons aged 15 or older have MPF, and when looking specifically at persons aged 15 or older who have two or more biological children, approximately one in five have MPF (Monte, 2017, 2019). In Canada, 5.3% of men and 7.5% of women aged 25 to 64 have children with more than one partner, representing 10.6% of men and 13.1% of women who have at least two children (Fostik & Le Bourdais, 2020). These snapshots underestimate how many

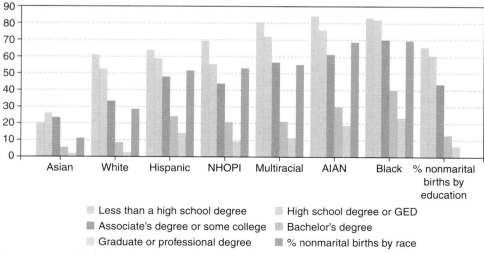

FIGURE 3-3 Percentage of Births by Race and Education That Were Nonmarital: United States, 2018
Notes: NHOPI is Native Hawaiian or Pacific Islander; AIAN is Native American or Alaska Native.
Source: Data from Vital Statistics Birth Data, 2018.

adults will experience MPF because many of the respondents have not yet completed their fertility and may go on to have biological children with different partners. In the SIPP data, the proportion of adults with MPF increases up to 14.9% among adults ages 40 to 49 years who are more likely to have completed their fertility, and proportions decrease in older age groups (Monte, 2019). This suggests a cohort effect, where MPF is becoming more common among younger cohorts of Americans. Other data sources confirm that younger cohorts are transitioning to MPF at earlier ages than previous cohorts and point to increasing rates of MPF as these cohorts age (Guzzo, 2014).

Similar to other diverse family structures, MPF is more common among some racial/ethnic minorities. Asians and Whites are less likely to experience MPF than Blacks, Hispanics, and all other races or race combinations (Monte, 2019). On average, adults with MPF tend to be less educated, be less likely to be married, have higher rates of poverty, and have more biological children on average, even when compared to those with single-partner fertility who have at least two biological children (Guzzo, 2014; Monte, 2019). Individuals with MPF also tend to enter parenthood differently than those with single-partner fertility who also have at least two biological children. In both Canada and the United States, those with MPF have their first birth at a younger age, are less likely to have an intended first birth, and are less likely to be living with the other biological parent when they had their first birth (Fostik & Le Bourdais, 2020; Guzzo, 2014; Monte, 2019).

MPF is related to lower levels of parental well-being and connections with children. Compared to other men and women aged 25 to 32 with two or more children, men and women with MPF have higher rates of depression, are less likely to be happy in their role as a parent, and are less likely to feel close to their children (Guzzo, 2014). This same study found that, for men aged 40 to 44 years with two or more children who did not live with them, men with MPF whose children are spread across more households are less likely than men with single-partner fertility to think they are doing a good job or very good job as a father.

Assisted Reproductive Technology

Childbearing is now a possibility for couples who previously were told that fertility and childbearing were not an option. Today, technological advances allow previously infertile couples, same-sex couples, and women with chronic illnesses or disabilities to conceive and carry a pregnancy to birth. These new technologies have changed family composition and structure as families negotiate complex technical procedures, consider possibilities of donated ovum or sperm, and add children to their family where the possibility did not exist without the technology (Smock & Greenland, 2010).

Assisted reproductive technologies (ART) involve fertility treatments where both the egg and the sperm are handled outside the body and fertilized eggs are transferred to a woman's body. The number of births annually using ART has been growing in Canada and the United States: even as the number of multiple births from these procedures is decreasing (Canadian Assisted Reproductive Technologies Register Plus [CARTR Plus], 2019; Sunderam et al., 2019). Still, only about 2% of births in the United States in 2016 were a result of ART (Sunderam et al., 2019; Hamilton et al., 2017) and in Canada, ART treatments in 2016 resulted in 6,514 live births (CARTR Plus, 2019), representing approximately 1.7% of births during this time (Statistics Canada, 2020b). The use of ART is often time-consuming and expensive, making it more accessible to families with more time and financial resources (Smock & Greenland, 2010). When clinics first began offering ART in the early 1980s, single women, lesbians, and gay men were often excluded. This discrimination persisted, prompting the Ethics Committee of the American Society for Reproductive Medicine (2006, 2009, 2013) to issue a statement in 2006, and reiterate it in 2009 and 2013, that all requests for assisted reproduction should be treated equally, regardless of gender, sexual orientation, or marital status.

Lesbian couples using ART must decide who will carry the pregnancy, who will supply the egg, whether to use a known or unknown sperm donor, and the donor traits and characteristics that are important (Greenfeld & Seli, 2013). Some lesbian couples choose Co-IVF, where one partner becomes the biological mother by supplying the egg and the other partner becomes the birth mother by carrying the pregnancy (Yeshua et al., 2015). Gay male couples must decide whether to use a known or anonymous egg donor, find a surrogate, and decide who will provide the sperm (Greenfeld & Seli, 2013). In some cases, both men choose to become biological fathers by fertilizing different eggs with each of their sperm and transferring an embryo from each of them to the surrogate, producing children that are half-siblings due to a shared egg donor (Greenfeld & Seli, 2011). While gay men using ART typically choose anonymous egg donors where there is no expectation of an ongoing relationship (Greenfeld & Seli, 2011), they often develop close relationships with the surrogate during treatment and pregnancy, and many maintain ongoing relationships for years after the birth (Fantus, 2020).

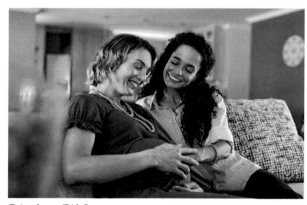

© istock.com/Ridofranz

Single men and women and heterosexual couples experiencing infertility that use ART may also have to grapple with decisions about donor eggs, donor sperm, and surrogates. These decisions have the potential to bring other people into the family, which adds complexity. With the rise of the internet and donor sibling registries, and more recently commercial genetic testing, donor-created families can search for and connect with genetic kin. A growing number of parents who share biologically related children from using the same donor are connecting through online forums where they can share information about their children and exchange socioemotional support (Hertz & Mattes, 2011). Many of these relationships move offline and result in face-to-face meetings and ongoing relationships (Hertz et al., 2017). Some parents even come to consider their child's donor siblings as part of their nuclear family, and a majority consider a donor sibling and their parents to be extended kin if they have communicated with them or met them in person. Offspring are twice as likely as their parents to consider donor-siblings

they met as part of their nuclear family (42%), and more than 20% consider identified donor siblings as part of their nuclear family even if they had never met or communicated with them. Only a small proportion of offspring consider their donor-siblings' parents part of their nuclear family, even if they had met them, and in contrast to their parents, less than half consider them part of their extended family.

The role of ART in changing family structures is a clear example of changing attitudes and changing diversity in the definition of family and parenting. Nurses will continue to care for and support families as they pursue strategies to become parents. While technology has helped many families realize their goal to become parents, this process often includes years of complex decision making, grief at lost pregnancies, and legal and policy dilemmas that follow families throughout their journey.

Adoption

Adoption is another option for families who seek parenthood. There are three ways to adopt in Canada and the United States: public adoption of a child in the care of a provincial or state child welfare authority, private domestic adoption, and international adoption. While adoptions have been present for generations, the number of domestic adoptions in the United States peaked, following a surge after World War II. Most adoptions at that time were through public agencies, and most were domestic and racially matched. During the time period prior to 1970, most couples preferred to adopt newborns, and adoption agencies could be very selective in who they allowed to adopt, giving preference to normative families, who were often religious and followed a breadwinner model. Adoptions were often secretive, silenced by the stigma of illegitimacy and infertility, with birth and adoptive family identities unknown to the other party and many children never being told that they were adopted. Following reliable contraception, the passing of *Roe v. Wade*, and acceptance of single parenting, the domestic adoption rate decreased. This trend led to a sharp increase in international adoptions and adoptions of children with disabilities (Adoption.org, 2020).

In post–World War II Canada, until the early 1970s, as many as 95% of residents of unwed maternity homes and 74% of unwed women giving birth outside these facilities surrendered their babies for adoption, whereas today only about 2% of babies born out of wedlock are given up for adoption (Standing Senate Committee on Social Affairs, Science and Technology, 2018). Societal pressures against so-called illegitimate children, preference for the rearing of children in homes with two married parents, and the high demand for adopted babies contributed to what has been described as forced adoption practices in Canada during this time, particularly among White women (Andrews, 2018). In the United States, for births prior to 1973, about 20% of babies born to never-married White women were relinquished for adoption, whereas less than 1% of babies born between 1996 and 2002 to never-married women were given up for adoption, regardless of race (Jones, 2009). This trend has led couples to seek alternatives to adopting domestic newborns, including international adoptions, adoptions of older children, and adoptions of children with disabilities.

Recent trends in the United States have shown growth in the number of public adoptions of children older than the newborn period (children adopted through a child welfare agency). Not only did the number of children adopted increase annually (from 55,536 in 2015 to 66,035 in 2019) but an even greater number of children were also waiting to be adopted for whom parental rights of all living parents had been terminated (from 62,320 in 2015 to 71,335 in 2019) (U.S. Department of Health and Human Services, 2020). Children adopted through a public agency had an average age of 6.4 years and waited approximately 12 months from the termination of parental rights to adoption. Half of these children were White, 18% were Black, and 20% were Hispanic (U.S. Department of Health and Human Services, 2020).

A majority of publicly adopted children were adopted by a married couple (68%), and one in four were adopted by a single female. Just over half were adopted by their unrelated foster parent, and 36% were adopted by a relative. Almost all of these adopted families (93%) received an adoption subsidy (U.S. Department of Health and Human Services, 2020). This subsidy makes adoption more accessible to lower-income families. Not surprisingly, families who adopt through foster care are much more likely to have household incomes at or below 200% of the poverty level than families who adopt privately or internationally (Ishizawa &

Kubo, 2014). Some prospective adoptive parents prefer not to adopt from foster care given the age and racial composition of the children available for adoption and concerns about the lasting impact of abuse or neglect that resulted in their removal from their biological parents (Ishizawa & Kubo, 2014; Raleigh, 2016).

A lack of a single administrative source that tracks adoptions makes adoption trends challenging to track (Kreider, 2020). Government data is often available annually on the number and source of international adoptions, as well as public adoptions through child welfare agencies, but data on private domestic adoptions is typically not available (Raleigh, 2016). Beginning in the 2000 U.S. Census and subsequent American Community Surveys, "adopted son or daughter" was added as a relationship category for identifying how each person in the household is related to the primary respondent. This categorization does not allow for distinguishing between different types of adoption; misses respondents who choose not to identify a child as adopted; and may even capture informal adoptions, where someone has taken on primary responsibility for the care of a child without legally adopting them (Kreider & Lofquist, 2014).

International adoptions peaked in 2004, with adoptions occurring from Central America, India, China, Korea, Vietnam, Romania, and Russia. Many of these countries have increased their limits on allowable adoptions outside their country. Overall, the number of adopted children has declined since 2004 (Kreider, 2020). Using American Community Survey data from 2013 to 2017, 12.1% of children less than 18 years of age who were identified as adopted were international adoptions (Kreider, 2020), down from 13.6% of adoptions using data from the 2009–2011 American Community Survey (Kreider & Lofquist, 2014). Changes in the policies of other countries that make it harder to adopt or that restrict international adoptions (sometimes specifically by Americans), the implementation of operating standards outlined by The Hague Convention and Intercountry Adoption Act in 2008, and restrictions placed by the U.S. government on adoptions from specific countries have all contributed to the decline in international adoptions (Kreider, 2020). Changes in some countries have significantly limited the ability of single and same-sex couples to adopt internationally. For example, China, where most children adopted internationally in Canada and the United States originate, allows intercountry adoption only by married heterosexual couples and single women if they meet specific age, income, and family context requirements; lesbian, gay, bisexual, transgendered, or intersex individuals or same-sex couples are not permitted to adopt under any circumstances (U.S. Department of State, 2020). The COVID-19 pandemic is restricting international adoption even further, and it is unclear what the long-term effects will be (Fronek & Rotabi, 2020).

Trends and attitudes toward transracial adoption (TRA) have also fluctuated over time. Historically, children from underrepresented races were frequently removed from their families and placed in institutional settings, such as boarding schools. Only when demand for White babies exceeded the supply did private adoption agencies begin to include children from underrepresented racial groups, older children, and children with disabilities in any significant number (Fogg-Davis, 2002). White/Black TRAs increased in the 1950s and 1960s in the United States as adoption agencies and White families embraced ideals of racial integration and color blindness (Fogg-Davis, 2002). However, in the 1970s, underrepresented groups organized a backlash against this practice; they viewed TRA as a form of racial and cultural genocide. Public and private domestic TRAs subsequently declined, and policies and practices prioritizing same-race foster care placements and adoptions were established (Lee, 2003). Yet international TRAs continued to grow during this time.

An unintended consequence of same-race preferences was a growing number of children from underrepresented groups in the child welfare system waiting for, and often not finding, a permanent home due to the mismatch between the race of families seeking to adopt and the race of children waiting to be adopted. The Multiethnic Placement Act (MEPA) enacted in 1994, and the 1996 amendment that added provisions for the removal of barriers to interethnic adoption were designed to facilitate permanent placements of minority children by (1) prohibiting entities that receive federal financial assistance and are involved in foster care or adoption placements from delaying or denying placement on the basis of race, and (2) requiring states to recruit proactively foster or adoptive parents that reflect the racial and ethnic

diversity of the children in that state in need of homes. Transracial placement in adoption through the child welfare system increased slightly after these changes, from 11% in 1995 to 15% in 2004 (Hansen & Simon, 2004).

Approximately 29.1% of adopted children under the age of 18 years in the United States are of a different race than their adoptive parent(s), and 36% differ on Hispanic origins (Kreider, 2020). Most TRAs involve non-Hispanic White parents, not only because most individuals adopting are non-Hispanic White but also because minority individuals and couples are less likely to adopt a child of a different race or ethnicity (Raleigh, 2016). Same-sex couples and single individuals are also more likely than heterosexual married couples to adopt across race, not necessarily because they have less of a preference for same-race adoption but more likely because of restrictions in the adoption marketplace that encourage them to broaden their selection criteria (Raleigh, 2012).

While race should not be the sole factor limiting TRA, "adoption policy and practice should be sensitive to the effects of a race-conscious society on individual children in need of adoption" and their families (Fogg-Davis, 2002, p. 2). Because of the large numbers of transracial adoptive families, nurses are encouraged to continue their learning about the outcomes for families across time. There was a time when parents who were a different race than the child they adopted were told to assimilate the child into their own race and culture, and some families continue to do this. There has been an emphasis more recently on the importance of racial-ethnic socialization in the child's culture for ethnic identity and long-term well-being, yet adoptive parents differ in their awareness of racial-ethnic and cultural socialization (Montgomery & Nickolas, 2018). Nurses should be sensitive to these differences and help connect parents to resources that will help them understand the benefits of racial-ethnic and cultural socialization for their child.

The secrecy surrounding adoption is also eroding with implications for birth and adoptive families. Open adoptions are now common, with birth and adoptive families maintaining varied levels of contact and involvement over time (Farr et al., 2018). Technological advancements and policy changes are also allowing adult adoptees to identify and connect with their birth families. Many states and provinces are recognizing the rights of children to know the identities of their biological parents and making previously sealed adoption records available, and not always with the consent of the birth parents (Baffer, 2019). Commercial DNA testing has also made it possible for many adopted children to identify their birth parents even without the use of official records. The relationships between children and their birth families after reuniting in adulthood and the implications of these reunions warrant further study.

Stepparents

The definition of a stepfamily has shifted over time. Traditionally, a relationship in which the married partner of the biological parent was not the biological parent of one or more children in the family constituted a stepfamily (Kreider & Lofquist, 2014). More recently, a variety of terms have been used to categorize relationships between children and biological parent partners, whether those partners are married or cohabiting, or unmarried partners living elsewhere. The language used seems to be determined by each family based on the negotiation of relationships and relational boundaries within the household, and often these relationships are determined by the acceptance of the child(ren) of the stepparent as a family member (Kreider & Lofquist, 2014). Brown et al. (2015) argue that measures focusing solely on the child's relationship to the parent misses families with more complex and varied family structures, such as families in which there are half-siblings, and stepsiblings who may not reside in the same household. Brown et al. (2015) defines these family arrangements as "complex families," which, in addition to the presence of half-siblings and stepsiblings, may contain stepparents, unmarried partners, or cohabiting partners.

Historically, stepfamilies were formed after the death of a biological parent. For stepfathers, this meant taking on the role of earning a living to support nonbiological children. For stepmothers, it meant managing the household and rearing nonbiological children (Ganong & Coleman, 2018). By the mid-1970s, as divorce rates rose, stepfamily structures also increased, now due more to divorce than to widowhood. Today, nonmarital childbearing also contributes to the formation of stepfamilies. About 16% of women and 14% of men become stepparents when they get married for the first time, and this is twice as common for Black adults than White adults (Carlson, 2020). While this statistic captures children who both live in the home with the stepparent and those who only visit that home, it misses those children who have stepparents when their biological parent enters a cohabiting union with a nonbiological parent.

As aging North Americans have divorced at higher rates, the potential for late-in-life stepfamilies has also increased (Papernow, 2018). These families face similar challenges as do stepfamilies that form earlier in the life course, including struggles with child loyalties and grief related to marital dissolution of biological parents, tensions related to parenting decisions, defining and forming relational bonds and roles, and ex-spouse interactions. Besides these challenges, late-in-life stepfamilies experience unique challenges such as navigating elder caregiving responsibilities and tasks, estate planning, and end-of-life decisions (Papernow, 2018). For aging family members, especially those in which repartnerships have dissolved or ended in widowhood or divorce, former stepchildren may not provide the same level of care as biological children (Carr & Utz, 2020).

HOUSEHOLD COMPOSITION AND LIVING ARRANGEMENTS

Propelled by demographic family trends including later age of marriage, and increasing rates of cohabitation, divorce, nonmarital births, multipartner fertility, and blended families, household composition and living arrangements have also changed. The growing complexity of families, as well as fluctuations in other factors that influence living arrangements (e.g., availability of affordable housing), have contributed to a growing disconnect between who we live with and who we consider family. While household composition and family structure frequently overlap, nurses should consider them as separate sources of individual risk and protective factors.

Household Size and Composition of Private Households

The most complete information we have on household composition comes from census data.

A census involves collecting information on every member of a population and is very costly when done at the national level. In the United States, a national census of the population is completed in years that end in 0 (every ten years), whereas in Canada, a national census is conducted in years that end in 1 or 6 (every five years). The United States also collects data similar to the long form of the decennial census every year through the American Community Survey, but only a fraction of the population is captured (about 3.5 million households instead of all households). Still, data from this nationally representative survey provides reliable estimates of the population and insights into how it is changing between census years.

Countries differ in how they define a household or a family, and these definitions change over time (Willekens, 2010). This can make comparisons across countries and even within a country over time challenging and imperfect. Even within a country at a given point in time, the definitions of *household* and *family* can differ depending on the source and purpose of the data. Consequently, it is always a good idea to look closely for any differences in definitions across the data sources being compared, even when data is coming from the same source but from a different time point or compiled for a different purpose. Box 3-1 provides details on how households are categorized in the United States and Canadian censuses and notes key differences.

Unless institutionalization is temporary, data on private households does not capture those living in institutional settings such as student dormitories;

hospitals; correctional facilities; group homes; homeless shelters; military housing; and residences for older adults, including nursing homes and assisted living facilities. Statistics on institutional settings are typically reported separately from private households, and this section will focus on the household composition of private households.

In both the United States and Canada, the proportion of private households that house families and the average household size have been on a slow but steady decline for more than 50 years. Table 3-1 presents information on the composition and average size of private households in the United States from 2000 to 2020, and Table 3-2 presents the same information for Canada from 2001 to 2016, demonstrating the most recent trends available. Average household size in Canada is similar to the United States (2.4 and 2.5, respectively). While household sizes may have increased slightly during times of economic hardship (Fry, 2019), these changes were not sustained and the longer-term trend in both countries continues to be a slow decline in average household size.

Given the differences in how Canada and the United States categorize households, direct comparisons of household types are not meaningful, with one exception: both countries measure one-person, nonfamily households the same way. The most recent data available from Canada (2016), and the United States (2020), show 28.2% of private households in both countries were comprised of a single occupant. One-person households became the most common household type in Canada in 2016, up from 7.4% in 1951 (Statistics

Table 3-1 Private Household Composition: United States, 2000–2020	2000	2005	2010	2015	2020
Nonfamily households	31.2	32.2	32.9	34.4	34.9
One-person household	25.5	26.6	26.7	28.0	28.2
Nonfamily household	5.7	5.6	6.2	6.4	6.7
Family households	68.8	67.8	67.1	65.6	65.1
Married couple without minor children	28.7	28.3	28.8	28.9	30.1
Married couple with minor children	24.1	22.9	20.9	19.3	18.4
Lone-parent family with minor children	8.9	9.1	9.1	8.8	7.7
Other family households	7	7.6	8.3	8.6	8.9
Average household size	2.6	2.6	2.6	2.5	2.5

Sources: Data from United States Census Bureau. Historical Households Tables, HH-1, HH-4 and Historical Families Tables, FM-1.

BOX 3-1

Sources to Obtain Information on Demography and Public Health

**Current Population Surveys
(U.S. Census Bureau, 2019)**

Many of the statistics discussed in this chapter draw on information from the *Current Population Surveys* (CPS) collected by the U.S. Census Bureau.

- This is a continuous survey of about 60,000 households, selected at random to be representative of the national population.
- Each household is interviewed monthly for two 4-month periods. During February through April of each year, CPS collects additional demographic and economic data, including data on health insurance coverage, from each household.
- This Annual Demographic Supplement is the most frequently used source of data on demographic and economic trends in the United States and is the data source for the majority of statistics presented in this chapter regarding changes in families.

**National Center for Health Statistics, 2019
(CDC, 2021)**

Several large health-related surveys are conducted by the National Center for Health Statistics.

- *National Health Interview Survey* (NHIS): NHIS is a large, continuous survey of about 43,000 households per year, covering the civilian, noninstitutionalized population of the United States. NHIS is the major source of information on health status and disability, health-related behaviors, and health care utilization for all age groups.
- National Health and Nutrition Examination Survey (NHANES): NHANES collects data using examinations, mental health questionnaires, dietary data, analyses of urine and blood, and immunization status from a random sample of Americans (about 10,000 in each 2-year cycle). NHANES also collects some basic demographic and income data. The survey is another source of data on risk factors impacting health status

in the population and particularly among specific age groups and racial/ethnic groups.
- National Survey of Family Growth (NSFG): The NSFG is the primary source of information on marriage and divorce trends, pregnancy, contraceptive use, and fertility behaviors and the ways in which they vary among different groups and over time. Birth and death certificates sent by hospital and funeral homes to state offices of vital events registration provide the raw material for calculating fertility and mortality rates and life expectancy. The data are collected from the states and analyzed by the national Center for Health Statistics.

Decennial Census

For estimates for small subgroups of the population, demographers often used data from the so-called long form of the decennial census, which collected data from one-sixth of all households.

- The census collects a range of economic and demographic information, including incomes and occupations, housing, disability status, and grandparent responsibility for children.
- The census cannot match the detail found in more specialized surveys. For example, only four short questions measure disability for children; surveys designed for precise and complete estimates of disability have dozens of such questions. Since 2004, the American Community Survey replaced the sample data from the census and now provides a more continuous flow of estimates for states, cities, counties, and even towns and rural areas for which estimates were made only once a decade.

National Population Health Survey, Canada

In Canada, the National Population Health Survey has interviewed a panel of respondents every 2 years since 1994 to track changes in health-related behaviors, risk factors, and health outcomes.

Sources: Centers for Disease Control and Prevention. (2019). Health, United States, 2019: The annual report on the nation's health. https://www.cdc.gov/nchs/index.htm; Statistics Canada. (2020). National Population Health Survey. https://www.statcan.gc.ca/eng/survey/household/3225; U.S. Census Bureau. (2019a). About the Current Population Survey. https://www.census.gov/programs-surveys/cps/about.html; U.S. Census Bureau. (2020b). Decennial Census of Population and Housing. https://www.census.gov/programs-surveys/decennial-census.html

Canada, 2017g). In the United States, the most common household type still belongs to married couples without co-resident minor children, which has comprised approximately 30% of households since the 1960s (U.S. Census Bureau, 2020g). However, the proportion of sole occupancy households

in the United States has been steadily increasing for decades (U.S. Census Bureau, 2020c), just like in Canada.

The proportion of United States households containing a married couple has been in steady decline in the United States for the past 70 years.

Table 3-2	Private Household Composition: Canada, 2001–2016			
	2001	**2006**	**2011**	**2016**
Nonfamily households	29.4	30.5	31.7	32.3
One-person household	25.7	26.8	27.6	28.2
Nonfamily household	3.7	3.7	4.1	4.1
Family households	70.6	69.5	68.3	67.7
Couple without children	24.2	25.1	25.5	25.8
Couple with children	31.5	29.9	27.6	26.5
Lone-parent family	8.9	8.9	8.9	8.9
Multigenerational	2.5	2.7	2.7	2.9
Other family	3.4	3.3	3.6	3.6
Average household size	2.6	2.5	2.5	2.4

Sources: Data from Statistics Canada, Censuses of the Population, 2001, 2006, 2011, 2016.

In 1950, almost 80% of U.S. households contained a married couple, but by 2010, the majority of households did not (U.S. Census Bureau, 2020g). Some of the decrease in the past 20 years has been offset by a rise in households containing cohabiting couples, but even taking this into account, the share of U.S. households containing a co-resident couple in a committed relationship has declined.

Until 1980, the number of households containing married couples with minor children outnumbered those of married couples without minor children. Since then, the share of households with a married couple and minor children dropped from 30.9% to 18.4%. Overall, the proportion of households in the United States with minor children has declined from approximately one in three in 2000, to one in four in 2020 (see Table 3-1). Delayed childbearing, declining fertility rates, increases in childlessness, and population aging all contribute to this trend. During this time, the proportion of households with an unmarried parent and minor children increased until it peaked at 9.3% in 2012 and has been decreasing ever since (U.S. Census Bureau, 2020a).

The share of private households in Canada comprised of a couple and no one else is slowly growing, while the share of households containing only a couple and their children is shrinking. These trends are primarily due to the aging of the population, delays in childbearing among young adults, and more couples becoming empty nesters as their children leave home (Statistics Canada, 2017b). If current trends continue, it will not be long before there are more couple-only households without children than couple households with children. Taken together, couple-only households (with or without children) make up a majority but a declining share of private households. This reflects an overall decline in the proportion of adults who are married or cohabiting. Currently, almost four out of five co-resident couples (with or without children) are married, although the proportion of couples who are married continues to decline (Statistics Canada, 2017e).

The proportion of households comprised of lone or single-parent families has remained steady since 2001 at just under 9%, but the proportion of multigenerational households, or households with other family members, some of which contain lone parents, is increasing. While the share of private households in Canada that were multigenerational in 2016 was only 2.9%, this is currently the fastest growing household type and represents the living arrangement for 6.3% of the population living in private households (Statistics Canada, 2017b). In places in Canada where there are large Aboriginal communities, such as Nunavut and the Northwest Territories, or large immigrant populations, such as Ontario and British Columbia, multigenerational households are more common (Statistics Canada, 2019c).

Household size and composition are important because they are crude indicators of the caregiving demands and resources of its members. Nurses are increasingly likely to encounter patients who are living alone and have no one to help them in the home should they become seriously ill.

Living Arrangements of Children

The living arrangements of children have also changed over time, with more children living in diverse households, including with lone parents, stepparents, grandparents, and/or same-sex parents. These living arrangements reflect changes in values, beliefs, and attitudes toward acceptable ways to parent children.

Married and Cohabiting Biological or Adoptive Parent Households

Approximately 73% of children under the age of 15 years in Canada, and 64% of children under the age of 18 years in the United States, are currently living with both biological or adoptive parents, a majority of whom are married (Payne, 2019b; Statistics Canada, 2017j). As families have become more complex, so has the diversity observed in the living arrangements of children, and considerable variation exists along several factors including geographic region, race/ethnicity, socioeconomic status, and religious affiliation (Bohnert et al., 2014; Payne, 2019a; Pew Research Center, 2019; Statistics Canada, 2017b). Asian children are the most likely to be living with their married biological parents (82%), followed by White children (69%), and Hispanic children (57%), while a minority of Black children (32%) currently live in this family structure (Payne, 2019b).

A smaller proportion of children in the United States (4%) are living with both their nonmarried biological parents (Payne, 2019b). Racial/ethnic differences are not as dramatic with this structure, which captures the living arrangements of 4% of Asian and non-Hispanic White children, and up to 6% of Hispanic children.

Snapshots of living arrangements also show variation by the age of children, with younger children most likely to be in families with married or cohabiting biological parents, and the incidence of stepfamilies and lone-parent households increasing with age (Bohnert et al., 2014). This reflects the instability present in the living arrangements of children that change over time as their family circumstances change. While all families are at risk of changing, some family structures have higher risk of instability, with children born into cohabiting or lone-parent households at greater risk of future transitions than those born to married parents.

Same-Sex Parent Households

For same-sex couples, there are four primary pathways to parenthood, which include stepparenting, adoption, the use of ART, or partnering with someone who has followed one of the previous pathways (Moore & Stambolis-Ruhstorfer, 2013). In both Canada and the United States, same-sex couples are less likely to have children living with them compared to opposite-sex couples (12.0% versus 51.4% and 16.1% versus 38.1%, respectively) (Statistics Canada, 2017e; U.S. Census Bureau, 2019d). The sex of the same-sex couple is also associated with the likelihood of having children. North American female same-sex

couples are more likely to have children in their household than male same-sex couples (24% compared to 7.2%, respectively) (U.S. Census Bureau, 2019d). In Canada, among same-sex couples with children, female parent couples are also more likely to have children than male same-sex couples, and they are less likely to be married than male parent couples (49.7% versus 59.8%) (Statistics Canada, 2017e). When considering paths to parenthood, it is estimated that 10% of children raised by same-sex parents are adopted; same-sex couples are six times more likely to foster a child, and they are four times more likely to adopt a child compared to opposite-sex couples. While the most likely path to parenthood for same-sex parents remains adoption or stepparenting, increasing numbers of same-sex parents are seeking surrogates, sperm donors, or technology to provide opportunities to include biological ties to their child. These paths to parenthood increase the complexity as couples negotiate who carries the child, who donates sperm or ovum, and what role sperm donors or surrogate mothers play in the life of the child (Cote & Lavoie, 2009).

Measuring the exact number of children living in same-sex couple homes or in homes with at least one LGBTQ+ parent has been difficult due to the stigma surrounding sexual minorities and a resulting reluctance to participate in research or census studies. Given that challenge, it is estimated that between 2 to 3.7 million children under the age of 18 years have an LGBTQ+ parent, and 200,000 children are being raised by a same-sex couple (U.S. Census Bureau, 2017). In Canada, about 12% of same-sex couples had children living with them compared with 51% of opposite-sex couples. This accounts for 10,020 children from birth to age 14 years living with same-sex parents. Similar to the United States, more male same-sex parents were married compared to female same-sex parents (Statistics Canada, 2016).

Same-sex parents may have concerns about raising children due to the potential for discrimination. Research initially hypothesized that same-sex couples would face the same challenges that other underrepresented families faced when preparing their children for discrimination. LGBTQ+ individuals face higher rates of job discrimination, loss of employment, discrimination by health care providers and other service providers such as police and firefighters, and harassment and threats by others (Oakley et al., 2017). Because of these hardships, many worried that the children of same-sex parents would face similar discrimination. Oakley and colleagues (2017) studied 106 same-sex families (29 gay couples and 27 lesbian couples) and found that the children fared better when their parents included cultural socialization into the LGBTQ+ culture, prepared their children for bias, taught appropriate mistrust of those opposed to LGBTQ+ culture and parenting, and taught egalitarianism and the value of diverse family structures. They found, along with other researchers, that LGBTQ+ couples are more than capable parents, and the children develop and socialize at least as well as comparable opposite-sex parents' children. The authors emphasized that children's outcomes are more dependent on teaching family values than on any one specific family structure (Oakley et al., 2017).

Blended/Stepfamily Households

In Canada, 9.8% of children under the age of 15 years are living in a stepfamily (Statistics Canada, 2017j). However, the most common stepfamily arrangement is a child living with both biological parents and half-siblings (3.6%), followed by a simple stepfamily where a child is living with one biological parent and one stepparent and no half or stepsiblings (3.1%), and complex stepfamilies involving a stepparent and half- or stepsiblings (2.9%). The proportion of children who are living in a stepfamily in the United States is about 9%, with half being in married versus cohabiting stepfamilies (Carlson, 2020).

In contemporary families, stepparents no longer replace biological parents but serve supplemental and somewhat ill-defined roles within the newly formed family (Ganong & Coleman, 2018). As stepfamily structures have become more accepted and more prevalent, research has focused more on understanding stepfamily dynamics and outcomes, negotiations over roles and boundaries, stepfamily dynamics within LGBTQ+ families, and stepfamilies throughout the life course (Ganong & Coleman, 2018). Challenges in demographic research continue, with researchers now having trouble finding large-enough sample sizes, particularly of stepfamilies consisting of racial minorities.

Outcomes for stepfamily members are mixed, yet negative outcomes tend to outweigh positive benefits among reviews of the literature. Sanner, Russell, et al. (2018) found that complex family structures are more likely to experience negative outcomes in parental involvements, conflict, and feelings of family belonging. Furthermore, children within these families are more likely to exhibit antisocial behaviors, drawbacks in educational achievement, increased depressive symptoms, increased family transitions, and detriments to economic well-being. However, stepfamilies may also experience financial benefits and less sibling conflict than biological and full-sibling families (Brown et al., 2015; Sanner, Russell, et al., 2018). These findings may reflect outlying factors such as social class and marital status of parents and the increased emotional distance between halfsiblings and stepsiblings compared to full siblings. In addition, gendered family roles and normative family structures may affect the ability of a stepfamily to form strong relational ties. Within stepfamilies with adult children, the stepmother's role is secondary to the biological mother's role unless the biological mother is deceased (Houdt et al., 2020). Stepfather support does not seem to be affected by the presence of the biological father, and overall stepfathers tended to provide more support than biological fathers. These findings reflect the central importance of the biological mother's role and the more flexible and less child-centered role of fathers, both biological and nonbiological (Houdt et al., 2020).

The most consistent finding among all ages of stepchildren and the timing of repartnership is that the strength of stepfamily functioning and stepfamily relationships is contingent upon the intentional work the family does in defining family roles and relationships during family formation (Coleman et al., 2015; Houdt et al., 2020; Papernow, 2018; Sanner, Coleman, et al., 2018; Sanner, Russell, et al., 2018). If the family works to build relationships between stepparents and stepchildren through support, patience, and respect of biological parent roles and relationships, stepfamilies are more likely to experience closer and longer-lasting bonds, even after dissolution of stepfamily partnerships. Coleman et al. (2015) found that when children consider a stepparent a family member and felt close to the stepparent, the likelihood that the relationship would remain intact after marital dissolution was higher.

Conversely, children were more easily able to walk away from those stepparenting relationships when the sense of connection and closeness were ill-defined or distant. Furthermore, negative disclosures from biological parents toward former stepparents also affect the likelihood of maintained and close relationships between stepparents and children. This holds true for intergenerational stepfamily ties such as between step-grandchildren and step-grandparents. Findings supported other research that shows that the longevity and strength of stepparent relationships with stepchildren or step-grandchildren are highly contingent on the strength of the relationship prior to marital dissolution and on the efforts by biological parents to maintain connections with former step-grandparents (Sanner, Coleman, et al., 2018).

Multigeneration and Skipped-Generation Households

Contemporary grandparenting is complex and varied. Grandparents maintain relationships with grandchildren in a variety of contexts, including nonresidential, residential, custodial, long-distance, and transnational grandparenting (Meyer & Kandic, 2017). Grandparents may reside in the same home as grandchildren within multigenerational households or they may live in skipped-generation households in which a grandparent is the primary caregiver without the presence of either of the grandchild's parents (Casper et al., 2017). Recent research shows that 20% of North Americans live in multigenerational households that include two or more adult generations such as grandparents, their children, and their grandchildren (Cilluffo & Cohn, 2017). Multigenerational households have been on a steady rise since hitting a low of 12% of the population in the United States in 1980 (Cilluffo & Cohn, 2018). In 2011 in Canada, nearly 600,000 grandparents aged 45 years and older lived with their grandchildren, representing 8% of grandparents in this age group (Statistics Canada, 2015). From the child perspective, approximately 7% of Canadians aged 24 years or younger that were living in a census family were living with their grandparents. Most were also living with two parents (62%), but 29% had only one parent in the household and 9% were living with grandparents without either parent present. It is important to note that grandparenting contexts are not static and may change over

time. Co-residential grandparent arrangements may fluctuate, particularly in families with single parents, given that they may enter into a variety of living arrangements throughout the life course (Casper et al., 2017).

Grandparenting contexts frequently vary by socioeconomic class, race, and culture. Multigenerational households are more common among Native American, Indigenous, Asian, and African American families (Casper et al., 2017; Cohn & Passel, 2018; Luo et al., 2012; Statistics Canada, 2019c). However, African American and Native American families are more likely to have grandparent-led or grandparent-maintained families, while Latino and Asian American families are more likely to provide care and support for aging grandparents (Casper et al., 2017). Twenty-nine percent of Asian American families, 27% of Hispanic American families, and 26% of African American families live in multigenerational households compared to 16% of European American families (Cohn & Passel, 2018). African American grandparents are more likely to head skipped-generation households than grandparents of other races (Luo et al., 2012). Immigration status may also contribute to increasing multigenerational household trends, with foreign-born grandparents more likely to live in multigenerational households with their grandchildren than native-born grandparents (Cohn & Passel, 2018; Statistics Canada, 2019d). In the aftermath of the Great Recession of 2007–2009, co-residential grandparent households increased significantly because housing security crumbled for families with children (Casper et al., 2017; Cohn & Passel, 2018).

Consistent with gendered caregiving roles throughout the life course, grandmothers tend to provide more care to grandchildren than grandfathers. Grandmothers tend to outnumber grandfathers in co-residential living arrangements, reflecting the increased mortality rate of men as they age (Casper et al., 2017). A review of the literature finds that grandfathers are as interested in being involved in the lives of their grandchildren, yet they struggle to move out of traditional gendered patterns of care (Stelle et al., 2010). A somewhat contradictory finding by the U.S. Census Bureau shows that grandfathers are more likely to be caregivers for their grandchildren than grandmothers as grandparents age (Roberts & Ogunwole, 2018). More research is needed to understand the dynamics and complexities of grandfather and grandchildren relationships.

Additional characteristics involved in grandparenting arrangements include age of grandparents, number of grandchildren, economic security of grandparents, and additional caregiving responsibilities of grandparents. Younger grandparents who live closer to grandchildren tend to provide more hands-on and frequent care, while older grandparents tend to provide more material support (Casper et al., 2017). Grandparents who maintain households for their grandchildren tend to be younger and employed in the labor force (Casper et al., 2017; Luo et al., 2012). As the number of grandchildren increases, grandparents are more likely to provide some type of grandchild care (Luo et al., 2012).

Grandparents and parents with different levels of financial security have different grandparenting experiences. European American grandparents tend to provide more material assistance and babysitting than ethnic minority grandparents (Luo et al., 2012). As the intensity of grandparent caregiving increases, the financial impact of grandparenting also increases. Poverty rates for African American grandmothers in skipped-generation households tend to be higher (Casper et al., 2017). In addition, as grandparents attend to various caregiving responsibilities outside the grandparent-grandchild relationship, this also changes the dynamics of grandparenting. Grandparents with their own minor children in the household are less likely to provide care to grandchildren (Luo et al., 2012).

Much like research focusing on grandfathering experiences, there is a dearth of literature for LGBTQ+ grandparenting experiences (Stelle et al., 2010). This is an important avenue for further research because sexual orientation or gender identities may affect the relationship that grandchildren have with their grandparents and the ways in which grandparents express their caregiving roles with grandchildren.

The advantages and disadvantages of grandparent-maintained or co-residential grandparenting arrangements are mixed (Casper et al., 2017; Meyer & Kandic, 2017). Grandparents caring for grandchildren allow parents to work in paid employment outside the home while not paying for the increasing costs of outsourced child care, which is of particular importance for low-income families and single parents (Statistics Canada, 2019d). Grandparents also provide a cultural link to past generations, familial history, and cultural knowledge. Meyer and Kandic (2017) found that grandparenting has emotional and physical benefits, with grandparents expressing increased levels of joy in maintaining relationships and caring for their grandchildren as well as increased exercise and better diets to provide good examples for their grandchildren.

The types and intensity of grandparenting responsibilities may determine caregiving outcomes. Grandmothers who provide child care (such as babysitting) for grandchildren report better self-rated health and well-being compared to grandmothers who do not provide babysitting care for their grandchildren (Hughes et al., 2007). More demanding child care and reduced resources, however, were associated with a higher prevalence of negative outcomes for grandparents (Hughes et al., 2007; Meyer & Kandic, 2017). These differing outcomes may demonstrate the strain of poverty and the overall health of grandparents as they take on the tasks of child care rather than inconsistency in the benefits of being an involved grandparent.

As medical professionals interact with a variety of family structures, it is important to recognize the unique living and parenting situation for each family that seeks health care. Parents may intentionally choose for grandparents to be a more integral part of their grandchild's life to secure ties to their culture or generational past. Parents may face challenging financial situations with little choice but to rely on grandparents to provide child care to grandchildren. Parents may also be unable or unwilling to care for their children due to drug addiction, lack of material resources, or transnational living status. In these various situations, medical professionals must consider legal guardianship status, family decision-making procedures, and living arrangements when treating children. When working with older adults, it is important for nurses to gather background information regarding the caregiving tasks and responsibilities of patients, current living arrangements, and the timing of living arrangement transitions to better understand the potential stress, benefits, and access to familial support of older patients.

Single- or Lone-Parent Households

Whereas many lone parents used to be widowed, those are now in the minority, with most lone parents being divorced and a growing proportion being never-married (Bohnert et al., 2014). The retreat from marriage, increases in the financial independence of women, and nonmarital child-bearing have all contributed to an increase in the proportion of children who are living with a single parent. Looking at the proportion of lone-parent households does not adequately convey the prevalence of this living arrangement for children. In 2016, 19.2% of Canadian children under the age of 15 lived with a lone parent (Statistics Canada, 2017j). In the United States, approximately 23% of minor children live in a lone-parent household, the highest rate in the world (Pew Research Center, 2019). This figure varies considerably by race, with almost half of Black children living with a lone parent and approximately one in four Hispanic or multiracial children living in lone-parent families, compared to 11% of Asian children and 16% of non-Hispanic White children (Payne, 2019b). While female-headed lone-parent families receive the most attention, approximately 19% of lone-parent families in Canada and 18% in the United States are headed by males (Statistics Canada, 2017j; U.S. Census Bureau, 2020e).

Foster Care

Approximately 0.5% of Canadian children under the age of 15 years are living in foster care (Statistics Canada, 2017j). In the United States, in 2019, more than 670,000 children (approximately 1%) were served by the foster-care system, representing a slight decline over the previous three years (U.S. Department of Health and Human Services, 2020). The most common placement setting was in a nonrelative foster family (46%), followed by a relative foster family home (32%).

There continues to be an overrepresentation of African American and Native American children in the United States in the child welfare system, with 35% of children in foster care being African American, even though they make up only 15% of the child population, and 2% being Native American, even though they make up only 1% of the child population (National Conference of State Legislatures, 2020). Canada also has an overrepresentation of minority children in foster care. For example, while Aboriginal children represented less than 8% of all children under the age of five years in 2016, they accounted for more than half (51.2%) of all children in this age range living in

foster care, and less than half had at least one foster parent who was Aboriginal (Statistics Canada, 2017k).

Efforts to reduce unnecessary foster-care placements by identifying permanent placements for children in foster care through reunification, guardianship, and adoption contributed to a decline in foster-care entries between 2005 and 2011. However, since 2012, entries into foster care have been increasing. This increase is partially attributable to increases in reported child abuse and neglect related to parental drug use and corresponds with national trends in opioid use (Meinhofer & Angleró-Díaz, 2019). Children raised by relatives is desired over unrelated foster care because several studies report improved childhood outcomes with kinship placement over foster placement. The benefits include increased likelihood of siblings staying together, improved behavioral and mental health, improved permanency with fewer transitions, and improved child well-being. In 2017, 2.5 million children in the United States were being parented by relatives without a biological parent in the home (Epstein, 2017).

Homelessness

In January 2018, point-in-time data collection on homelessness from a single night found that one-third of documented homeless individuals in the United States belonged to a homeless family with children (Henry et al., 2018). Ethnic and racial minorities are overrepresented among homeless families. Approximately three in 10 people in families experiencing homelessness in the United States were Hispanic or Latino Americans, and five in 10 were African Americans. Point-in-time estimates from a single night suggest that overall homelessness among families with children has been declining since 2007; however, in seven states, the number of people in families experiencing homelessness has increased during this time. These figures undoubtedly underestimate the number of families experiencing homelessness. Only 5% of documented homeless people in families with children in the United States report experiencing chronic homelessness, so data collected on one day of the year is missing all the families who experienced homelessness between data collection points. There is also the hidden homeless population; people who live temporarily with others often do not access homeless supports and services and, as a result, are not counted in attempts to document the number of homeless.

The proportion of sheltered homeless people that are children in homeless families is higher in the United States than in Canada. In Canada, only 4.2% of shelter users were children from birth to age 16 years with an adult, whereas 27.6% of sheltered homeless people in the United States were children from birth to age 17 years with an adult (Gaetz et al., 2016; Henry et al., 2018). In addition, Indigenous people are overrepresented among homeless shelter users in Canada, and homelessness among older adults is on the rise in both countries.

Household Transitions and Multiple Households

Snapshots of families and living arrangements of children fail to capture the prevalence of household instability. Approximately 3% of children in the United States experienced a transition in 2017 involving shifting co-residence with a biological or stepparent, and among those 3%, one in three experienced multiple transitions (Scherer & Mayol-García, 2020). Transitions into and out of different types of families, the timing of these transitions, and relationships with family members before and after these transitions have both direct and indirect effects on physical and mental health for parents and children (Fomby & Osborne, 2017; Umberson & Thomeer, 2020).

Demographers noted the divergence between the concepts of family structure and household composition (Smock & Schwartz, 2020). As a result, looking at members of the household, particularly when relationships are defined only in relation to the head of household, never fully captures the complexity of these families. Growing rates of nonmarital fertility, cohabitation, divorce, and remarriage mean children are also increasingly connected to significant others who do not live in the household, including parents, stepparents, half-siblings and stepsiblings. MPF, by definition, creates complex families that span multiple households. Specifically for families living with minor children, approximately one in four involve MPF, where at least one parent (including stepparents and adoptive parents even if they are not biologically related to the co-resident child) has biological children with more than one person (Monte, 2019). In the case of families where a lone parent lives with minor children and does not have a spouse or cohabiting partner in the household, 30.5% have MPF, and 43.6% of families where cohabiting couples live with minor children have MPF (Monte, 2019).

Further complicating our measurement of the living arrangements of children is the increasing phenomenon of children literally belonging to more than one household. Shared custody, where children spend at least 25% of their time with each parent, is now the most common postdivorce custody arrangement in most states (Meyer et al., 2017). This parenting arrangement is no longer related to the age and gender of the child but rather to the income of the households, with higher-income households more likely to divide custody more equally. All shared-custody families are disadvantaged by social policies that recognize only one home for the child in determining eligibility of benefit levels for social programs, and even income taxes force families to decide which household will be able to claim the child as a dependent (Berger & Carlson, 2020).

Living Arrangements of Young Adults

Young adults experience the highest frequency of transitions in living arrangements, and a majority are continuing to live with their parents longer, while some return to the parental home during times of hardship. In both the United States and Canada, just over one-third of young adults (aged 20 to 34 years in Canada and aged 18 to 34 years in the United States) are living with at least one parent (Statistics Canada, 2017g; Vespa, 2017). The rates of co-residence with parents are even higher at younger ages of adulthood. Even prior to the COVID-19 pandemic that has resulted in more families sharing a household (Garcia & Paciorek, 2020), more than 60% of those aged 20 to 24 years in Canada and 18 to 24 years in the United States were living with at least one parent (Fry, 2019). This is believed to be influenced in part by high student loans and high housing costs (Mather et al., 2019). Young adult co-residence with parents is more common among young adults who are males, visible minorities, students, unemployed, and first- and second-generation immigrants (Fry, 2019; Milan, 2016). While there are many benefits to parent–adult child co-residence, returning to the parental home after living independently is associated with worse mental health for both the adult child and the parent that are not associated with the circumstances leading to the transition (Caputo, 2019).

Paradoxically, the share of young adults in Canada ages 20 to 34 years living alone; with roommates; or with other relatives who were not a partner, parent, or child has also increased slightly (20.3% to 23.4%) (Statistics Canada, 2017g). While the share of young adults simultaneously living with a parent and a family of their own (partner, or child, or both) remained relatively steady at 2.5%, the most dramatic change in living arrangements was the decrease in the proportion living with a partner and/ or a child independently from their parents, which dropped from 49.1% to 41.9%.

Living Arrangements of Older Adults

For adults ages 60 years and older in Canada and the United States who live in private households, almost half (47%) lived with only their spouse, 26% lived alone, 19% lived with their children (some of them still minors), and 7% lived in extended family households (Pew Research Center, 2019). There are distinct gender differences among those who live alone. As the population ages, women increasingly outnumber men, reaching a ratio of two females to every male by the time they reach 85 years or older (Roberts & Ogunwole, 2018). In Canada, 33% of women aged 65 years and older live alone, compared to 17.5% of men (Statistics Canada, 2017b). Consequently, for aging women living alone, injuries and accidents may go unnoticed until an informal or formal caregiver checks in on the care recipient, if such a relationship is established. A smaller yet related and significant trend among aging North Americans is what has become known as orphaned elders: older adults with no immediate family close by to provide support. About 3% of older adults are believed to be elder orphans, with a further 21% determined to be at risk (Roofeh et al., 2020).

As they age, older adults have a diminished likelihood of living within a private household because many of them move to institutional (long-term care) settings. Among those aged 65 to 74 years old in the United States, 1.4% lived in group quarters defined as adult correctional facilities, nursing facilities/skilled nursing facilities, or other health care facilities/residential schools for people with disabilities (Roberts & Ogunwole, 2018). The risk for living in a residential or institutional setting increased with age. For those aged 75 to 84 and 85 years and older, 3.2% and 10.6%, respectively, lived in these settings. Even though a majority of older adults lived at home, only 9.8% of the 115 million housing units in the United States are considered "aging-ready" (Vespa et al., 2020).

Family Roles and Responsibilities

Not only have there been dramatic changes in the size and composition of families but there has also been an evolution in the division of work and child-care responsibilities within families. These changes in the roles and responsibilities are partly a direct result of women increasing their participation in the workforce and increases in lone parenting, divorce, and caregiving across family development.

Women's Labor Force Participation and Economic Equality

Women's entry into the labor force has weakened patriarchal control and increased financial independence for women, allowing them more freedom and opportunity to avoid, postpone, or leave marriages (Ruggles, 2015). In both the United States and Canada, there has been considerable convergence in the labor force participation rates for men and women since the 1970s (Drolet et al., 2016; England et al., 2020). This convergence in the United States was mostly due to dramatic increases in women's labor force participation, from 48% to 73%, but also due to declines in men's labor force participation, from 91% to 84%, by 2019, which was driven by lower employment rates among men with a high school diploma or less (England et al., 2020). If only workers aged 25 to 54 years are considered, the gender gap between male and female labor force participation rates in 2015 was smaller in Canada (8.9%) than in the United States (14.4%) (Drolet et al., 2016). In the past 20 years, reductions in the gender gap in the United States have primarily been due to the declining rates of labor force participation among men, while in Canada the reduction is due to more advances in women's labor force participation (Drolet et al., 2016).

Canadian female labor force participation rates lagged behind their American counterparts until

1989, when both countries saw 74% employment among women ages 25 to 54 years, followed by a period of stagnation (Drolet et al., 2016). Explanations for this stall include increases in overtime hours for men, women's marital status, persistent gendered divisions of household labor, and the motherhood penalty for women (Bavel et al., 2018; Budig & England, 2001; Cha & Weeden, 2014). In the late 1990s, the labor force participation rates for women began to increase again in Canada but not in the United States (Daly et al., 2018). Economic analysts believe that greater access to parental leave programs and subsidized child care in Canada explain much of this divergence and that more women in the United States would join the labor force if similar policies and comparable supports were available (Drolet et al., 2016).

Marital status and the presence and ages of children affect women's likelihood of participating in the labor force. The younger the children are in the home, the less likely a mother is to be working. Approximately 66.4% of married mothers with children under the age of six years participate in the labor force, and mothers with children under the age of three years have the lowest labor force participation rates, at 62.2% (U.S. Bureau of Labor Statistics, 2020). In both countries, the younger the children in the home, the less likely the mother is to be working, but Canadian mothers are more likely to be in the labor force than their counterparts in the United States, even among mothers with children under the age of three years (70% versus 62%) (Drolet et al., 2016). Marital status, combined with parental status, is also a factor in female labor force participation. Seventy-two percent of mothers with children under the age of 18 years participated in the labor force in 2019, but only 69% of *married* mothers participated in the labor market (U.S. Bureau of Labor Statistics, 2020). Families with greater economic resources are more likely to be married, so married women with young children may have more opportunities to opt out of the labor market due to increased financial security within the home. In contrast, single-headed households led by women are less likely to have any other source of income other than their earned wages. More than 65% of opposite-sex married couples with minor children in the United States are dual-earner couples, but approximately one in four couples (one in three if children under the age of six years are present)

follow a traditional male single-earner household model, and one out of 25 couples shift from that tradition with only the mother working in the labor force (U.S. Census Bureau, 2020j). Looking at all couples with children under the age of 16 years in Canada, nearly 70% are dual-earner households, one in five are male single-earner households, and about one in 20 are female single-earner households (Uppal, 2015).

Both the United States and Canada continue to fight the gender gap in pay between men and women. Mothers in the United States make .69 for every dollar that fathers make, which means that mothers make an average of $18,000 less per year than fathers for similar jobs. The gap is even higher for women of color (Gurchiek, 2019). The median salary of full-time employed men is 18.5% higher than the median salary of full-time employed women in the United States, and it is 17.6% higher in Canada (Organisation for Economic Co-operation and Development [OECD], 2020). This gap exists even though women have surpassed men in educational attainment in both countries (U.S. Census Bureau, 2020f). While some of this difference can be explained by employment sector segregation and gender discrimination in pay and career advancement (England et al., 2020), penalties associated with motherhood and other family caregiving responsibilities also play a substantial role. Women frequently reduce work hours, take unpaid family leave, bypass promotions, change jobs, or leave the labor force altogether to accommodate childbearing and other caregiving responsibilities, and employer discrimination against mothers is also a factor (Gough & Noonan, 2013). Men are also more likely to work overtime and receive a wage premium for doing so (Cha & Weeden, 2014), something women are often unable to do because of family obligations.

The labor force participation of North American women has recently been dealt a terrible blow by the COVID-19 pandemic. Unlike previous recessions, the pandemic has had a greater impact on the employment of women compared to men, partly because the sectors hardest hit were female-dominated industries but also because a greater proportion of women who lost their jobs dropped out of the labor force and stopped seeking employment compared to men (Desjardins & Freestone, 2021; Landivar et al., 2020). Women with minor children, especially single women, have fared worse than their male counterparts and women without minor children. Many women are dropping out of the labor force or reducing hours in response to additional child-care responsibilities that disproportionately fell to women when in-person schooling and day care closed. Mothers more than fathers took on the burden of distance learning for their children (U.S. Census Bureau, 2020d).

Division of Household Labor

As women have been taking a more active role in the labor force, men have been taking a more active role inside the home. While the distribution of housework and child care has become more egalitarian since the 1970s, full sharing of these tasks has yet to be achieved (Moyser & Burlock, 2018; Perry-Jenkins & Gerstel, 2020; Preisner et al., 2020). According to the 2019 American Time Use Survey, men spend close to 1.5 more hours at work per weekday, on average, than women, and women spend about 1.75 hours more per weekday on household tasks and unpaid care work than men (U.S. Bureau of Labor Statistics, 2019a, 2019b). Despite younger cohorts expressing more positive acceptance of egalitarian gender roles between partners, the vestiges of the traditional gender ideology hold strong in the United States (Bavel et al., 2018).

Sexual underrepresented, transgender, and gender nonbinary parents tend to exhibit more equitable divisions of household labor (Tornello, 2020); however, in heterosexual, cisgender relationships, women continue to spend more time than men doing housework, regardless of employment status (Perry-Jenkins & Gerstel, 2020). Gendered beliefs about housework translate into higher expectations for cleanliness from women, and women are judged more harshly than men when these standards are not met (Thébaud et al., 2019). As such, we observe women spending more time on housework than men even when they live alone (Moyser & Burlock, 2018).

Compared to men, women spend more time multitasking; are more likely to be combining housework and/or child care; and are more likely to experience negative effects, stress, psychological distress, work-family conflict, and family time guilt from multitasking (Offer & Schneider, 2011). While mothers and fathers report greater subjective well-being when engaged in activities with children, compared to without, women report less happiness, more stress, and greater fatigue when engaged in activities with their children than do men (Musick et al., 2016). Overall, what appears to matter most for work and relationship satisfaction, individual well-being, and child adjustment is not the actual division of labor but perceptions of fairness, with women suffering more than men when expectations are not met (Perry-Jenkins & Gerstel, 2020).

Paradoxically, in both the United States and Canada, men and women spend significantly more time on child-care tasks now than in the 1980s, with the gender gap widening slightly as the increase in the amount of time spent by women outpaced the increases by men (Moyser & Burlock, 2018). This coincides with the push toward intensive forms of parenting, particularly intensive mothering, since the mid-1990s in both countries (Hays, 1996). This form of parenting practice requires that mothers spend an intense amount of time, mental energy, and finances on the rearing of children in an effort to provide the best foundation for the future growth and success of children. Increases in time spent in child rearing by U.S. parents began in the mid-1990s, with the increase being twice as large for highly educated parents, and it was driven primarily by increased time spent on school-age children (Ramey & Ramey, 2009). This timing corresponds with a rising wage premium for a college education and increasing competition for placement at good schools in the United States.

Despite increases in time spent with children over the last three decades, over 46% of fathers and 23% of mothers with minor children feel they are not spending enough time with their children (Nomaguchi & Milkie, 2020). In addition, 50% of working fathers and 56% of working mothers say it is difficult for them to balance the responsibilities of their job and their family. This difficulty comes in the form of feeling rushed, not being able to devote as much time as they would like to family life or personal leisure, and experiencing reduced well-being due to multiple demands on their time and energy (Nomaguchi & Milkie, 2020).

Fathers' Roles and Responsibilities

Fathers are increasingly taking on a more prominent role in the lives of their children, from the moment children are conceived to mentoring throughout adult development. While fathers' involvement is not yet on par with the amount of time mothers spend in child rearing, fathers' roles are evolving to be more than just financial providers for their children and increasingly involve the caretaking and nurturing of children (Pew Research Center, 2013a). In the mid-1980s, only one in three Canadian fathers reported providing care for their children, and by 2015 this figure had increased to approximately one in two fathers (Statistics Canada, 2019c). In 2006, Quebec introduced a parental insurance plan that allowed fathers to claim paternal leave from employment upon the birth of their child. Before this plan was introduced, about 27.8% of fathers claimed or intended to claim parental leave. In 2015, almost 86% of fathers either claimed or intended to claim parental leave upon the birth of their child (Statistics Canada, 2017c).

Positive paternal involvement is associated with a number of beneficial outcomes for children, including fewer problem behaviors, better mental and physical health, and enhanced cognition (Allport et al., 2018; Slaughter et al., 2019). However, the extent and nature of father involvement in parenting is strongly influenced by marital status, living arrangements, socioeconomic status, sexual orientation, MPF, and culture (Monte & Knop, 2019; Pew Research Center, 2013a). Alongside increased involvement of fathers, family demographic trends have resulted in more fathers being absent from the home, leading some researchers to describe a "tale of two fathers" to highlight the countervailing trends of fathers becoming more active but also more absent (Livingston & Parker, 2011). Nurses can facilitate paternal involvement by focusing on the mother-father-child triad rather than the mother-child dyad at medical appointments, encouraging father presence during prenatal and child wellness checks when appropriate, engaging with fathers when they are present, encouraging fathers' involvement in childbearing and child care, and facilitating cooperative coparenting (Allport et al., 2018).

DEMOGRAPHIC THEORIES OF CHANGE

Demographers study population-level trends by looking collectively at changes in individual and family behaviors. Demographic theories attempt to explain observed changes at the population level by looking at the broader economic and social contexts that individuals and families are embedded in and identifying similarities across countries that would demonstrate similar trends. The *First Demographic Transition* that was identified was the reduction in fertility and the associated reductions in mortality that accompanied industrialization and modernization. However, this theory could not explain why fertility was dropping below replacement levels in some countries and could not account for other sweeping changes observed in these same countries. The framework of a *Second Demographic Transition* is being used to understand below-replacement-level fertility, delayed marriage and childbearing, the retreat from marriage and higher rates of cohabitation, the increase in nonmarital births, new patterns in living arrangements, and family instability more broadly (Zaidi & Morgan, 2017). According to this framework, economic and cultural changes together explain these shifts in family size and structure. Most recently, musings of a *Third Demographic Transition* characterized by a low-fertility native-born population and a high-fertility racial and ethnic immigrant population are emerging (Lichter & Qian, 2018). This section of the chapter outlines the macro-and exo-level changes over the past 70 years that are shaping the second, and possible third, demographic transition in the United States and Canada. Awareness of the impact of these broader societal factors on families provides insight into current and future challenges for families as Canada and the United States continue to experience changes in work, educational attainment, the economy, gender and family norms, social policy, advancements in technology, and public health crises.

Technological, Economic, and Social Conditions

Economics, employment, and educational achievements influence financial independence and security, time use, and overall well-being, all of which can influence decisions about family structure and transitions, including marriage, divorce, having children, and living arrangements. Dramatic fluctuations in the economic climate over the past 70 years and the changing nature of work have shifted family demographic trends in both Canada and the

United States, and they have exacerbated family inequality, especially in the United States.

Postwar economic growth and prosperity in Canada and the United States provided strong wage growth and low unemployment that was sustained into the 1950s and 1960s (Farley, 1996; Ruggles, 2015). Under these economic conditions, a man with only a high school education could find well-paying, stable employment that allowed him to purchase a home and support a family (Farley, 1996; Ruggles, 2015). Widespread confidence in the ability to support a family contributed to high rates of marriage, marriage at younger ages, and larger family sizes than those observed in subsequent decades (Vanorman & Jacobson, 2020). High demand for workers during this time also facilitated the entry of married women into the labor force and led to a shift from the dominance of the male-breadwinner family to dual-earner families (Ruggles, 2015).

The 1950s, 1960s, and 1970s were a socially turbulent and transformative time in American history, with various movements to reject the status quo and overhaul normative structures. The civil rights movement made progress in dismantling the Jim Crow laws that legalized racial segregation. The gay rights movement that later evolved into the LGBTQ+ movement increased the visibility of sexual minorities and the decriminalization of consensual sodomy. Second-wave feminism, the women's liberation movement, and the sexual revolution emerged, and passionate activists pursued equal rights and opportunities for women as well as greater personal freedom. Popular culture mediated public displays of sexuality through music, magazines, film, and television, challenging societal norms regarding sexual relationships (Schaefer, 2014). More effective birth control options became available, and activists fought for greater access, giving both married and unmarried women more control over their fertility and allowing them to pursue educational and occupational goals without having to sacrifice sexual relationships (Heer & Grossbard-Shechtman, 1981).

In addition to the technology revolution that changed the nature of work and economic prospects, the sexual revolution expanded the acceptance of sexual relations outside marriage, the women's movement loosened the marriage mandate for women and opened opportunities for education and employment outside of the home,

and the youth movement of the 1960s and 1970s disparaged adulthood and promoted a sustained youthful and carefree lifestyle (Arnett, 2014). While earlier cohorts were eager to join the ranks of adulthood and take on those responsibilities, young adults became less eager for this status and freer to explore different possible paths in the years that opened up between childhood and settling down into stable "adult" roles in love and work. This has resulted into a new phase of the life span, between the ages of 18 and 25 years (and sometimes 29 years) that has become known as emerging adulthood. This new developmental time is characterized by instability, identity exploration, self-focus, immense possibilities, and feeling somewhere between adolescence and adulthood. The pathways through this stage are diverse and shaped by gender, sexuality, race, culture, and socioeconomic conditions as well as changing social and economic environments and childhood characteristics determined by the experiences of one's parents (Bea & Yi, 2019; Olmstead, 2020).

During the 1970s and 1980s, the economy began to shift away from manufacturing toward services and technology-based sectors, the influence of labor unions declined, globalization and outsourcing of jobs began to increase, and there was more competition for jobs as the baby boom generation entered into the labor market (Farley, 1996; Ruggles, 2015). These factors contributed to rising inflation and unemployment, and stagnated or decreased wages, especially for less-educated workers. The proportion of American adults age 25 years and older with at least some college education doubled between 1970 and 1990 (U.S. Census Bureau, 2020f). During this time, marriage rates declined, signaling a retreat from marriage. Fewer people were getting married and those who did were doing so at an older age. The median age at first marriage began to increase dramatically, and families became smaller. Ruggles (2015) estimates that about half of the change in marriage rates between 1960 and 2013 can be attributed to a decline in the economic circumstances of young men compared to their fathers and that about half of the observed differences between Black and White men can be explained by race differences in this deterioration.

While the 1990s witnessed a return to a robust economy with economic growth and low inflation and unemployment, the benefits were not experienced equally across all segments of the population (White & Rogers, 2000). Whites, the college educated, women, and dual-earner families experienced the most gains, contributing to increasing family inequality based on race, education, and family structure. This relative security for families changed when the Great Recession, which began in December 2007, led to dramatic increases in the ranks of the unemployed and underemployed (Christiano et al., 2014). Both male and female participation in the labor force was affected by this economic shock. The Great Recession also led to secondary changes in families not directly reflected in employment rates or the amount of money in one's savings account. For example, Cherlin et al. (2013) found that fertility rates declined by around 10% and was more marked in states where unemployment was the highest. The rates of intergenerational co-residence also increased as young people opted to live with their parents for longer periods of time until the economy stabilized (Cherlin et al., 2013). The reduction in divorce rates observed during this time subsequently recovered, but the impact on marriage and cohabitation appears to have followed current long-term trends (Schneider, 2017). The implications of the Great Recession for families and the continued residual effects can be seen today, as well as recent changes in family's economic status due to the COVID-19 pandemic.

The COVID-19 pandemic began to affect family well-being in February 2020 as the world reacted to the rapid spread of this coronavirus. From February to November 2020, the unemployment rate initially surged to 20% in the United States following a massive lockdown of nonessential businesses. Following the reopening of many businesses in June 2020, the unemployment rate has fluctuated between a low of 3.5% in Nebraska to a high of 14% in Hawaii. Families of color and those working for low wages in the service industries have been overrepresented in the unemployment rates, with rates twice as high as White individuals and those working in moderate- to higher-wage positions. This pandemic has caused growing insecurity for families, including 16% of families with children not having enough to eat (this rate is 20% for Black families and 18% for Hispanic families); 14% of families have a reduced income secondary to loss of employment, reduced employment, lost working hours due to having to take care of children out of school or day care, health concerns, and/or unpaid quarantine requirements (Center on Budget and Policy, 2020).

Early data on COVID-19 and marriage rates show a significant decline in marriages during 2020; increased stress in one in three marriages; and, contrary to reports in the popular media, a decline in divorce rates (Wilcox et al., 2020). Approximately one in three women report a change in their plans to have children because of the COVID-19 pandemic, either delaying pregnancy or choosing to have fewer children (Lindberg et al., 2020). This was even more likely among women with lower household income (37%) and women who identified as queer (46%), non-Hispanic Black (44%), or Hispanic (48%). Full understanding of the implications of COVID-19 for families will take decades of research. In addition, the impact of recessions and national and international health crises will continue to emerge in research because these events will continue to influence the timing of family transitions (i.e., marriage, divorce, employment trends, living arrangements, and childbearing). Other changes in our society have threatened the family's ability to obtain employment with wages sufficient to support family members. For example, advancements in technology have eliminated many jobs. From 2016 to 2018, the fastest rate of decline was found in jobs eliminated secondary to automation. This trend is affecting women the most in areas of bookkeeping and retail sales (Stettner, 2019).

More than 150 years of data have demonstrated that access to good-paying jobs has influenced who gets married, the age at which people can afford to get married, and the prevalence of multigenerational households (Ruggles, 2015). The changing nature of work has influenced the types of jobs available and the amount of education needed to obtain stable employment with sufficient income to support a family. Good jobs with decent wages, benefits, and job security have increasingly involved higher levels of education. Pursuing higher levels of education delays entry into the labor market, delays marriage and childbearing, and requires a higher level of individual and family debt due to the expense of higher education in the United States. As higher education has become more necessary and pervasive, it has also become more expensive. Nearly half of recent postsecondary graduates in Canada report student debt, with the median amount varying from less than $15,000 for students completing a two-year degree to $60,300 for professional degree holders (Galarneau & Gibson, 2020). In the United States, close to one in five adults ages 30 to 44 (22%) have outstanding student loans, as do 4% of adults age 45 and older (Cilluffo, 2019). Student debt in both countries continues to burden students for years, extending the economic impact, hampering financial independence, influencing living arrangements, and shaping decisions regarding marriage and family (Velez et al., 2019).

In addition to the significant financial burdens associated with postsecondary education and delayed entry into the labor market, the changing nature of work and multiple economic downturns have made it challenging for young people across the education spectrum to find stable employment that is self-fulfilling and meets their financial aspirations (Cooper & Pugh, 2020). The employment-based private health insurance system in the United States coupled with limited access to public health insurance puts young adults at high risk of not having access to health insurance. In 2010, the Affordable Care Act introduced a parental insurance coverage extension that allowed parents to include their adult children under age 26 years on their health insurance plan. This improved coverage for this age group across racial/ethnic groups, but the benefits were highest for Whites, and racial/ethnic disparities in coverage and access persist (VanGarde et al., 2018).

Overall, reliance on parental resources during emerging adulthood has become common, even for young adults who have achieved some measure of financial independence (Bea & Yea, 2019). This further perpetuates inequalities in young adults based on the financial ability of their parents to help and relationship quality among parents and adult children. Young adults who experience low socioeconomic status (SES) benefit less from direct cash transfers and may rely more on in-kind support such as co-residence and child care than young adults in higher SES families, and young adults who are estranged from their parents for a variety of reasons most often get neither (Fingerman & Yahirun, 2015). Young adults from lower SES backgrounds, immigrants, and racial/ethnic minorities may also be called upon to support their parents or extended family members financially.

Changing Family and Gender Norms and Attitudes

Revolutions prompt changes in behavior, and greater acceptance of these changes in behavior allows more people to change their behavior, shifting attitudes even further and thus creating a feedback loop that plays a critical role in the process of family change (Ruggles, 2015). As an example, the contraceptive revolution in the 1960s provided greater availability of effective birth control options that gave women more control over their fertility, increasing opportunities previously unavailable to most women because of the need to care for large families. Women were able to choose alternatives to child rearing and began to pursue educational attainment and labor force participation (Bahn et al., 2017). As more women furthered their education and participated in the labor force, growing acceptance made it easier for more women to follow this path.

Family Norms and Attitudes

Significant shifts in American attitudes about gender roles, sexual relationships, and family formation and dissolution were observed in the 1960s and 1970s. Negative attitudes toward remaining single or childless declined, and people became more tolerant of premarital sex, abortion, cohabitation, and divorce. Consistent with cultural and ideation shifts in other parts of the Western world, a move away from conformity and an increasing emphasis on personal freedom and self-fulfillment also occurred during this time (Lesthaeighe, 2010; Thornton, 1989). It became acceptable to delay marriage and instead seek personal fulfillment through educational and career aspirations, reserving marriage as a capstone event or rite of passage signaling the achievement of other markers of adulthood (Cherlin, 2009). Among cohabiting partners who are not engaged but want to get married someday, a majority cite their own (56%) or their partner's (53%) financial situation as reasons they are not engaged or married, and 44% give the reason for not being married as not being far enough along in their career (Horowitz et al., 2019). Marriage became more about individual satisfaction, legitimizing the dissolution of unfulfilling marriages that do not meet these expectations. Most Americans believe that divorce is preferable when the marital couple is consistently unhappy and feel that it is better for children than having a conflictual and unhappy parenting relationship model (Taylor et al., 2007). Yet one in four Americans still do not agree that divorce is morally acceptable, with regular church attenders remaining the most morally opposed (Dugan, 2017).

Social acceptance of childbearing out of wedlock has been more gradual because illegitimate births were heavily stigmatized in the past. In post–World War II Canada until the early 1970s, as many as 95% of residents of unwed maternity homes and 74% of unwed women giving birth outside these facilities surrendered their babies for adoption; today only about 2% of babies born out of wedlock are given up for adoption (Standing Senate Committee on Social Affairs, Science and Technology, 2018). Societal pressures against illegitimate children, preference for the rearing of children in homes with two married parents, and the high demand for adopted babies contributed to what has been described as forced adoption practices in Canada during this time, particularly among White women (Andrews, 2018). The stigma against births outside marriage persists but is weakening. In 2015, 66% of Americans felt that more single women having children without a partner was bad for society, but only 48% felt that more unmarried couples raising children was bad for society, suggesting that the greater acceptance of nonmarital births is directed toward births to cohabiting couples and not toward single individuals (Livingston, 2018).

For most Americans, getting married and having a child are no longer important indicators of becoming an adult (Vespa, 2017), and the average age at first marriage and first birth continues to increase. The stratified context of emerging adulthood has increased the diversity in family formation pathways, but a few trends are pervasive. With regard to parental status, becoming a parent during emerging adulthood is becoming more concentrated among individuals with lower levels of education and racial/ethnic minorities (Martin et al., 2019), and nonmarital pregnancy is more likely to lead to cohabitation than to marriage (Sassler & Lichter, 2020). Recent studies indicate that, as cohabitation has become more prevalent, its association with marriage has diminished, particularly among those with less education (Sassler & Lichter, 2020). Approximately two-thirds of Americans view cohabitation as a step

toward marriage, but this is more common among those with a bachelor's degree (50%) compared to those with a high school degree or less (28%) (Horowitz et al., 2019). In Canada, cohabitation is increasingly becoming an alternative to marriage rather than a stepping-stone (Wright, 2019).

Before same-sex marriages became legal across all parts of the United States and Canada, most same-sex couples lived in common-law or cohabiting relationships, and many hid their status from the public view. As attitude shifts grew with greater acceptance of same-sex couples and a growing desire for same-sex couples to afford the same benefits as married couples, many same-sex couples traveled to locations that provided legal same-sex marriages. Marriage outside the couples' state or province was often in name only, as the location in which they lived more often did not recognize these unions. These actions and the long-fought advocacy to change the laws that prevented these couples from entering into a formal and legal marital relationship demonstrate the importance of the institution of marriage and the personal meaning attached to it by couples and society at large.

Despite legal recognition and the growing numbers of same-sex marriages, many Canadians and those living in the United States still hold negative views of same-sex marriage. Recent public opinion polls have estimated that 10% of Canadians and 28% of those living in the United States oppose the right of same-sex couples to marry (Canseco, 2019; Public Religion Research Institute [PRRI], 2020). Renewed attacks by two Supreme Court justices on the court's same-sex marriage ruling, coupled with changes to the membership of the U.S. Supreme Court in late 2020, are also promoting anxiety among members of the LGBTQ+ community, who fear that their right to marriage could be in jeopardy.

Gender Norms and Attitudes

Gender norms are socially constructed expectations for acceptable and appropriate behavior based on biological sex that are embedded in both formal and informal institutions and reproduced through social interactions (Cislaghi & Heise, 2019). Americans became more egalitarian in their attitudes toward sex roles in the 1960s and 1970s, and this trend continued into the 1980s, but progress slowed in the 1990s (Scarborough et al., 2018; Thornton, 1989). Support for women's labor force participation, even among mothers, continued to expand, but further progress regarding equality in the home did not (Scarborough et al., 2018). A cultural logic of egalitarian essentialism emerged that embraced gender equality outside the home, but it retained essentialized notions of motherhood, requiring women to maintain the traditional role of primary caregiver regardless of their responsibilities outside the home.

Gendered expectations for work and family responsibilities influence decisions about family because they create different costs and rewards for different family relationships based on gender. Expectations of caregiving for women affect their academic and career opportunities. Differences in life expectancy and health in later life coupled with gendered expectations for caregiving influence older women's decisions about repartnering in later life, with many women choosing to remain single or opting for Living Apart Together (LAT) relationships. Conventional research on couples has focused on co-residential unions; however, a growing body of research is investigating couples who do not live together as a new family form. For older adults, LAT relationships are stable alternatives to living with a partner and are more common than cohabitation in this age group (Brown & Wright, 2017; Connidis et al., 2017).

North American society is just beginning to recognize individuals who are transgender or who are gender nonbinary, either because they choose not to identify as male or female or because they view their gender as fluid and constantly changing. In Canada, approximately 75,000 people identify as gender diverse or transgender (Jaffray, 2020). Meerwijk and Sevelius (2017) estimate that there are approximately 1 million transgender adults in the United States. Transgender people and gender minorities experience higher rates of nonintimate partner violence due to their gender identity than cisgender people, and they report higher levels of suicidal ideation and diagnosis related to mood disorders than cisgender people (Jaffray, 2020). However, relatively little is known about families of nonbinary gender persons.

McGuire et al. (2016) reviewed multiple theoretical and empirical studies about transgender family dynamics and found that these families must navigate the challenges associated with gender socialization both within and outside the family in larger social institutions. This requires family members to navigate new identity nomenclature and decision making regarding gendered practices such as housework, sexual interactions, and child-rearing practices. Family members may elect to "do gender" in some spaces while "undoing gender" within the intimacy of trusted family relationships (McGuire et al., 2016). These families may experience significant transitions and challenges, but they may also be able to develop important skills and resiliency in the face of such challenges.

A barrier to research on couples and families with members who identify as gender nonbinary, gender fluid, gender neutral, transgender, or other gender identities is that most data sources do not ask questions to identify these individuals in the data. Gender identity conversations have occurred fairly recently on a large scale in social-political discourse in the United States, and nomenclature and feelings of safety for those being surveyed is still a primary question in its formative stages (Holzberg et al., 2018). Sexual orientation and gender identity (SOGI) survey questions must cover a wide array of identities and distinctions, and the language used must be readily understandable by this heterogenous group (Holzberg et al., 2018). In addition, due to the sensitive nature of this data, people may be unwilling to share it with census workers. The Canadian census approved use of the terms gender diverse (D), cisgender (C), and transgender (T) in January 2018, and they will be implemented in the 2021 Census (Statistics Canada, 2018).

Social Policies

Institutions reflect the status quo in society and provide opportunities and constraints that shape behavior accordingly. As has been discussed, various factors can affect the ability of individuals to abide by the status quo, and new behaviors can emerge as individuals adapt to these circumstances. Early adopters of behaviors typically experience a difficult path because they are often stigmatized and denied various rights and protections when their behaviors are not sanctioned by society. However, societal attitudes gradually shift over time in response to new family behaviors, and these changes in attitudes can eventually lead to institutional changes (Ruggles, 2015). Examples of this include the reduction of legal barriers to divorce with the implementation of no-fault divorce laws, the legalization of abortion and increased access to contraception, and the legalization of same-sex marriage. As institutions change to reduce barriers and become more accommodating or supportive of family diversity, more individuals adopt the behaviors (Ruggles, 2015).

Family policies by design affect family behaviors. However, other types of social policies, while not explicitly intending to do so, create opportunities and constraints that result in unintended consequences for families and frequently exacerbate existing social inequalities (Berger & Carlson, 2020). For example, systemic racism and social policies contributed to mass incarceration that disproportionately affected Black men in the United States, and mass incarceration contributed to higher rates of noncustodial parenthood and MPF among Black families (Sykes & Pettit, 2014). The public health impact of incarceration also extends beyond the incarcerated and has been linked to negative health effects for female partners and children of incarcerated men (Wildeman & Wang, 2017).

Social policies surrounding the economic health of individuals and families, and policies made during times of economic downturn, including wars, diseases, crime, and business and political challenges, have an impact on family well-being. The social influence trickles across systems to affect individual families, including the decision to move, work, marry, divorce, have children, spend time with career pressures or family needs, and continue to change attitudes that allow and support diversity.

Other Demographic Trends

Concurrent with sweeping technological, economic, social, cultural, and policy changes were two other demographic trends that are shaping the Canadian and American families and the population as a whole. These changes include life expectancy and immigration and related racial and ethnic diversity.

Life Expectancy

Life expectancy is an estimate of the number of years a person can expect to live based on the mortality rates for a specific population. Active life expectancy, also known as health expectancy, is an estimate of the number of years a person can

expect to live disability free, but what is meant by *disability free* depends on how it is calculated (Saito et al., 2014). These two indicators, life expectancy and active life expectancy, have important implications for families because longer and healthier lives mean more opportunities for vertical family relationships and the postponement of disability-related care needs.

The overall trend has been an increase in life expectancy over time. In 1948, the United States and Canada had similar life expectancies (67.25 and 67.27 years, respectively), and while both countries have experienced a relatively steady increase since then, the gains have been greater in Canada. As of 2020, the national life expectancy for males in Canada was 80 years, compared to 76 years in the United States (Statista, 2021). Researchers attribute these trends of increasing life expectancy to advances in preventative medicine. Increases in the use of vaccinations; decreases in infectious diseases; delays in cardiovascular deaths; and widespread adoption of preventative health programs such as smoking cessation, alcohol reduction, and the promotion of physical activity have contributed to delayed mortality (Klenk et al., 2016). The diverging life expectancies of the United States and Canada are largely explained by higher levels of obesity in the United States, and in Canada, universal access to health care and lower levels of social and economic inequality, especially among older adults. Obesity has been rising steadily in the United States for decades, with estimates from 2015 to 2016 categorizing nearly 40% of adults as obese (National Center for Health Statistics [NCHS], 2019). Canadian rates of obesity have remained relatively stable at around 27.25% since 2015–2016 (Statistics Canada, 2019b).

These national trends obscure significant socioeconomic, gender, and racial disparities in life expectancy in both countries. In Canada and the United States, education and income are both positively associated with longer life expectancy and health-adjusted life expectancy, and research suggests that the disparities across education and income groups are growing (Bushnik et al., 2020; Montez et al., 2019). Education and differences in life expectancy are also prominent in the United States (Montez et al., 2019).

Gender differences in life expectancy are a nearly universal phenomenon around the world, and women's life expectancy has exceeded men's in the United States and Canada for more than a century. Figure 3-4 shows life expectancy in the United States and Canada in 2017. In Canada, women have a four-year advantage in life expectancy over men. In the United States, the female advantage is slightly larger and varies by race, with non-Hispanic Black females having a 6.6-year advantage over their male counterparts, non-Hispanic White females having a 4.9-year advantage, and Hispanic females having a 5.2-year advantage. Notable racial differences in life expectancy also exist in Canada, where the nonindigenous population has a ten-year advantage in life expectancy over First Nations and Inuit populations, and a five-year advantage over Metis populations (Tjepkema et al., 2019).

This gender difference in life expectancy has important implications for families. The U.S. Census Bureau projects that the sex ratio in 2020 will be 84 men for every 100 women among 65- to 84-year-olds, and 56 men for every 100 women among those 85 years and older (Mather et al., 2019). This means that older women are more likely to be widowed, live alone in later years, and have fewer prospects for remarriage than older men. Older women are also less likely to have a spouse caregiver available to support them in later years. Not having a spouse, living alone, and living

longer also contributes to higher levels of poverty among older women.

A concerning trend in both Canada and the United States is the recent stagnation, and in some cases declines, in life expectancy. The primary cause of this trend is the increase in accidental deaths related to drug overdose (Statistics Canada, 2019f; Woolf & Schoomaker, 2019). Opioid overdose deaths were six times higher in 2017 than in 1999 (Kochanek et al., 2017; Hedegaard et al., 2017). Since the 1990s, drug overdose deaths have been rising. Deaths related to drug overdoses rose at a rate of 3.2% annually from 2007 to 2014 and accelerated to an average of 15.5% per year from 2014 to 2017 (National Center for Health Statistics, 2019). In 2018, deaths from overdose declined for the first time in 28 years in the United States (Hedegaard et al., 2020), but it is too early to tell if this is the beginning of a new trend or not.

Together with improvements in life expectancy have come improvements in the disability rates at older ages, so that North Americans are not only living longer than in the past but also enjoying more years of life without chronic illness or disabilities. However, recent trends related to obesity and other lifestyle health behaviors are contributing to a reversal of this trend among some populations. Census data indicates that 69% of aging Americans suffer some type of disability, compared to less than 9% of those under the age of 65 (Roberts & Ogunwole, 2018). The leading cause of disability in those over the age of 65 years is related to ambulatory challenges, followed by hearing and cognitive disabilities. For those aged 85 years and older, cognitive limitations, the ability to care for oneself, and inability to live independently are significant challenges.

Longer life expectancy brings opportunities for extended family relationships. In the early 20th century, less than a quarter of infants had four grandparents alive (Casper et al., 2017). As medical technology and preventative health care has advanced, North Americans are living longer and healthier lives, which has increased opportunities for grandparents to have intact and robust relationships with their grandchildren. By 2030, demographers estimate that close to 70% of 8-year-olds will have at least one living great-grandparent (AARP, 2019). In 2017, there were over 7.5 million grandparents aged 45 years and older in Canada, the highest number recorded since the inception of

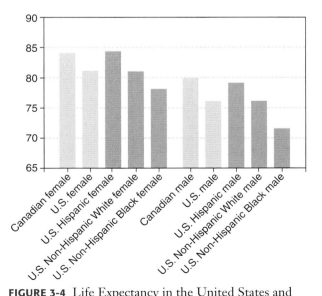

FIGURE 3-4 Life Expectancy in the United States and Canada by Sex, and by Sex and Race in the United States Only, 2017 *Sources: Data from United States Life Tables, 2017, National Vital Statistics Reports; Statistics Canada, Life Tables, 2016/2018.*

the General Social Survey (Statistics Canada, 2019c). Furthermore, the average age of grandparents has increased by three years since 1995, with most grandparents becoming first-time grandparents at age 50 years (AARP, 2019; Statistics Canada, 2019c).

Longer life expectancy coupled with lower replacement-level fertility results in an aging population. In 2016, roughly 15% of the U.S. population were aged 65 years or older, while in Canada, this number is closer to 18%, and both countries are projected to continue aging (Roberts & Ogunwole, 2018; Statistics Canada, 2019d). By 2030, one in five Americans will be over the age of 65 years, older adults will outnumber children, and the United States will shift from a youth-dependent population to an aged-dependent population (Vespa et al., 2017).

Immigration and Racial/Ethnic Diversity

Immigration policies shape families by influencing the size and characteristics of the immigrant population. Approximately 22% of the Canadian population and 14% of the U.S. population are foreign born (Budiman, 2020; Statistics Canada, 2017d). Despite political rhetoric, most of the immigrant population in the United States is in the country legally (77%), representing about 3% of the total U.S. population (Budiman, 2020), and the number has been declining since 2005 (Passel & Cohn, 2019). In the United States, one of the results of the Immigration and Nationality Act of 1965 has been immigration dominated by family reunification, which is relatively unique among Western countries (Cohn, 2015), and different than Canada, where only one in four immigrants are sponsored by families (Statistics Canada, 2017d).

Some of Canada's immigration policies, such as the foreign domestic worker program, favor lone female migrants, causing sex-ratio imbalances among immigrant populations that, when coupled with interracial marriage patterns, have contributed to the rise in lone-parent Black families in Canada (Livingstone & Weinfeld, 2015). It is important to note that the composition and experience of Black Canadians is very different from that of Black Americans, so assumptions about Black Canadians based on their American counterparts should be avoided. Despite being the third largest visible minority in Canada (Statistics Canada,

2017d), Black Canadians make up a much smaller portion of the population (only 2.5%). More than half are recent immigrants or first generation; most have Caribbean roots, though a growing minority are from Africa; and most have not had to contend with the same domestic legacy of slavery as African Americans (Livingstone & Weinfeld, 2015).

In addition to immigration being a primary driver of population growth (Cilluffo & Cohn, 2017; Statistics Canada, 2020a), first- and second-generation immigrants tend to be younger and have higher levels of fertility, significantly influencing natural increase. As a result, racially diverse families make up larger percentages of the population than ever before and continue to grow. Around 22% of Canada's population is comprised of visible minorities (up from 4.7% in 1981), mostly South Asian or Chinese, and only 30% are Canadian born (Statistics Canada, 2017d). If current trends continue, one in three Canadians will be a visible minority by 2036 (Statistics Canada, 2017f). The United States is more racially diverse than Canada. Approximately 72% of the U.S. population is non-Hispanic White, 13% is non-Hispanic Black, 18% is Latino/Hispanic (any race), 6% is of Asian descent, and less than 5% are other races or identify as multiracial (U.S. Census Bureau, 2019e). It is projected that, by 2045, most of the population will no longer be non-Hispanic White (U.S. Census Bureau, 2019b). Thus, multicultural awareness and cultural sensitivity will be increasingly important for nurses (Sharifi et al., 2019).

The very act of immigrating physically separates and reunites families. Immigration can have a disruptive or solidifying impact on immigrants and their families as they contend with new socioeconomic circumstances; cultural and language differences; and discrimination based on nativity or other related factors such as race, language, or religion (Livingstone & Weinfeld, 2015; Van Hook & Glick, 2020). Language and cultural barriers are stressful and can alter the roles of immigrant family members. Children of foreign-born parents must often act as language and cultural brokers for their parents (Berger Cardoso et al., 2018). In recent decades, anti-immigration rhetoric and laws have negatively affected the health of both citizen and noncitizen Latinx populations in the United States (Vargas et al., 2017). Undocumented families and mixed-citizenship-status families also experience fear of deportation and family separation, and face additional vulnerabilities in parenting their children (Berger Cardoso et al., 2018).

Whether citizens or immigrants, cultural factors as well as systemic racism and discrimination can have a significant impact on the day-to-day lives of minority families. More than three-quarters of Black and Asian Americans say that they have experienced some form of discrimination or unfair treatment due to their race or ethnic identity, and those with darker skin tones are at greater risk than those with lighter skin tones (Horowitz et al., 2019). Experiences of discrimination and unfair treatment can have profound influences on the ways that marginalized minority parents raise their children and interact with the health care system. Nomaguchi and Milkie (2020) found that Black mothers experienced more parenting strain of their school-age children than White mothers, and as their children grow, they must have more conversations with their children regarding discrimination and racial profiling by the various social institutions in which they interact. Immigrant and minority parents also express more aggravation in parenting than U.S.-born non-Hispanic White parents (Yu & Singh, 2012), likely reflecting the additional stressors and hardships these families experience.

Implicit racial/ethnic bias and discrimination in health care are well documented (Hall et al., 2015). In addition to affecting outcomes due to treatment within the health care system, these interactions can increase the likelihood that minorities will distrust medical authorities and forgo or delay medical treatment for themselves and their children. As medical professionals engage with racially and ethnically diverse families, they must consider potential language or cultural barriers, and the vulnerability of different citizenship statuses. Nurses may need to collaborate with important family members to provide translation of services and treatment and to understand that children in the translator role may not know translations for advanced medical terminology. Health care providers need to be aware of their internal racial biases through intentional and focused reflection on their own early socialization experiences regarding racial and ethnic differences, and medical institutions should be prepared to provide the training needed for such reflections.

WHY DEMOGRAPHY MATTERS AND IMPLICATIONS FOR NURSES

Family demography takes a systemic view of family life, highlighting significant changes in family formation, dissolution, and functioning that have produced the varied and complex forms of contemporary families. Demographic theories link these changes to evolving technological, economic, social, and cultural conditions that alter family structures and the differing risks and rewards associated with them over time. As the composition of families and the contexts surrounding them change, an understanding of these relationships provides clues to how these changes will affect the composition of families in the future and how family inequality may be alleviated or exacerbated as a result.

Demography Highlights Family Diversity and Complexity

As the demographic statistics in this chapter highlight, families are becoming increasingly complex and diverse. Health care providers should take a holistic approach to understanding the family structures of the families that they work with. For example, Houdt et al. (2020) suggested that the best way to understand stepfamily dynamics is to glean the perspectives of both the parents and children involved in stepfamily and complex family situations. Asking the question of who has legal guardianship and authorization rights is becoming more and more important, and past norms cannot be assumed. Asking follow-up questions, such as, "Is there a parent or set of parents that the children demonstrate having stronger relationships?" can help guide treatment plans. Due to the likelihood of several health care providers being involved with some parts of families across households, it is important to ask who family members trust with important medical and health care information. Seltzer (2019) also suggests that researchers and family practitioners understand that family members and important family relationships may not all live and be within the same household; conversely, co-residential family members may not have deep and meaningful relationships, and fragile family relationships can, and sometimes frequently do, lead to family structure changes throughout the life course.

Demography Gives Clues to Current Risks and Resources Available to Different Families

Notable differences in the level of formal and informal support and sanctioning of different types of families exist, including differences in social acceptance, institutional supports, economic risks and resources, and the availability of informal caregivers.

Social Stigma and Institutional Supports

Non-normative family structures often face social stigma and lack institutional supports, which can have negative effects on families. As certain family forms become more common and accepted, social stigma is reduced, and institutions adapt by building in supports and accommodations, weakening the harmful effects associated with these structures over time. For example, studies of the impact of being socially rejected have emerged over the past two decades, since the first legalized marriage of same-sex partners in Massachusetts in 2004 and legal union in Vermont in 2000. Health disparities were well documented in LGBTQ+ individuals before this time, including physical health risks from decreased preventive care, decreased access to health care, and provider biases, to increased mental health concerns, including higher rates of depression and suicide and substance abuse. Following the passing of laws to legalize same-sex marriages, couples have reported improved health in a number of studies. The improvement stems from increased access to health insurance, decreased split between authentic self and false self from hiding sexual orientation, increased hope, increased empowerment, decreased depression and suicide rates, decreased substance abuse, and improved family ties following legal marriage (Tuller, 2017). Research is continuing as national data follow trends across time and compare same-sex couples that marry versus those that stay single or in a cohabiting relationship. Of interest is that research on the rate of dissolution of same-sex marriages is unfolding, and early studies indicate that same-sex marriages are less likely than opposite-sex marriages to end in divorce (Miller, 2013). However, if homonormativity increases social pressure for same-sex relationships to mimic heterosexual relationships and get married, future same-sex couples may not be as committed as early adopters, and the advantage in marital stability originally observed may erode over time.

Institutions often lag behind social behaviors and attitudes, reinforcing the status quo by penalizing some family structures and privileging others. Despite similar trends in cohabitation in Canada and the United States, the implications of these trends are very different between these two countries because of differences in the rights and obligations afforded to unmarried partners (LaPlante & Fostik, 2016). The Supreme Court of Canada ruled in January 2013 that provinces and territories have the right to determine if common-law couples have the same rights and obligations as married couples, such as the separation of assets upon dissolution of the relationship and spousal support if warranted. In all provinces and territories, except Quebec, common-law marriages have the potential to be equivalent to legal marriages (LaPlante & Fostik, 2016). This is very different in the United States, where no such ruling by the Supreme Court exists, and individual states have very different laws regarding common-law unions. Even though two-thirds of Americans feel that cohabiting couples should experience the same rights to health insurance and tax benefits as married couples (Horowitz et al., 2019), rights such as these are not protected by laws and policies the way they are in Canada.

Across the federal government of Canada, the standard definition of a common-law relationship is continuous cohabitation for at least one year in a conjugal relationship between adults over 18 years of age. However, considerable variability exists across provinces and territories. In some provinces (such as British Columbia and Alberta), common-law couples that live together for a specified period of time (two to three years) or have a child and live together (Alberta) automatically have the same rights and responsibilities as married couples, and in other provinces (such as Manitoba and Nova Scotia), the couple has to register their relationship in order to take advantage of some privileges. Quebec, in contrast, specifies that married partners and unmarried partners receive equal treatment by the state and third parties, and children are treated the same regardless of whether their parents are married. If the couple is unmarried and without children, the individuals can keep their property separate and are not entitled to support payments (LaPlante & Fostik, 2016).

Cohabitating households can pose unique challenges for health care providers, especially in the United States. Because cohabitating relationships are not legally sanctioned in most states, partners must be careful to have medical power of attorney granted to their partners and sign consent forms to share medical information if desired. Updated wills are also necessary if the cohabitating partner is to retain any of the couple's assets or custody of children if a partner were to die (Erskine, 2021; Manning, 2015).

Economic Risks and Resources

Demography matters because different family structures experience different economic risks and resources. Women still have not achieved economic parity with men, so female-headed households are at greater risk of poverty than male-headed households, and dual-earner households are at the lowest risk of poverty. Women's lower participation in the labor force and lower lifetime earnings, coupled with longer life expectancy, increase the risk that women will be living alone and in poverty in old age.

Poverty and family structure are highly correlated with race in the United States. White families with children experienced poverty rates of 11% in 2017, compared with 33.1% for African American/Black, 26.3% for Hispanic/Latino, 25.4% Native Hawaiian/Pacific Islander, 32.7% Native American/Alaska Native, and 10.8% for Asian families with children (Kids Data Center, 2020a). These numbers increase greatly for single-mother households: 24% of non-Hispanic White single-mother households live in poverty, compared with 65% of African American/Black, 41% of Hispanic/Latino, 53% of Native American, and 15% of Asian/Pacific Islander (Kids Count Data Center, 2020b).

In Canada, one in five children live in poverty (Canada Without Poverty, 2021). Canadian lone-parent families with children younger than 18 years are much more likely to have low incomes and thus are more likely to be poor. Among children living in female lone-parent families, 21% were low income, whereas 7% of children lived in poverty if their lone parent was their father. One in two Status First Nations children lives in poverty. Overall, one in seven children lived in poverty in the United States in 2018, which is higher than most developed nations. A majority of these children come from working families. Even more alarming is that the youngest children are at the highest risk for living in poverty. This is the time important brain development is occurring, which has been shown to be negatively affected by poverty (Children's Defense Fund, 2019; Children International, 2020). More alarming, 40% of children in the United States will spend at least one year living in poverty. The risk for poverty is well-documented, leading to increased preventable health issues; food insecurity with related physical and mental health problems; being a victim to violence, crime, and drugs; and being at risk for dropping out of high school (Children International, 2020).

Overall, current demographic trends suggest a continuing trend of diverging destinies, where more affluent families experience cumulative advantages, and families with low levels of education and economic resources experience cumulative disadvantages. These trends extend across generations, constraining economic mobility and reinforcing the intergenerational transmission of poverty and privilege (Lerman et al., 2017). Cavanagh and Fomby (2019) suggest a growing trifurcation of families, with education as a primary factor in determining advantage. The "truly advantaged" are overwhelmingly the highly educated, who delay marriage and childbearing; are less likely to have nonmarital relationships and MPF; and are more likely to get married, stay married, and raise their children in marriage. The "truly disadvantaged" are predominantly the least educated, many without even a high school degree, who experience childbearing and raising children outside of marriage or cohabiting unions. The "moderately advantaged" are largely those with a high school degree or some college who are not as economically advantaged as earlier generations with the same level of education; they demonstrate the most heterogeneity, trying to maintain standard family forms in cohabitation if not in marriage, but they experience more family instability. However, this typology neglects significant gender and racial/ethnic differences that are also a reflection of systemic sexism and racism that provide different opportunities and constraints for people of different genders and races.

Both Canada and the United States have tried to fight poverty with a variety of social programs to increase employment, provide subsidies for food and shelter, and increase awareness of racial and gender inequalities. Chapter 4 goes into more detail on the attempts through social policies to decrease poverty in families. Nurses are encouraged to be aware of family income levels, family structure, and community and federal resources that can help families living in poverty.

Caregiving

Demography provides insight into the pool of potential caregivers for dependent family members as well as the populations at greatest risk of unmet needs. As the baby boomer generation reaches the ages of 65 years and older, caregiving support will be more important than ever. The U.S. Census Bureau (2019e) estimates that by 2034, there will be 77 million people aged 65 years or older, and only 76.5 million under the age of 18 years. This will mark the first time in U.S. history that older people will outnumber children. This will affect families on a large scale considering the current dependency ratio within North America. A dependency ratio is the combined size of dependent populations (those under the age of 15 years and those 65 years and older) compared to the size of the population between 16 and 64 years old (Rogers & Wilder, 2020). In 2019, the dependency ratio was 53.7, meaning that for every 100 working-age people, there were almost 54 dependent-age people in the United States. In other words, more than half of the U.S. population is dependent on the remaining 46% of the population. By the time all baby boomers reach age 65 years, which is estimated to happen in 2030, this dependency ratio could climb to between 65% and 75%, indicating that two-thirds to three-quarters of the U.S. population would be dependent on the remaining one-third to one-quarter of Americans. In Canada, trends are similar. Those over the age of 65 years have outnumbered children in Canada since 2015. Older Canadians account for 18% of the population, while youth account for 15.9% of the population (Statistics Canada, 2020a). In short, caregiving responsibilities will shift dramatically over the next several decades.

Home health care services were the most-used long-term care service in 2015 to 2016, while hospice services are the next most commonly used for adults aged 65 years and older (NCHS, 2019). About 25% of the home health patients and 16.3% of adult day services users were aged

85 years and older (NCHS, 2019). Expenditures related to medical care for aging populations are significant. The average cost of a nursing home is $290 per day, or $8,821 per month, and unaffordable for the majority of families in the United States (Genworth, 2021). Almost one-third of aging families cannot afford a nursing home for even one year (West et al., 2014). This leaves many families relying on unpaid care from family members and friends.

As previously outlined, the cost associated with providing care for aging populations is expensive, ranging from a national average of $570 monthly for an in-home health aide to $6,870 monthly for a room in a private nursing care facility, making paid care out of reach for most aging families (West et al., 2014). Canada's government provides some financial support to families who provide care, in the form of federal tax credits or other governmental programs, yet only 14% of those who provided care for aging spouses or parents received this type of financial assistance (Hango, 2020). Many North Americans must rely on private insurance, public health insurance options, purchased long-term care insurance, or a combination of these to afford long-term care expenses. A majority (89%) of those aged 50 and older prefer to remain at home as long as possible compared to residing in an assisted living or long-term care facility (AARP Public Policy Institute, 2009).

To fill the gap between paid, formal care are informal, unpaid caregivers. Informal caregivers are comprised of spouses, adult children, other family members, and friends who provide support and care to aging members of society. Caregiving tasks can range from providing day-to-day socialization outlets for seniors to more intense medical-related tasks. These tasks can take significant amounts of time and energy on the part of the caregiver (Polenick et al., 2017). In 2020, 21.3% of Americans (53 million) served as caregivers to dependent adults or dependent children with special needs (AARP, 2020a). In Canada, about 30% of its 7.8 million caregivers expressed a desire for additional support, particularly financial support from the Canadian government, to continue their work as informal care providers (Hango, 2020). Researchers have found that unmet caregiving support needs were higher for women aged 35 to 65 years, reflecting the social norm that women are more likely to serve in caregiving roles than men, and this age group is more representative in caring for both children and aging parents simultaneously (Hango, 2020). In 2016, the National Academies of Sciences, Engineering, and Medicine found that women spend an average of 6.1 years (almost 10% of their adult lives), providing care to others compared to men, at 4.1 years (7%). In same-sex relationships, both men and women seem to be more equitable and cooperative in providing supporting to aging family members (Reczek & Umberson, 2016).

The emotional and physical burden of this unpaid caregiving support weighs heavily on caregivers, which can affect their physical health over time (National Academies of Sciences, Engineering, and Medicine, 2016). One-quarter to one-third of caregivers with unmet caregiving needs (such as emotional, physical, and financial support) reported being dissatisfied with life, that their days were moderately to extremely stressful, or that they have fair to poor mental health (Hango, 2020). In addition, the role of caregiver can have collateral effects on marriages and relationships. Penning and Wu (2019) found that the psychosocial costs of caregiving can have a destabilizing effect on marriages, particularly if the caregiver is female and provided care before the age of 45 years. However, caregivers who received some kind of support reported lower occurrences of this same type of stress or dissatisfaction with life; thus, it is not caregiving in itself that leads to caregiving stress or burden but caregiving coupled with lack of support (emotional, physical, or financial) (Hango, 2020).

Caregiving is not relegated only to those of the working-age population. Older adults provide care to their spouses, peers, and even their own elders. Carr and Utz (2020) found that people aged 75 years and older are one of the most rapidly growing groups of caregivers in the United States. Most of these elder caregivers average 34 hours per week on care tasks, 10 more hours than younger caregivers (AARP, 2020b). Older caregivers are particularly vulnerable in managing the co-occuring stress of caregiving as well as their own medical and social needs (Carr & Utz, 2020).

Demography Gives Clues to Future Changes and Challenges

Families have historically promoted the health and well-being of their members, and continue to do so. Families also serve an important function as a private safety net for each other, relying on each other for physical and economic support when a member becomes ill and helping them recover and remain healthy (Seltzer, 2019). This is even more critical in the United States, which has a relatively weak social safety network compared to other countries, including Canada (Cho, 2017). The Canadian system also has areas of difficulty, however, such as disparities in health care for vulnerable families in rural areas, and the impacts of these shortcomings are magnified during times of social and economic upheaval (Hillel, 2020). Future changes in social and economic conditions and the institutionalized support for different family forms will directly and indirectly affect the composition of future families, their well-being, and their ability to support each other. A few examples of trends to watch include the future of access to abortion and effective birth control, criminal justice and immigration reform, and programs and policies related to student-loan forgiveness.

Given the fundamental importance of families for sustaining the health and well-being of their members, any change in family connections can weaken the family's ability to support vulnerable family members, especially children and older adults (Seltzer, 2019). One concern is the availability and willingness of family to support future cohorts of older adults. Given current trends, a greater number of men and women will reach older adulthood without a significant partner or children. In addition, those with a significant partner will be less likely to be married or living with them, and connections with adult children may be weaker due to higher levels of family instability and MPF.

Demographic theories provide insights into the mechanisms of population-level changes in family structure and functioning. This understanding highlights the significance of the aging Canadian and American populations. Continuing education about the changing needs and circumstances of this population will be essential for all nurses, and the demand for nurses who specialize in working with older adult populations will undoubtedly increase. Demographic trends also project a more culturally diverse population in the near future for both countries, as racial and ethnic minorities and first- and second-generation immigrants make up an increasing share of the population. These populations can have different expectations for, and availability of, support from family members and varying levels of access to, and trust in, the health care system.

SUMMARY

Families change in response to socioeconomic conditions, cultural changes, and shifting demographics such as the aging of the population and immigration. North America has gone through significant changes in the last few decades resulting in changes in family structure, function, and processes. Families have also grown more diverse.

- Rapid changes in family size and structure have occurred in the United States and Canada over the last 70 years. These changes have been propelled by technological advancements and evolving social and economic conditions that have transformed gender and family norms, values, and policies.
- The number of marriages decreased and occurred at later ages; cohabitation became more common, as did nonmarital births; women chose single parenting more than ever before and delayed or rejected childbearing and child rearing; families became smaller; women sought higher education and worked in the labor force in nontraditional roles at record levels; divorce rates climbed; and same-sex marriages were legitimized. While not all Americans approved of these changes in attitudes and behaviors, the general North American culture changed.
- During these historic changes, immigration shifted in the United States and Canada from a majority of immigrants from European countries to increasing numbers of immigrants from Central America, Mexico, Asia, and Africa. Life expectancy increased.
- The economy of the United States and Canada shifted from post–World War II to economic downturns during the oil crisis of the 1970s to the Great Recession of 2007–2009, to the current COVID-19 recession. These events and more have continued to challenge traditional attitudes, beliefs, and behaviors, especially within and surrounding families.
- Within the field of nursing, understanding the complexities of family demographic trends provides a foundation for implementing best practices in patient interaction, diagnosis, treatment, and care. Nurses will better understand the relevant structural and institutional factors that intersect with diverse family structures and populations.
- It is important to note, however, that demography is not destiny. In other words, just because a trend or phenomenon exists at a macro level of the population, one should not assume that individuals or specific families within that community share the same experience. For example, while most families living in the United States have access to clean water, that is not true for some 1.6 million families who do not have access to safe plumbing (Riggs et al., 2017). Understanding family demography provides a starting point where nurses can develop a curiosity about a specific patient for which they are caring, sensitizing nurses to important individual and family factors while providing a broader context for understanding the specific circumstances of each family.

chapter 4

Families and Health Policy

The Intersection of Family Policies, Health Disparities, and Health Care Policies

Tammy L. Henderson, PhD, CFLE

Deborah Padgett Coehlo, PhD, C-PNP, PMHS, CFLE

Laura Fairley, MN, RN, CHPCN(C)

Shan Mohammed, RN, MN, PhD

Chuck Lester, MPH

Critical Concepts

- The health outcomes of families continue to be challenged by health disparities that result from deeply rooted social issues, including racism and stigma, as well as by a variety of factors, including poverty; restricted access to health care resources; and a complex political system of cultural beliefs and policies that affect individuals, families, and communities at all levels of societies.

- The integration of Jones's Levels of Racism Theory and Bronfenbrenner's Ecological Systems Theory provides a deeper understanding of the complexities of family development and the impact of policies on family health.

- Providing health care to families based on a human rights and legal perspective may promote health equity by transforming and developing policies, programs, and laws that inhibit the limited or restricted access to health care services to families.

- Policy decisions made by societies or governments, including what constitutes a legal relationship and how health care and other policies are delivered, profoundly affect families and their health.

- The meanings that a family, the government, or the health care system attaches to the definition of *family* shape the person's health by determining access to government-funded programs.

(*continued*)

Critical Concepts—cont'd

- Social determinants of health—meaning where an individual or family lives, learns, and works; their social address (e.g., race, ethnic, gender, national origin, age, residential tenure, sexual orientation, ability, body size, and more); their access and use of resources; and the intentional or unintentional influence of policies, and social meanings and norms—shape the health and development of individuals, families, and communities.

- Social policies go beyond family policies that promote marriage, procreation, and reproduction and refer to laws, programs, and directives that promote, protect, and provide for families' education, health, economic, housing, social justice, and other familial needs.

- Social policies are currently being challenged in the United States because of conflict over racism, prioritizing health versus the economy, the importance of the environment on health, and the ongoing debate of private versus public health care.

- Competing views about and goals toward individual responsibility and personal behaviors, the government's role, and the meanings attached to laws also require a careful examination of social policies, family health, and the field of family nursing.

- Currently, there are no policies that guarantee the right to health care in the United States except for the social insurance programs of Medicare, Medicaid, and Children's Health Insurance Program (CHIP) and need-based programs and policies.

- Canada has provided comprehensive, federally funded health care access for physicians' services, hospital care, and diagnostics since 1966. Similar to the United States, families have the option of federally and province-funded health care services and/or private insurance.

- For effective outcomes, health policies and health promotion programs must consider the social determinant of health as the foundational concepts.

- Today, most frontline nurses in the United States and Canada function in the acute-care setting, which historically provides a limited understanding of the social determinants of health and related limitations in client advocacy. Advancing health care will require a cultural shift toward increasing opportunities and related education for the nursing profession to play a key role in education, practice, and advocacy for vulnerable populations across practice settings.

INTRODUCTION

Family and social policies provide nurses with a unique opportunity to unmask the influence of family health through multiple systems and to understand the complexity of positive and negative cultural, historical, economic, and political influences that intersect with nursing care of families. Family policies focus on promoting, safeguarding, and bolstering families in the areas of family creation, relationships, economic support, child rearing, education, health care, and caregiving (Bogenschneider, 2014). Social policies, on the other hand, are broader sets of laws and programs aimed at addressing social, economic, and culturally defined concerns (Herrick, 2013).

Understanding the foundation for the concepts underlying the substance of this chapter regarding the intersection of family and social policies, health, social determinants of health, and health disparities is important for understanding the nurse's role in participating in the development, advocacy, and implementation of family policies that affect family health. Policies contribute to and/or determine the health status, health care delivery, and health equity of a person, community, and group.

Social policies influence social determinants of health and in turn direct the health of individuals, families, and communities (World Health Organization [WHO], 2021). WHO (2021) defines *social determinants of health* as "conditions in which people are born, grow, work, live, and age, and the wider set of forces and systems shaping the conditions of daily life. These forces and systems include economic policies and systems, development agendas, social norms, social policies and political systems" (paragraph 1). More specifically, health determinants include a person's demographic characteristics, such as race, ethnicity, genetics, and age, which cannot be changed, and a person's education, place of employment, and use of resources, which can and do change. Social determinants organize the world and shape societal responses, include changeable (e.g., eating and physical activities) and unchangeable factors (e.g., early childhood experiences and environmental conditions) (U.S. Department of Health and Human Services [USDHHS], 2021).

Social determinants also include physical, social, educational, and economic environments, which further break down into income, housing, education, employment, access to health care, public safety, transportation, and availability of community-based resources, which can all be classified as changeable or unchangeable depending on policies and cultural constructs (WHO, 2021). Health determinants have a strong, deep-seated influence on the development of families and will continue to contribute to health in community systems.

The Parable of the Drowning People

Imagine yourself and a fellow nurse going on an outing to a beautiful natural pool at the foot of a magnificent waterfall. While sitting on the beach area, you observe a person fall down the waterfall and immediately struggle not to drown. You and your colleague quickly jump in the water, pull the victim to shore, and provide lifesaving care. Soon after you stabilize the first victim, you see another person falling down the waterfall and into the pool, crying for help. So you return to the water to save this new victim, but you find that, each time you save the person in the water, a new one falls down the waterfall until you and your friend are close to exhaustion. As another person falls into the pool, you leave the water and begin to walk up the long path to the waterfall. When your friend asks with incredulity why you are leaving, you tell them, "I'm headed upstream to figure out why people keep falling down the waterfall." Once upstream, you see a series of bridges. Many are in passable shape but some of them have gaping holes, which are causing people to fall as they try to cross the bridges. While all of the bridges could use some repairs, it becomes obvious that there are some bridges that are almost completely failing and need immediate attention to prevent more people from dying. You make a decision to work on the repairs, while your colleague continues to save drowning people.

While this parable is most often told to illustrate the concept of primary prevention, it makes an ideal framework for the discussion of family policy and nursing. The families you work with may often have immediate and overwhelming needs. But it is important to be mindful of the power that nurses have as advocates to change not just individual behavior to enhance health or to treat illness at the individual levels but also to be a change agent in correcting flaws in the environment that contribute to health and illness.

The Ecology of Health

Social determinants of health require a careful examination of health disparities, whether changeable or unchangeable. Health disparities arise from the complex interaction between social policies across ecological systems and include systems of oppression, such as institutional racism, personally mediated racism, and internalized racism (Jones, 2020).

- Ecological systems refer to the integration of individual (micro), family (meso), community (macro), and exo (larger government, culture, and environment) systems across time (chrono) (Bronfenbrenner, 2005).
- Institutional racism refers to differential access to resources and opportunities that impede the health and well-being of individuals, families, and communities (Jones, 2014).
- Personally mediated racism refers to prejudice (e.g., differential assumptions) and discrimination (e.g., negative actions) practiced by individuals, families, and communities across societies that

undermines the humanity of others (Jones, 2014).

■ Internalized racism refers to the acceptance and adoption of socially constructed negative messages about one's abilities, character, lower status, and the resulting loss of civil and social rights (Jones, 2020).

Health care policies continue to be debated in the United States and Canada, with ongoing discussions of appropriate resources to changeable versus unchangeable health disparities, cultural discrimination of marginalized groups, just disbursement of resources, attention to scientific evidence versus political ideas, unjust biases, and financial influences. In this chapter, health policies are explored in the context of the definition of family, theories proposed by Jones (2014, 2020) and Bronfenbrenner (1995, 1996, 2005), social determinants of health, and health disparities and the nurse's role in participating in the development of, advocating for, implementing, and evaluating family policies that enhance positive health care and resulting positive health outcomes without discrimination against marginalized groups of people. Finally, this chapter explores nursing involvement in the development and promotion of health literacy, health equity, and family policy. At the completion of this chapter, family nurses will have a broader understanding of social and family policy and how it can contribute to or mitigate health disparities, social determinants of health, and overall health outcomes. Armed with this knowledge, nurses can assist families in adopting health promotion and disease prevention strategies and be more familiar with family policies that can assist families in achieving a higher state of well-being. Family nurses will be prepared to advocate for families in their everyday care and to participate in professional organizations, communities, and nations to adopt policies that minimize disparities and maximize access to resources. This in turn will contribute to improving health of families and their members.

DEFINITION OF FAMILY POLICY

Family policy includes explicit and implicit laws, codes, programs, and policies that are designed to promote, safeguard, and protect children, families, and communities (Bogenschneider, 2014). Sometimes, however, the intended and/or unintended consequences of these laws, codes, programs, and policies actually serve to harm some of the very children, families, and communities they purport to protect. This is particularly true for Black and Indigenous children and families, and Hispanic families, as well as LGBTQ+ families.

The notion of family is not explicitly noted in the U.S. Constitution. Federal, state, and local governments are charged with protecting the individual rights of citizens. Individual rights must be balanced against the common good of all citizens. The evolution of family policies has been debated, and such debate has included the right of governments to make family policy in spite of that right not being explicitly defined in the U.S. Constitution and in state constitutions.

Family policies support and help parents and families effectively manage paid work and family caregiving, reduce poverty, and improve adults' and children's well-being (Hengstebeck et al., 2016). Policies, laws, and programs influence everyday life, including a person's ability to form intimate and legal partnerships; render economic support to family members; manage reproduction; parent and care for children; and engage in family caregiving of infants, children, spouses, siblings, older adults, and individuals with illness and/or disabilities (Bogenschneider, 2014).

Family and social policies intersect in legal decisions and programs. For example, the U.S. Supreme Court determined in *United States v. Windsor* (2013) that the 1996 Defense of Marriage Act (DOMA) was unconstitutional because it treated couples differently based on their sexual orientation, which violates equal protection of a person's liberty rights and undermines equitable access to health care and other benefits offered to legally recognized married couples. Therefore, DOMA represents a familial and social concern.

From an ecological perspective, family nurses' understanding of family and social policy advances their capacity to promote health equity and advocate for healthy families. Social policies reach beyond family policies that promote marriage, procreation, and reproduction (Center for American Progress, 2021) to laws, programs, and directives that promote, protect, and provide for families' education, health, economic, housing, social justice, and their other needs. Pertinent social policies focused specifically on health in the United States include Medicare, Medicaid, the Patient Protection and Affordable Care Act of 2010, and CHIP.

Definition of Family in the United States

Today's nursing family policy advocacy role is shaped by the social and legal meanings of family, although *family* is not included in the U.S. Constitution. Policy decisions made by a society or government about families and how they are legally defined, and the meaning of what constitutes a legal relationship, have a profound effect on families and their health care options, health outcomes, and general well-being. The meaning of and protections afforded to U.S. families have emerged from legislative, administrative, and judicial decision making. For example, the fundamental right to personal and family relationships and the right to life, liberty, and the pursuit of happiness (liberty interests) are woven into the U.S. Constitution and U.S. Supreme Court decisions (*Loving v. Virginia*, 1967; *Moore v. the City of East Cleveland*, 1977). In the case of *Loving v. Virginia* (1967), the U.S. Supreme Court determined that the Virginia law that prohibited Blacks and Whites from marrying violated the marital autonomy rights, among other rights, of Richard and Mildred Loving.

For the most part, *family* has been socially defined as two heterosexual parents with children, creating the cultural expectation for the traditional family in the United States (Hansen, 2019) and carving out a hierarchy of legal protections. In the decision of *Moore v. City of East Cleveland* (1977), the U.S. Supreme Court determined that an intergenerational household—a grandmother, her son, and two grandchildren—functioned similar to a traditional family. Therefore, this family deserved to live in an area zoned for single-family units. This functional definition of family is complemented by structural meanings such as single-parent, blended, divorced, and long-term foster families or same-sex partners and cohabiting couples. The U.S. Census Bureau (2020) defines *family* as two or more people living together who are related by birth, marriage, or adoption. Although this definition expands policies that support families, individuals living together as a family but without legal protection based on this definition remain

vulnerable. For example, two adults living together but not married cannot obtain the same benefits as two adults who are legally married, particularly in the areas of taxes, housing rights, health care, and reproductive rights.

Contemporary demographic trends reflect shifts in the meaning of families that correspond to the growth of intergenerational and other diverse families. In 2015, an estimated 5.8 million children younger than 18 years of age in the United States resided with a grandparent, and 2.6 million grandparents were responsible for the basic needs of one or more grandchildren younger than 18 years of age (U.S. Census Bureau, 2016). In the *United States v. Windsor* (2013) decision, the U.S. Supreme Court determined that Section 3 of DOMA, which narrowly defined "marriage" as the legal union "between one man and one woman as husband and wife" and "spouse" as "a person of the opposite sex who is a husband or a wife," was unconstitutional. DOMA stigmatized, legally disadvantaged, and differentially treated heterosexual and same-sex couples, violating the individual right to marriage and personal relationships. In essence, the law violated the Fifth Amendment's guarantee of equal protection under the law, which was similarly protected in *Loving v. Virginia* (1967).

Looking specifically at the context of health care, members of a family can be given or denied access to health insurance, housing, and social and health programs based on whether they meet the federal definition of *family*. In the United States, the Administration for Children and Families is part of the USDHHS, which oversees federal programs that support the economic and social well-being of children and families, such as Temporary Assistance to Needy Families, the Healthy Marriage Initiative, and Head Start. But because of how families are legally defined, many individuals who consider themselves part of a family unit would be ineligible for these programs. The meanings that a family, the government, or the health care system attaches to *family* also shape the health of the person by determining access to government-funded programs.

Defining *Family* in Canada

Similar to the United States, Canada's social and legal definitions of *family* play a critical role in individuals' abilities to gain access to essential health and social services, economic resources, and government-funded programs. Historically, legal definitions of *family* in Canada have reflected deeply entrenched practices of privileging biology and/or genetics as so-called true markers of family, and they were constructed in a way that excluded families that did not fall within the realm of the nuclear, heterosexual, and monogamous archetype (Bruineman, 2019). This served to perpetuate the erasure of nonbiological or chosen, queer, polyamorous, single-parent, skip-generation, and transnational families (Bruineman, 2019).

Over the last 30 years, Canada has seen a significant shift in family demographics, including (Statistics Canada, 2020a):

- an increase in the number of couples (both same-sex and heterosexual) living in common-law relationships (56% married and 15% common law in 2017). The rate of common-law relationships is three times the rate found in 1981 (6.3%).
- a decreasing fertility rate (251 live births per 1,000 women aged 20 to 40 years in 2015 compared to 218 live births per 1,000 women aged 20 to 40 years in 2019).
- an increasing rate of women's employment. (The women's employment rate has grown from 21.6% of women in 1950 to 82% of women in 2015.)
- an increasing number of lone-parent families (1,629,163 in 2016 compared to 1,779,502 in 2020).
- an increasing number of transnational families through immigration (an average of 250,000 immigrants from 2004 to 2015, with a jump to an average of 299,000 over the next five years).
- an increasing number of both multigenerational families and skip-generational families (37.5% growth from 2001 to 2016) (Battams, 2017).
- an increasing number of aged family members (currently at 5.9 million people, which is up 20% since 2011) (Vanier Institute of the Family, 2020; Statistics Canada, 2020a).

These demographic shifts have fueled a surge of new wide-ranging needs to which the federal and provincial governments have had to respond, necessitating a broadening of the legal and social parameters of what constitutes *family* in Canada.

While there is no direct reference to *family* in the Canadian Constitution's Charter of Rights and Freedoms, the concepts of both marital status and family status are enshrined in the Canadian Human Rights Act of 1977, as well as most of the provincial/territorial Human Rights Codes (Canadian Centre for Diversity and Inclusion, 2018). These laws prohibit actions that discriminate against Canadians based on their family status in a protected social area, which may include housing, employment, education, health care, and social services. They also protect individuals against harassment based on one or more of the grounds of discrimination such as age, race, gender, and sexual orientation. The Canadian Human Rights codes provide the legal framework to facilitate broad legislative reforms to a range of provincial and federal policies directly affecting families.

These reforms include the legal recognition of common-law/adult interdependent relationships in every province and territory across the country, whereby nonmarried partners are entitled to the same rights and benefits as a married couple (Government of Canada [GOC] 2018); the legalization of same-sex marriage in 2005; the legalization of stepchild and joint adoption by same-sex/queer couples in every province and territory by 2011 (GOC, 2018); the legalization of naming of more than two parents on a child's birth certificate in recognition of polyamorous families, certain queer families, and coparenting families in British Columbia, Newfoundland, and Ontario by 2019 (Bruineman, 2019); and the expansion of the legal definition of *kin* in provincial child welfare legislation to include someone who is considered by the child to be family, including biological family members, a godparent, friend, teacher, or neighbor (Ontario Association of Children's Aid Societies, n.d.).

These legislative reforms to legal definitions of *family* within a Canadian context reflect a broader social and cultural shift away from focusing on *who* constitutes a family toward what a family *does* as its defining feature. Consistent with Bogenschneider's (2014) notions of families functioning as partnerships, economic support, child rearing, and caregiving, the focus is on what families in Canada do as captured in the Vanier Institute of the Family's (2021) functional definition of family. The Vanier

Institute of the Family, a nonprofit agency dedicated to understanding the diversity and complexity of families in Canada, identifies a family as "any combination of two or more persons who are bound together over time by ties of mutual consent, birth and/or adoption or placement and who, together, assume responsibilities for variant combinations of some of the following" (page 1; paragraph 2):

- physical maintenance and care of group members
- addition of new members through procreation or adoption
- socialization of children
- social control of members
- production, consumption, distribution of goods and services
- affective nurturance—love

This definition foregrounds the similarities between families, regardless of gender, sexuality, genetic makeup, and/or marital status of each family's members. By moving away from what families look like to what families do, policymakers in Canada can think more broadly and inclusively about the challenges faced by modern families in Canada, in all their iterations, as they relate to fertility assistance, parental leave benefits, child and family benefits, disability supports, child-care subsidies, caregiving benefits, spousal/partner benefits and pensions, income assistance, and child custody. This has major implications for the development of new policy and program initiatives that can better meet the needs of the diverse population.

THEORETICAL BACKGROUND FOR THE INTERSECTION OF POLICIES, HEALTH DISPARITIES, AND FAMILY HEALTH

A discussion of the intersection of policies and family health cannot be fully understood without understanding theoretical models that help explain the complexity of health outcomes across diverse groups, families, and communities, including the intersection of social determinants of health and health disparities. These are best understood by comparing two theories: Jones's (2000) Three Levels of Racism Theory and Bronfenbrenner's (1984,

1995, 1996, 2005) Ecological Systems Theory. The term *racism* can include all groups that are stigmatized, because race is not a biological structure but a socially constructed idea created and accepted by people (Jones, 2014). It can include other isms that stigmatize by religion, gender, sexual orientation or identity, body size, socioeconomic status, or ability.

Jones's Three Levels of Racism Theory

Jones's Three Levels of Racism Theory emphasizes the importance of looking at racism from a complex view of institutional prejudices and related policies and practices; community and cultural reinforcement of those prejudices, including practices such as segregation; and internal beliefs that those forces are justified. Jones (2000) describes these three levels of racism in her model: institutional, personally mediated, and internalized.

Institutional racism refers to deferential access to resources and opportunities, including health care, education, gainful employment, healthy food and clean water, adequate housing, and living in a healthy environment. Each of these resources and opportunities in turn affects health and is commonly listed as a health determinant. Institutional racist practices are often normalized by a particular society and often protected by laws and policies within that society.

Personally mediated racism refers to prejudice and discrimination practiced by individuals, families, and communities across societies (Jones, 2020). Prejudice refers to differential assumptions about the "abilities, motives, and intentions of others" (Jones, 2000, p. 2) according to their identified, stigmatized group affiliation. Discrimination refers to the action toward the differentiated groups that negatively affects their well-being. These actions include lack of respect, unwarranted suspicion (i.e., not sitting next to a person based on prejudiced beliefs), devaluation (i.e., not choosing a qualified person for a job based on the person's stigmatized characteristics), and scapegoating (i.e., punishing an entire group of people based on the rumored actions of one in the group). See *A Documented History of the Incident Which Occurred at Rosewood, Florida, in January 1923* (Dye, 1997) for a clear example of this process. This tragedy involved an entire town being burned and an undocumented number of Blacks killed based on a rumor that a White woman was sexually assaulted by a Black man. The incident occurred in 1923 and yet it took until 1994 for any retribution to be awarded to the nine survivors.

Internalized racism refers to stigmatized individuals accepting negative messages about their abilities and their inherent lower status, leading to loss of civil and social rights (Jones, 2020). Many individuals who are placed in a stigmatized group begin to accept labels placed on them by other groups and accept disparities in resources as their due. This pattern is similar to a woman being raped and then blaming herself for the rape, labeling herself as asking for it based on, for example, the clothes she was wearing at the time of the rape.

Jones (2000, 2014, 2020) provides clear metaphors to illustrate the negative impact of each of the three levels of racism on health. Her first metaphor describes the difference in perception of moths as they fly in and out of colored lights. The metaphor emphasizes that the moths do not change in color or ability as they fly but rather the surrounding lights change the perception of their appearance. This is similar to certain groups of people that are stigmatized in one setting yet welcomed and valued in another setting based on perception rather than any inherent change in the identified group. For example, a Native American man is welcomed within his cultural celebrations, but he may be shunned in a predominantly European American celebration, even though the individual did not change between these two settings.

Jones's second metaphor is that of a closing restaurant. The people already in the restaurant can enjoy the resources, yet those locked on the outside can only observe the enjoyment. This is often illustrated by a stigmatized group being unable to access a service but being able to observe the privileged groups enjoying that resource, such as quality health care or access to stable housing.

Finally, the most compelling metaphor Jones offers is noticing the difference in growth of two plants. One plant is given rich soil and an abundance of water to grow, and the other plant is given poor soil and barely enough water to survive. The first plant will obviously flourish, whereas the second plant will grow slowly and never reach its true potential. If one is observing these two plants and not considering the impact of the environment on the difference in growth, one could easily decide that the first plant was inherently superior. This metaphor describes the common practice of observing an oppressed group of individuals who are surrounded by an unhealthy environment and assuming that they are inherently inferior to those growing up in a rich and healthy environment (Jones, 2014). This is commonly described as blaming the individual for societal and environmental problems or blaming the individual for unchangeable factors rather than supporting changeable factors. This is especially important because policies can hinder individual growth (e.g., block quality child care from low socioeconomic groups) rather than supporting growth through social and environmental changes (e.g., supporting quality child care for all).

Using Jones's model to consider domestic violence can illustrate why many women struggle to get the support they need to leave their abusive partner and end the cruelty (National Domestic Violence Hotline, 2020). From an *institutional level*, many women around the globe are believed to be the property of the men in their families. As property, they have no voice to change or challenge those men's actions. Many countries prohibit women from working outside the home or leaving the home without a male family escort. Even in the United States, many women are totally dependent on a partner's income and lack experience or education to work outside the home and support themselves and their children. Laws against domestic violence have improved in the last 40 years, but they continue to limit the institutional support of women needing to leave an abusive home safely and still have enough resources to care for herself and her children.

Personally mediated racism is apparent by the limited and often crowded shelters that women live in as they struggle to rebuild their lives and care for their children after leaving an abusive partner. Communities often shun abused women and label them as weak, asking for their abuse, or neglecting their children by staying in an abusive home too long. Legal assistance to pursue prosecution and protection from the abusive partner is often impossible to obtain due to the cost or the long wait if it is offered without cost. Women are often accused of neglecting their children by failing to protect them from abuse, and thus they fear losing their children to their abusive partner or foster care. These challenges often leave a woman feeling that she has no choice but to stay in an abusive home.

Finally, *internalized racism* can lead an abused woman, as an all-too-common example, to believe she deserves her abuse (National Domestic Violence Hotline, 2020). She may be taught that women have less value than men and that a good partner endures the deserved abuse. She may blame herself for not knowing how to stop the abuse or not standing up to the abusive partner. The inferiority of females when compared to males is one of the most dangerous, socially constructed concepts passed on across generations and cultures. The assumption that women need to be protected by men due to inferiority is not based on science but rather a strong societal desire to keep women oppressed (Jones & Clifton, 2018). This belief system perpetuates the pattern of women staying in an abusive relationship out of fear: a woman may be killed if she leaves and feel that people will think she is crazy to be fearful, despite many women being killed soon after they try to leave an abusive partner. Interventions for women of diverse or vulnerable groups cannot stop at the individual level; rather, they should include advocating for increased and improved community resources; community awareness and educational programs; local, state, and national family policies that change the environment that allows domestic violence to thrive; and continually changing the inaccurate social construct that women are inferior to men and deserve the abuse due to this inequality.

Using Jones's model to understand and change policies is valuable for nurses. If family nurses consider the three levels of racism or other isms, they are more likely to identify trends undermining the health of patients and participate in changing policies that continue to oppress vulnerable populations. Nurses can intervene on individual, institutional, and community levels by promoting change through health education, involvement, and resistance to racism as an accepted value. Understanding Jones's model and how her model interacts within the ecological systems is a way to understand where to place health promotion across systems.

Bronfenbrenner's Ecological Systems Theory

Bronfenbrenner's Ecological Systems Theory describes the interacting systems between micro-, meso-, macro-, and exosystems, and adds the system of time, or the chronosystem. The microsystem or individual system includes internal systems (i.e., the most intimate system of development or health status of the individual). The mesosystem refers to the family system, including roles, responsibilities, boundaries, and communication patterns within the family and toward the outside world. The macrosystem represents the surrounding community, including neighborhood culture and structure, schools, parks, churches, and other community resources. The exosystem embodies the larger government and culture, including laws and policies. The chronosystem signifies changes across time.

When considering policy development, the use of an ecological model has broadened our focus from an individualist model to a multisystem model (Eriksson et al., 2018). Historically, the United States made a major shift in overall health through policies that focused on improved sanitation, air quality, and local environments (exosystem) as well as overall access to health care. With the growth in biomedical science, however, there was a shift away from broad environmental policies to individual health care policies (microsystem). Life expectancy grew an average of three years per decade as biomedical research improved the treatment for hypertension, diabetes, heart disease, and cancer. This trend caused a marked increase in the development of the current individual insurance program rather than social programs to pay for health care.

A microsystem approach, which focuses on the individual's approach to personal health, includes taking responsibility to maintain health, finding providers to treat health problems, and paying for care to support health. To be most successful in changing behaviors that lead to health determinants, individuals benefit from support, rather than blame. These changeable and unchangeable characteristics include behavioral or social determinants. Changeable behavioral determinants include activities such as eating habits, smoking, substance use, physical activity, and coping skills. Unchangeable behavioral determinants include challenges such as physical and mental disabilities, early childhood experiences including adverse events, trauma, and environmental conditions such as poverty and war that have an impact on individuals. By focusing only on the microsystem level, the risk of also blaming the individual for health problems (i.e., blaming the individual for obesity rather than changing social policy surrounding marketing of food, school lunches, lack of outdoor space, etc.) is high. Therefore, it is important to consider other systems and to look at the complex interplay between the multiple systems affecting family health.

From a macro level or community level in the United States, the COVID-19 pandemic provides an excellent example of the multiple system model and the intersection of race, ethnicity, and access to quality care. For example, the health experiences of Navajo people, rural residency, and the COVID-19 pandemic provide an excellent context for exploring a macro- or community-level influence on the outcomes of health in this population during this pandemic. The Navajo Reservation is a sprawling, 27,000-square-mile tract with land in Arizona, Utah, and New Mexico. Around 156,823 Native people live on the reservation with just 12 health care facilities. Navajo people suffer disparate rates of chronic illness, such as diabetes, heart disease, and obesity compared to national averages. Significantly, the Centers for Disease Control and Prevention (CDC) indicates that all of these illnesses represent an increased risk of severe illness for people who contract COVID-19 (Navajo Nation Health Survey, 2020).

As of October 2020, the Navajo Reservation had 11,298 confirmed cases and 574 deaths attributed to the COVID-19 virus (Navajo Department of Health, 2020). The Navajo Nation's per capita case rate of 7,204 cases per 100,000 people ranked higher than all but 40 of the 3,141 counties in the United States (CDC, 2020b), making the Navajo Nation's death rate of 366 per 100,000 higher than New York City during the height of their struggle with the pandemic and higher than that of Wuhan at the height of the outbreak in China (Doshi et al., 2020). The recommended changes at a macrosystem level to address this health crisis are to increase quality of and access to health care, increase internet access, and increase health education programs on the reservation (Doshi et al., 2020).

Another important aspect of policy is understanding and research on the impact of the macrosystem on family health among populations in Canada. If a family resides in a macrosystem, meaning a community, marked with poverty, their health is shaped by that environment. For example, type 2 diabetes is on the increase and is more likely in communities with lower incomes compared to communities with higher incomes and in ethnically diverse groups compared to European Canadians (Tenkorang, 2017). Communities with residents who have lower incomes often have higher proportions of immigrant populations and people using social assistance programs (Tenkorang, 2017).

The intersection of the macrosystem factors (e.g., people living below the federal poverty threshold) and individual behaviors provides a more holistic view of the issue. While health promotion efforts involving diet and exercise to address obesity have a significant influence on disease rates, these efforts often require sufficient resources. Because of a lack of resources, preventive measures, such as keeping a healthy weight, are much less likely in groups with lower income (Tenkorang, 2017).

Aboriginal people, for example, developed diabetes when they started to eat Western foods instead of their traditional diets. Tenkorang (2017) found that, across gender and ethnic groups, diabetes rates were higher among persons living in lower-income neighborhoods, confirming that the reasons for this disparity are complex and multilayered and include lifestyle changes within different communities. Multilayer factors include the lack of needed resources for a healthy lifestyle, such as access to healthy foods; inability to pay for prescription drugs; lower incomes; unhealthy environments; racial or ethnic discrimination; and ongoing stress and trauma (Tenkorang, 2017).

Researchers have also found evidence, in a study of 215 older adults, that worry and chronic stress, which lead to high cortisol levels, increase the risk of chronic disease (Herriot et al., 2018). Other researchers have found a similar trend in children and adolescents with chronic conditions (Reaume & Ferro, 2019). Chronic stress disproportionately affects most diverse ethnic groups, who are often subject to discrimination, violence, early death by accidents and homicide, and the constant worries attached to life with low incomes (Omariba, 2015). When people must cope with the added expenses of the illness, stress increases, creating a cycle of exacerbating chronic illness. As stated earlier, the social determinants that create health disparities are multilayered, complex, and mutually reinforcing within multiple ecological systems.

At the exosystem level, family and social policies affect the ability of individuals and families to access, afford, and benefit from resources. This chapter focuses on those exosystem policies that hinder or help families thrive.

Application of Theoretical Models to Policies

Both Jones's Three Levels of Racism Theory and Bronfenbrenner's Ecological Systems Theory consider the individual; families; communities; and the broad economic, social, cultural, and physical environment. The use of each model improves our understanding, treatment, and promotion of health care and pertinent familial and social policies. These models emphasize the importance of recognizing environmental impact on health, such as Jones's metaphor of the plants growing differently depending on the health of their environments, and the consideration in Bronfenbrenner's Ecological Systems Theory of multiple systems interacting together, all of which affect family health and include the environmental system (exosystem). The social determinants of health and health disparities demonstrate the intersection of policies with the application of the Ecological Systems Theory and Jones's Levels of Racism Theory.

THE INTERSECTION BETWEEN SOCIAL AND FAMILY POLICIES AND HEALTH DISPARITIES

Family policies are explicit and implicit laws, codes, and programs developed to promote and protect children, families, and communities (Bogenschneider, 2014). Social policies, on the other hand, are broader laws and programs created to tackle socially, economically, and culturally defined concerns (Herrick, 2013). The differences in family and social policies tend to blur when policies, laws, codes, and programs are enacted to protect social rights, including health, food and water, education, housing, employment, and a healthy environment. Civil rights legislation protects a citizen's right to participate in political decisions (i.e., voting and

public forums), legal rights, and civil protection; social rights are controversial because of a generational belief that social rights are largely the responsibility of the individual (Levitsky, 2013). We suggest that these laws converge in that laws, policies, codes, and programs influence families and address social, economic, and health concerns. In fact, policies have been developed for the purpose of preventing health problems on a societal scale (i.e., immunization programs and clean water policies) and to *mitigate* health disparities. This section of the chapter explores examples of policies that have had an impact on family health and on health disparities.

Social Determinants and Resulting Health Disparities

Health disparities are a continuing problem in the United States, causing negative health outcomes for individuals, groups, and families. Because of this continued problem, Congress ordered the Institute of Medicine (IOM) to investigate and develop a report on the subject. The landmark IOM (2003) report, *Unequal Treatment: Confronting Racial and Ethnic Disparities in Health Care*, detailed the long-standing and deeply rooted inequalities in health care directly related to race and ethnicity. Despite the IOM providing a comprehensive review of the contributing factors to health disparities and recommendations to promote health equity, health disparities still continue. For instance, Blacks in the United States continue to experience higher rates of death from heart disease and cancer than Whites, and children of color who live in urban areas are more likely to have asthma than children living in less population-dense areas as well as White children in both rural and urban communities (U.S. Health and Human Services Office of Minority Health, 2018; CDC, 2017). These health disparities continue to correlate with the following: certain environments that lack adequate resources (such as limited access to health care); exposure to environmental toxins in impoverished environments; personal behaviors related to substance abuse, inadequate nutrition, and lack of physical exercise; and lack of treatment for mental illnesses (IOM, 2012; CDC, 2017). In the IOM (2003) report, the authors apply Jones's Three Levels of Racism Theory and Bronfenbrenner's Ecological Systems Theory to explore social determinants of continued health disparity that briefly are explored via the intersection of poverty with housing, homelessness, the gender gap, and the consequences for children living in poverty in the United States and Canada. Afterward, the authors deconstruct social determinants of health and health disparities by examining chronic illnesses, obesity, type 2 diabetes, addictions, asthma and other lung diseases, and COVID-19 as examples of continuing health disparities across America.

Poverty in the United States and Canada

Social determinants of health are interrelated and mutually reinforcing. Poverty influences other social determinants that have a negative impact on family health, such as housing, food and job security, education, and lifestyle choices. Racism continues to influence strongly who is a victim to poverty and can be analyzed by examining multiple interacting ecological systems. The social determinants of poverty, housing, homelessness, and the gender gap illuminate the interrelationships of social determinants for health and health disparities.

It is impossible to discuss individual lifestyle choices, for example, without discussing family cultures; community access to education about healthy lifestyles; and governmental policies that fund and support, through family policies, healthy lifestyle promotion. Likewise, poor-quality housing or overcrowding—a result of poverty—affects health by contributing to stress (individual, or micro level) and safety issues (micro and macro levels). When considering chronic illnesses such as asthma, using medications can decrease symptoms, but medications can be used only if the individual has access to health care. Mildew and dampness (community environment) might trigger asthma and be beyond an individual's or family's ability to correct. Unemployment or employment insecurity, which can result in poverty, limits the choice of affordable housing, and living in a low-resource community further adds to unhealthy lifestyle choices. For example, areas where affordable housing is located tend to lack public transportation and grocery stores; therefore, citizens using low-income housing end up having less access to fresh fruits and vegetables, which makes shopping for and eating healthy foods difficult. The only choice for these families is often to buy unhealthy processed foods from local variety stores, frequently at high prices (Burrows, 2018).

Poverty, another social determinant of health, creates serious issues when it comes to housing and can result in homelessness for many families who live below the poverty level. There are 2.5 million children experiencing homelessness in the United States, which is one in every 30 children (American Institute for Research, 2020). Homeless children are three times more likely to have been born to a single mother than their nonhomeless counterparts (Bassuk et al., 2015). According to Bassuk et al. (2015), the major causes of homelessness in children include:

- national high poverty rate
- lack of affordable housing
- racial disparities
- challenges of single parenting
- history of a traumatic experience, especially domestic violence

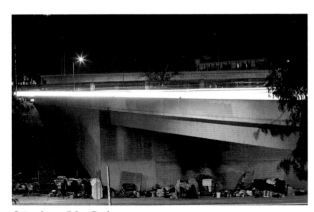

© istock.com/MattGush

In fact, one of the most significant outcomes for young children who experience homelessness is the potential for devastating changes in the brain that can interfere with learning, emotional self-regulation, cognitive skills, and social relationships (Bassuk et al., 2015). Therefore, family nurses work with families with children that are experiencing homelessness to help them find emergency shelter and essential services, and follow these children and families as they progress to permanent housing. Nurses need to be skillful in conducting comprehensive assessments, including screening for mental health concerns and developmental delays, domestic violence, food insecurity, lack of a medical home (comprehensive primary care provider), and cultural values and beliefs that have an impact on access to care. Nurses can advocate for programs that support family security, such as programs that allow single-parent mothers to receive job training and workplace skills. Nurses also help mothers find safe and quality child care for their children (e.g., Head Start programs). Family nurses also need to help these parents learn parenting skills so they can build strong healthy relationships with their children.

In 2018, more than 38.1 million North Americans lived in poverty in the United States (Poverty USA, 2021). Fifteen million children, or 21% of children, currently live in poverty in the United States (National Center for Children in Poverty, 2019). As explored further in the following sections on race and gender, Black families and Black female heads of household disproportionately account for those living at or below the poverty level. Blacks earn 61% ($31,969) of what non-Hispanic White individuals earn ($52,423). Women continue to earn 80% of what men earn overall (American Association of University Women, 2017). Women of color, especially single mothers, however, represent the highest groups of families living in poverty in the United States (Creamer & Mohanty, 2019).

In 2018, the federal government of Canada released "Opportunity for All—Canada's First Poverty Reduction Strategy," which contained long-term commitments to guide public policy to reduce poverty. This policy document comes late in Canada's long-standing history of poverty and income inequality, despite being a high-income and resource-rich country. Similar to the United States, Canada experiences income disparity. Based on after-tax household income, Canadians in the top 10% of incomes accounted for 23.0% of total income in Canada in 2018, whereas the bottom 40% of the population represented 20.8% of total income (Statistics Canada, 2020b). Income inequality in Canada is shaped by gender discrimination, racism, geographic area, and other social factors. For instance, racialized women in Canada earned 59 cents for every dollar that nonracialized men earned, while nonracialized women earned 67 cents for every dollar that nonracialized men earned (Block et al., 2019).

Children and families often experience the negative health impact of income inequality and poverty. Universal health insurance may offer a protective effect in Canada against being born with poor health status. As children age, however, income-related health inequities appear to widen and are not mediated by universal health care. In Canada, parental income has a substantial impact on children's health through its effects on developmental mechanisms such as nutrition intake, access to educational resources, and neighborhood disadvantage (Wei & Feeny, 2019).

Poverty, Health Care, and Health in the United States and Canada

In the United States, the availability of employment-based health coverage declined from 64.4% in 1997 to 56.5% in 2010; however, by 2015, the rate had climbed to 90.9% owing to the Affordable Care Act (Barnett & Vornovitsky, 2016). This increase has provided more citizens and their dependents with health coverage, but many are faced with high-deductible plans and high monthly premiums. The highest number of families covered by health insurance remains those with employer-covered care, at 56% of the population. Yet many employers are requiring higher shared costs of health insurance from their employees. A study of 4,000 employers with employees making median-level incomes was conducted to evaluate trends of employee and employer contributions to health insurance between 2008 to 2018 in the United States (Collins et al., 2019). The authors noted that the burden of health insurance costs for families is influenced by four main factors, including the total premium costs, the share paid by employers versus employees, the size of the deductibles, and the families' overall annual income. The average family's expenditure on health insurance rose from 7.8% in 2008 to 11% in 2018. This increase outpaced the increase in median income for families. While rates varied across states, families paid from $3,862 to $6,597 per year for health insurance and from $1,308 to $2,447 for deductible expenses. These expenses are often unaffordable to families earning low wages who do not qualify for Medicaid but cannot afford health insurance premiums due to other high-priority expenses, including housing and food (Collins et al., 2019).

The number of families living in poverty and covered by government-funded programs has steadily grown to 37% of the population. With this continued growth in health care coverage for families in the United States, we are still faced with 29 million children not covered by health insurance, with a majority of those children being African American or Hispanic (Barnett & Vornovitsky, 2016). The cost of health coverage is well beyond the means of those living in or close to the poverty level. Meanwhile, the public debate on an appropriate level of support for families who lack basic housing, food, health services, or social stability continues.

Multiple factors may worsen the influence of poverty on health outcomes, including access to resources, health literacy, gender, ethnicity, and education. All these factors are considered major contributors to poor health, particularly cardiovascular disease and type 2 diabetes (CDC, 2020b), higher blood pressure, mental illness (Mental Health Commission of Canada, 2021), and poorer adherence to medications (CDC, 2020b). For example, children who live in poverty, especially during the early years or for an extended period of time, are at significant risk of poor health outcomes and developmental delays (American Academy of Pediatrics, 2016).

U.S. citizens who live in poverty are at higher risk of developing chronic illness and mental illness, especially depression (CDC, 2018). Even a nominal copay of $2 has been shown to decrease the number of visits to a physician for those living in poverty (USDHHS, 2015). This results in poorer health care and related negative health outcomes. It is important that nurses and other health care providers support policies that help to eradicate poverty and the resulting health disparities.

Assigned Sex at Birth and Gender

The assigned sex at birth and gender is a social determinant everywhere, with women and gender minorities experiencing disparities in access to resources and well-paying jobs (Bleiweis, 2020; Nath, 2018). Women and other genders earn less than men when performing the same job, which is approximately 80% of men's wages (American Association of University Women, 2017), yet they are more likely than men to be heads of single-parent households. In fact, gender is one of the factors that

exacerbates poverty and in turn contributes to even greater health disparities. Gender affects health care in other ways as well. For example, women who are at risk of heart disease are 11% less likely than men to have been told they are at risk and receive counseling about risk modification (Leifheit-Limson et al., 2015). Women with ischemic heart disease are more likely to be underrecognized and treated than are men (Graham, 2016). Women are also less likely to receive adequate pain management (Hoover, 2021).

Health Disparities in the Lesbian, Gay, Bisexual, Transgender, and Queer or Questioning (LGBTQ+) Population

Arguably one of the most significant areas of current increased awareness and relevance to family health in North America relates to families in which one or more members identify as lesbian, gay, bisexual, transgender, queer or questioning (LGBTQ+). These families characterize a growing number of households in the United States (U.S. Census Bureau, 2015). Some estimates from these data suggest that there has been as much as a 51.8% increase in the number of formal same-sex households from the previous decade, although the prevalence in the overall population is still quite small, at approximately 1.5% of U.S. households. Approximately 17% of these households have children, with a majority being biological children (U.S. Census Bureau, 2015). This prevalence is significant because, with the federal definition of family currently changing, these couples and parents face several challenges with insurance access, financial benefits and death planning, decision-making abilities, and other key policy-related family health challenges.

The number of Canadians who identify as LGBTQ+ is estimated to be 3% to 5% of the population, although this is likely a vast underrepresentation of the size of the actual population (Rainbow Health Ontario [RHO], 2020). While Canada has made significant progress over the past 20 years in passing legislation that protects the rights of LGBTQ+ populations, disparities in social and health outcomes persist. Heteronormative, monosexual, and/or cis-normative language and assumptions continue to dominate the realms of policy development, education, and social/clinical health services delivery. Both LGBTQ+ Canadians and Americans encounter homophobic/biphobic/transphobic forms of discrimination, harassment, and violence in schools, the workplace, health care environments, and often in their social circles and/or families of origin when they come out (RHO, 2020). While Canadians have more options for legal recourse than their American counterparts, the physical, material, and social implications of these forms of discrimination and violence are similar on both sides of the border.

Individuals who identify as LGBTQ+ experience significant differences in health-seeking and health-promoting behaviors as a result of their erasure from programs, policies, and practices. They are far more likely to delay accessing health care for an acute medical need. They are less likely to receive preventive screenings such as mammograms, PAP smears, and/or colonoscopies. They are far less likely to receive and/or seek relevant sexual health education. They are far less likely to receive reproduction-related education and counseling (RHO, 2020). These factors, in conjunction with the negative impact of ongoing experiences of stigma and discrimination, produce a wide range of specific health disparities, including increased rates of anxiety, depression, and suicidality; suicide completion; traumatic injuries; substance use; involvement in teen pregnancy; sexually transmitted infections such as syphilis and HIV; and increased rates of particular cancers and other chronic conditions (RHO, 2020).

Researchers have shown that family support has a significant impact on the mental health outcomes for LGBTQ+ youth, dramatically reducing the incidence of suicidality and suicide completion (RHO, 2020). To combat these individual and family health problems, San Francisco State University completed a significant family-based intervention project to assist families to develop skills and attributes of acceptance, particularly among families with high degrees of religiosity (Ryan et al., 2010). Their Family Acceptance Project provided an entire evidence-based family intervention plan and resources available to the general public, along with links to peer-reviewed research aimed to assist families. Efforts such as these that aim to assist families at the individual and community levels, in combination with systems of health research, provide an important link between family policy development and LGBTQ+ individual and family health issues.

Race and Ethnicity

Socioeconomic disparities, such as lower income levels and poor access to high-quality jobs, contribute directly to health disparities, which disproportionately affect racial and ethnically diverse individuals, including people of Indigenous and First Nation status (Muhammad et al., 2019). Recent Canadian data show that the health of non-European immigrants of color deteriorates over time, whereas the health of European immigrants is superior to that of Canadian-born residents. Hispanic and Latino men are three times as likely to contract HIV as White men, and Latino populations are disproportionately affected by HIV, accounting for nearly 20% of new infections in the United States (CDC, 2015). Other examples of disparities based on race and ethnicity are as follows: Blacks, Native American, and Puerto Rican infants have higher death rates than White infants; Blacks, Hispanics, Native American, and Alaska Natives are twice as likely to have diabetes than non-Hispanic Whites; and Hispanic and Black older adults are less likely than non-Hispanic Whites to receive influenza and pneumococcal vaccines (CDC, 2015).

In addition, racial and ethnic disparities in access to and quality of health care are persistent and contribute to negative health outcomes among communities of color. In a large sample study assessing multiple measures of perceived racial and ethnic discrimination among individuals of color in Chicago medical settings, 40% of participants reported discrimination that affected the quality of the care they received, limited the time they spent with providers, and resulted in them not being involved with decision making (Benjamins & Middleton, 2019). Other recent studies indicate that although diverse and vulnerable populations are more likely to require health care, they are less likely to receive health services. Even when access is equal, diverse vulnerable populations are far less likely to receive surgical or other therapies, giving nurses an opportunity to advocate for clients who are faced with discrimination in the system and ensure that they receive the same care and treatment as everyone else (CDC, 2015).

Chronic Illness

Chronic illness is a determinant that leads to health disparities, especially in the face of poverty, and often results in poor quality of life and increased financial strain. This is heightened for persons who have no or limited access to health care and other resources. In severe cases, chronic illness leads to the inability to work and therefore forces persons who are ill to rely on the social safety net. Despite improvements in treatment and management strategies for chronic illness and the resulting improvements in both quantity and quality of life, social determinants continue to place disadvantaged populations at risk of poor outcomes from chronic illness. The presence of chronic illness is itself a determinant that leads to health disparities for and between families. If one family member is ill, then the whole family is affected and often must pick up the financial and care burden. This is true for the United States and Canada, where many medications and access to home care, for example, are not covered by universal health care. The following section explores several common chronic illnesses (type 2 diabetes, substance use and abuse, asthma and other lung diseases) and the ways that they are influenced by one's race, ethnicity, economic status (namely poverty), residency, age, or gender. While these conditions are not the only chronic illnesses that are influenced by factors increasing health disparities, all of these conditions would benefit from a systems and individualized approach to care.

Obesity in the United States and Canada

One of the most disturbing trends in health across North America over the past decade has been the increase in the proportion of the population that is overweight or obese. Obesity is defined as a body mass index (BMI) at or above the 95th percentile of the sex-specific BMI, according to the CDC's BMI-for-age growth charts (CDC, 2020b). BMI is calculated as weight in kilograms or pounds divided by the square of height in meters or feet/inches. Individuals struggling with obesity are more likely than those of recommended BMIs to suffer from heart disease, stroke, diabetes, gallstones, sleep apnea, and some types of cancer (CDC, 2020).

Hypertension, musculoskeletal problems, and arthritis tend to be more severe in people who are obese. Obesity increased little in the U.S. population between the early 1960s and 1980. Fifteen percent of North American adults were obese in the mid- to late 1970s. Since 1980, however, obesity has increased dramatically in the United States. Between 1999-2000 through 2017-2018, the prevalence of obesity increased from 30.5% to 42.4% and the prevalence of severe obesity increased from 4.7% to 9.2% (CDC, 2021). The highest prevalence of obesity in adults was among non-Hispanic Black adults (49.6%), followed by Hispanic adults (44.8%), non-Hispanic White adults (42.2%), and non-Hispanic Asian adults (17.4%) (CDC, 2021).

It should be noted that changing the narrative about obesity is extremely important. Losing weight is no longer considered a measurement of willpower but rather a complex multisystem approach to a chronic illness. Researchers, for example, have identified multiple genes responsible for obesity and have identified multiple other chronic conditions associated with obesity. Social stigma and shaming a person for having obesity is another form of ism and prevents compassionate and effective care (Ryan et al., 2018).

Along with these changes, the breastfeeding rates in the United States continue to increase, from 71% of mothers breastfeeding their newborns in 2000 to 84% in 2017 (CDC, 2020a). One of the benefits to breastfeeding is a reduced risk for obesity later in life. Although the American Academy of Pediatrics (2021) recommends breastfeeding for the first six months of life, only 50% of mothers continue to breastfeed their babies this long. The rate of breastfeeding also declines with income, with 95% of mothers in the United States breastfeeding if their income is above 400% of the federal poverty level (FPL) compared to 71% of mothers breastfeeding if their income is below the FPL. Other factors affecting breastfeeding rates include higher rates with higher education and older mothers (CDC, 2020a).

Although the modest improvement in obesity rates is a positive change, childhood obesity remains of deep concern because one in eight children remain obese, with one in five Black children and one in six Hispanic children being obese. Boys and girls have been historically about equal in their likelihood to be overweight, but between 2007 and 2008 a higher percentage of boys (21.2%) were obese than girls (17.3%). Mexican American and African American teenagers are more likely to be overweight than are non-Hispanic White teenagers. Between 2007 and 2008, the percentage of overweight Mexican American teenagers was 24.2% compared with 22.4% for Blacks and 17.4% for Whites (Federal Interagency Forum on Child and Family Statistics, 2014). Obesity costs the United States health care system an estimated $147 billion a year, and those costs are climbing based on the projection that nearly half of adults will be obese by 2030 (Ward et al., 2019). The rising costs of obesity also impact indirect costs associated with morbidity and mortality which can be difficult to estimate, including losses from work productivity, short- and long-term disability, absenteeism, permanent work loss, and premature death (Goettler et al., 2017).

Obesity and Canadian Children

Obesity rates are lower in Canada than in the United States, but Canadian rates have also increased rapidly in recent years. Approximately 24% of Canadian adults were obese in the period from 2007 to 2009 (Shields et al., 2011). In contrast with the United States, men in Canada were more likely to be obese than women. Trends in the incidence of obesity are now similar for both; between 2007 and 2009, 24.3% of men and 23.9% of women were obese in Canada (Shields et al., 2011).

Obesity among Canadian children has nearly tripled in the last three decades (Government of Canada, 2019). However, the numbers may be coming down due to health promotion efforts, from 35% of children aged 2–17 who were overweight or obese in 2004 to 30% of children aged 5–17 in 2018 (Government of Canada, 2019). Of these children who had excess weight, 28.5% were boys and 16.9% were girls. Children who are obese experience many physical health conditions and socioemotional challenges, which demonstrates the links between health and overall development. Children who suffer from overweight and obesity are at higher risk for asthma, type 2 diabetes, and heart disease (Government of Canada, 2019). In addition, children who are obese are bullied and teased more than other children and often suffer from isolation, depression, and lower self-esteem (Sutin et al., 2018). Childhood obesity is a well-known precursor to obesity in adulthood.

Recommendations to Address Obesity

As noted, the most common recommendations for the treatment of obesity across America have focused on individual behavioral changes, including increased physical exercise and changes in dietary intake or healthy eating. Although healthy diets and exercise are part of the solution to the obesity epidemic, a broader view that encompasses macro-level community approaches and exo-level or government interventions also are being explored. Communities are enhancing bike and walking trails with added green space to encourage exercise, funding of childhood and adult sports through community programs, and making grassroots changes to school meals in an attempt to change obesity rates at the community level. During the Obama administration, changes in school-provided meals with improved nutrition were put into effect through the Healthy, Hunger-Free Kids Act of 2010. While the recommendations were based on evidence that increased fruits and vegetables; increased whole grains; and a limit on high-fat and flavored milk, sodium, and high-fat snacks would contribute to decreasing obesity rates and malnutrition in children, the Trump administration rolled back these changes in 2018 (Kogan, 2019).

Researchers have documented the success of other community-based interventions to combat obesity rates, yet professionals continued to focus on microsystem, or individual, interventions. For example, Melius (2015) reviewed 51 articles in social work journals looking for evidence that community-based interventions were being supported and evaluated. Her conclusions were that social workers continue to focus on individual interventions with very little effort to support community or policy-based changes. In preparation for this chapter, a thorough search of the literature to find research conducted by nurses on interventions for obesity rates at a community or policy level found similar results.

It is important to consider social and policy factors that contribute to body size, including lack of access to healthy foods, unsafe neighborhoods with limited facilities for physical exercise, and cultural beliefs and attitudes about weight and health, in order to begin making needed and lasting changes at a family policy level. Overall, we know that losing weight reduces and sometimes corrects many health disorders, including type 2 diabetes; cardiovascular diseases; joint deterioration and pain; reproductive complications; and other complications from surgeries and other medical conditions, including COVID-19. Correcting obesity also helps to treat mental health disorders, such as depression and anxiety from low self-esteem, and institutional and personal racism from public rejection, decreased employment opportunities, and increased risk for poverty (Ryan et al., 2018). Interventions cannot stop at individualized interventions alone. Nurses have to look at policy changes at the local and national levels, including filling in the gap in research, and helping to change community and social policies to augment individual care.

Type 2 Diabetes

The prevalence of type 2 diabetes in both Canada and the United States has been steadily increasing over the last 20 years and is disproportionately affecting communities living in poverty or people from diverse ethnic and racial communities. African Americans, Hispanic/Latinos, and Asian populations all have a higher incident rate of type 2 diabetes compared to White populations (Meng et al., 2016). Indigenous peoples living in Canada are among the highest-risk populations for diabetes and related complications (Diabetes Canada, 2018). These realities show the complex, multilayered relationships between poverty, racism, and poor health status.

Researchers have shown that a diet in high-glycemic index foods can increase the risk of developing type 2 diabetes (Diabetes Canada, 2018). High-glycemic foods are carbohydrates that are easily and quickly used by the body for energy, leading to a faster rise in blood sugar and insulin secretion from the pancreas. Over time, the spikes and dives in blood sugar caused by these foods can impair the body's ability to produce and/or respond to insulin, causing type 2 diabetes. Foods with a high glycemic index are often processed foods, such as white bread, breakfast cereals, white pasta, and potato chips. Diabetes prevention and health promotion efforts focus on encouraging people to make healthier choices in the grocery store and at mealtimes and to select whole-grain foods and fruits and vegetables. However, processed food is often much cheaper to purchase than whole foods, limiting the choices people with limited economic means can make in the supermarket (Diabetes Canada, 2018). This has caused a nutritional divide across income lines that puts people with lower income at greater risk for developing this chronic disease.

Similarly, health promotion efforts encouraging exercise to prevent type 2 diabetes presuppose that individuals have access within their communities to green spaces and community centers that are geographically and socially accessible. North American researchers have found that even when neighborhoods have accessible parks, residents are less likely to utilize the space for leisure activities if they feel unsafe due to gang or drug activity (Chien et al., 2017). Walkability, pedestrian safety, pollution, built amenities, and safety all play a role in whether green spaces in urban environments are used by community members. U.S. and Canadian parks near or in urban, impoverished communities have also been found to be smaller and have fewer amenities (Parks Canada, 2019). This shows how the ability to choose an active lifestyle is mediated and constrained by particular social and socioenvironmental realities, highlighting the impact of social constructions of race, class, and residency on health inequities.

Researchers have found evidence that worry and chronic stress, which lead to high cortisol levels, play a role in chronic disease (Herriot et al., 2018). Chronic stress disproportionately affects most diverse and ethnic groups, who are often subject to discrimination and the constant worries attached to low incomes. When people have to cope with the added expenses of the illness, it increases stress further, creating a cycle and exacerbating chronic illness. For example, the experience of racial discrimination for Indigenous adults in Canada is associated with a linear increase in chronic stress; having Indigenous cultural continuity had a protective effect on lowering chronic stress (Currie et al., 2020). As stated earlier, the social determinants that create health disparities are multilayered, complex, and mutually reinforcing.

Substance Use and Abuse

The prevalence of legal and illegal drug use, the particular drugs used, and the methods in which they are taken vary considerably based on a person's race, ethnicity, residence or neighborhood, social and economic factors, and region of the country. Substance use and abuse presents family nurses with the challenge of understanding the prevalence of the problem, recognizing the social determinants of and inequities regarding health, and the laws surrounding various drugs. Nurses also have the capacity to identify effective treatment approaches. In 2013, an estimated 24.6 million North Americans, or 9.4% of the population, over the age of 12 reported using an illicit drug in the last month (National Institute on Drug Abuse, 2015). The use of marijuana has increased from 14.5 million (5.8% of those over the age of 12) to 19.8 million (7.5% of those over the age of 12). Methamphetamine use is on the rise, with an increase from 353,000 in 2010 to 1.6 million people in 2017 (National Institute on Drug Abuse, 2018). Drug use is highest in people between 18 and 20 years of age, with 22.6% of the population reporting drug use (National Institute on Drug Abuse, 2018). However, drug use is increasing in those who are in their fifties and sixties, which is thought to be related to baby boomer population (National Institute on Drug Abuse, 2018).

In this section, we review the use of alcohol, marijuana, and opioids, emphasizing the socially acceptable use of alcohol that complicates the controversies in the United States surrounding marijuana, and the opioids addiction among White North Americans. Although drinking by underage persons from 12 to 20 years initially declined between 2002 and 2013, from 28.8% to 22.7%, the rate has increased significantly, to 39.7% of this age group over the next six years (National Institute on Drug Abuse, 2020). Binge drinking is more common among men (30.2%) compared to women (16.0%). Alcohol and substance abuse have serious consequences for individual health. Individuals who engage in excessive drinking are more likely to suffer from high blood pressure and to develop chronic diseases, such as liver cirrhosis, pancreatitis, and different types of cancers (National Institute on Drug Abuse, 2020). Excessive drinking also affects psychological health. In addition, substance abuse causes unintentional injuries produced by car accidents, drowning, falls, and other types of incidents (National Institute on Drug Abuse, 2020).

The Opioid Crisis in the United States

The current opioid epidemic stands as a powerful reminder that health disparities arise from inadequate and inappropriate policies and includes people from diverse racial, ethnic, economic, and educational backgrounds. Opioids are a class of drugs that includes heroin and prescribed pain relievers, including oxycodone, hydrocodone, codeine, morphine, fentanyl, and other combinations and extended-release formulations (e.g., OxyContin) (American Society of Addiction Medicine, 2016).

The opioid crisis of today, which has caused a decrease in life expectancy since 1998, began in the mid-1990s due to a series of health care policies that led to the unintended consequence of a national epidemic of addiction, related health problems, and death due to opioid addictions. Many believe that the epidemic started with the 1996 recommendation by the Joint Commission on Accreditation of Healthcare Organizations that pain be monitored as a fifth vital sign. This recommendation led to the approval two years later by the Food and Drug Administration of the opioid pain reliever OxyContin (oxycodone hydrocholoride—extended release), which in turn added to the rapid increase in opioid prescriptions and related addictions. OxyContin is used to treat pain 24 hours per day as an extended-release formula rather than as a short-acting pain medication that typically lasts three to four hours, in an attempt to decrease the abuse potential.

During the same period, insurance companies were limiting the coverage of behavioral pain therapy, and pharmaceutical companies were evolving the delivery systems for their pain medication to increase the potential of extended-release medications. In addition, physician incentive programs designed by pharmaceutical companies to encourage prescribing opioid medications, and a large number of physicians who prescribed opioid medications at dangerous rates, including (1) prescribing for chronic rather than acute pain, (2) providing more opioid medication than what was needed, and (3) using opioid prescriptions to treat intermittent and/or mild to moderate pain that would be better managed through other medications and nonpharmaceutical methods (i.e., position changes and heat/ice), helped fuel the epidemic. This growth in opioid addictions resulted in a staggering increase in overdoses and long-term health problems associated with opioid addiction.

One of the groups most affected during the early stages of the epidemic were White women with private-care physicians (Dasgupta et al., 2018). By 2015, over 2 million North Americans were addicted to prescription pain relievers compared to 591,000 heroin use disorders (American Society of Addiction Medicine, 2016). White women were more likely to be prescribed addictive opioid medications for chronic pain and at higher doses than White men. Forty-eight thousand women died of prescription pain opioid overdoses between 1999 and 2010 (American Society of Addiction Medicine, 2016). Similarly, Black males were found to be prescribed more opioids than other ethnic groups for chronic pain (Dasgupta et al., 2018.). Native Americans also have a high rate of opioid addiction and related deaths compared to other ethnic groups. Regardless of race, opioid use and abuse is a "disease of despair" with a combination of negative events, such as chronic pain, economic disadvantage, depression, and complex illnesses such as obesity, that further increase the risk of opioid misuse (Dasgupta et al., 2018).

Around 2010, the first efforts to limit the medical use of opioids and the reformulating of medications to make them less likely to be misused led to a second wave of the epidemic. This wave saw a precipitous rise in the number of heroin overdoses as people who had become dependent on opioids became more tolerant of medical dosing and the supply of prescription medications became scarce. Individuals abusing opioids turned into individuals abusing heroin to avoid painful withdrawal symptoms from prescription opioids (Dasgupta et al., 2018). In fact, four of five heroin users started out misusing prescription painkillers (American Society of Addiction Medicine, 2016; CDC, 2013).

The response to the opioid epidemic in suburban and rural White communities stands in stark contrast to the so-called war on drugs of the 1970s and 1980s. The war on drugs focused on increased law enforcement and resulted in mass arrests and incarceration of racial minorities. Interventions tended to treat addiction as a series of poor choices on the part of the drug user rather than treating the underlying causes and the medical condition (Mendoza et al., 2016). This approach is strikingly different from the one employed during the current epidemic, which includes a variety of prevention and harm reduction efforts, including prescription drug monitoring programs, takeback programs, widespread distribution of opioid overdose reversal medications, and Good Samaritan laws (Dasgupta et al., 2018).

Today, opioid-related deaths continue, and addiction to opioids is not dropping as planned. Analysis of why this epidemic continues despite multilayered policies instituted in efforts to stop the epidemic includes the realization that our health care system in North America continues to function on volume rather than depth of care, and it labels addiction more as a crime and character flaw than as a negative health syndrome. If we replaced efficiency in care and rapid treatment of pain with acknowledgment of the complexity of treating suffering or, even better, the importance of compassion (Dasgupta et al., 2018), we would be better able to apply evidence-based treatment programs. Methadone treatment programs, access to experts in the field of addiction in both urban and rural areas, continued attention to at-risk groups with associated correction of needed structural changes, increased access to treatment centers, and prolonged needed care protocols are all potential opportunities to address the opioid epidemic.

Asthma and Other Lung Diseases

According to the American Lung Association (2020), approximately 9% of adults and children in the United States report a diagnosis of asthma, and the incidence of asthma is increasing with similar reports from Canada. Direct health costs for treating asthma are estimated to be $10 billion annually. Asthma is the leading chronic illness among children and is the third leading cause of hospitalization for children younger than 15 years of age (American Lung Association, 2020). Asthma is associated with poor-quality physical environments such as regions with increased air pollution and substandard housing. Triggers for a major asthma attack include secondhand tobacco smoke, dust, pollution, cockroaches, pets, and mold. Less common triggers include exercise, extremes of weather, food, and hyperventilation (National Center for Environmental Health, 2017).

In adults, chronic obstructive pulmonary disease (COPD) and lung cancer are serious chronic diseases that shorten life and decrease its quality. Lung diseases, like all other diseases, are associated with social determinants such as poverty, as well as with considerable health care costs. For example, lung cancer is the most diagnosed cancer in Canada and is the leading cause of cancer death; more Canadians die of lung cancer than colorectal, breast, and pancreatic cancers combined (Canadian Cancer Society, 2020). In Canada, First Nations and Indigenous people are more likely to be hospitalized for a respiratory tract infection and for asthma than non-Indigenous people (Carrière et al., 2017). In the case of asthma, having a lower household income increased the rate of being hospitalized. For all Canadians, people with lower income are more likely to be diagnosed with lung cancer and more likely to be diagnosed at a later stage of disease than people with a higher income (Canadian Cancer Society, 2020).

Cancer and Heart Disease

In the United States, it is estimated that four persons out of 10 will develop cancer in their lifetime. In recent years, with improved detection and treatment, many cancers are now cured or, similar to HIV infection, can become chronic diseases that people live with for many years. In Canada, the top three causes of deaths are cancer, cardiovascular diseases, and cerebrovascular disease. Twenty-nine percent of all deaths in Canada are from heart disease (Statistics Canada, 2017). As persons with chronic illnesses live and work within their communities, they need to learn how to self-manage their conditions (see Chapter 10 for more about self-management in chronic illness). Nurses have a large role to play here as advocates and coaches when they care for individuals and families within the context of their physical and social environments. Part of the nurse's role when helping clients with chronic diseases is teaching health literacy.

Avoiding Growing Health Care Disparities

In addition to the chronic health conditions discussed previously, there are several areas within health care that can be addressed with supportive health policies designed to support vulnerable individuals and families while reducing risk for health disparities.

Elder Care

The current growth of the Baby Boomer population (born between 1946 and 1964) is one of the most significant trends in the history of the United States. While policy makers have had decades to plan, it is not clear that sufficient support will be available to meet the needs of the aging population (Mather et al., 2015). In 2016, the population of people aged 65 or over in the United States was 49.2 million (Roberts et al., 2018) and the number of Americans aged 65 or over is predicted to nearly double from 52 million in 2018 to 95 million by 2060 (Population Reference Bureau [PRB], 2021). The older adult population is also growing in diversity. Between 2018 and 2060, it is also predicted that the older non-Hispanic White population will drop from 77% to 55% (PRB, 2021).

About half of the people over 65 years (68%) in 2016 lived in family households (Roberts et al., 2018). Of those aged 65 years and older, 70% of men and 44% of women were married (Roberts et al., 2018). For the oldest age group of over 85 years, only 15% of women remained married (Roberts et al., 2018).

The provision of care to the elderly is growing both as a family responsibility and as a profession. More women are caregivers than men. Policies such as the Family and Medical Leave Act are written as gender neutral, but women experience a general expectation that they will be the caregivers regardless of the burden that such a role places on them. Lay caregivers are unpaid, which benefits social programs, especially Medicare and Medicaid. Home care in Canada is also poorly funded, and the Canadian economy benefits enormously from free labor by family members. This home care by family members has negative health outcomes for the caregivers. For example, women who provide lay home health care experience much greater levels of stress than their other family members, as well as more alienation from those outside the home (Revenson et al., 2016). Families continue to need respite care and increased home health nursing and other supports to ease caregiver burdens. Recently, some parts of Canada introduced compassionate-care benefits, which apply when the death of a family member is expected within the next 6 months. Day care for older adults and increasing funding for community-based care in the home would make it easier for older people to stay out of costly institutional care and increase their quality of life. This type of care has to include house calls by doctors, nurses, physical therapists, and other health care providers if clients are unable to go to appointments. It also has to focus on home safety (Change Foundation, 2013). Community-based care in the home could go a long way toward reducing health disparities imposed by chronic illness by providing access to optimal care for vulnerable older persons. This is another example of why it is so important to look past micro- and macrosystem care and include exosystem policies that reduce health disparities in our aging populations.

Women's Reproductive Health

Women's reproductive health is another area where shifts in social policy and programs could help stem health disparities, both in the United States and Canada. Access to birth control, including barrier methods, hormonal methods, long-acting reversible methods, and permanent sterilization, are currently mediated, to varying degrees, by the state, religious institutions, professional regulatory bodies, and each country's respective health care system. The complex interplay of competing interests, values, and policies places innumerable barriers to accessing timely and appropriate reproductive and sexual health care for women. For example, nearly half of the pregnancies in the United States are unintended (Kaitz et al., 2019), yet Medicaid policies related to publicly funded tubal ligations have not changed since 1978 (Borrero et al., 2014). Medicaid requires all women who qualify for coverage to complete the consent to sterilization section of the Medicaid Title XIX form at least 30 days and no more than 180 days before undergoing the procedure. While it is possible to waive the 30-day requirement, a minimum of 72 hours is required between the request and the procedure. This prevents women who desire sterilization immediately following birth to be denied access to this procedure in the direct postpartum period.

Similarly, some pharmacists have refused to fill prescriptions for contraceptives, including emergency contraception, stating that doing so is in direct conflict with their moral and personal beliefs (The Guttmacher Institute, 2017). In these circumstances, women's legal right to access prescription medications is overridden by pharmacists' religious and/or moral beliefs. The Guttmacher Institute (2017) identified 45 states that have a policy allowing health care providers, including nurses and pharmacists, who conscientiously object to the delivery of reproductive health services to refuse this care to patients, without the legal requirement to refer to another provider who will. These policies severely constrain women's access to choices regarding their reproductive health.

In 2014, approximately 30% of women in the United States had an abortion before the age of 45 (Jones & Jerman, 2017). The total number of abortion providers declined 4% from 2008 to 2011. Forty-four laws to limit access to abortions were implemented from 2008 to 2010 in 18 states. That number increased to over 400 laws across several states to limit abortions by 2020 (Ellman, 2020). These laws served to stigmatize abortion and contribute to a climate of fear among women. While the rates of abortion have continually declined from 2009 to 2020, the biggest decline is in female individuals under the age of 18 years (Kortsmit et al., 2020).

In contrast, the Supreme Court of Canada ruled in 1988 that Canada's abortion law was unconstitutional, violating a pregnant person's charter rights to life, liberty, and security of person. It was struck from the federal criminal code at this time, leaving Canada free of any criminal law restricting abortion. This court decision redefined abortion as a medical procedure, leaving Canada as one of the few countries in the world that has no abortion restrictions enshrined in law. Since decriminalization, estimated abortion rates in Canada suggest there are approximately 100,000 abortions per year, the vast majority occurring in the first 12 weeks of pregnancy (Shaw & Normal, 2020). Nationally collected data shows that access to these services varies widely from province to province, with extremely limited to no abortion services available in the eastern provinces and the northern territories to a high number of abortion services available in Quebec, Ontario, and British Columbia (Shaw & Norman, 2020). Many women (for example, undocumented immigrants) must travel long distances to obtain an abortion and/or pay hundreds of dollars out of pocket for the procedure if they do not have provincial health care coverage. These geographic and cost barriers continue to pose significant challenges to equitable access to abortion services in Canada.

COVID-19: A System Under Stress

The risk of serious illness and death due to the Sars-CoV-2 (COVID-19) virus is now well known. Health care providers are at a higher risk than the general public due to their close proximity and increased exposure to ill patients (Kambhampati et al., 2020). COVID-NET, a national program designed to survey laboratory-confirmed COVID-19 cases in 99 counties and 14 states in the United States, found that out of 6,760 individuals who tested positive for COVID-19 and were hospitalized, 438 were health care providers (HCPs). Of interest is that the highest proportion of infected HCPs were nurses, at 36% of this sample (Kambhampati et al., 2020). The next highest group of infected HCPs were nurses' aides, at 8%, and physicians, at 5% of this sample. Of these nurses, 89% had an underlying condition, with 73% being obese. Despite the average age (49 years) of these nurses being younger than the identified vulnerable age of over 60 years for COVID-19 infection, 28% were treated in intensive-care units, and 4% died. Nurses across the country have shared their stories of being in one of the highest at-risk occupations and their experiences of being frontline HCPs in a system in crisis. Their care is guided by a strong commitment to care for their patients, despite the risk to themselves, their family members, and their friends from cross exposure. Nurses are not only faced with the ethical dilemmas of risking the health of themselves and those close to them, but they are also faced with being a nurse during a pandemic that has many other risks. A study of 13 qualitative studies looking at nurses' responses to providing care during respiratory pandemics over the past 20 years revealed several themes that hold true during the COVID-19 pandemic (Fernandez et al., 2020):

1. Nurses are expected to take on the risk of exposure more than other health care providers, including physicians.
2. Nursing shortages caused by many nurses leaving the workforce due to fear of exposure and being vulnerable (i.e., being older, having underlying conditions, or having vulnerable family members) and the infection rate and hospitalization rate surpassing nursing availability result in nurses working longer hours, working outside their area of expertise, and working with fewer days off. This burden results in sleep deprivation and heavy workloads.
3. Nurses face fear of litigation from having to ration care due to staff and equipment shortages and related inadequate care.

Because knowledge about the contagion changes rapidly, policies change rapidly, leaving nurses with inadequate information and training to provide quality care.
4. Nurses face isolation from family and friends as they try to protect these loved ones from exposure.

What this study did not mention is the vicarious trauma so many nurses are reporting during the COVID-19 pandemic. This vicarious trauma is caused by watching large numbers of patients dying and dying alone without family support. Nurses are facing death in emergency rooms, hospital hallways, makeshift medical units, and intensive care units. Nurses are exhausted with working long hours; facing death every day; and constantly worrying about personal health, family health, and broad community and global health while the public doubts the very existence of the pandemic (Remnick, 2020). Many nurses cry in anguish as protesters resist CDC recommendations to wear masks, wash hands, and social-distance because they live the consequences of ignoring these guidelines. Federal and state policies that distribute personal protective equipment (PPE), distribute ventilators and other medical equipment, support or discourage CDC guidelines, restrict or open high-risk businesses, and fund vaccine development and distribution directly affect nurses' emotional, psychological, spiritual, and physical health. Despite the risks to nurses, most nurses continue to work overtime to care for their patients, despite risks to themselves and their close family and friends. Nurses as a group illustrate the importance of unified federal and state programs to minimize health risks to vulnerable populations.

Although Canada's response to the pandemic has differed from that of the United States, COVID-19 has highlighted the impact of privatization, health care funding policies, and the lack of a coordinated public health response on Canadian families. Between 62% and 82% of deaths from COVID-19 in Canada were residents of continuing-care homes, which include long-term care facilities, nursing homes, and supportive living facilities (Holroyd-Leduc & Laupacis, 2020). Compared to the hospital sector, which is almost exclusively publicly funded, privately managed and for-profit continuing care existed in Canada well before the pandemic. As COVID-19 began to spread widely across the country, many continuing-care organizations failed to change their staffing models (e.g., mandating that employees work only in one home), provide pandemic pay, ensure basic protective equipment, and alter the physical layout of facilities (e.g., erecting physical barriers) (Armstrong et al., 2020). Privately run continuing-care facilities in Canada managed COVID-19 more poorly than publicly run organizations because of their lack of accountability, lack of regulation, and for-profit aims, which led to public outrage. The COVID-19 crisis may represent a turning point for Canadians who will need to reflect on their commitment to supporting publicly funded continuing and long-term care.

Health Literacy

Health literacy is identified in the *Healthy People 2030* objectives as the degree to which individuals have the ability to find, understand, and use health-related information that they can use to make informed decisions about their health (USDHHS, 2020). This definition has been expanded to include individual and community knowledge, decision-making ability, problem-solving skills, critical reflection, and the ability to know about and use community resources that enhance health outcomes (Jimenez, 2018). For example, health literacy includes the ability to understand and carry out instructions for self-administered medical treatments and make the decision of when, how often, and if a medication should be taken; make lifestyle adjustments to improve health status; make decisions related to health care for self, family members, and the community; and understand when and how to access appropriate and timely health services. Health literacy is one of the social determinants that is a major contributor to health disparities because it mediates both individuals' access to and use of critically important health information. Health literacy is a product of health promotion and education efforts, which change across time, with changes in accessibility of resources, funding, and opportunity. Health literacy also changes with expertise, cultural influences, the age of individuals, and the longevity of communities (Jimenez, 2018).

Low health literacy is a significant problem in both Canada and the United States. IOM found that approximately 9 out of 10 adults have difficulty understanding health information (IOM, 2011). Fifty-five percent of working-age adult Canadians, and 88% of people over the age of 65, have inadequate health literacy skills (Canadian Public Health Association [CPHA], 2014). Several factors may influence an individual's health literacy in North America, including one's socioeconomic status, level of education, age, linguistic competency in English, and cognitive abilities. Adults living below the poverty level have lower health literacy than those living above the poverty line. Those who have not graduated high school, those whose first language is not English, or those who are neuro-atypical similarly have lower health literacy than their counterparts. These disparities illuminate the connections between education opportunities, employment, and social engagement with the cultivation of both basic and higher-level cognitive and social skills.

Low health literacy has been linked to lower adherence to healthy lifestyles, lower participation in health-screening programs, poorer management of chronic disease, poorer adherence to medical regimens and protocols, less participation in community groups, less use of primary-care services, and increased use of emergency and urgent-care services (CPHA, 2014). All of these result in poorer health outcomes, including higher incidences of chronic disease, increased medication dosing and scheduling errors, increased complications associated with chronic disease, and increased morbidity and mortality from health conditions experienced by the elderly (CPHA, 2014).

Health literacy is one of the social determinants that contributes to health disparities. Although a relationship between health disparities and health literacy has been established, it is complex. Up to 60% of individuals living in Canada are unable to understand, obtain, or access information in order to make positive health decisions on their own. Older adults, immigrants, and unemployed people have been found to have higher rates of health illiteracy compared to other groups (ABC Life Literacy Canada, 2021). Individuals with low health literacy do not understand health information, which affects their health outcomes disproportionately because they seek fewer health screenings, use urgent or emergency care, experience errors in medication dosing and scheduling, lack alternatives in treatment regimens, and are unable to access accurate health-related information.

As educators and advocates, nurses must consider the health literacy of the patients and families whom they serve (Coleman et al., 2017). Explaining health-related concepts in plain language helps to ensure that patients understand the information correctly. Nurses may also assist families with filling out complicated forms when they are applying for social support or filing insurance claims.

THE URBAN/RURAL DIVIDE

Rural communities pose a growing challenge to the health and well-being of their residents. The rural challenges facing Canada will be used as an exemplar of factors influencing health disparities in rural areas across America. The number of individuals residing in rural and remote communities across Canada has declined significantly over the past 100 years and currently represents only 18% of the Canadian population. A higher proportion of these rural dwellers are concentrated in the Atlantic provinces and the Northern Territories, particularly Prince Edward Island and Nunavut (Statistics Canada, 2017). Rural dwellers include those living in nonmetropolitan cities (less than 10,000 people), small towns, sparsely populated regions, and remote communities that have limited or no road access. Most remote communities in Canada are Indigenous communities, comprised of First Nations, Metis, or Inuit peoples. Their cultural practices, spoken languages, spiritual beliefs, and traditional foods are incredibly diverse. These communities must rely on boats, trains, and planes to access resources in the late fall, winter, and early spring seasons when flooding, snow, and ice make roads impassable.

Demographic information about Canada's rural and remote populations are regionally specific, although there are a few notable trends. Many rural communities are aging and losing their young people to larger metropolitan areas. The national census data show that people between 15 and 29 years of age make up less than 17% of rural populations compared to 20% of urban populations (Statistics Canada, 2017). The exception to this trend is Nunavut, which has the youngest population in Canada and an exceptionally small elderly population. The outmigration of young people from rural and remote communities is attributed to the pursuit of postsecondary education and/or better employment opportunities in urban centers. This is causing household size to decrease in rural communities, on average, by almost one-quarter. In 1981, the average household was three persons, but it is now much closer to two persons per household (Morris et al., 2020). This decrease in average household size threatens to erode the informal social fabric of rural communities that has been found to serve as a protective factor against social isolation and loneliness for many (Smith-Carrier, 2019). Offsetting this trend has proven challenging for municipal and provincial governments. While Canada continues to welcome hundreds of thousands of immigrants and refugees each year, a relatively small percentage of immigrants settle in rural communities, preferring to stay in larger urban centers that have more settlement services and programs (Patel et al., 2019).The federal government recently implemented a pilot program aimed at attracting immigrants to a select number of rural and northern communities, but this program remains in its infancy and has not yet released any outcomes data (GOC, 2019).

The primary economic activities of Canadian rural and remote communities are wide-ranging and regionally specific, spanning agriculture, natural resource extraction (fishing, forestry, petroleum, and mining), manufacturing, and tourism, among others. The job market in rural Canada has become increasingly precarious as larger factory farms have replaced smaller family farms, long-standing mines have closed, the number of manufacturing jobs has declined, and climate change has affected natural resource industries. Current employment opportunities in rural and remote parts of Canada are often part-time, low-wage, and contractual or seasonal, with limited to no health/pension benefits, leaving many to struggle to make ends meet (Smith-Carrier, 2019). Annual incomes of rural dwellers have been found to be 14% lower than the national average. The threat of financial insufficiency is further compounded by the significantly higher costs of living in low density and/or remote geographic locations, particularly for electricity, water, and food. Calls to reform the federal employment insurance program, nationalize electricity support programs, and expand the federal nutrition north Canada subsidy program to ease the cost of living for rural dwellers have gone unheeded.

It is no surprise, then, that there is high prevalence of working Canadians living in poverty in rural communities and experiencing concomitant food insecurity. Almost two-thirds of all food-insecure households in Canada are reliant on salaries and wages. Poverty and food insecurity have been found to affect disproportionately remote Indigenous communities in the northern territories of Canada. The First Nations Food, Nutrition, and Environment Study found that 48% of households in remote Indigenous communities across Canada are food insecure, which is four times higher than the national average of 12% (Chan et al., 2014). This study also found that the price of food in areas more than 50 kilometers away from major urban centers is two to three times higher, making a nutritious diet out of reach for many. The realities of climate change, including thinning ice and changing migration patterns due to weather changes, are making the supplementation of purchased foodstuffs with locally procured food (through hunting, fishing, foraging, and agricultural practices) increasingly difficult (Howard & Edge, 2013).

The consequences of the social, economic, and material realities of rural and remote communities is that their populations have higher incidences of chronic disease, mental illness and suicidality, injury, nutritional insufficiency, and lower life expectancy rates than their urban counterparts (Bosco & Oandasan, 2016). Many rural and remote communities experience chronic shortages of family doctors and nurse practitioners, forcing residents to travel long distances to access primary care, emergency services, and/or medical specialists. Health care delivery is primarily focused on downstream effects, or the treatment of illness or crisis intervention, rather than health promotion, disease prevention, or rehabilitation (Smith-Carrier, 2019). While inroads have been made in improving access to medical care through telemedicine and e-health innovations, there remains a significant digital divide along geographic and socioeconomic lines in Canada. In 2018, the Canadian Radio Television and Telecommunications Commission (CRTTC, 2018) found that 63% of rural households did not have access to internet services at the speed required to participate in the modern digital economy. In northern Indigenous communities, this number was found to be even higher, at 75% (CRTTC, 2018). This

has particularly stark implications in the context of the COVID-19 pandemic, when Canadians are being asked to flatten the curve by working from home, having their children educated remotely, and acquiring goods/accessing services online instead of in person. Without high-speed Wi-Fi, these measures become an impossibility for rural dwellers, increasing their vulnerability not only to this highly communicable disease but also to increasing economic, social, educational, and informational gaps (Open Media, 2020).

In addition to challenges caused by living in rural areas, Indigenous peoples may be susceptible to the health inequities caused by the migration to urban areas because of the history of colonization and the Canadian government's failure to uphold its legal commitment to support Indigenous health across multiple settings. Indigenous people who live in urban settings represent the fastest growing segment of the Indigenous population. The 2016 census found that 39% (Single Nations) to 43% (Aboriginal) Indigenous individuals lived in metropolitan communities (Statistics Canada, 2016). Results of a population survey suggest a decline in health care use and self-reported health status for Indigenous peoples related to urbanization (Wrathall et al., 2020). This decline may be related to jurisdictional disputes about health care coverage, systemic racism, and a lack of equity-oriented health services. For example, a survey of Indigenous health users in Toronto, Canada's largest city, suggest that 28.5% experienced discrimination by a health care provider and that 27.3% perceived that their health needs were not met (Kitching et al., 2020).

Relationships to land and nature, which is a determinant of health for many Indigenous peoples, have been viewed as challenging to achieve in an urban context with shrinking green and public spaces, growing commercialization, and environmental degradation (Hatala et al., 2019). However, there is a growing contemporary movement of Indigenous grassroots organizations seeking to recover and return to land-based practices and to return to urban spaces to healing, wellness, and belonging. This movement is supported by the emergence of Indigenous-run, community-based organizations across the country, such as the Metis First Nations Friendship Centre in Saskatoon, which exemplifies the distinctiveness of urban Indigenous identities (Neale, 2017). Such organizations often require formal and ongoing support from the Canadian government to keep their programming.

There have been some rural health policy reforms in Canada to support rural health, although much has yet to be done to support rural communities. For example, in 2017 the Canadian Collaborative Taskforce launched a Rural Road Map for Action (RRM) that reinforced the importance of education for health professionals and rural-specific health care practice models and launched a pan-Canadian rural research agenda. At the same time, few of these policy initiatives addressed the impact of the social determinants of health on rural health and the lack of research in this area (Garasia & Dobbs, 2019). The urban/rural divide in Canada remains an opportunity for further research and practice development.

HEALTH CARE POLICIES

Health Care Policies in the United States

Providing health care to families based on human rights and legal perspectives has been proposed as a strategy to promote health equity by transforming and developing policies, programs, and laws that counter the limited or restricted access of health care services to families. Social insurance and universal health care programs are modeled internationally and are generally funded through taxes. The United States has focused on providing health care through primarily private insurance companies accessed through individuals' employment and subsidized by public insurance policies for those in economic hardship positions. Political parties have made several attempts to increase public insurance to offset the large number of families left uninsured, using varying goals and values (Herrick, 2013).

President Theodore Roosevelt was one of the first presidents of the United States to attempt to enact a national health care policy, in the early 1900s (Physicians for a National Health Program, 2016). President Franklin D. Roosevelt expanded this effort by mimicking insurance plans that protect against adversity. The first social insurance policy was the Old-Age, Survivors, and Disability Insurance (OASDI) that was signed into law by President Franklin D. Roosevelt and commonly called the Social Security Act of 1935. The Social Security Act was the government's direct response to the Great Depression and offered minimum income to unemployed and retired workers. The federal government also provided survivor benefits to widows and children and services for older adults, persons who were blind, and children with disabilities. Other money was set aside for vocational therapy, public health care in rural areas, and educating public professionals.

Later, in 1939, President Roosevelt attempted to pass the Wagner National Health Act, which was taken out of the Social Security Act. Despite the collapse of the Wagner National Health Act, the study of health care remained in the Social Security Act. The passage of this New Deal policy marked one of the greatest contributions to a universal health care program in the United States. Following the enactment of the Social Security Act of 1935, the Truman administration added the Old-Age and Survivors Insurance section of this act, which provided 60 days of hospital insurance per year for retired adults ages 60 and older (Oberlander & Laugesen, 2015). It took the country until the 1960s to reexamine health care concerns at the national level. The Medicare and Medicaid Services enacted in 1966 were similar to national health care services provided to citizens in other Western countries, excepting a lower eligibility criterion, and a continued reliance on private insurance for employed workers (Kaiser Family Foundation, 2015).

Contemporary Medicare and Medicaid Services

The U.S. Centers for Medicare and Medicaid Services (2021) is the government agency in the United States with responsibility for Medicare, Medicaid, the State Children's Health Insurance Program (CHIP), the Health Insurance Portability and Accountability Act (HIPAA), and the Clinical Laboratories Improvement Amendment (CLIA). Medicare is a health insurance program for people 65 years and older, certain younger people with disabilities, and those with end-stage renal disease (ESRD). Medicare covers more than 55 million persons on an annual basis (Kaiser Family Foundation, 2015), with a growth from 19 million in 1966 to 52 million in 2012. The recent increase in the growth of Medicare recipients can be explained in large part by the number of baby boomers now aging into Medicare benefits (Kaiser Family Foundation, 2015).

There are four parts to Medicare:

- Part A provides inpatient hospital care, care in nursing facilities, hospice care, and a limited amount of home-care services (U.S. Centers for Medicare and Medicaid Services, 2021).
- Part B of the Medicare program covers some of the costs associated with physician and outpatient care, medical supplies, and preventive services.
- Known as Medicare Advantage Plans, Part C is a nongovernmental plan. Private companies hold contracts with Medicare, offering Parts A and B services. Humana Medicare Advantage is an example of a health maintenance organization that provides health insurance under contract to Medicare recipients. Other advantage plans may be organized as preferred provider organizations, private fee-for-service plans, special needs plans, and Medicare medical savings account plans.
- Part D, prescription drug coverage, is another feature of Medicare. Medicare .gov (at https://www.medicare.gov/part-d/) outlines some of the plans used to cover prescription drug costs, such as Medicare private-fee-for-services and Medicare medical savings account plans. To put prescription drug costs in context, Schondelmeyer and Purvis (2016) report that brand-name drugs used for a prolonged period of time may cost an average of $5,800 per year. For the average older adult who takes 4.5 prescription drugs on a monthly basis, the annual cost of prescription drugs may be as high as $26,000 per year. Medicare beneficiaries are allocated $24,150 for prescription drugs.

The enactment of Medicare moved health care for vulnerable populations from the responsibility of state and local governments and charitable organizations to the federal government. Medicaid, in contrast, is a federal–state partnership health insurance program for eligible groups with lower income. Different from Medicare, which is managed by the federal government, Medicaid is managed by individual states. Medicaid is not a social insurance program. It offers health care to persons living in poverty by physicians *who accept patients who rely on Medicaid*. Discussed later in this chapter, an expansion of Medicaid was a feature of the Patient Protection and Affordable Care Act (PPACA) of 2010 (or Affordable Care Act [ACA]). The federal government outlined a provision to assist citizens whose incomes fell below 138% of the federal poverty level. This would equate to $12,060 for individuals and to $24,600 for a family with four members (U.S. Centers for Medicare and Medicaid Services, 2021). Looking at the influence of the expansion of Medicaid, McMorrow et al. (2017) reported a decline in the uninsured rate for individuals whose income was below the poverty line, and childless from 45.4% in 2013 to 16.5% in 2015.

In addition to Medicare and Medicaid, CHIP was enacted in 1997 to address the lack of health insurance coverage for children who did not qualify for Medicaid (U.S. Centers for Medicare and Medicaid Services, 2021c). Similar to Medicaid, this program represents a federal–state government partnership. States have three options for implementing CHIP: (1) creating a new health care program for children, (2) building on the current Medicaid program, or (3) using some combination of these two options. According to the federal fiscal year (FFY) statistical enrollment data system report for 2019, more than 35 million children were covered by Medicaid, with an additional 9.7 million receiving health care via the CHIP program (Medicaid.gov, 2020). Overall, children's enrollment in Medicaid and CHIP decreased by 1.6% between FFY 2018 and FFY 2019, with fewer children enrolled in Medicaid (decrease of 2.1%); by contrast, there was an increase of 0.2% who were enrolled in CHIP (Medicaid.gov, 2020).

To continue to promote the well-being of children, the federal government reauthorized the CHIP program from October 1, 2017 through September 30, 2023, providing annual allotments that increase the Healthy Kids Act funding from $21.5 billion in 2018 to $25.9 billion in 2023 which will cover costs in all states (Brooks, 2018).

Also, worth noting is the Prenatal Care Assistance Program (PCAP), which targets pregnant women who meet certain income requirements and are eligible for part of the Medicaid system.

The PCAP program includes prenatal care; delivery services; postpartum care up to 2 months after the birth of the baby; referral to the Women, Infants, and Children (WIC) program; and infant care for 1 year (U.S. Department of Agriculture, 2021).

In the United States, most government health care programs are managed and delivered by individual states, with only partial monetary support by the federal program. Thus, the burden on state budgets is enormous. Some unique programs have been implemented to help individual states bridge this gap in the cost of health care coverage.

Affordable Care Act (ACA)

The United States continues to strive toward a more affordable and accessible health care system. ACA had the goal of universal health care for every citizen. The objectives of this act included:

1. decreasing the number of uninsured U.S. citizens
2. decreasing health care costs in the United States
3. improving the efficiency of health care
4. decreasing discrimination by insurance companies based on preexisting conditions
5. improving health care outcomes (Levitsky, 2013)

The intent of this act was to ensure that every American citizen be covered by health insurance through the workplace, the federal or state government (i.e., Medicare and Medicaid services), or private purchase of insurance. The ACA also ensured a Patient Bill of Rights that placed restrictions on denying insurance based on preexisting conditions and mandated that no insurance company could increase annual rates above 10% per year. The act also provided free services for expectant mothers, contraceptive care, domestic violence screening and treatment, and well-women's health care. Finally, CHIP was expanded to every state and included free well-child checks, vaccinations, vision examinations, behavioral assessment and care, and screening for autism for low-income children. Beginning in 2013, the approximately 40 million uninsured U.S. citizens were able to access health coverage through the Health Insurance Marketplace, a set of government-regulated and standardized health care plans that allowed those without insurance to submit one application to choose from multiple private-sector policies. The selection was based on their individual eligibility and ability to pay the set monthly premiums (Levitsky, 2013).

Despite much legislative and legal wrangling, the ACA was upheld by the U.S. Supreme Court in 2012, and implementation efforts began in 2013 (Kaiser Family Foundation, 2012). Although the ACA achieved its intended goals, it did not specifically intend to decrease (nor did it succeed at decreasing) health disparities as many hoped it would. Rather, the goal of U.S. citizens having access to health care insurance was achieved. The outcome still left many without the ability to pay for needed services beyond limited preventative care and without affordable health care to treat acute and chronic conditions unless they qualified for Medicaid. Even those who qualified for Medicaid or Medicare often could not find a provider willing to take state or federally funded insurance, and high deductible rates set by the insurance companies were a burden to most outside Medicare and Medicaid services. A clear distinction to consider is that access to health insurance does not guarantee access to quality, affordable, and equitable health care.

Despite the progress brought by these recent changes to the health care system, the United States continues to face health disparity. The long-standing lack of universally available health care has resulted in a return to trying to establish a health care system that meets the needs of the citizens, the insurance companies, and the providers.

Currently, there are no policies that guarantee the right to health care in the United States except for the social insurance program of Medicare and need-based programs and policies. These include Medicaid services laws prohibiting denial of health care based on discriminatory grounds. An example of this is the Emergency Medical Treatment and Active Labor Act (EMTALA), which ensures that hospitals cannot refuse to treat anyone who comes to the emergency room for care regardless if they can pay or if they have insurance coverage; however, this act has remained an unfunded mandate since its creation in 1986 (American College of Emergency Physicians, 2021). EMTALA does not guarantee diagnosis and ongoing treatment, but rather stabilization of symptoms, with the assumption that the individual will receive comprehensive care from a primary-care provider or outpatient specialist (American College of Emergency Physicians, 2021).

For family nurses, another important model of care to consider is family-focused care. This model of primary care includes the family as the client and recognizes the importance of addressing all family members when caring for an individual with health care needs. This is especially important for children with special health care needs (CSHCN) because family-focused care has been shown to improve health outcomes across time (Barnard-Brak et al., 2017). In a study conducted in California neonatal intensive care units (NICUs), parents reported challenges with receiving family-centered care, particularly those who were families of color and families with low socioeconomic status (Sigurdson et al., 2020). The investigators proposed that intentional efforts to improve family-centered care should emphasize mutual trust and power-sharing no matter what intervention is utilized (Sigurdson et al., 2020). The importance of family-focused health care cannot be overstated. Similar to many other areas of health disparity, however, underrepresented groups continue to struggle with access to high quality, equitable health interventions, leading to continued negative health outcomes.

Health Care Policies in Other Countries

Other countries, including countries in South America, South Africa, Europe, and Asia, support laws and national policies with funding to protect civil rights, political rights, and social welfare rights. Social welfare rights include security, housing, education, clean water, food, and *health care.* In spite of programs that not only cover universal health care but also face challenges such as access and treatment of HIV/AIDS, prescription medications, reproductive health care, and comprehensive preventive health care, national health care costs in these nations are consistently lower than those in the United States. The United States is unique with its ongoing struggle with whether health care should be governed by citizens' social rights versus market value and fiscal profits for those administering or providing health care. In spite of the majority of the public consistently stating that health care should be a right, there have not been any policies that reflect this opinion. Another fear that prevents universal health care policies from being passed in the United States is that, because of the expense of universal health care, health care would be rationed, which is a result of the outcome of other rationing programs across history, including rationing of food and gas during World War II and rationing of gas with long gas lines during the oil crisis of 1976. Health care, however, is already rationed through pricing, employment, and access.

Health Care Policies in Canada

By way of contrast with the United States, Canada has supported widespread, federally funded health care access for physicians' services, hospital care, and diagnostics since the 1966 Medical Care Act (Martin et al., 2018). The act has had a major influence on family policy affecting health care. It ensures that, on a national level, hospital care, doctor's visits, and diagnostic services are accessible to everyone without charge. Many people also have additional extended benefit plans through their employers for medication coverage, dental care, and other health care. Persons who are on social assistance programs, such as welfare or disability pensions, as well as those receiving old-age pensions, have additional publicly funded coverage for essential medications and basic dental care. However, these additional benefits do not extend to those working for low wages with no additional benefits and who often cannot afford their medications (Pilkington et al., 2011). Although some provincially funded coverage is available for this group, obtaining it is very difficult; it is only meant for dire situations of need and disqualifies most who work for low wages. Therefore, many families may prioritize the choice to pay the rent or mortgage or to feed their families instead of purchasing medications. Health Canada (2019), a federal government agency, released a report entitled "A Prescription for Canada" to advocate for national pharmacare and to emphasize that Canada is the only country in the world with universal health care that does not provide universal coverage for prescription drugs. National pharmacare is estimated to improve access to lifesaving medications, standardize how people obtain drugs, and ultimately reduce the overall costs of health care by billions of dollars.

Although universal health care exists in Canada, it does not cover all aspects of health. Similar to other Western countries with universal health care, there remains a gap in health care delivery for those who lack private insurance. Provinces and municipalities in Canada provide long-term care for persons in need, but access to care is a challenge because of an insufficient number of facilities and providers. Some provinces have sometimes attempted to implement user fees for doctor and emergency department visits. Because of immense public pressure, the federal government has thus far stepped in to stop this practice. One policy severely curtailing federal health care funding for refugees was implemented in 2012 by the federal government, leaving this vulnerable and often traumatized group unprotected (Service Canada, 2012). At the time, this move was seen as a major injustice by the public as well as by physicians' and nurses' associations because of the increase in the number of people seeking asylum in Canada. This act was also criticized by hospital groups and community health centers, who have voiced a strong and unified opposition to this policy. In 2016, the Liberal government, led by Prime Minister Justin Trudeau, restored federal funding for refugee health and instituted the Interim Federal Health Program (IFHP), which provides limited, temporary coverage for people not eligible for Canadian Medicare. Although public funding in refugee health has increased overall since 2016, others have advocated for increased investments in underserved areas such as maternal care, mental health, and medical language interpreters (Piccininni & Kwong, 2019).

Health Promotion Policies

Health promotion generates health improvements through multiple approaches, including research, public education, changes in the physical and social environment, regulation of disease- and injury-promoting activities or behaviors, and improved access to high-quality health care through policies that mitigate disparities and promote equity. For effective outcomes, policies must consider social determinants of health as foundational concepts that have an impact on and influence health.

At the urging of the U.S. Surgeon General, the U.S. federal government published a national agenda for health promotion titled *Healthy People 2000* that identified 319 objectives for health promotion and set measurable goals for achieving them. An updated national framework, *Healthy People 2030*, includes goals for a standardized approach to assess changes in behaviors that determine health outcomes. Numerous tables in the statistical yearbooks published by the National Center for Health Statistics form a scorecard for this national health promotion effort. Many of the objectives address health behaviors such as physical activity and exercise; tobacco, alcohol, and drug use; violent and abusive behaviors; safer sexual practices; and behaviors designed to prevent or mitigate injuries.

Ensuring access to health and illness care services is one way to improve the health of individuals and families. Health promotion efforts aimed at the first five years of life are known to reduce the population-level burden of disease (Trinh-Shevrin, 2015). Using upstream preventative care approaches, children should receive necessary immunizations and should be evaluated on a regular basis for normal growth and development. It is also important that adults be adequately immunized and screened for hypertension, diabetes, and cancer at appropriate ages and intervals. The Canadian government introduced the Healthy Kids Strategy (Ontario Healthy Kids Panel, 2013) with a focus on health promotion of children, including support before and during pregnancy and during the early years, and initiatives to promote healthy eating and building healthy environments for children in their communities. The approach is to address health in young children to improve their longer-term health outcomes.

Although much emphasis has been on the roles that parents play in ensuring that their children receive needed services, many adults also have responsibilities for the health care of aging parents. Adults with both children and aging parents that are dependent for support struggle with access to health care and management of illnesses, and they therefore experience a particularly difficult burden in today's world. They are referred to as the sandwich generation and are in danger of caregiver burnout (Boyczuk & Fletcher, 2016). Adequate supports for families are needed so they do not have to shoulder the burden of care alone. Suggestions for promising approaches are health coaches, particularly registered nurses (RNs), who develop a trusting relationship with their clients and act as advisers and resources for the clients.

The RN Health Coach introduced in the United States in 2013 used this model and demonstrated positive results (Change Foundation, 2013). Similar nursing roles are being developed and integrated throughout the provincial health care systems across Canada, with a particular focus on supporting families with aging members. These nurse navigators support patients and families through all aspects of their care, including coordination of primary care with physicians and ensuring timely services and safe transitions through all aspects of the health care system.

Promoting health literacy for patients, groups, and communities is often framed as a practice requirement for nurses in Canada and the United States. For example, the nursing regulatory body of Ontario, the College of Nurses of Ontario (2020) expects nurses to "identify learning needs with clients and apply a broad range of educational strategies towards achieving optimal health outcomes" (p. 8) as an entry-to-practice competency. However, there are a limited number of specific health literacy course offerings in university health-related degree programs in Canada (Vamos & Yeung, 2016). In addition, there are currently no formal certification programs or regulatory expectations for retraining in health literacy for nurses in Canada or the United States. The absence of formal training for nurses and other health professionals may reflect the lack of formal governmental policy on health literacy at the federal, provincial, and territorial levels in Canada (Vamos et al., 2019). The United States faces similar challenges, with little formal training on health literacy past nursing education curriculums at colleges and universities. And, similar to Canada, nurses in the United States are expected to provide health education to individuals, families, and groups (Loan et al., 2018). Health literacy remains an important facet for the everyday work of nurses across multiple clinical settings and forms an opportunity for professional practice growth and development.

Nurses can employ a number of evidence-based strategies while working with individual clients and families to ensure that their clients' health literacy needs are being addressed proactively. Print health materials distributed to clients should be written at the sixth-grade reading level (Haas et al., 2018). The wording should be simple, it should be written in short sentences, and there should

be accompanying illustrations (Haas et al., 2018). When orally communicating health information to clients and families, nurses should employ plain language and not medical terminology, which may be easily misunderstood. Complex information should be broken up into smaller segments to enhance understanding and prevent informational overload. Nurses should frame health communication/teaching as a dialogue and encourage their clients to ask context-specific questions and troubleshoot anticipated challenges together (Coleman et al., 2017). Nurses should also use the teach-back method to assess a client's comprehension and retention of provided health information and then address any knowledge gaps (Nesari et al., 2019). Finally, nurses should support clients and families in identifying credible, evidence-based sources for health information on the internet.

THE NURSE'S ROLE IN ADVOCACY IN FAMILY POLICIES

An important role of the nurse is to advocate for family policies to promote the health of clients and families, particularly those who are disadvantaged. As holistic-care providers, nurses are in an excellent position to inform the public, including politicians, about what policies are needed and why, and to negotiate for, and help clients and families obtain, the best possible resources established by these policies.

Nursing Today

Nurses comprise a significant segment of the United States and Canadian health care workforce and must be active leaders in improving the access to and quality of health care. Today most front-line nurses in the United States and Canada function primarily in the acute-care setting, a practice that supports a limited perspective and understanding of the social determinants of health and an associated limitation in advocacy. This limited involvement, however, is changing as the transformation of health care thanks to the ACA in the United States has taken place, and care in both countries has moved more and more from institutions into the community.

In 2011 IOM released a report outlining key recommendations for preparing the nursing workforce to meet the needs of the population: *The Future of Nursing: Leading Change, Advancing Health*. This landmark report described the need to harness the power of nurses to realize the objectives set forth in the ACA by transforming the health care system from one that focuses on the provision of acute-care services to one that delivers health care where and when it is needed, ensuring access to high-quality preventative care in the community. The IOM committee explained that nurses will need to be full partners in redesigning efforts, to be accountable for their own contributions to delivering high-quality care, and to work collaboratively with leaders from other health care professions by taking responsibility for identifying problems, devising and implementing solutions to those problems, and tracking improvements over time to ensure the health of the population (IOM, 2011). Increasing evidence shows that improvements in policies in childhood education, child poverty, healthy work environments, social safety, and healthy living environments make a difference in decreasing health disparities. If nurses could advocate more on behalf of the poor, oppressed, and vulnerable populations in these areas, then progress would be faster (Williams et al., 2018). Despite being leaders in health care, few nurses are involved with policy development and political advocacy.

Nurses and nursing organizations in Canada have viewed collective activism, political lobbying, and health policy work as part of their professional responsibilities. Nurses have used their status as the largest and most trusted group of health professionals to advance policies that promote high-quality family health and social equity and the key roles that nurses can play to achieve these goals. The Canadian Nurses Association, a federal nursing organization, took a bold step in the role of nurses in addressing health and social disparities. The Canadian National Expert Commission report (2013), *A Nursing Call to Action: The Health of Our Nation, the Future of Our Health System* "recommends . . . the use of a cost-effective, wellness-based model that places greater emphasis on primary care, health promotion and the prevention and management of chronic diseases" (p. 6) (Canadian Nurses Association, 2021). In addition, it suggests that care be moved as much as possible from acute-care facilities to community sites. Provincial professional nursing organizations such as Registered

Nurses' Association of Ontario (RNAO) have used social and mass media, advertising campaigns, and open letters to politicians to bring public awareness to important health issues, engage voters, and make key suggestions for improved health policy. RNAO has led political campaigns on a number of health issues such as hiring more long-term staff, mandatory naloxone training for staff, climate change, and promoting patient safety.

Advancing health care requires a cultural shift in the expectations of the nursing profession regarding education, practice, and advocacy for vulnerable populations. In Canada, Pilkington et al. (2011) found that, even in community-based health care centers, many nurses failed to account for the clients' social and housing conditions when planning health education and care because these concepts were not included in the standard nursing assessment forms. The allotted time spent with clients was mostly focused on traditional health teaching about lifestyle changes despite the fact that these same nurses indicated that assessment of access to necessary resources was a critically important component for success in meeting clients' needs to promote their health. This trend emphasizes the need for nursing educators to reexamine how nurses can better understand social and family policy to improve the health care of their clients.

Nurses must look beyond health behaviors and medications as primary interventions and instead look at and treat underlying social issues, including:

- poverty and the lack of employment security
- unequal access to health care
- the lack of education and health literacy
- the stigma of mental illness, obesity, and HIV infection
- racism and social exclusion
- individual, family, and community stress
- the lack of social support and isolation
- food insecurity and the lack of quality nutrition

ACA listed many stipulations that directly affect the nurse's role in care and the salient need for nurses to become actively involved in family policy. For example, ACA required all adults to have a primary-care provider by 2014. This requirement put a strain on the health care system because family practice physicians were in short supply. Nursing leaders stepped up and advocated increased investment in funding education for advanced nurses with the goal of nurses being able to meet the need of primary-care access. ACA increased funding to those who provided care to underserved populations. Nurses increased their efforts to document their care of underserved populations, thereby increasing funding for nursing care across both urban and rural populations (Mahoney & Jones, 2013).

Hewison (2007) described an organized method for policy analysis to be used by nurse managers. The method involves a process by which a summary of the policy is developed, including its origin and status; a history and link to other policy initiatives are provided; and themes and elements of nursing practice affected by the policy are listed (Hewison, 2007). Once the analysis is concluded, the nurse can take a position on whether the policy meets the needs of the constituency. Today, the National League for Nursing compels nurses to become engaged in civic policies because of nurses' knowledge of diversity, caring, and integrity, which makes them prime professionals to make a difference. Nurses can be active participants and leaders in health care reform and increasing government support for nursing education (National League for Nursing, 2021). Nurses with strong policy analysis skills are critical to improving health for all citizens and to closing the health disparities gap.

Professional nurses with an interest in learning more about their role in the family policy arena can find resources through professional associations or can extend their knowledge by taking continuing education courses in health care policy. One example is the Washington Health Policy Institute conducted by George Mason University in Arlington, Virginia. Nurses and other health care providers spend one week learning about health and family policy, strategies to advocate for at-risk populations, and how to influence policymakers. Similarly, in Canada, the Canadian Nurses Association and provincial associations such as RNAO also offer information, workshops, and training for nurses to gain skill in health care policy development. Family policies are a major contributing factor to the mitigation of health disparities. Nurses have the ability to influence policy on many levels and thereby improve the health outcomes of the most vulnerable populations.

Nursing Policy, Research, and Education

Many important policies are at the institutional level where nurses work. Nursing practice, research, and education should reflect this orientation.

Nurses Influencing Family Policy

The implications of becoming involved in the development of family policy in the context of nursing care of families are limitless, especially in community and institutional settings. Nurse involvement in policy development can constitute a wide range of activities, from the micro level, by asking open-ended questions about sexual orientation; to the meso level, by asking about housing and food security or environmental safety in the community; to the macro level, where nurses can inform institutional policies in the workplace; to the exo level, where nurses may petition government representatives regarding development of needed policies, modification of harmful policies, or correcting for absent policies.

Nurses can influence policy from the initial assessment of families in clinics and hospitals to discharge planning for return to the community, including open exploration of potential support and resources. With the latter, nurses can avoid the omission of needed resources and any assumptions that resources are automatically available. Specific strategies for nurses to get involved in influencing policy from the micro to the exo level include:

- joining committees in your institution to change relevant policies (e.g., include questions regarding available resources in assessment forms; make sure needed resources are available before discharge; ensure follow-up after discharge or referrals)
- joining professional associations and advocating for needed family policies
- writing to or phoning elected representatives regarding needed policies or changes to those that are harmful
- joining community advocacy groups, such as those requesting affordable day care
- joining boards of directors for agencies, such as social housing and community health centers (CHCs)

Examples of ways that nurses can become more engaged in social and family policies are identified in Table 4-1.

Nursing Research

Nursing research has already developed useful tools and frameworks for providing nursing care to overcome cultural barriers and under difficult circumstances. The development of community-based participatory research models provides a methodology for studies more respectful of the potentially diverse views of family in a community. This approach requires the nurse researcher to establish a relationship with the community in which the study is to occur *before* the development of the research question. By sharing all stages of the research process with members of the community, nurse scientists can use this collaborative approach to examine health disparities that are mitigated directly by community improvement based on the results of the study.

Adopting this level of respect for reshaping nursing studies about family helps nurses gain a more complete understanding of health care for all types of families. This approach is particularly important as trends in care move away from acute-care institutions toward community-based care delivery in both the United States and Canada. Nurses are particularly well positioned to participate in policy changes and program development in collaboration with an interdisciplinary team, including their clients and families.

Nursing Education

As discussed previously, there is currently very little inclusion of family policy development and advocacy work in nursing curricula. Opportunities for learning experiences in settings that have established services for vulnerable populations provide the nursing student with clinical situations in which to practice assumption-free assessment skills and learn about diverse life situations and

Table 4-1	Suggested Roles for Nurses Under Major Policy Categories	
IMPORTANT POLICIES THAT IMPACT HEALTH	**NEED**	**NURSING ROLE WITH POLICY**
Early childhood education	Children from low-income homes are at risk for developmental delays and are enrolled in preschool less often than children from higher-income homes.	Collaborate with early intervention and early childhood programs to advocate for increased funding opportunities, community education and support, and universal access to quality child care and prekindergarten programs for families.
Child poverty	Children rely on their parents for health care and education. Parents who live in poverty struggle more with providing quality education and health care for their children. Food insecurity, poor housing, low employment rates, low-quality and inaccessible child care all have an impact on childhood health outcomes that in turn have an impact on health in adulthood.	Support policies that provide food security for children, such as free quality meals at school. Support programs that provide economic opportunities for parents. Participate in programs that help educate parents and children.
Youth development	Positive youth programs decrease delinquency, drug use and abuse, and the numbers of unintentional accidents, and they improve mental health.	Support youth programs, especially those that encourage parent involvement. Support policies that help fund positive youth programs. Collaborate with schools and other youth programs to increase education and accessibility to youth programs.
Health of families	Determinants of health are negatively affected by oppression of vulnerable groups, poverty, poor housing, low income, rural geography, and poor access to quality education and health care.	Support policies that provide quality health care for all individuals. Support policies that provide food security and safe housing for families. Support families being able to care safely for family members. Support policies that help families live in a healthy environment.

Source: Adapted from Williams, S. D., Phillips, J. M., and Koyama, K. (2018). Nurse advocacy: Adopting a health in all policies approach. *OJIN: The Online Journal of Issues in Nursing, 23*(3), Manuscript 1.

needs. Homeless shelters, services for LGBTQ+ adolescents, shelters for victims of intimate partner abuse, outreach centers for sex workers, and street syringe and needle exchange programs all reach a disproportionate share of individuals whose family experiences are not the idealized norm. By working with clients and other health care providers, nurses can ensure the maximum benefit of such policies on the needs of families, communities, and society (National League for Nursing, 2021).

The inclusion of health policy in nursing education has the potential to increase the sensitivity of nurses to social and health policy issues. Nurses must understand that it is not sufficient to provide care in isolation from the forces that increase risk for disease or limit access to medical services. Electives in history, economics, and political science further inform nurses' understanding of policy. IOM recommends that nurses engage in lifelong learning, thereby speaking to the need for nurses to engage in professional practice that

strives to stay current about issues in health care and the influences of public policy on the delivery of that health care (IOM, 2011). Nurses at all levels must be able to understand current affairs; join nursing and other advocacy organizations; and participate in local, state or provincial, and national political processes. Nurses should be educated to take on responsibility for advocating for equity and social justice to help develop family-friendly policies.

Clearly, nurses can have a strong impact on family policies that affect the health of the citizens they serve. The American Nurses Association Code of Ethics addresses social policy in Provision 8: "The nurse collaborates with other health professionals and the public to protect human rights, promote health diplomacy, and reduce health disparities" (Lachman et al., 2015). This provision recommends that nurses work in conjunction with community organizations and legislative policy at the state and national level.

Case Study: Smith Family

Heather is a 19-year-old female diagnosed with bipolar disorder. She was recently hospitalized for 10 days because she experienced a manic episode with psychotic symptoms. During her hospitalization, she admitted stopping her medications because she could no longer afford the high cost, and her parents' insurance had a high deductible that would not cover her medications until that deductible was met. Since her hospitalization, however, the deductible was met and she was now interested in taking the medications again and stabilizing her mood. During the discharge planning, Heather met with her psychiatrist, mental health nurse, and her parents.

Heather's history includes being diagnosed with depression at age 13 years, with a trial on sertraline (Zoloft) for 2 years. Although her depression symptoms went into remission, her parents noted that she became increasingly agitated and argumentative. During her sophomore year in high school, she became involved with a "rough crowd" and started using marijuana daily, with periods of depression lasting months followed by weeks of argumentative behavior, poor sleep, and rapid mood shifts. She also started failing her classes, which her parents noted was unusual because she had been identified as a talented and gifted child in elementary school. Her parents sought treatment from a new psychiatrist at that point, and Heather was diagnosed with bipolar I disorder. She tried several mood stabilizers and was finally stabilized on paliperidone (Invega) titrated to 6 mg per day. During her senior year in high school, she stopped taking her medications because she believed she was stable and no longer needed medication. She quickly became agitated and started believing she was talking directly to characters on the television. She also stole her parents' credit card and purchased more than $2,000 worth of items that she later admitted she did not want or need. She agreed to go back on her medication, and her symptoms stabilized over the course of 3 weeks. Heather did well on her return to school and, through credit recovery, graduated from high school. She attended the local community college for 1 year and was starting her second year when she decided to stop her medications again because of the high cost. Her parents both complained about having to pay $880.83 per month to cover her medications (GoodRx, 2017). They noted that their current insurance, offered by Heather's father's employer, cost the family $600 per month and had a $10,000 deductible. Heather noted that she had applied for disability services and Medicare health coverage because of her diagnosis of bipolar I disorder, but she was denied because of her successful functioning in school when she was stable. She also tried to apply for Medicaid services in light of her low income as a student and her bipolar diagnosis, but she was denied because she had creditable insurance through her father's employer. She stated that she did not want to be a burden on her parents, already felt guilty asking them to help her

Case Study: Smith Family—cont'd

with her tuition and living costs, and did not want to also ask for money to cover her medication costs. Heather's parents asked what could be done to help them afford the high cost of keeping Heather stable. Heather's father anxiously pointed out that the hospital bill thus far was $7,595 and covered only 9 days; that amount did not include the cost of medications during the hospital stay. He lamented that his high-deductible insurance plan was the best they could afford at this time.

The nurse asked the Smith family what their goals were, both individually for Heather and as a family. Heather stated that she wanted to complete her college degree in old English literature and eventually teach at a university. She was hoping to obtain her doctorate degree in Victorian literature eventually. She said she worried that her diagnosis of bipolar disorder would interfere with that plan because she could not imagine being able to pay for her medications. She now understood how critical it was to take her medications; otherwise, she would be disabled and unable to complete school or be successful at any job. Heather's parents agreed with Heather's goals and stated that they too were worried that successful treatment of her disorder was not affordable.

Heather's psychiatrist stated that she believed the paliperidone (Invega) was the best option for successful treatment of Heather's bipolar disorder because of her psychotic symptoms with mania. She also noted that Heather's previous psychiatrist had appropriately tried less expensive mood stabilizers (i.e., risperidone, lithium) but because of intolerable side effects (tremors, weight gain, and abnormal thyroid function) and breakthrough manic symptoms, these medications were discontinued, and Heather was given paliperidone, with good results. Until she stopped taking her medication, Heather was stable and doing well in school and with relationships, and she was getting along well with her parents.

Heather's family history included being the only child of her biological parents. (See Figure 4-1, the Smith family genogram, and Figure 4-2, the Smith family ecomap.) Her parents denied any history of depression, anxiety, or bipolar disorder, but her father noted that his brother was also diagnosed with bipolar disorder and spent most of his life in and out of inpatient care. Heather's mother noted that her mother suffered from depression and anxiety but was stable on an antidepressant medication. Heather was close to her biological grandparents but did not have any contact with her paternal uncle. She noted that her mother was also an only child. Heather stated that she had a boyfriend whom she had been dating for the past 2 years. He was also a student who was studying biology at the community college. She stated that she had a stable group of friends and spent time several days per week with these friends. She said that she no longer used drugs or alcohol because she recognized the negative effects of drugs and alcohol on her mood stability. Heather stated that she was also seeing the counselor at the community college weekly to help her learn strategies for mood regulation.

The nurse helped the family prioritize steps to ensure that Heather's goals and the family's goals would be supported. The policies that affected this family the most included:

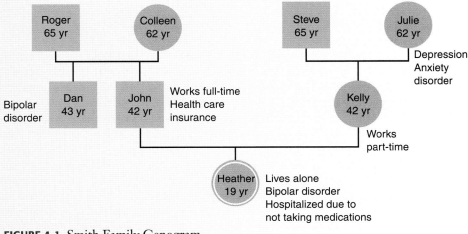

FIGURE 4-1 Smith Family Genogram

(continued)

Case Study: Smith Family—cont'd

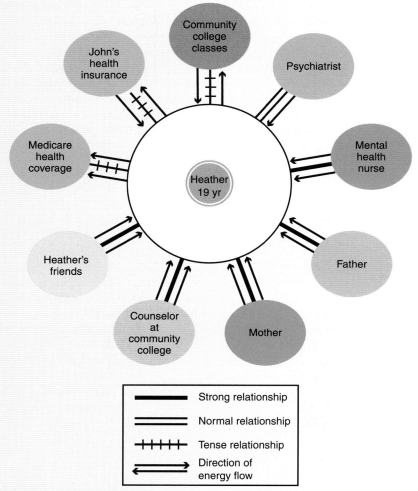

FIGURE 4-2 Smith Family Ecomap

- *Medicare eligibility mandates coverage for disabled individuals.* Heather, unfortunately, did not meet the criteria for being disabled because she functioned well when she was on her medication. She could stop medication, and if her functionality declined, she would then qualify for Medicare; however, this option would not support her goals of striving for a successful career. Heather stated that she would rather look for other options to fund her medication.
- *Medicaid eligibility mandates coverage for certain groups of vulnerable populations, including those living in the federally accepted poverty range.* Although the ACA increased the numbers of individuals eligible for Medicaid coverage, those with creditable insurance through an employer are not eligible. As long as Heather was covered under her parents' insurance plan, she would not qualify for Medicaid benefits. The family analyzed whether it would be more cost effective not to take Heather as a tax deduction as a dependent and cancel her insurance versus continuing her coverage but having to pay for her mental health care, including medications. They decided to visit their accountant to discuss these two options. Heather stated that she would feel more comfortable if she qualified for Medicaid and that she had done some research and learned that Medicaid does cover the cost of paliperidone (Invega) (GoodRx, 2017). She also learned that Medicaid would cover the cost of counseling should she decide to transfer her counseling services to the county mental health clinic.
- *Employer-supported insurance programs offer employees a discount on their monthly premiums.* Even with this discount, however, families spend an average of $6,422 per year on health care costs, including insurance premiums and

Case Study: Smith Family—cont'd

high-deductible expenditures (Common Wealth Fund, 2016). Although each state is different, the percentage of health care costs compared to the family income ranges from a low of 6.8% in Massachusetts to a high of 14.7% in Mississippi (Common Wealth Fund, 2016). ACA allowed children to remain on their parents' plans until they are age 26 years. Although this allows young adults the opportunity to have health insurance, the high deductibles associated with most employer-based programs continue to place a burden on most families, including those with young adult children.

• *Many community and national programs attempt to ease the burden of high-cost prescriptions for most individuals.* These programs are often offered through community agencies or pharmaceutical companies. Of interest is that many of these medication discount programs are given only to those with private insurance. Heather's nurse found out that Heather qualified for a discount program that would reduce her medication costs by 50% (GoodRx, 2017).

Heather is one of many individuals with a chronic condition who face the dilemma of how to treat symptoms given the continued high cost of health care. Although hospitalization is significantly more expensive than outpatient care and stabilizing medications, many, such as Heather, end up in the emergency department or in inpatient care because of inability to pay for outpatient care and medications. Family policies provide health care coverage for many, but not all. In addition, many chronic conditions place individuals in a stigmatized group, further hindering their ability to access care. Mental health disorders are a large group of chronic conditions commonly stigmatized. Heather was lucky to have a mental health nurse interested in family policies who would help better stabilize Heather's symptoms and help her reach her goals. Future efforts are needed to ensure that all individuals and families, including young adults, are not burdened with high-cost health care that, in the end, may cause an increase in chronic disabilities rather than supporting successful functioning in the community.

Questions for reflection on the nursing care of the Smith family:

1. Reflect on Heather's access to health care and what resources she has to manage her chronic condition. If you, someone in your immediate family, or a close friend were faced with managing a chronic condition, what resources would you have to do this?
2. As you review Heather's family health history and her social support (family genogram and family ecomap), what gaps do you see for support that might benefit Heather now or in the future?
3. What resources are available in your local community that support young adults who are managing bipolar disorder or another chronic illness?
4. What can nurses do to support individuals and families when they report challenges with accessing prescription medications?

SUMMARY

This chapter began with a well-known parable regarding the dilemma of saving drowning people versus fixing the problem that causes people to fall in the water in the first place. By analyzing the causes of health disparities and poor health outcomes, and understanding and advocating for positive changes in these policies, nurses have the opportunity to improve the challenging conditions that people are experiencing. This chapter focused on family health policies and how continued health disparities continue to leave many vulnerable populations with inadequate and unequal health care. As nursing care shifts from institutions into the community, nurses who want to deliver the most effective family-focused care need to return to historical role models in nursing, with leaders working hard to provide health care to those in need. They need to become knowledgeable about the influence of the political and social structures that are facilitating or hindering health promotion and particularly affecting those vulnerable families affected by racism and exclusion. When promoting health and mitigating disparities, nurses have to be aware of and keep in mind the following:

- Health disparities arise from complex, deeply rooted social issues, including racism and stigma.
- Health disparities are directly related to the social and political structure of a society, which gives rise to the determinants of health.

- The social determinants of health include poverty; housing; education; employment and food security; access to health care; presence of chronic illness; gender; and being a member of an ethnic, racial, or other oppressed group.
- The three levels of racism—institutional racism, personally mediated racism, and internalized racism—provide a foundation for understanding the causes and potential solutions of health disparities.
- Interventions at the micro, meso, macro, and exo levels are important in addressing changes to family policies.
- All social determinants of health intersect and mutually reinforce each other.
- Social determinants are the root causes of illness and health because they affect lifestyle possibilities and limitations and access to health care resources.
- The policy decisions made by a society or government about families, what constitutes a legal relationship, and how health care is delivered have a profound effect on families and their health.
- In the past, the profession of nursing had a well-defined role in advocating for vulnerable populations. In the last century, nursing involvement in the development of health policy has declined because of a focus on medical diagnosis and acute, individual care rather than on whole individuals and families in their environmental and social contexts.
- Nurses today need to get involved in policy development at institutional and societal levels to promote health and well-being for families.
- Nursing professionals can benefit from theoretical and practical education about family policy issues that are broad and complex and that deeply affect the health of the family.
- Family nursing practice has the potential to improve the health of all families, regardless of definition and composition, with close collaboration with clients and interdisciplinary health care teams.
- Nursing education should include teaching policy development and advocacy.
- Nursing research should include collaborative, community-based participatory research with families to best meet families' needs because they are the experts of their own lives.
- Nurses are in a unique and key position to make a difference in the health of families.

chapter 5

Family Nursing Assessment and Intervention

Paul S. Smith, PhD, RN, CNE

Delene Volkert, PhD, RN, CNE

Critical Concepts

- Families are complex social systems with which nurses interact in many ways and in many different contexts; thus, the use of a logical systematic family nursing assessment approach is important.

- In the context of family nursing, the creative nurse thinker must be aware of possibilities, be able to recognize the new and the unusual, be able to decipher unique and complex situations, and be inventive in designing an approach to family care.

- Nurses determine the theoretical and practice lens(es) through which to analyze the family event.

- Knowledge about family structures, functions, and processes informs nurses in their efforts to optimize and provide individualized nursing care that is tailored to the uniqueness of each family system.

- Nurses begin family assessment from the moment of contact or referral.

- Family stories are narratives that nurses construct in framing, contextualizing, communicating, and interpreting their family clients' needs as they exercise clinical judgment in their work.

- Interacting with families as clients requires knowledge of family assessment and intervention models, as well as skilled communication techniques so that the interaction will be effective and efficient for all parties.

- The family genogram and ecomap are both assessment data-gathering instruments. The therapeutic interaction that occurs with the family while diagramming a genogram or ecomap is itself a powerful intervention.

- Families' beliefs about health and illness, nurses and other health care providers, and themselves are essential for nurses to explore in order to craft effective approaches to family interventions and to promote health literacy.

- Families determine the level of nurses' involvement in their health and illness journeys, and nurses seek to tailor their work and approach accordingly.

(continued)

■ Nurses and families who work together and build on family strengths are in the best position to determine and prioritize specific family needs; develop realistic outcomes; and design, evaluate, and modify a plan of action that has a high probability of being implemented by the family.

■ The final step in working with families should always be for nurses to engage in critical, creative, and concurrent reflection about the family, their work with the family, and their own professional practice.

One of the most difficult and challenging aspects of working with families for nurses is how not to compare, judge, or assume what is the best action for the family or client based on their personal experience with their own families. The way in which a nurse interacts with another person sets in motion a multitude of possibilities. The nurse who stops to prepare mentally before interacting with a family becomes fully present for that family before entering the room, which brings the best of self, or *therapeutic self*, to that interaction. Using therapeutic self in interactions places the other's illness story at the focal point of care. Maintaining curiosity about the other's experience, thoughts, life, and needs allows the exploration of varied possible outcomes. The nurse who is open to diverse experiences welcomes the other as a partner in care. This way of practicing family nursing is known as relational inquiry (Doane & Varcoe, 2015; Varcoe & Doane, 2018).

In this chapter, family assessment is explored in the context of relational inquiry, and an emphasis is placed on family-centered care (FCC) principles that will guide interactions between families and the nurse providing care. This chapter will also explore various family nursing assessment models as well as instruments used when working with families.

RELATIONAL INQUIRY IN FAMILY NURSING PRACTICE

Relational inquiry family nursing practice is oriented toward enhancing the capacity and power of people and families to live a life that is meaningful to them from their own perspective. Although this may involve treating and preventing disease or modifying lifestyle factors, the primary focus is to enhance peoples' well-being as well as their capacity and resources for meaningful life experiences.

Thus, relational inquiry focuses very specifically on how *health is a sociorelational experience* that is strongly shaped by contextual factors.

> *Like a scientific inquiry, inquiry-based nursing practice involves being in that in-between relational space of knowing/not knowing, being curious, looking for what seems significant, examining the interrelatedness between the elements as well as the relevance of those interrelationships in the experiential moment and also acting toward them. (Doane & Varcoe, 2015, p. 6)*

Families, health, and family nursing are understood to be shaped by the historical, geographical, economic, political, and social diversity of the particular person's/family's context. By purposefully working with this diversity, nurses are prepared to account for the contextual nature of people's/families' health and illness experiences and how their lives are shaped by their intrapersonal, interpersonal, and contextual circumstances in order to provide the most appropriate care. There is an ongoing need for nurses to collaborate with families in order to promote health, to support families who are coping with illness, and to provide assistance to families as they navigate complex health care systems (Smith & Jones, 2016).

Understanding and working directly with context provides a key resource and strategy for responsive, health-promoting family nursing practice. Context is not something outside or separate from people; rather, contextual elements (e.g., socioeconomic circumstances, family and cultural histories) are literally embodied in people and within their actions and responses to particular situations (Varcoe & Doane, 2018). Having an appreciation for the range of diverse experiences and how the dynamics of geography, history, politics, and economics shape those experiences allows nurses to provide more effective care to particular families, better understand the stresses and challenges that families face, and better support families to draw on their own capacities.

Context is considered something that is integral to the lives of people, as something that shapes not only people's external circumstances and opportunities but also their physiology at the cellular level (Varcoe & Doane, 2018). In other words, context is embodied. For example, if a person is born into a middle-class, English-speaking, Euro-Canadian family, the very way that person speaks—accent, intonation, vocabulary—is shaped by that context. The way that a person's body grows is influenced by the nutritional value of the food and quality of water available, the level of stress in the family, the family's quality of housing, and the opportunities for rest and physical activity. Similarly, the person's sense of self and expectations for his or her life are shaped by the circumstances into which the person is born. The individual's success in education will depend not only on what educational opportunities are available but also on how the person comes to that education—for example, how well fed or hungry, well rested or tired, or confident and content he or she is—and the economic resources available that shape which school the person attends. It will also be affected by how education is valued within the person's family or community. Thus, a person's/family's multiple contexts cannot be understood as being outside or separate from one's self or even as necessarily under one's control. Rather, people and families embody their circumstances, and their circumstances embody them. Although people have some influence over their circumstances, such influence generally is more limited than we would like to imagine. In addition, the contextual elements, and the experiences to which those elements give rise, live on in people. That is, past contexts go forward within people, shaping how they experience present and future situations.

People are both influenced *by* their context and live *within* contexts (Varcoe & Doane, 2018). Throughout nursing careers, nurses provide care in specific contexts, and families live in their own diverse contexts. Consciously considering the interface of these differing contexts and how they are shaping families' health and illness experiences is vital to providing responsive, health-promoting care. Also foundational to this process is the need to inquire into how context shapes the life of a nurse and his or her practice. This self-reflection enables nurses to choose more intentionally how to draw on those influences to enhance responsiveness to the needs of families. For example, many nurses practice in health care settings where they are surrounded by well-educated and financially stable professionals. This context contrasts with many clients who may lack education and live in low-income and unstable housing because of financial instability. When a nurse recognizes this difference, care can then include sensitivity to the disparity between these two contexts.

Through a relational inquiry lens of family nursing, nurses look for how people, situations, contexts, environments, and processes are integrally connecting with and shaping each other. Nurses step outside their personal experience of family and actively engage in conversations to uncover the family illness story (Wright & Leahey, 2019). The illness story differs from the medical story. The medical story is about the patient who has the disease or health problem and includes signs and symptoms, medications, treatment regimen, and prognosis or trajectory of illness. The family illness story is how the family and each of its members live through the experience of the illness or health event. "Relational practice is a humanely involved process of respectful, compassionate, and authentically interested inquiry into another" (Doane & Varcoe, 2015, p. 200).

Without a careful consideration of context and its influence on families' health and illness experiences, nurses typically draw uncritically on stereotypes in ways that limit possibilities for the families they serve. By inquiring into the context of families, nurses can provide optimal responsive, ethical, and appropriate care. Through relational inquiry, nurses connect across differences and work with family members by providing options and choices to help them determine the best decisions for them and their family in this situation at this point in time. Relational inquiry is the foundational value inherent in all aspects of family nursing but especially for assessment and specific, tailored family interventions.

FCC principles should be applied in all interactions between families and nurses or other health care providers. According to the Institute for Patient- and Family-Centered Care (IPFCC, n.d.), the core principles of FCC are respect and dignity, information sharing, participation, and collaboration. The goal of FCC is to increase the mutual benefit of health care provision for all parties, with a focus on improving the satisfaction and outcomes of health care for families and advocating for families to share in decision making and maintain their control (IPFCC, n.d.). By utilizing these principles in all aspects of the family nursing approach, from assessment through intervention and evaluation, nurses can facilitate exchanges of shared expertise, which lead to better holistic health outcomes.

THERAPEUTIC APPROACH TO WORKING WITH FAMILIES

During the initial interaction with families, it is critical for nurses to introduce themselves to the family, meet all the family members present, learn about the family members not present, clearly state the purpose for working with the family, outline what will happen during this session, and indicate the length of time the meeting will last. Taking these actions demonstrates respect for family members and their unique story. To continue with this precedent, the nurse needs to develop a systematic plan for the first and all subsequent family meetings. This focus on respect, dignity, and collaboration in initial meetings helps to establish relationships that are therapeutic. Effective, satisfying partnerships between nurses and families are critical as they work together toward health-related goals.

Nurses who use a therapeutic approach to family meetings have found that their focus on FCC increases and that their communication skills with families become more fluid with experience (Franck & O'Brien, 2019). When nurses use therapeutic communication skills with families, the families report feeling a stronger rapport with the nurse, an increased frequency of communication between families and the nurse occurs, and families perceive these nurses to be more competent (Arkorful et al., 2020).

Conducting family meetings requires not only skilled communication strategies but also knowledge of family assessment and intervention models. Nurses use a variety of data collection and assessment methods to help gather information systematically and efficiently. Therefore, it is important that the instruments be carefully selected so that they are family friendly and render information pertinent to the purpose of working with the family.

FAMILY NURSING ASSESSMENT

Central to the delivery of safe and effective family nursing care is the nurse's ability to make accurate assessments, identify health problems, and develop appropriately unique plans of care. Each step in working with families, whether applied to individuals within the family or the family as a whole, requires a thoughtful, deliberate reasoning process. Nurses decide what data to collect and how, when, and where those data are collected. Nurses determine the relevance of each new piece of information and how it fits into the emerging family story. Before moving forward, nurses decide whether they have obtained sufficient information on problem and strength identification or whether gaps exist that require additional data gathering.

Nurses must always be aware that "common" interpretations of data may not be the "correct" interpretations in any given situation and that commonly expected signs and symptoms may not appear in every case or in the same data pattern presentation. The ability of nurses to be open to the unexpected and to be alert to unusual or different responses is critical to determining the primary needs confronting the family. Nurses should be able to perceive what is not obvious and to understand how this family story is similar to or different from other family stories.

The family nursing assessment includes the following steps:

- *Assessment of the family story*: The nurse gathers data from a variety of sources to see the whole picture of the family experience.
- *Analysis of the family story*: The nurse clusters the data into meaningful patterns to see how the family is managing the health event. The family needs are prioritized using a family reasoning web.
- *Design of a family plan of care*: Together, the nurse and family determine the best plan of care for the family to manage the situation.
- *Family intervention*: Together, the nurse and family implement the plan of care incorporating the most family-focused, cost-effective, and efficient interventions that assist the family to achieve the best possible outcomes within an agreed-upon time line.
- *Family evaluation*: Together, the nurse and family determine whether the outcomes

are being reached or partially reached, or need to be redesigned. Is the care plan working well, does a new care plan need to be put into place, or does the nurse/family relationship need to end?

- *Nurse reflection*: Nurses engage in critical, creative, and concurrent reflection about themselves and their own family experiences, the family client, and their work with the family.

Engaging Families in Care

Background and First Contact

Nurses encounter families in diverse health care settings for many different kinds of problems and circumstances. Every family has a story about how the potential or actual health event influences its individual members, family functioning, and management of the health event. Nurses are charged with gathering, sifting, organizing, and analyzing the data to craft a clear view of the family's story. Nurses filter data gathered in the story through different views or approaches, which affects how they think about the family as a whole and about each individual family member. For example, a family that is faced with a new diagnosis of a chronic illness would have different needs than a family that is faced with a member dying of an end-stage chronic illness. Nurses might use different strategies if the patient is in the acute hospital setting, in an assisted living center, or living at home.

The underlying theoretical approach used by the nurses working with families influences how they ask questions and collect family data. For example, if the family is worried about how its 2-year-old child will react to a new baby, such as in the Bono family case study presented later in this chapter, the nurse may elect to base the assessment and interventions on a family systems theoretical view or the developmental family life cycle theoretical view. Refer to Chapter 2 for a detailed discussion of working with families from different theoretical perspectives.

Data collection, which is the first part of assessment, involves both subjective and objective family information that is obtained through direct observation, through examination, or in consultation with other health care providers. In all cases, family assessment begins from the first moment that the family is referred to the nurse. Following are some circumstances in which a family is referred to a nurse:

- A family is referred by the hospital to a home health agency for wound care on the feet of a client with diabetes.
- A couple seeks advice for managing their busy life with three children as the mother returns home from the hospital following an unplanned cesarean section.
- A family calls the Visiting Nurse Association to request assistance in providing care to a family member with increasing dementia.
- A school nurse is asked by the school psychologist to conduct a family assessment with a family who is suspected of child neglect.
- A physician requests a family assessment for a child who has nonorganic failure to thrive.
- A family with a member with critical-care needs is asked to make decisions about life-sustaining treatments in the intensive-care unit.

Making Community-Based Appointments

As soon as a family is identified, the nurse begins to collect data about the family's story. Sources of data that can be collected before contacting a family for a home or clinic appointment are listed in Box 5-1. Specifically, the nurse needs to know the following information:

- the reason for the referral or requested visit
- the family knowledge of the visit or referral
- specific medical information about the family member with the health problem
- strategies that have been used previously
- insurance sources for the family
- family problems identified by other health providers
- family demographic data, when available, such as the number of people and ages of family members or basic cultural background information
- the need for an interpreter

Before contacting the family to arrange for the initial appointment, the nurse needs to decide whether the most appropriate place to conduct the appointment is in the family's home or in the clinic or office. The type of agency where the nurse works may dictate this decision. Advantages

---

BOX 5-1
Sources of Preencounter Family Data

- *Referral source:* includes data that indicated a problem for this family, as well as demographic information.
- *Family:* includes family members' views of the problem, surprise that the referral was made, reluctance to set up the meeting, and avoidance in setting up the appointment.

- *Previous records:* records in the health care system or that are sent by having the client sign a release-for-information form, such as process logs, charts, phone logs, or school records.

---

and disadvantages of a home setting and a clinic setting are listed in Table 5-1.

Contacting the family for the appointment provides valuable information about the family. It is imperative that the nurse be confident and organized when making the initial contact. Information that is important for the nurse to note is whether the family acts surprised that the referral was made, shows reluctance in setting up a meeting, or expresses openness about working together.

The family also gathers important information about the nurse during the initial interaction. For example, family members may notice whether the nurse takes time to talk with them, uses a lot of words they do not understand, or appears organized and open to working with the family. To facilitate the best possible outcomes in engaging families for the first time to learn about their health and illness story, effective nurses consider the family and its needs as central to starting a successful collaboration. This relationship of trust begins from the moment of first contact with families. Box 5-2 outlines steps to follow when making an appointment with a family.

BOX 5-2
Setting Up Family Appointments

When organizing family appointments:
- Introduce yourself.
- State the purpose of the requested meeting, including who referred the family to the agency.
- Do not apologize for the meeting.
- Be factual about the need for the meeting but do not provide details.
- Offer several possible times for the meeting, including late afternoon or evening.
- Let the family select the most convenient time that allows the majority of family members to attend.
- Offer the services of an interpreter, if required.
- Confirm the date, time, place, and directions.

Table 5-1   Advantages and Disadvantages of Home Visits Versus Clinic Visits

HOME VISIT	CLINIC VISIT
Advantages	
• Opportunity to see the everyday family environment.	• Conducting the family appointment in the office or clinic allows for easier access to consultants.
• Observe typical family interactions because the family members are likely to feel more relaxed in their physical space.	• The family situation may be so strained that a more formal, less personal setting will facilitate discussions of emotionally charged issues.
• More family members may be able to attend the meeting.	
• Emphasizes that the problem is the responsibility of the whole family and not one family member.	
Disadvantages	
• Home may be the only sanctuary or safe place for the family or its members to be away from the scrutiny of others. Therefore, conducting the meeting in the home would invade or violate this sanctuary and bring the clinical perspective into this safe world.	• The clinic or office may reinforce a possible culture gap between the family and the nurse.
• The nurse must be highly skilled in communication, specifically setting limits and guiding the interaction, or the visit may have a more social tone and not be efficient or productive.	

Family Assessments in Acute-Care Settings

Nurses in acute-care settings encounter the families of their individual patients on a daily basis. The degree to which nurses feel comfortable and the degree to which they demonstrate clinical competence engaging families varies widely. The short length of stay in acute-care hospitals and the increasing population of people with chronic illnesses who need help with symptom management of both their acute health problem and their chronic illness mean that nurses in acute-care settings often feel there is little time to engage families effectively. Lack of time has been identified by nurses as the primary barrier to engaging families, though there are many other barriers as well, including nurse bias, safety concerns, and negative nurse attitudes about working with families (Carthon et al., 2019). It is critical that nurses gain skill and comfort with families in acute-care settings because families are the primary caregivers following the discharge of their family members. Families need the help of nurses in order to learn how to complete effective postdischarge care tasks, engage in shared decision making with health care providers, understand the current health status of their ill family member, balance admission and postdischarge family life demands, assist during critical events such as resuscitation, and solve ethical dilemmas that arise in the care of their loved one. With this extensive list of needs, it is essential that nurses in acute-care settings engage families intentionally and effectively.

Nurses in acute-care settings encounter several challenges, including caring for several acutely ill persons simultaneously, managing the informational needs of interdisciplinary providers, and coping with a host of distractions that often keep nurses away from the bedside. Therefore, nurses who seek to engage families, complete family assessments, and implement family interventions must be highly efficient and creative. Several specific strategies and tools must be used to accomplish a meaningful and effective experience. Refer to Chapter 16 for an in-depth discussion of acute-care family nursing needs and to Chapter 17 for information about families where patients are older adults.

Using Interpreters With Families

It is critical for the nurse to determine whether an interpreter is needed during the family meeting because the number of families for whom English is a second language is increasing. With the growing immigrant population in the United States that needs health care, hospitals are struggling to meet the needs of families who are limited in English proficiency (Schwei et al., 2018). Language barriers have been found to complicate many aspects of patient care, including comprehension and adherence to plans of care, and may result in poor health outcomes (Azam & Watson, 2017). Language and communication barriers have been found to contribute to adverse health outcomes, compromised quality of care, avoidable expenses, dissatisfied families, and increased potential for medical mistakes (Hurtig et al., 2018). Thus, it is essential that nurses who are not bilingual use interpreters when working with non-English-speaking families. Even though health care providers may know the benefits of using an official interpreter, many choose not to use them, with one main reason being that it takes more time (Gutman et al., 2018).

The types of interpreters that nurses solicit to help work with families have the potential to influence the quality of the information exchanged and the family's ability to follow the suggested plan of action. The most common types of interpreters used are bilingual family members or friends, called *ad hoc family member interpreters*, or *child language brokers* when using children. The problems with using family members as interpreters are that they have been found to buffer information, alter the meaning of the content, or make the decision for the person for whom they are interpreting (Paradise et al., 2019; Palmer & Kresevic, 2014). The ad hoc family member interpreter also has been found to lack important language skills, especially when it comes to medical interpretation, and this is especially true when children are used as interpreters (Paradise et al., 2019; Palmer & Kresevic, 2014). If the ad hoc family member interpreter is a child, the information that is being discussed may be frightening or the topic may be too personal and sensitive (Kamara et al., 2018; Palmer & Kresevic, 2014). Therefore, it is not ideal for nurses to use a family member for interpretation, especially if another choice is available.

The use of a qualified medical interpreter is the preferred approach for interpretation. However, it is not sufficient that a person speaks a specific language; it is also important to consider the interpreter's ethnic origin, religious background, gender, language or dialect, social group, clothes, appearance, and attitude. If a qualified medical interpreter cannot come to the meeting in the family home, the nurse should plan to use a speaker phone or video remote option (e.g., Zoom©) so that the professional interpreter can be involved in the conversation with the family. One of the problems with using an interpreter on the phone is that interpreters do not have the advantage of seeing the family members in person and cannot observe nonverbal communication. Also, the nurse should be aware that using a telephone interpreter introduces another outside person into the family setting, which may be perceived as impersonal by the family.

FAMILY NURSING ASSESSMENT MODELS AND INSTRUMENTS

Nurses practicing family nursing use a variety of tools. The following three family assessment models have been developed by family nurses. The Family Assessment and Intervention Model and the Family System Stressor-Strength Inventory (FS³I) were developed by Berkey and Hanson (1991). Friedman developed the Friedman Family Assessment Model (Friedman et al., 2003). The Calgary Family Assessment Model (CFAM) and Calgary Family Intervention Model (CFIM) were developed by Wright and Leahey (2019). These three approaches vary in purpose, unit of analysis, and level of data collected. Table 5-2 presents a detailed comparison of the essential components of these three family assessment models.

Family Assessment and Intervention Model

The Family Assessment and Intervention Model is based on Neuman's Systems Model (Kaakinen & Tabacco, 2018). According to the Family Assessment and Intervention Model, families are subject to tensions when they are stressed. The family's reaction depends on how deeply the stressor penetrates the family unit and how capable the family is of adapting to maintain its stability. The lines of resistance protect the family's basic structure, which includes the family's functions and energy resources. The family core contains the patterns

of family interactions and strengths. The basic family structure must be protected at all costs or the family ceases to exist. Reconstitution or adaptation is the work the family undertakes to preserve or restore family stability. This model addresses three areas: (1) health promotion, wellness activities, problem identification, and family factors at lines of defense and resistance; (2) family reaction and instability at lines of defense and resistance; and (3) restoration of family stability and family functioning at levels of prevention and intervention.

The FS³I is the assessment and intervention tool that accompanies the Family Assessment and Intervention Model. The FS³I is divided into three sections: (1) family systems stressors—general, (2) family stressors—specific, and (3) family system strengths.

Nurses can assess family stability by gathering information on family stressors and strengths. The nurse and family work together to assess first the family's general overall stressors and then specific family problems. Identified family strengths indicate the potential and actual problem-solving abilities of the family system. A plus to the FS³I approach is that both quantitative and qualitative data are used to determine the level of prevention and intervention needed. The family is actively involved in the discussions and decisions. This assessment and intervention approach focuses on both family stressors and strengths and provides a theoretical structure for family nursing.

Friedman Family Assessment Model

The Friedman Family Assessment Model is based on the structural-functional framework and developmental and systems theory. This assessment model takes a macroscopic approach to family assessment by viewing families as subsystems of the wider society, which includes institutions devoted to religion, education, and health. The family is considered an open social system, and this model focuses on the family's structure, functions (activities and purposes), and relationships with other social systems. The Friedman Family Assessment Model is commonly used when the family-in-community is the setting for care (e.g., in community and public health nursing). This approach enables family nurses to assess the family system as a whole, as a subunit of the society,

Table 5-2	Comparison of Family Assessment Models Developed by Family Nurses		
Name of model	Family Assessment and Intervention Model and the Family System Stressor-Strength Inventory (FS³I)	Friedman Family Assessment Model	Calgary Family Assessment and Intervention Model
Citation	Berkey and Hanson (1991)	Friedman, Bowden, and Jones (2003)	Wright and Leahey (2019)
Purpose	Concrete, focused measurement instrument that helps families identify current family stressors and builds interventions based on family strengths	Concrete, global family assessment interview guide that looks primarily at families in the larger community in which they are embedded	Conceptual model and multidimensional approach to families that looks at the fit of family functioning, as well as effective and behavioral aspects
Theoretical underpinnings	Systems	Developmental	Systems
	Family systems	Structural-functional	Cybernetics Communication Change Theory
	Neuman systems	Family stress-coping	
	Model	Environmental	
	Stress-coping theory		
Level of data collected	Quantitative	Qualitative	Qualitative
	Ordinal and interval	Nominal	Nominal
	Qualitative		
	Nominal		
Settings in which primarily used	Inpatient	Outpatient	Outpatient
	Outpatient	Community	Community
	Community		
Units of analysis	Family as context	Family as client	Family as system
	Family as client	Family as component of society	
	Family as system		
	Family as component of society		
Strengths	Short	Comprehensive list of areas to assess family	Conceptually sound
	Easy to administer		
	Yields data to compare one family member with another family member		
	Assess and measure focused presenting problem		
Weaknesses	Narrow variable	Large quantities of data that may not relate to the problem	Not concrete enough to be useful as a guideline unless the provider has studied this model and approach in detail
		No quantitative data	

and as an interactional system. Box 5-3 delineates the general assumptions of this model (Friedman et al., 2003, p. 100).

Structure refers to how a family is organized and how the parts relate to each other and to the whole. The four basic structural dimensions are role systems, value systems, communication networks, and power structure. These dimensions are interrelated and interactive, and they may differ in single-parent and two-parent families. For example, a single mother may be the head of the family, but she may not necessarily take on the authoritarian role that a traditional man might in a two-parent family. In turn, the value systems, communication networks, and power structures may be quite different in the single-parent and two-parent families because of these structural differences.

Function refers to how families meet the needs of individuals and meet the purposes of the broader society. In other words, family functions are what a family does. The functions of the family historically are discussed in Chapter 1, but the following specific family functions are considered in this approach:

- passing on culture, religion, and ethnicity
- socializing young people for the next generation (e.g., to be good citizens, to be able to cope in society through education)
- providing sexual satisfaction and reproduction
- providing economic security

BOX 5-3

Underlying Assumptions of Friedman's Family Assessment Model

Friedman's Family Assessment Model includes the following underlying assumptions:

- A family is a social system with functional requirements.
- A family is a small group possessing certain generic features common to all small groups.
- The family as a social system accomplishes functions that serve the individual and society.
- Individuals act in accordance with a set of internalized norms and values that are learned primarily through socialization.

Source: Friedman, M. M., Bowden, V. R., & Jones, E. G. (2003). *Family nursing: Research, theory & practice* (5th ed.). Prentice Hall/Pearson Education.

- serving as a protective mechanism for family members against outside forces
- providing closer human contact and relations

The Friedman Family Assessment Model form consists of six broad categories of interview questions: (1) identification data, (2) developmental stage and history of the family, (3) environmental data, (4) family structure (i.e., role structure, family values, communication patterns, power structure), (5) family functions (i.e., affective functions, socialization functions, health care functions), and (6) family stress and coping. Each category has several subcategories (Friedman et al., 2003).

Friedman's assessment was developed to provide guidelines for family nurses who are interviewing a family. The guidelines categorize family information according to structure and function. Friedman's Family Assessment Model Form exists in both a long form and a short form. The long form is quite extensive (13 pages); it may not be possible to collect all the data in one visit, and all the categories of information listed in the guidelines may not be pertinent for every family. Similar to other approaches, this model has its strengths and weaknesses. One problem with this approach is that it can generate large quantities of data with no clear direction about how to use all the information in diagnosis, planning, and intervention. The strength of this approach is that it addresses a comprehensive list of areas for assessing the family. The short assessment form has been developed to highlight critical areas of family functioning. The short form, which is included at the website fadavis.com, outlines the types of questions the nurse can ask.

CFAM

CFAM blends nursing and family therapy concepts that are grounded in systems theory, cybernetics, communication theory, change theory, and a biology of recognition. The following concepts from general systems theory and family systems theory make up the theoretical framework for this model (Wright & Leahy, 2019, pp. 21–44):

- A family system is part of a larger suprasystem and is also composed of many subsystems.
- The family as a whole is greater than the sum of its parts.

- A change in one family member affects all family members.
- The family is able to create a balance between change and stability.
- Family members' behaviors are best understood from a perspective of circular rather than linear causality.

Cybernetics is the science of communication and control theory, and it differs from systems theory. Systems theory helps change the focus of one's conceptual lens from parts to the whole. By contrast, cybernetics changes the focus from substance to form and attempts to emphasize the design and function of any system, which would be inclusive of families. Stafford (2017) compared the cybernetic functioning of a family to a computer: at the core are individual components; however, these components function as a whole through a continuous feedback loop. When the feedback is positive, indications are that the system is operating as expected; if the feedback is negative, there is some type of breakdown within the system. Wright and Leahey (2019) drew two useful concepts from cybernetics theory:

- Families possess self-regulating ability.
- Feedback processes can simultaneously occur at several system levels within families.

Communication theory in this model is based on the work of Watzlawick and colleagues (1967, 1974). Communication represents the way that individuals interact with one another. Concepts derived from communication theory used in CFAM are as follows (Wright & Leahey, 2019):

- All nonverbal communication is meaningful.
- All communication has two major channels for transmission: digital (verbal) and analogical (nonverbal).
- A dyadic relationship has varying degrees of symmetry (similarity) and complementarity (divergence, contrast, or complementary characteristics).
- All communication has two levels: content and relationship.

Helping families to change is at the very core of family nursing interventions. Families need a balance between change and stability. Change is required to make things better, and stability is required to maintain order. Several concepts from change theory are important to this family nursing approach (Wright & Leahey, 2019):

- Change depends on the perception of the problem.
- Change is determined by structure.
- Change depends on context.
- Change depends on coevolving goals for treatment.
- Understanding alone does not lead to change.
- Change does not necessarily occur equally in all family members.
- Facilitating change is the nurse's responsibility.
- Change occurs by means of a "fit," or meshing, between the therapeutic offerings (interventions of the nurse) and the biological, psychological, sociological, cultural, and spiritual structures of family members.
- Change can be the result of a myriad of causes.

Figure 5-1 shows the branching diagram of CFAM (Wright & Leahey, 2019, p. 48). The assessment questions that accompany the model are organized into three major categories: (1) structural, (2) developmental, and (3) functional. Nurses examine a family's structural components to answer these questions: Who is in the family? What is the connection between family members? What is the family's context? Structure includes family composition, sex, sexual orientation, rank order, subsystems, and the boundaries of the family system. Aside from interview and observation, strategies recommended to assess structure include the genogram and the ecomap.

The second major assessment category in the CFAM approach is family development, which includes assessment of family stages, tasks, and attachments. For example, nurses may ask, "Where is the family in the family life cycle?" Understanding the stage of the family enables nurses to assess and intervene in a more purposeful, specific, and meaningful way. There are no actual instruments for assessing family development, but nurses can use developmental tasks and stages as guidelines.

The third area for assessment in CFAM is family functioning. Family functioning reflects

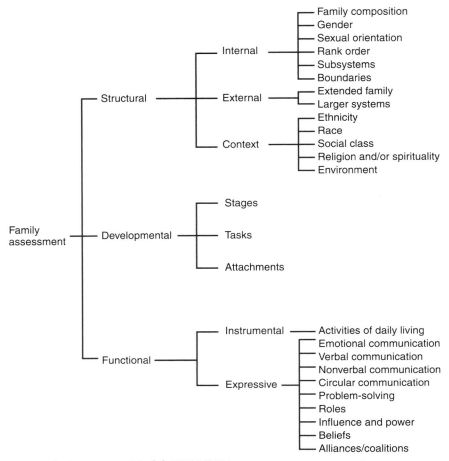

FIGURE 5-1 Calgary Family Assessment Model (CFAM) Diagram *Sources: Shajani, Z., & Snell, D. (2019).* Wright & Leahey's Nurses and families: A guide to family assessment and intervention *(7th ed.). F. A. Davis.*

how individuals actually behave in relation to one another, or the "here-and-now aspect of a family's life" (Wright & Leahey, 2019, p. 116). Aspects of family functioning include activities of daily life, such as eating, sleeping, meal preparation, and health care, as well as emotional communication, verbal and nonverbal communication, communication patterns (the way communication and responses are passed back and forth between members), problem solving, roles, influence and power, beliefs, and alliances and coalitions. Wright and Leahey indicate that nurses may assess in all three areas for a macroview of the family, or they can use any part of the approach for a microassessment. Wright and Leahey developed a companion model to CFAM called CFIM. This intervention model provides concrete strategies by which nurses can promote, improve,

and sustain effective family functioning in the cognitive, affective, and behavioral domains. The strength of CFAM and CFIM is that they are conceptually sound models that incorporate multiple theoretical aspects into working with families. The strength of this approach is also its weakness because it is difficult to implement in acute-care settings unless you are intimately knowledgeable about the model and the interventions. Silva Correa et al.'s (2019) qualitative study in Brazil used CFAM to assess nontraditional families and found its use was beneficial for nurses to understand family dynamics and to identify the needs of family units in all types of families. Leahey and Wright (2016) have offered their own narratives and reflections on the use of CFAM/CFIM and how this model allows for application when working with families.

Family Assessment Instruments

There are approximately 1,000 family-focused instruments that have been developed and used in assessing family-related variables (Touliatos et al., 2001; Westmoreland et al., 2009). Box 5-4 lists family nursing instruments that have been developed by family nursing scholars. The selection of the appropriate instrument to use can be complex. A simple questionnaire or instrument can sometimes be completed in just a few minutes, while others can take hours to administer, score, and interpret. No one instrument for data collection on family history or experience is relevant in all contexts for all purposes (Wilson et al., 2012). To select the most appropriate assessment instrument, be sure that the instrument has the following characteristics:

- written in uncomplicated language at a fifth-grade level
- only 10 to 15 minutes in length to be useful in most clinical settings (rather than research settings)
- relatively easy to score
- valid data on which to base decisions
- sensitive to sex, race, social class, education level, and ethnic background, and tested on diverse populations

Regardless of which assessment or measurement instrument is used, families should always be informed about how the information gathered through the instruments will be used by the health care providers.

BOX 5-4

Family Nursing Instruments Developed by Family Nurse Scholars

Family Functioning Variables

Feetham Family Functioning Survey (FFFS)	• Suzanne Feetham, United States (e-mail: stfeetham@gmail.com) • Hohashi, N., Honda, J., & Kong, S. K. (2008). Validity and reliability of the Chinese version of the Feetham Family Functioning Survey (FFFS). *Journal of Family Nursing, 14*(2), 201–223. • Hohashi, N., Maeda, M., & Sugishita, C. (2000). Development of the Japanese-language Feetham Family Functioning Survey (FFFS) and evaluation of its effectiveness. *Japanese Journal of Research in Family Nursing, 6*(1), 2–10. [in Japanese] • Roberts, C. S., & Feetham, S. L. (1982). Assessing family functioning across three areas of relationships. *Nursing Research, 31*(4), 231–235. • Sawin, K. J., & Harrigan, M. P. (1995). Well-established self-report instruments: Feetham Family Functioning Survey (FFFS). In K. J. Sawin & M. P. Harrigan (Eds.), *Measures of family functioning for research and practice* (pp. 42–49). Springer.
Family Management Measure (FaMM)	• Kathleen Knafl, Janet Deatrick, Agatha Gallo, United States (website: http://nursing.unc.edu/research/office-of-research-support-and-consultation/family-management-measure/) • Knafl, K., Deatrick, J. A., Gallo, A., Dixon, J., Grey, M., Knafl, G., & O'Malley, J. (2011). Assessment of the psychometric properties of the Family Management Measure. *Journal of Pediatric Psychology, 36*(5), 494–505.
Family Functioning, Health, and Social Support Instrument (FAFHES)	• Paivi Åstedt-Kurki, Marja-Terttu Tarkka, Eija Paavilainen, Kristiina Lehti, Finland (e-mail: paivi.astedt-kurki@uta.fi) • Åstedt-Kurki, P., Tarkka, M.-T., Paavilainen, E., & Lehti, K. (2002). Development and testing of a family nursing scale. *Western Journal of Nursing Research, 24*(5), 567–579. • Åstedt-Kurki, P., Tarkka, M.-T., Rikala, M.-R., Lehti, K., & Paavilainen, E. (2009). Further testing of a family nursing instrument (FAFHES). *International Journal of Nursing Studies, 46*(3), 350–359.
Family Health Routines (FHR)	• Sharon Denham, United States (e-mail: sdenham@mail.twu.edu) • Kanjanawetang, J., Yunibhand, J., Chaiyawat, W., Wu, Y.-W. B., & Denham, S. A. (2009). Thai family health routines: Scale development and psychometric testing. *Southeast Asian Journal of Tropical Medicine and Public Health, 40*(3), 629–643.

(continued)

BOX 5-4

Family Nursing Instruments Developed by Family Nurse Scholars—cont'd

Assessment of Strategies in Families–Effectiveness (ASF–E)	• Marie-Luise Friedemann, United States (website: https://friedemm.info/index.php/assessment-of-strategies-in-nursing/development) • Friedemann, M. L., Cardea, J. M., Harrison, M., & Lenz, E. R. (1991). An instrument to evaluate effectiveness in family functioning. *Western Journal of Nursing Research, 13*(2), 220–241. • Friedemann, M. L., & Smith, A. A. (1997). A triangulation approach to testing a family instrument. *Western Journal of Nursing Research, 19*(3), 364–378.
Iceland-Expressive Family Functioning Questionnaire (ICE-EFFQ)	• Eydis Sveinbjarnardottir, Erla Kolbrun Svavarsdottir, & Birgir Hrafnkelsson, Iceland (e-mail: eks@hi.is) • Sveinbjarnardottir, E. K., Svavarsdottir, E. K., & Hrafnkelsson, B. (2012a). Psychometric development of the Iceland-Expressive Family Functioning Questionnaire (ICE-EFFQ). *Journal of Family Nursing, 18*(3), 353–377.
Iceland-Expressive Family Functioning Questionnaire (ICE-EFFQ)	• Margrét Gisladottir, Erla Kolbrun Svavarsdottir, Iceland (e-mail: eks@hi.is) • Gisladottir, M., & Svavarsdottir, E. K. (2016). Development and psychometric testing of the Iceland-Family Illness Beliefs Questionnaire. *Journal of Family Nursing, 22*(3), 321–338. • Svavarsdottir, E. K., Looman, W., Tryggvadottir, G. B., & Garwick, A. (2017). Psychometric testing of the Icelandic Health Care Practitioner Illness Beliefs Questionnaire among school nurses. *Scandinavian Journal of Caring Sciences, 32*(1).
F-COPES	• McCubbin, H. I., Thompson, A., & McCubbin, M. A. (1996). *Family assessment: Resiliency, coping and adaptation-inventories for research and practice*. University of Wisconsin.
Survey of Family Environment (SFE)	• Naohiro Hohashi & Junko Honda, Japan (e-mail: naohiro@hohashi.org) • Hohashi, N., & Honda, J. (2012). Development and testing of the Survey of Family Environment (SFE): A novel instrument to measure family functioning and needs for family support. *Journal of Nursing Measurement, 20*(3), 212–229.

FAMILY NURSE/FAMILY CARE VARIABLES

Family Nursing Practice Scale (FNPS)	• Peggy Simpson, Canada; Marie Tarrant, Hong Kong (e-mail: peggysimpson01@gmail.com) • Simpson, P., & Tarrant, M. (2006). Development of the Family Nursing Practice Scale. *Journal of Family Nursing, 12*(4), 413–425.
Family Nurse Caring Beliefs Scale (FNCBS)	• Sonja Meiers, Patricia Tomlinson, Cynthia Peden-McAlpine, United States (e-mail: smeiers@winona.edu) • Meiers, S. J., Tomlinson, P., & Peden-McAlpine, C. (2007). Development of the Family Nurse Caring Belief Scale (FNCBS). *Journal of Family Nursing, 13*(4), 484–502.
Families' Importance in Nursing Care: Nurses' Attitudes (FINC-NA)	• Eva Benzein, Pauline Johansson, Kristofer Arestedt, Agneta Berg, Britt-Inger Saveman, Sweden (e-mail: eva.benzein@lnu.se; britt-inger.saveman@nurs.umu.se) • Benzein, E., Johansson, P., Årestedt, K. F., Berg, A., & Saveman, B.-I. (2008). Families' importance in nursing care: Nurses' attitudes—an instrument development. *Journal of Family Nursing, 14*(1), 97–117. • Saveman, B.-I., Benzein, E. G., Engström, A. H., & Årestedt, K. (2011). Refinement and psychometric re-evaluation of the instrument: Families' Importance in Nursing Care—Nurses' Attitudes. *Journal of Family Nursing, 17*(3), 312–329.
Parents' Perceptions of Care (PPC)	• Hanna Maijala, Tiina Luukkaala, Paivi Åstedt-Kurki, Finland (e-mail: paivi.astedt-kurki@uta.fi) • Maijala, H., Luukkaala, T., & Åstedt-Kurki, P. (2009). Measuring parents' perceptions of care. Psychometric development of a research instrument. *Journal of Family Nursing, 15*(3), 343–359.
Family Nurse Presence Scale (FNP)	• Sandra Eggenberger, United States (e-mail: sandra.eggenberger@mnsu.edu)

BOX 5-4

Family Nursing Instruments Developed by Family Nurse Scholars—cont'd

Iceland-Family Perceived Support Questionnaire (ICE-FPSQ)

- Eydis Sveinbjarnardottir, Erla Kolbrun Svavarsdottir, Birgir Hrafnkelsson, Iceland (e-mail: eks@hi.is)
- Bruce, E., Dorell, A., Lindh, V., Erlingsson, C., Lindkvist, M., & Sundin, K. (2016). Translation and testing of the Swedish version of the Iceland-Family Perceived Support Questionnaire with parents of children with congenital heart defects. *Journal of Family Nursing, 22*(3), 298–320.
- Sveinbjarnardottir, E. K., Svavarsdottir, E. K., & Hrafnkelsson, B. (2012b). Psychometric development of the Iceland-Family Perceived Support Questionnaire (ICE-FPSQ). *Journal of Family Nursing, 18*(3), 328–352.

Sources: Bell, J. (2019). *Family nursing research instruments developed by family nurses* (Blog Post). https://janicembell.com /family-nursing-research-instruments-developed-by-family-nurses/; and Sawin, K. J. (2016). Measurement in family nursing: Established instruments and new directions [Guest editorial]. *Journal of Family Nursing, 22*(3), 287–297.

Family Genogram and Family Ecomap

Two family data-gathering instruments that should be used in working with families are the family genogram and the family ecomap. Both are short, easy instruments used to perform assessment and gather essential family data while engaging the family in therapeutic conversation. Genograms and ecomaps provide health care providers with visual diagrams of the current family story and situation (Kaakinen & Tabacco, 2018). Information gathered from both the genogram and ecomap helps guide the family plan of action and the selection of intervention strategies. One of the major benefits of using these two instruments when working with families is that family members can feel and visualize the amount of energy they are expending to manage the situation, which in itself is therapeutic for the family (Freeman, 2018).

The use of genograms and ecomaps among nurses and other health care providers is growing, and these useful tools are being applied in several practice and research contexts. Genograms, used historically in the context of genetic prediction and counseling, have been applied alongside ecomaps as primary assessment and decision-making tools in acute centers (Leahey & Svavarsdottir, 2009; Svavarsdottir, 2008). Examples of how other health care providers have used these tools include enhancing health promotion (Kehoe & Kehoe, 2008), increasing provider cultural competence and spiritual assessment of families (Hodge & Limb, 2010), and assessment of child social support systems (Baumgartner et al., 2012). It is clear that generating and annotating visual data in these diagrammatic forms will be increasingly useful to nurses caring for families in many settings and contexts.

Family Genogram

The *family genogram* is a format for drawing a family tree that records information about family members and their relationships for at least three generations (McGoldrick, 2016; McGoldrick et al., 2008). In addition, the genogram captures significant nonblood kin who are considered family, as well as pets. This type of diagram offers a rich source of information for planning intervention strategies because it displays the complexity of a family visually in a way that provides a quick overview. Family genograms help both nurses and families to see and think systematically about families and the impact of the health event on family structure, function, and processes.

The three-generational family genogram had its origin in Family Systems Theory (Bowen, 1985; Bowen & Kerr, 1988). People are organized into family systems by generation, age, sex, or other similar features. How a person fits into his or her family structure influences the family's functioning and relational patterns, and what type of family he or she will carry forward into the next generation. Bowen (1985) incorporated Toman's (1976) ideas about the importance of sex and birth order in shaping sibling relationships and characteristics. Families repeat themselves through the generations in a phenomenon called the *transmission of family patterns* (Bowen, 1985). What happens in one generation repeats itself in the next generation; thus, many of the same strengths and problems are played out from generation to generation. These include psychosocial, physical, and mental health issues.

Nurses establish therapeutic relationships with families through the process of asking questions while collecting family data. Families become more engaged in their current situation during this interaction as their family story unfolds. Both the nurse and the family can see the big picture historically on the vertical axis of the genogram and horizontally across the family (McGoldrick, 2016; McGoldrick et al., 2008). This approach can help families see connectedness and help identify potential and missing support people.

The diagramming of family genograms must adhere to specific rules and symbols to ensure that all parties involved have the same understanding and interpretations. It is important not to confuse family genograms with a family genetic pedigree. A family pedigree is specific to genetic assessments (see Chapter 8), whereas a genogram has broader uses for family health care practitioners. Genograms may assist nurses to offer a more comprehensive, holistic nursing care perspective (Charnock, 2016; Gallagher, 2013). Creative blended models built on these ideas are emerging in practice, with innovative applications such as the use of color coding for enhancing multimodal understanding of children and families (Driessnack, 2009).

Figure 5-2 provides a basic genogram from which a nurse can start diagramming family members during the first, second, and third generations

(McGoldrick et al., 1999). Figure 5-3 also depicts the genogram symbols used to describe basic family membership and structure; family interaction patterns; and other family information of particular importance, such as health status, substance abuse, obesity, smoking, and mental health comorbidities (McGoldrick et al., 2008). The health history of all family members (e.g., morbidity, mortality, and onset of illness) is important information for family nurses and can be the focus of analysis of the family genogram. An example of a family genogram developed from one interview is contained in the Bono family case study that follows.

The structure of the interview conducted to gather the genogram information is based on the reasons why the nurse is working with the family. For example, if the context of creating a genogram is that of obtaining a health history aimed at uncovering family patterns of illness, the nurse may wish to explore more fully the health history of each generational family member. On the other hand, if the context of the nursing care is determining the nature of social relationships and roles among family members to craft an acute-care plan of discharge, the nurse may wish to focus the interview more closely on determining who is directly in the home and how their relationships function to aid in the recovery of the ill family member. A suggested format for conducting a concise, focused family genogram interview is outlined in Box 5-5. Most families are cooperative and interested in completing their genograms, which becomes part of their ongoing health care record. The genogram does not have to be completed at one sitting.

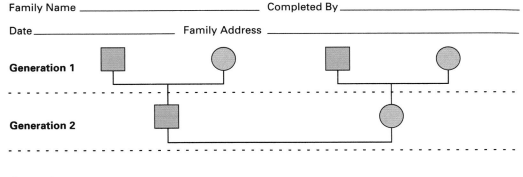

FIGURE 5-2 Basic Genogram Format

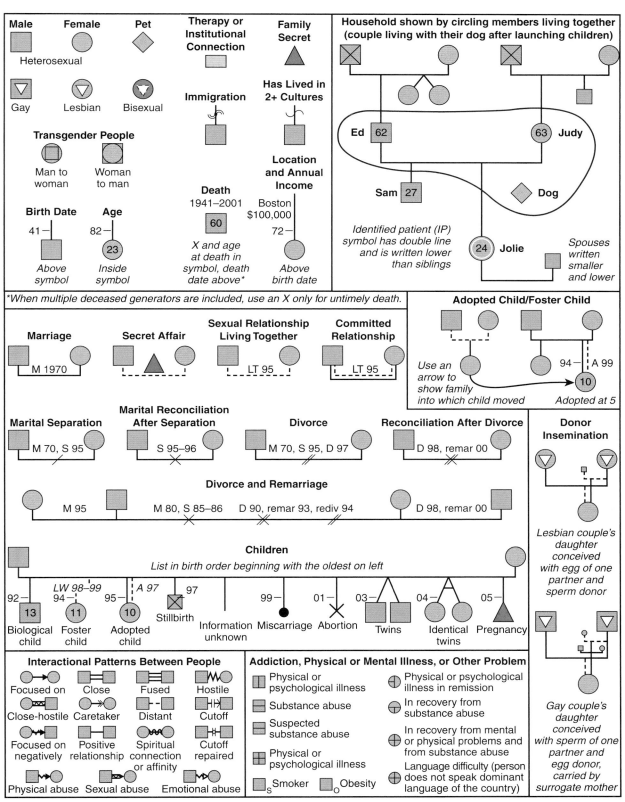

FIGURE 5-3 Genogram Symbols *Sources: McGoldrick, M., Gerson, R., & Petry, S. S. (2008).* Genograms: Assessment and intervention *(3rd ed.); and McGoldrick, M., Gerson, R., & Schellenberger, S. (1999).* Genograms in family assessment *(2nd ed.); with permission from W.W. Norton.*

BOX 5-5

Family Genogram Interview Data Collection

During a family genogram interview, do the following:

- Identify who is in the immediate family.
- Identify the person who has the health problem.
- Identify all the people who live with the immediate family.
- Determine how all the people are related.
- Gather the following information on each family member.
  - age
  - sex

- correct spelling of name
- health problems
- occupation
- dates of relationships: marriage, separation, divorce, living together, living together/committed
- dates and age of death
- Seek the same information for all family members across each generation for consistency and to reveal patterns of health and illness.
- Add any information relative to the situation, such as geographical location and interaction patterns.

As the same or a different nurse continues to work with a family, data can be added to the genogram over time in a continuing process. Families should be given a copy of their own genogram, with an explanation of the process and the interpretation of the family's history.

Family Ecomap

A *family ecomap* provides information about systems outside the immediate nuclear family that are sources of social support or that are stressors to the family. The ecomap is a visual representation of the family unit in relation to the larger community in which it is embedded (Kaakinen & Tabacco, 2018) and of the relationship between an individual family and the world around it (McGoldrick et al., 2008). The ecomap is thus an overview of the family in its current context, picturing the important connections among the nuclear family, the extended family, and the larger community.

The blank ecomap form consists of a large circle with smaller circles around it (Figure 5-4). A simplified version of the family is placed in the center of the larger circle to complete the ecomap. This circle marks the boundary between the family and its extended external environment. The smaller outer circles represent significant people, agencies, or institutions with which the family interacts. Lines are drawn between the circles and the family members to depict the nature and quality of the relationships and to show what kinds of energy and resources are moving in and out of the immediate family. Straight lines show strong or close relationships; the more

pronounced the line or the greater the number of lines, the stronger the relationship. Straight lines with slashes denote stressful relationships, and broken lines show tenuous or distant relationships. Arrows reveal the direction of the flow of energy and resources between individuals and between the family and the environment. Ecomaps not only portray the present situation but also can be used to set goals; for example, to increase connections and exchanges with individuals and agencies in the community. See the Bono family case study later in this chapter for an example of a completed ecomap.

The value of using a genogram and ecomap in family nursing practice is extensive. By creating a visual picture of the system in which the family exists, a family is better able to envision alternative solutions and possible social support networks (Freeman, 2018). Ecomaps help patients in palliative care identify who is important and who they desire to have involved in their lives (Gallagher, 2013). Family genograms have been used by nurses in diverse cultures: for example, in Brazil to work with children who have special needs (Neves et al., 2013); in Brazil, as identified in a systematic review of Brazilian use of family genograms and ecomaps (Nascimento et al., 2014); in Iceland, while working with families, children, and adolescents in active cancer treatment (Svavarsdottir & Sigurdardottir, 2013); and in Sweden, where spiritual ecomaps were used as a component of care (Hodge, 2015). In addition, the process of this data collection itself helps to expose a clearer picture of the supportive or unsupportive family relationships that are part of a family system (Neufeld

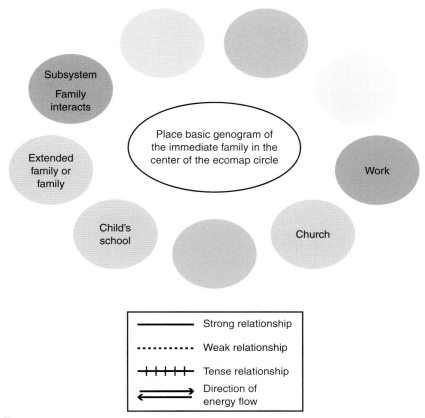

FIGURE 5-4 Blank Ecomap

et al., 2007). This information enhances understanding of the family's social network with its caregivers (Rempel et al., 2007).

Family Health Literacy

The definition of *health literacy* has evolved. The following definition is the most comprehensive and explanatory:

Health literacy is linked to literacy and entails people's knowledge, motivation, and competence to access, understand, appraise, and apply health information in order to make judgments and decisions in everyday life concerning healthcare, disease prevention and health promotion to maintain or improve quality of life during the life course. (Sorensen et al., 2012, p. 3)

Concepts of health literacy include the comprehension of medical words, the ability to follow medical instructions, and the understanding of the consequences when instructions are not followed (Rutherford et al., 2018). Many health care providers have limited ability to identify patients with low health literacy, so the Agency for Healthcare Research and Quality (AHRQ) suggests that health care providers use health literacy guidelines for low literacy with all patients (Brega et al., 2015). AHRQ has an online toolkit (see www.ahrq.gov/professionals/quality-patient-safety/quality-resources/tools/literacy-toolkit/index.html) that is an excellent resource for all health care providers. Nurses who understand the concept of health literacy can provide education, materials, and other supports such as videos or websites that are accessible to the family.

Health literacy is an important measure for health care providers because lower health literacy is strongly associated with poor health outcomes (Berkman et al., 2011; Dickens & Piano, 2013; Federman et al., 2014; French, 2015; Parnell,

2014; Watts et al., 2017). Health literacy plays a primary role in people's ability to gain knowledge, make decisions, and take actions that result in positive health outcomes (Dickens & Piano, 2013; Sorensen et al., 2012), especially when managing a chronic illness (Dickens & Piano, 2013; Watts et al., 2017).

Multiple approaches to helping patients understand their health and health care needs have been designed. Table 5-3 includes tips for successful oral education. Box 5-6 outlines guidelines for improving readability and visualization of written material.

Nurses need to approach assessment of a family's health literacy with sensitivity and understanding. It is a crucial element to consider during the analysis of the family story and in the development of the family action plan.

ANALYSIS OF THE FAMILY STORY

One of the challenges of data collection is organizing the individual pieces of information so that the big picture, or whole family story, can be understood and analyzed. To understand the family picture, the nurse must consolidate the data that were collected into meaningful patterns or categories. This process helps the nurse visualize the relationships between and among the patterns to uncover how the family is managing the situation. Diagramming the family and the relationships between the data groups assists in identifying the most pressing issues or problems for the family. If the family and nurse focus on solving these major family problems, the outcome will have a ripple effect by positively influencing other areas of family functioning.

Table 5-3	Tips for Successful Oral Education	
LANGUAGE ELEMENTS	**RECOMMENDATIONS**	**EXAMPLE**
Use the active voice.	• The subject of the sentence is performing the action.	• You will take your medications with breakfast. *Not:* The medications are taken at breakfast.
Converse: be interactive.	• Limit long monologues.	• What questions do you have for me? (Ask this several times in the teaching session.)
Be considerate toward listeners.	• Announce topics.	• Aspirin. Aspirin helps stop heart attacks.
	• Periodically call the learner by name.	• Rosie, could you tell me what you ate yesterday?
	• Convey information in little stories.	• I know a woman named Charisse who forgot to take her Plavix for 3 days, and then wham, she got chest pain and came back to the emergency room. And guess what? The metal coil they just put in her heart had blocked off and caused another heart attack!
Give "need to know" rather than "nice to know" information.	• Reinforce important information (such as the prescription regimen).	• Take your water pill every morning, right after breakfast. *Not:* Your diuretic works on the distal loop of Henle.
	• Limit information on pathophysiology.	• When you leave the hospital today, I want you to remember to make your follow-up appointment, take your Plavix every day, and call us if you have any chest pain.
	• Provide information in three to five chunks in each session.	
Focus on the patient.	• Contextualize the information being taught.	• In the morning, get out of bed, go to the bathroom, and then weigh yourself. Do this every day, before you eat or drink anything for breakfast.
	• Use everyday language familiar to the patient.	• Fast food is really bad for your health.
Be mindful of language complexity.	• Speak in short sentences (fewer than 15 words).	• If you have chest pain, go to the emergency room.
	• Use words with fewer than three syllables.	• Drink a lot of water with these pills.
	• Decrease medical jargon.	• Your water pill will make you pee a lot.

Source: Dickens, C., & Piano, M. R. (2013). Health literacy and nursing: An update. *American Journal of Nursing, 113*(6), 52–57, Wolters Kluwer Health, Inc. with permission.

BOX 5-6

Guidelines for Improving Readability and Visuals of Written Materials

Criteria	Specifications
Typography	• Use bold or underlined headers. • Use sans serif or serif 12- to 14-point fonts. • Do not use all caps for headers. • Use white space around your main content area. • Use high-contrast colors (black on white).
Layout	• Put the most important information first. • Limit bullet points to three to seven items at a time. • Turn sentences into lists. • Create headings with subheadings.
Language	• Explain how to perform the action, *not* the mechanism of action. • Limit use of the words *not, don't,* or *unless.* • Select familiar words and use them frequently. • Provide specific action steps. • Keep paragraphs short. • Use active, *not* passive, voice. • Use words with one or two syllables when possible. • Limit the use of jargon or scientific language. • If you have to use medical jargon, define the word. • Provide text at the fifth-grade or lower reading level.
Graphics	• Use captions that explain each graphic. • Place illustrations adjacent to text on the page. • Do not use shading or graying. • Do not use cues, such as circles or arrows. • Use photographs to portray real-life events and emotions. • Use culturally relevant images. • When showing a sequence, number the images.

Source: Dickens, C., & Piano, M. R. (2013). Health literacy and nursing: An update. *American Journal of Nursing, 113*(6), 52–57, Wolters Kluwer Health, Inc. with permission.

The family reasoning web (Figure 5-5) is an organizational tool to help analyze the family story by clustering individual pieces of data into meaningful family categories. The components of the family reasoning web have been drawn from various theoretical concepts, such as Family Structure and Function Theory, Family Developmental Theory, Family Stress Theory, and family health promotion models. This systematic approach to collecting and analyzing information helps structure the information collection process to ensure the inclusion of important pieces of information. The categories of the family reasoning web are as follows:

1. family routines of daily living (i.e., sleeping, meals, child care, exercise)
2. family communication
3. family supports and resources
4. family roles
5. family beliefs
6. family developmental stage
7. family health knowledge
8. family environment
9. family stress management
10. family culture
11. family spirituality

Once the data have been placed into the categories of the family reasoning web template, the nurse assigns a family nursing diagnosis to each category. "A nursing diagnosis is defined as a clinical judgment about individuals, families, or community responses to actual or potential health problems/life processes. Nursing diagnoses link information to care planning. Nursing diagnoses provide the basis for selecting nursing interventions to help achieve outcomes for which nurses are accountable" (Doenges et al., 2018, p. 10).

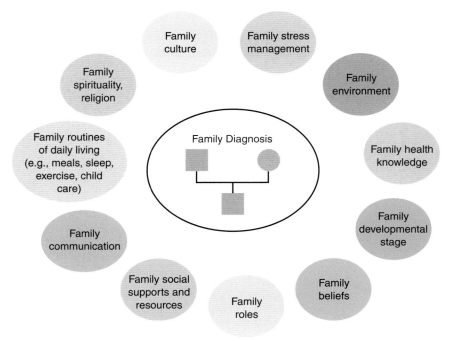

FIGURE 5-5 Family Reasoning Web Template

NANDA International Inc. (NANDA-I) has approved more than 200 nursing diagnoses that are used in multiple member countries. NANDA-I nursing diagnoses that are specific to families are listed in Box 5-7. If the pattern of family data in the specific category in the family reasoning web does not match one of the NANDA-I nursing diagnoses, nurses are encouraged to create a family nursing diagnosis that captures the family problem. Nursing diagnosis manuals are extremely important resources for nurses because family nursing diagnoses are readily linked with both the Nursing Intervention Classification (NIC) (Butcher et al., 2019) and the Nursing Outcomes Classification (NOC) (Moorhead et al., 2018) datasets. These resources provide many new ideas

---

BOX 5-7

NANDA-I Nursing Diagnoses Relevant to Family Nursing

Following are nursing diagnoses relevant to family nursing:

- ineffective childbearing process
- risk for ineffective childbearing process
- risk for impaired parent/infant/child attachment
- caregiver role strain
- risk for caregiver role strain
- ineffective role performance
- parental role conflict
- compromised family coping

- disabled family coping
- readiness for enhanced family coping
- dysfunctional family processes: alcoholism
- readiness for enhanced family processes
- interrupted family processes
- readiness for enhanced parenting
- impaired parenting
- risk for impaired parenting
- relocation stress syndrome
- ineffective role performance
- ineffective family therapeutic regimen management

Source: Doenges, M. E., Moorhouse, M. F., & Murr, A. C. (2018). *Nursing diagnosis manual: Planning, individualizing, and documenting client care* (6th ed.). F. A. Davis, with permission.

for family interventions and suggest focused family outcomes that can be explored with families.

Other diagnostic classification systems that can be used to identify problems include the Omaha System–Community Health Classification System (Martin, 2005; Omaha System, 2017), the *Diagnostic and Statistical Manual of Mental Disorders, Fifth Edition* ([DSM-5], American Psychiatric Association, 2013), and the *International Classification of Diseases, Tenth Revision, Clinical Modification* ([ICD-10-CM]; Centers for Disease and Control Prevention [CDC], 2020a). See Boxes 5-8 and 5-9 for examples of selected family diagnoses from the *DSM* and *ICD-10-CM* sources, respectively.

A rapidly growing system of diagnostic language relevant to nursing in North America is that of the World Health Organization (WHO) *ICD* companions, the *International Classification of Functioning (ICF)*, and its related child and youth version *(ICF-CY)* (WHO, 2018). This broad schema of classification focuses on making diagnostic statements of health impact in four domains: body structure, body function, activity and participation, and environment (WHO, 2018). Family nursing practice greatly involves the focus on the domains of activity and participation and on the environmental context of family life. Given that nurses' primary focus with individuals and families

---

BOX 5-8

Selected Family-Centered Diagnoses From *Diagnostic and Statistical Manual of Mental Disorders, Fifth Edition*

V61.9	Relational problem related to a mental disorder or general medical condition
V61.20	Parent-child relational problem
V61.10	Partner relational problem
V61.8	Sibling relational problem
V71.02	Child or adolescent antisocial behavior
V62.82	Bereavement
V62.3	Academic problem
V62.4	Acculturation problem
V62.89	Phase-of-life problem

Source: American Psychiatric Association. (2013). *Diagnostic and statistical manual of mental disorders (DSM-5)* (5th ed.). American Psychiatric Association Publishing.

BOX 5-9

Selected Family-Centered Diagnoses From *ICD-10-CM*

Z62.82	Parent-child conflict
F93.9	Childhood emotional disorder, unspecified
Z62.891	Sibling relational problem
Z63.8	Family disruption
Z63.5	Disruption of family by separation or divorce
Z30.09	Family planning advice

Source: Centers for Disease Control and Prevention. (2020a). *International classification of diseases, tenth revision, clinical modification (ICD-10-CM)*. https://www.cdc.gov/nchs/icd/icd10cm.htm

is the functional aspect of health in daily life, this system of categorizing and coding functional outcomes of health is compelling. The *ICF* and *ICF-CY* approaches are used with expanded focus in Europe and Canada particularly (Florin et al., 2013; Raggi et al., 2010).

After the categories have been assigned and a family nursing diagnosis has been determined, the next step in analyzing the family story is for the nurse and family to work together to determine the relationships between the categories. Arrows are drawn between the family categories to show the direction of influence if the data in one category influence the data in another category. By systematically working through all the relationships, the nurse and family clarify the important family problems or issues because they are the ones that have the most arrows indicating the strongest relationships to all other areas of family functioning. This step reveals the primary family problems.

Another dimension of the family story that is of importance to nurses is the dimension of beliefs. Family and family member beliefs about health, illness, health care providers, and even their own roles and processes are of great importance for nurses to assess in planning to provide optimal care. The Beliefs and Illness Model by Wright and Bell (2009) suggests that nurses should assess families' beliefs in several areas, specifically, family structure, roles, communication, and decision-making authority; beliefs about health and illness (how they are defined, why they occur, how they are managed); and beliefs about health care providers (their intentions, motivations, knowledge and the meaning of their presence and actions to the families and their health or illness experience). Individuals and families often behave based on their beliefs; thus, any attempt on the part of nurses to engage families in health promotion, health literacy, or health intervention in any setting requires an exploration of these key areas. After verifying all these findings with the family, the next step is to work with the family to understand their preferences for decision making and to design a family plan of care accordingly.

Shared Decision Making

Family nurses should explore how involved the family would like to be in the decision-making processes. Universal needs of families include consistency, clarity, comprehensive information, and

involvement in shared decision making with the health care provider (Elwyn et al., 2013; Légaré & Thompson-Leduc, 2014). One of the problems with the implementation of shared decision making is that individual health care providers may have a different definition and understanding of the components of this concept, as well as personal biases and beliefs about how individuals and families may or may not wish to participate (Elwyn et al., 2013). Shared decision making is not just informing the family of the decisions and keeping the lines of communication open, nor is it the health care providers determining what decisions the family can make. Shared decision making is defined as "a collaborative process that allows patients, or their surrogates, and clinicians to make health care decisions together, taking into account the best scientific evidence available, as well as the patient's values, goals, and preferences" (Kon et al., 2016). Patients and families vary in the process and degree to which they would like to be involved in decision making (Dy & Purnell, 2012; Légaré & Thompson-Leduc, 2014; Stiggelbout et al., 2015). Nurses should not assume that patients' or families' reluctance to engage in the decision-making process means that they do not want to be involved because reluctance could be related to several factors, such as a lack of self-efficacy (Légaré & Thompson-Leduc, 2014), poor understanding of health statistics (McCaffery et al., 2010), difficulty imagining future health state or events (McCaffery et al., 2010), and a belief that physicians are supposed to make these decisions (Hawley & Morris, 2017). In addition, some health care providers may feel more qualified to make decisions for a family than the family members and may therefore intimidate family members.

The amount of information families seek or need changes during the course of the health event, the stage of the illness, and the likelihood of a cure (Stiggelbout et al., 2015). Supporting the hypothesis that not all families and family members want full involvement in making health care decisions, Makoul and Clayman (2006, p. 307) outlined the following nine options for shared decision making:

- doctor alone
- doctor-led and patient acknowledgment sought or offered
- doctor-led and patient agreement sought or offered

- doctor-led and patient views/option sought or offered
- shared equally
- patient-led and doctor views/opinions sought or offered
- patient-led and doctor agreement sought or offered
- patient-led and doctor acknowledgment sought or offered
- patient alone

Studies have shown that some patients who elected to defer decisions to their health care provider want more involvement in making decisions after knowing more about their health situation (Stiggelbout et al., 2015). At the beginning of a health event that requires shared decision making, many patients and their family members do not have clearly defined preferences (Pieterse et al., 2013).

Several instruments have been designed to assist provider, patients, and families to work through their preferences and participate in decision making. One of the major concerns about use of these instruments is that they are not well tested for patients and families of minority race and ethnic backgrounds (Hawley & Morris, 2017) or with patients with lower health literacy (McCaffery et al., 2010). An option grid is one strategy for implementation of shared decision making (Elwyn et al., 2013). An option grid is developed by the family nurse and keeps health literacy principles at the fifth-grade level. Elwyn et al. specifically developed the grid format as a decision-making paper worksheet addressing common therapeutic approaches to specific health conditions where patients and families could view the benefits or drawbacks associated with different possible treatment decisions. On the worksheet, the most relevant, frequently asked questions about a specific condition make up the rows of the grid, and the specific options available for the decision make up the columns. Patients are given the paper grid, and the physician talks them through the options available to them. Table 5-4 provides an option grid that a nurse could design to help parents determine respite placement for their 12-year-old daughter who is medically fragile with severe cerebral palsy. This specific tool shows promise for nurses working with families because it not only represents the principles of FCC in practice, but it is also useful when families have difficulties understanding their options and the potential benefits or consequences associated with their choices.

Another approach to shared decision making is to use the Patient/Parent Involvement Information Assessment Tool (PINT) developed by Sobo

Table 5-4	Example of Option Grid	

The following is an example of an option grid for helping a family to decide about 1-week respite placement for their 12-year-old medically fragile child.

OPTION 1: HOME	OPTION 2: GRANDMOTHER'S HOME	OPTION 3: NURSING HOME
Child knows own home and is around familiar surroundings.	Child has been to grandmother's home only a couple of times because it is in a different city.	New setting for child.
Home is adapted to the child's needs and wheelchair.	Home is not adapted to the physical care needs of the child, such as wheelchair and bathing.	Setting can accommodate the child's special needs and wheelchair.
Caregiver would be the skills trainer who knows the child.	Caregiver is grandmother, who the child knows well and has spent considerable time with.	No personal relationship with caregivers in this setting. Grandmother could visit during the day.
Parents are comfortable with the child being with the skills worker during the day, but they do not have experience with this person at night.	Parents are comfortable with the child being with the grandmother. Grandmother has helped take care of the child for short times before, such as a weekend.	Parents do not have a relationship with the caregivers in this setting.
Cost: $250 a day for 7 days, for a total of $1,750. This would come out of the parents' pocket because insurance does not cover this care.	Cost: Nothing.	Cost: Covered by insurance.

(2004). PINT is a self-administered survey that can be kept in the medical record to facilitate and target information for communication between the health care team and the family. When collaborating in the care and meeting the needs of individuals and family members, nurses may ask the following two sample questions from PINT (Sobo, 2004, p. 258):

1. When possible, what level of information would you prefer to receive?

   ■ the simplest information possible
   ■ more than the simplest, but want to keep it on everyday terms
   ■ in-depth information that you can help me understand
   ■ as much in-depth and detailed information as can be provided

2. When possible, what decision-making role do you want to assume?

   ■ leave all decisions to the health care team
   ■ have the care team make the decisions about care with serious consideration of our views
   ■ share in the making of the decisions with the health care team
   ■ make all the decisions about care with serious consideration of the health care team advice

Shared decision making requires that health care providers tailor their communication, accommodate their talk to the level of the family, and present information in a way that allows the family to make informed choices.

FAMILY NURSING INTERVENTION

The family plan of action (or care) is designed by the nurse and the family to focus on the concerns that were identified in the family reasoning web as the most pressing or as causing the family the most stress. The plan should account for the family's preferences for decision making and should meet the family members' health literacy needs. The more specific the family plan of action and the interventions, the more positive the outcomes. The role of the nurse is to offer guidance to the family, provide information, and assist in

the planning interventions. Working with families from an outcome perspective helps to clarify what information and resources are necessary to address the family need. The following four points can help the family break the plan into action steps:

1. We need the following type of help.
2. We need the following information.
3. We need the following supplies or resources.
4. We need to involve or tell the following people about our family action plan.

For the purposes of clarity and evaluation, this plan should be a written document. The action steps or interventions should be clear and concise. The plan should outline specifically who needs to do what, by when, and also articulate the time frame in which the nurse will follow up. The last step of any family action plan should entail evaluation, with the nurse and family reflecting and sharing ideas about what worked well, what needs to continue to be addressed by the family, and avenues for seeking help in the future.

Working with families to improve health and adapt to illness is the primary goal of family health care nursing. Although there is direct evidence of the potential outcomes and effects associated with family nursing intervention, few studies have been conducted longitudinally or across multiple populations. What has been distilled from the literature on family health care intervention is that family intervention does seem to produce better effects than the usual, individual-focused medical care; greater effects have been shown in improving child health than adult health in some chronic conditions; and family-focused intervention examples found in childhood obesity efforts reveal the most compelling effects (Chesla, 2010).

Chesla (2010) also articulated that the means of interventions varied and ranged from simple home visits with the goal of coaching families to much more complex educational and skill-developing strategies. Nurses were involved in relationship-based interventions to improve family communication, problem solving, and skill building as they related to illness or health management. The more tools nurses tended to use to assist families (multi-modal) as part of their care plans, the better the outcomes seemed to be, particularly in managing complex health conditions that required numerous lifestyle changes. Family members were sometimes noted to be beneficiaries of interventions, experiencing unique and improved outcomes that were separate from the health of the patient (Chesla, 2010). More research is needed to demonstrate the impact of intervention strategies on individual and family health.

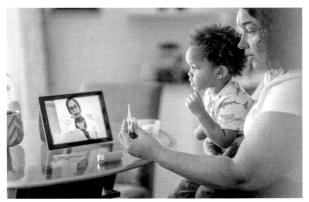

© *istock.com/FatCamera*

Nurses help by (1) providing direct care, (2) removing barriers to needed services, and (3) improving the capacity of the family to act on its own behalf and assume responsibility. Family nursing interventions can be directed toward improving the health outcomes of the member with the illness or condition, the family members' health-related outcomes of caregiving, or a combination of both. One of the important aspects of working with the family is the nurse–family relationship, which is an intervention in and of itself because families can experience a sense of strength, comfort, and confidence that can be therapeutic and useful (Friedman et al., 2003).

The nurse is responsible for helping the family implement the plan of care. The nurse can assume the role of teacher, role model, coach, counselor, advocate, coordinator, consultant, and evaluator in helping the family to implement the plan of care they jointly create. The types of interventions are limitless because they are designed with the family to meet its needs in the context of its family story. The three examples that follow illustrate different family nursing interventions in various contexts.

Brief Therapeutic Conversations in Acute Care

Brief therapeutic family conversations or interviews are an important family intervention (Bell, 2016) and have been linked to improved health outcomes (Street et al., 2009). These brief interviews could include nurses making introductions to family members, collecting focused data to complete simple genograms and ecomaps, and opening pathways of knowing about a family's self-defined needs and priorities (Wright & Leahey, 2019). Svavarsdottir et al. (2012) conducted a study measuring families' perceptions of nurse support and family members' own reports of family functioning. The study compared families who received brief family intervention interviews with nurses and those who did not. Predictably, families who received the nursing intervention interview reported feeling more supported than those who did not. Surprisingly, this finding was true for families with a child with an acute health crisis but was not true for those coping with chronic conditions. Expressive family functioning did not seem to change in the latter situation. Families of acutely ill children may experience significant benefits, however, when nurses take small amounts of time to enact simple family health care strategies (Svavarsdottir et al., 2012).

Home Visits and Telephone Support

Nursing visits to family homes are part of the early historical tradition of nursing and are appropriate to use today in family nursing. Gehring et al. (2017) utilized home visits when working with families whose children identified as obese in order to evaluate pediatric weight management. Of the 56 families, 89% were interested in having a home visit and felt this was helpful when working with their families (Gehring et al., 2017). Haber et al. (2020) found that when families were given oral health education during home visits, they incorporated this teaching into their child-care routines, with their children having significantly improved oral health outcomes.

Northouse et al. (2007) utilized a clinical trial design to provide three in-home support visits along with two follow-up telephone calls to partnered couples where men were living through prostate cancer treatment. In the study, both patients and partners who received the in-home visits and phone calls reported that their communication and relationship with one another improved. Nurses offered these families coaching in communication, facilitated discussions that identified the beliefs and needs of both partners, and helped the families make decisions about care tasks and life balance. The partners seemed to benefit by demonstrating improved quality of life, increased self-efficacy, and less overall caregiving negativity than partners who did not receive the intervention. In addition, some spouses continued to report these effects for up to 8 months following the intervention, suggesting that the act of providing access to nurses in the home and via telephone helped spouses long after the contact ended (Northouse et al., 2007).

Self-Care Talk for Family Caregivers

Nurses caring for families can intervene to promote health by helping families to identify potential health risks that stress the health of the family, such as when a 45-year-old father and husband with metabolic syndrome refuses to adhere to diet and exercise interventions. Parker et al. (2011) proposed a unique family nursing intervention for developing self-care motivation and implementation in family caregivers of people with high-acuity health needs; it is widely known that intensive periods of caregiving can result in worsening health of caregivers. In this intervention, family nurses made a series of six extended telephone calls that helped the family caregivers identify the barriers they faced in taking care of themselves. Using a theory-based framework, the nurses then assisted the caregivers to remove those barriers and implement self-care strategies to improve the caregivers' health. Clinical trial research is needed to demonstrate the efficacy and effectiveness of this intervention, but early evidence from similar approaches indicates that the ideas have promise for improving caregiver health. In addition, the relational nature of the intervention, supplied entirely by telephone, is creative and has implications for nurses serving families in a variety of settings, including those in rural locations. During the COVID-19 pandemic, the CDC (2020b) recommended increased use of telehealth modalities to provide low-risk screening, improve safety, and allow patients to engage in multiple types of therapies. Reimbursement for these resources was supported by insurers, including Medicare, during the pandemic. Koonin et al. (2020, para. 1) reported that "during the first quarter of 2020 the number of telehealth visits increased by 50%, compared with the same period in 2019, with a 154% increase in visits noted in surveillance week 13 in 2020, compared with the same period in 2019."

FAMILY NURSING EVALUATION

In making clinical judgments, nurses employ critical thinking to determine whether and to what extent they have achieved an outcome. The means of measuring desired changes in outcomes varies with the specific problem on which the action plan is focused. For example, if the family has identified that a primary focus problem is disrupted sleep routines for their young child with attention deficit hyperactivity disorder, the nurse may propose that the family create a simple chart to measure its new routine of sleep hygiene practices on a daily basis. The family determines that, at present, the child is not able to fall asleep with ease on any given night and sets a goal to have the child fall asleep with ease three nights a week initially. Using the simple daily charting concept, the nurse and family can easily look to the collected data at a specified time to determine if the goal has been met. The team makes the decision about whether to proceed as originally planned, to modify the family action plan, or to revisit the family story in total and possibly change the working diagnoses. As indicated previously, the critical reasoning approach of thinking about families and their needs is not linear; rather, it is circular. In practice, a constant flow occurs between the components of the family assessment and intervention strategy, with plans being continually changed and modified through reflection and evaluation.

Many reasons may underly a lack of success in meeting desired outcomes when working with families, some of which may be related to family factors, others to nurse factors, and others to additional environmental factors. Apathy and indecision are examples of potential family barriers (Friedman et al., 2003). Family apathy may occur because of value differences between the nurse and the family. The family may be overcome with a sense of hopelessness, may view the problems or bureaucracy as too overwhelming, or may have a fear of failure. Nurses also should consider whether they themselves impose barriers. Examples of nurse barriers to achieving desired family outcomes include discrepant values or beliefs from the family, resulting in a lack of follow-through on the part of the nurse; not listening to family concerns about the problems of importance, leading to two separate rather than one unified outcome goal; or even lack of time and resources needed for the nurse to address the family needs in a timely fashion. Examples of additional environmental factors that act as barriers to desired outcomes include a change in the prescription formulary that limits access to the effective drug of choice on a family's insurance plan, lack of access to an appropriate specialty care provider because of rural location, or the loss of a job by the primary wage earner in the family (Couch et al., 2013; Ezeonwu, 2018; Dolinar et al., 2019; Findholt et al., 2013). A more detailed list of possible barriers to family outcomes can be found in Box 5-10.

Aside from evaluating outcomes, another important part of the family evaluation is the decision when to end the relationship with the family. Sometimes care with a family ends suddenly. In this case, it is important for nurses to determine the forces that brought about the closure. The family may seek to end the relationship prematurely, which may require a renegotiating process. The insurance or agency requirements may place a financial constraint on the amount of time nurses can work with a family. Other times, the family–nurse relationship comes to an end more naturally, such as when the nurse and family together determine that the family has achieved the intended outcomes. Other times the family–nurse relationship ends due to the nurse's expertise with a particular family ending, such as a pediatric nurse transitioning a family to adult care. Whatever the reason for the end of the nurse–family relationship, it is crucial that closure be achieved between the parties.

Building closure and/or transition into the family action plan benefits the family by providing for a smooth transition process. Strategies often used in this transition include decreasing contact with the nurse, extending invitations to the family for follow-up, and making referrals when appropriate. If possible, this process should include a summary evaluation meeting where the nurse and family put

formal closure or termination to their relationship. Following up with a therapeutic letter can encourage families to continue positive adaptation. The therapeutic letter should include recognition of the family achievement, a summary of the actions, commendations to each family member, and an insightful question for the family to think about in the future that may provide the family with a future direction (Wright & Bell, 2009). An example of a therapeutic family letter is found in Box 5-11.

Nurse and Family Reflections

The final step in thinking critically about family nursing is for nurses and families to engage in vital, creative, and concurrent reflection about their work together. Engaging in individual and collaborative reflection has two purposes: to facilitate evaluation of progress toward the desired family outcomes and to increase expertise of the nurse.

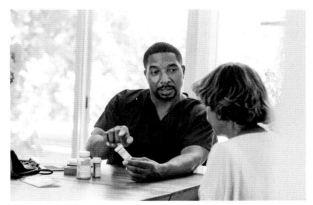

Source: © istock.com/SDI Productions

Evaluating Family Outcomes

The first purpose is for the nurse to reflect on the success of the family outcome in collaboration with the family as part of outcome evaluation.

BOX 5-10

Barriers to Family Outcomes

The following are barriers to family outcomes:

- family apathy
- family indecision about the outcome or actions
- nurse-imposed ideas
- negative labeling
- overlooking family strengths

- neglecting cultural or gender implications
- family perception of hopelessness
- fear of failure
- limited access to resources and support
- limited finances
- fear and distrust of health care system

BOX 5-11
Example of Therapeutic Family Letter

Dear W., H., and T.,

First, I want to thank all of you for allowing me the opportunity to get acquainted with your family. I appreciate your openness and willingness to talk with me.

During our time together, we discussed several issues that were important to your family. One of these issues was the ongoing possibility of H. losing his job because of the seasonal nature of his work. We explored the effects of potential job loss on a personal and family level.

H., you expressed some concern about your ability to provide adequately for your family. You indicated a personal constraining belief that a lack of steady employment meant that you were letting your family down and not providing for them. We discussed the idea that a paying job is only one part of the entire family support system that you provide. We explored some examples of noneconomic means of support, such as specific tasks related to farm chores, household management, and child care. If your job situation changes again, I hope you will find some of these suggestions helpful.

W., I was so impressed with your ability to juggle your caregiving job with home, farm, kids, and spouse. I can't think of many women who could handle all that with such strength and grace. With all that you do, it's not surprising that there isn't much time left over for your own personal endeavors. We discussed your constraining belief that you had to be responsible for everything. You envisioned the possibility of letting go of certain tasks

and suggesting ways to share other tasks more equitably among family members. If you and your family choose to implement some task-sharing ideas, I sincerely hope this will work for all of you.

T., you have mapped out a path to higher education and a future career. You have every reason to expect success. We briefly touched upon what "success" might mean for you and whether success depends on the university attended. I hope you will consider my thoughts in this regard. Whatever the outcome, you have the love and support of your parents.

Finally, I would like to commend all of you for your deep devotion to each other and for putting family first. You value family time, and you strive to communicate in a way that sustains your close relationship with each other.

I would like to invite W. and H. to consider a suggestion regarding making time for just the two of you. "Couple time" is easy to overlook when you are focused on creating a loving, stable home for E. and helping to launch T. into higher education. Please remember that you two are the solid foundation of your family; the stronger your relationship is, the stronger your whole family can be.

Because of our time spent together, I came away with the feeling that your family is exceptionally strong, deeply committed to one another, and fully capable of adapting to any of life's challenges. Thank you again for your time.

Best wishes to you and your family,
Nursing student signature here

Reflection entails the nurse thinking about her or his thought process relative to this family client. Nurses can link ideas and consequences together in logical sequences by using an "if (describe a situation) . . . then (explain the outcome)" exercise, which can help the family member articulate concerns. A comparative analysis approach of the family problem can be used to analyze the strengths and weaknesses of competing alternatives. The nurse may decide to reframe the family problem or priority need by attributing a different meaning to the content or context of the family situation based on testing, judgment, or changes in the context or content of the family story (Pesut & Herman, 1999). Although this process of reflecting with the family results in new cocreated evaluation and knowledge related to the collaborative work, the nurse can also engage in this comparative reflective reasoning individually in preparation for and as follow-up to the discussions with the family.

Increasing Nursing Expertise

The second purpose of reflection is for nurses to build on their expertise by reflecting on client stories and their practice with each family. In essence, nurses create a library of family stories so that each time they come upon a similar family story, they can pull ideas from previous experiences. This aspect of reflection assists nurses with pattern recognition.

Yet another, more individual purpose of reflection is to engage in self-reflection and self-evaluation. By using this critical thinking strategy, nurses learn from mistakes and cement patterns of action that assist them to advance in their nursing practice, from novice to expert family nurse.

The following family case study demonstrates critical reasoning about a family, assessment to identify concerns, and interventions to meet family needs.

Case Study: Bono Family

In preparation for her appointment with the Bono family in the mother-baby clinic, Jordan, a nurse working in a community clinic, reviews the chart notes written by the nurse-midwife about the family. Jordan sees that the Bono family is coming in for a 1-week well-baby checkup of newborn infant Hannah and a follow-up for Libby, the mother, after her cesarean section (C-section) delivery 7 days ago. The note from the receptionist indicates that Libby expressed some concerns with her effectiveness in breastfeeding Hannah. The appointment book notes that the whole Bono family is coming for this visit. Jordan notes that the Bonos are a nuclear family that consists of a married couple with two biological children. Figure 5-6 shows the Bono family genogram.

Knowing that this is a nuclear family coming in for a well-baby checkup, Jordan decides to use a Developmental and Family Life Cycle theoretical approach to this family with a new member. (See Chapter 2 for details about the Developmental and Family Life Cycle theoretical model.) Based on this approach, Jordan has many questions as she prepares for her appointment with the Bono family. The questions Jordan has about each family member and the whole family are presented below in bulleted lists after a brief description of each family member.

Libby Bono is a 35-year-old mother recovering from a cesarean section delivery 7 days ago. She does not have any existing health problems. Libby's roles in the family are primary child rearer, events planner, disciplinarian, and health expert. Libby is a hairdresser and is independently contracted with a hair salon. She has plans to take off 3 months for maternity leave.

- How might Libby's recovery from the C-section be affecting her roles in the family, especially with an active 2-year-old and a newborn?
- What are Libby's thoughts or plans for returning to work after her maternity leave?
- How is Libby adjusting to her expanded mother role?

Assess Libby for postpartum depression.

Matt Bono, 36 years old, works for a snack food company in sales and distribution. His primary roles in the family are decision maker, maintenance person, pioneer, and information provider. He reports feeling little attachment to his occupation and welcomes this new birth as a change in routine and an opportunity to consider a change in his place of employment. His current medical problems include type 2 diabetes and mild hypertension; both are well managed and controlled by oral diabetic and

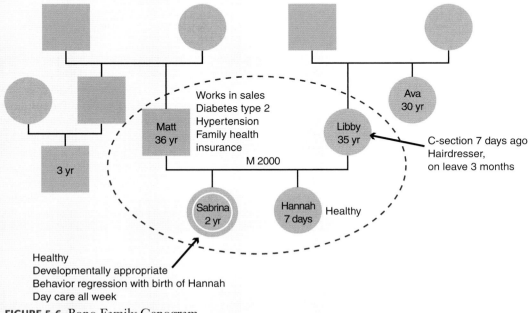

FIGURE 5-6 Bono Family Genogram

(continued)

Case Study: Bono Family—cont'd

antihypertensive medications. Currently, he is following the Weight Watchers® program to reduce his weight and to control the symptomatology experienced from his health conditions.

- How is Matt adjusting to the expanded role of father of two daughters?
- What are Matt's plans for employment, specifically about financial support for the family if he leaves his job? How would this affect health insurance for the family?

Sabrina Bono is a healthy 2-year-old girl who is developmentally appropriate. Psychologically, Sabrina is in the autonomy versus shame-and-doubt developmental stage. Her parents report that she often attempts to try new things on her own, and they frequently praise her efforts to promote independence. Her interest in potty training is developing but is still intermittent. Her immunizations are current. She normally goes to a day-care center that is close to her mother's work.

- How is Sabrina adjusting to the new baby?
- Is Sabrina showing any regression in her skills and abilities?
- Are each of the parents finding time to spend with Sabrina alone?
- How are the parents talking with Sabrina about her role as big sister?

Hannah Bono, 7 days old, was delivered after 42 weeks' gestation and was assessed as adequate for gestational age (AGA; 10th to 90th percentile), 53.75 cm and 3,966 g, with American Pediatric Gross Assessment Record (APGAR) scores of 8 at 1 minute and 9 at 5 minutes.

- Is Hannah developing on target for her age and gestational age at birth?
- How often is Hannah eating, and is she gaining weight?
- How is Hannah nursing?

The Bono family is a nuclear family that recently added a second child.

- What are the major concerns for the family at this time?
- Who in the family is having the most difficulty adjusting to the changes brought by the addition of a new family member?
- How is the family adjusting to these changes?
- Who or what are the support systems for this new family?

Bono Family Story

During the appointment, Jordan confirms that family life for the Bono family has changed. Hannah was found to be healthy and developmentally appropriate. Libby is healing well from the C-section, but she reported occasional discomfort when she "overdoes it." Libby's concerns about breastfeeding were easily relieved as Jordan validated her breastfeeding technique. An assessment for postpartum depression revealed that Libby is not demonstrating any signs of depression at this time. Throughout the examination of Hannah, the parents demonstrated overwhelming signs of bonding, such as talking with the infant and bragging about her beauty and temperament. During the appointment, Jordan noted that Sabrina was throwing toys and attempting to crawl onto her mother's lap while Libby was nursing Hannah. Sabrina would say, "Baby back" when she was upset. When Matt attempted to coddle or praise the baby, Sabrina became extremely angry with her father. They were not ignoring Sabrina, but they were not focused on her during the appointment. The parents' nonverbal actions showed frustration with Sabrina's behaviors. When asked, they reported that Sabrina has been very temperamental and inconsolable at day care. They reported that she had begun to show progress with toilet training before Hannah's birth but had now lost all interest.

Analysis of Bono Family Story

To help everyone see the larger family picture, Jordan uses the family reasoning web (see Figure 5-5). Based on the responses to the family reasoning web, Jordan uncovered the following family information for analysis:

- *Family routines of daily living:* Matt and Libby are both tired from Hannah's every-3-hour breastfeeding schedule. They share some of the responsibility for comforting Hannah and seeing to her needs. Meals have been challenging because Matt has had to assume this responsibility while Libby recovers from her C-section. At this time, they do not have extended family support. Sabrina is still going to day care but is evidencing difficulty there.

Case Study: Bono Family—cont'd

- *Family communication:* Communication has been identified as a strength for the couple. They have a shared decision-making style. They appear nurturing with their children. Sabrina is emotionally up and down. She is clingy with her father and ignores her mother except when she is breastfeeding Hannah. Sabrina was throwing toys when upset or frustrated. She periodically pointed to Hannah and said, "Take back."
- *Family supports and resources:* This family is fully covered under Matt's health insurance through his work. They have some family they can call on to help them. Ava, Libby's sister, volunteered to come for a visit and stay for 2 weeks. Matt's brother, his wife, and their 3-year-old child live in the same city. They have informally talked about sharing some child care. Both parents need to work to sustain their family lifestyle. Libby does not have benefits in her contracted hairdresser job. When she is off work, she does not make money. She does not have paid maternity leave. The couple planned for Libby to take 3 months off from work. The needs identified are for some immediate family support with everyday living and some financial concern at the end of the 3 months, given that the family had not planned for a longer period of reduced income.
- *Family roles:* All the family members are experiencing role ambiguity with their new roles. Matt and Libby are now parents of two daughters. Sabrina is a big sister, and Hannah is the new infant. Matt expressed some role overload because he is assuming many of the typical daily household chores of meals, laundry, food shopping, and primary care provider for Sabrina.
- *Family beliefs:* The Bonos strongly state that "family comes first." This was a planned pregnancy. They see themselves as loving parents. They express some confusion about disciplining Sabrina given her recent behaviors.
- *Family developmental stage:* This is a nuclear family in the family-with-toddler stage. They also have a new infant; therefore, they are in two developmental stages at the same time.
- *Family health knowledge:* The family expressed that it needed more help in knowing how to help Sabrina. The parents do not know how to work with Sabrina to help her adjust to being a big sister. They are confused with Sabrina's behavior of aggression, mood swings, clinging, and pointing at the baby and saying, "Take back." They feel that she has lost some of her skills. Health literacy does not appear to be an issue.
- *Family environment:* At this time, the Bonos have enough room in their home for a family of four. They live in a safe neighborhood, but they do not know their neighbors well.
- *Family stress management:* They express feeling stressed about Sabrina's behaviors. They are both tired. Sabrina is stressed, as evidenced by her behaviors and changes in behavior. They are dealing with the current situation on their own but are open to asking for help from family for immediate assistance with daily living routines. They are open to learning more about how to help Sabrina.
- *Family culture:* This family is Northern European American with an Italian-Catholic background. They are of working lower-middle-class socioeconomic status.
- *Family spirituality:* Both parents were raised Catholic but are not practicing their religion. They do not belong to a church. They describe themselves as spiritual.

The parents identified that both of them and Sabrina are having difficulty adjusting to the expansion of their family and the shift in their family roles. They state that they are most concerned with Sabrina's adjustment to the new baby and that they just do not know the best way to help her. They shared that they thought that because this was the "second time around," they believed they could be even better parents. They have been frustrated thinking about how to cope and what to do with two young children. The nursing diagnosis *Readiness for Enhanced Parenting* is related to the new role of parents of two children and is evidenced by the parents' subjective statements about parenting, Sabrina's reactions to the new baby, and parents asking for information and help on sibling rivalry.

Bono Family Intervention

The nurse, together with Matt and Libby, review the family genogram (see Figure 5-6), which helps the couple visualize the family. The parents decide that Ava is the best person to come to help at this time. They say they will talk later with Matt's brother and family about sharing some child care. They complete a family ecomap (Figure 5-7) to help assess what is creating stress and determine what could help alleviate family stress.

Jordan provides Matt and Libby with several educational packets about toddlers and new infants. She directs them to several online websites after she confirms that they have computer skills. They discuss ideas on how both parents can make personal

(continued)

Case Study: Bono Family—cont'd

time to spend with each daughter. They brainstorm ways to help Sabrina interact with Hannah but to keep Hannah safe from aggressive toddler behavior to a new sibling. They plan to talk with the day-care providers so they can be effective with their help for Sabrina. They will call Ava as soon as they get home to plan for her visit. Jordan makes a follow-up appointment with the Bono family for their next well-baby visit and to see how they are progressing with both children.

Bono Family Evaluation

Jordan plans a follow-up phone call to check in with Libby and Matt. At the next visit, Jordan will revisit the family action plan with Libby and Matt to see whether their priority family concerns remain the same, have decreased/increased, or have disappeared. Jordan plans to observe Sabrina's behaviors to see how she is coping and whether she is adapting in more positive ways. Jordan will talk with the parents to assess their anxiety level. Jordan will observe the parents and their interactions with both children.

Questions for reflection on the nursing care of the Bono family:

1. What approaches are recommended for working with families to identify and address their needs?
2. Are there specific communication strategies that would be effective when working with the Bono family?

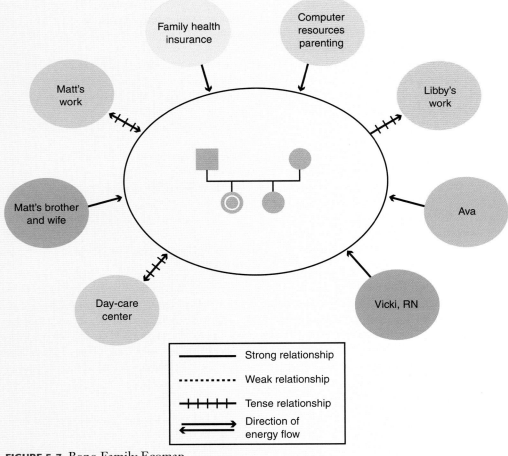

FIGURE 5-7 Bono Family Ecomap

SUMMARY

This chapter focused on family assessment which was explored in the context of relational inquiry. Family centered-care was emphasized to guide interactions between families and nurses providing care. The chapter also examined family nursing assessment models that are effective for nurses when working with families.

- Conducting a family assessment includes the following components: assessment strategies, including how to select assessment instruments; determining the need for interpreters; assessing for family health literacy; and diagramming family genograms and ecomaps.
- Family nurses must work in partnership with families as they build from a strengths model and not a deficit model.

- Using the family assessment approach outlined in this chapter, nurses and families together identify the family priorities.
- The family reasoning web is a systematic method for ensuring that families are viewed in a holistic manner, which also helps to keep the interventions oriented to family strengths.
- Family interventions must be tailored to each individual family, with consideration of the family's structure, function, and processes.
- By subscribing to and selecting a theory-based approach to assessment, and formulating mutually derived intervention strategies, families are more likely to be committed and follow through with family plans and interventions.
- Family nurses serve as the catalyst for assessment, intervention, and evaluation that are specific to family identified needs.

chapter 6

Environmental Health and Families

Gary Laustsen, PhD, FNP, RN, FAANP, FAAN

Morgan Torris-Hedlund, PhD, MPA, MS, CEN, PHNA-BC, NHDP-BC, FAWM

Critical Concepts

- Environmental health addresses physical, chemical, and biological factors external to a person.

- The external environment is the biotic (living), physical, and chemical factors that may affect human or population health.

- Ecosystems embrace the interactions, interconnections, and interrelationships between the components of a community.

- The ecological model of population health views human health as the center of multiple intersecting influences such as behavior; social, family, and community networks; living and working conditions; and the broader influences of national or global factors.

- Environmental justice is the fair treatment and meaningful involvement of all people regardless of race, color, national origin, or income, with respect to the development, implementation, and enforcement of environmental laws, regulations, and policies.

- The precautionary principle states that, in cases of serious or irreversible threats to the health of humans or ecosystems, acknowledged scientific uncertainty should not be used as a reason to postpone preventive measures.

- Environmental health risks (hazards) may originate from a number of environmental factors, including air, water, soil, and land quality; disease-carrying organisms; weather and climate; geological events; natural and human-created chemical toxins; and radiation.

- Disasters are the result of intricate, multifactor interactions in and between complex systems that interact with human health. A disaster is not an event but the consequences and effects of the event on people and social systems.

- The disaster management cycle is a process in which governments, businesses, and civil society plan for and reduce the impact of disasters, react during and immediately following a disaster, and take steps to recover after a disaster has occurred.

(continued)

- Food is obtained from natural environments and from anthropogenic sources, and food safety may be affected by biological, physical, and chemical food hazards that have an impact on family health.

- Environmental health threats can be found in the built and community environment. Threats to family health occur where family members work, play, and live, and nurses need to consider these different settings to determine exposure risks.

- A primary goal of environmental health policy should be to eliminate health disparities and the uneven burden that vulnerable populations feel from adverse outcomes.

- Environmental literacy, also known as ecological literacy or ecoliteracy, is an awareness about the environment and environmental problems, and the knowledge or methods to address those problems.

INTRODUCTION

This chapter looks at various aspects of environmental health and how aspects of environmental health may have an impact on family health. Environmental health topics are predominantly within the scope of public health nursing, although the concepts discussed in this chapter provide background information for any area of nursing practice. Because of the broad scope addressed by community or public health nurses, interventions to address a family's health that is affected by environmental health issues may occur at the individual family level or at the community/population level.

The chapter first presents an overview of environmental health concepts. The chapter then discusses some specific environmental health risks and looks at the general impact that various types of environmental pollution and climate change may have on family health. A brief overview of the impact of natural disasters (a type of environmental health hazard) is explored. Chemical, physical, and biological hazards are identified that have an impact on food safety and family health. Environmental health has a disproportionate impact on certain families and population groups. Various environmental justice issues are identified and discussed, and the role of nurses as family health advocates is explicated. Next, environmental health risks associated with the built and community environment are reviewed, and this discussion is followed by a section on the nurse's role in understanding and improving environmental health policy. The chapter ends with a discussion about the importance of advancing environmental health literacy for ourselves and for our clients.

ENVIRONMENTAL HEALTH CONCEPTS

Environmental health is an important aspect of human and family health. Although its importance is well recognized, the concept of environmental health does not have a clear and widely accepted definition. The social determinants of health (SDOHs) have rightly become recognized for their significant and broad impact on health. As also discussed in Chapter 19, SDOHs typically include access to education, social support services, cultural influences, housing availability and quality, neighborhood characteristics, and economic status. The physical environment is sometimes addressed within the scope of SDOHs. However, most environmental health practitioners prefer to consider the physical environment as a separate and unique determinant of health.

According to the World Health Organization (WHO), environmental health "addresses the physical, chemical and biological factors external to a person, and all the related behaviours" (Prus-Ustun et al., 2016, p. 3). Although there are other conceptualizations of environmental health, the WHO's definition is relevant and appropriate for our use in this chapter.

What are some other key concepts related to environmental health? The American Nurses Association (ANA, 2007) developed a document, *Principles of Environmental Health for Nursing Practice with Implementation Strategies*, and the Canadian Nurses Association (CNA, 2017) has a similar document: *Nurses and Environmental Health*. The ANA document is found in Table 6-1.

The ten principles outlined in the *Principles of Environmental Health for Nursing Practice with Implementation Strategies*:

are a call to action . . . [and] encourage nurses to gain a working understanding of the relationships between human health and environmental exposures and to integrate this knowledge into their practice. These principles are applicable in all settings where registered nurses practice and provide care and are intended to protect nurses themselves, patients and their families, other health care workers, and the community. (ANA, 2007, p. 4)

An understanding of the term *environment* is important when discussing environmental health. A person's genetic makeup and biochemical physiology are examples of internal environments that have an impact on health. This chapter will not specifically address internal environments, although

Table 6-1	American Nurses Association's Principles of Environmental Health for Nursing Practice

1. Knowledge of environmental health concepts is essential to nursing practice.

2. The precautionary principle guides nurses in their practice to use products and practices that do not harm human health or the environment and to take preventive action in the face of uncertainty.

3. Nurses have a right to work in an environment that is safe and healthy.

4. Healthy environments are sustained through multidisciplinary collaboration.

5. Choices of materials, products, technology, and practices in the environment that affect nursing practice are based on the best evidence available.

6. Approaches to promoting a healthy environment respect the diverse values, beliefs, cultures, and circumstances of patients and their families.

7. Nurses participate in assessing the quality of the environment in which they practice and live.

8. Nurses, other health care workers, patients, and communities have the right to know relevant and timely information about the potentially harmful products, chemicals, pollutants, and hazards to which they are exposed.

9. Nurses participate in research of best practices that promote a safe and healthy environment.

10. Nurses must be supported in advocating for and implementing environmental health principles in nursing practice.

Source: The American Nurses Association (2007).

they are critically important to the management of individual health. As a research-oriented science, epidemiology uses established methodologies to investigate the human health impacts from exposures to biologic, chemical, physical, and meteorological hazards.

"Ecosystems" is another key concept that focuses on the interactions, interconnections, and interrelationships between the components of a defined community. We are familiar with examples such as the rainforest ecosystem or the coral reef ecosystem, but we can also apply this concept to the health care ecosystem. Important aspects of ecosystems are that they are dynamic and complex, and they do not have precisely defined boundaries. *Ecology* is often simply defined as the study of ecosystems.

Connecting the concepts of environment, ecosystem, and ecology to environmental health is an ecological model of population health. In this model, human health is at the center of multiple intersecting influences such as behavior, social, family, and community networks; living and working conditions; and the broader influences of national or global factors (e.g., climate change). What is critical to understand is that, because humans are an integral part of their environments, the health of ecosystems is correlated with the health of human populations as well as the other biotic (animals, plants) components. Bronfenbrenner's Ecological Systems Theory (as described in Chapters 2 and 4) is another model promoting the interaction and interdependence of humans within the environment (Bronfenbrenner & Lerner, 2004) in addressing population and environmental health.

Another key concept in our discussion of environmental health is environmental justice. This term also has a variety of descriptions, but the U.S. Environmental Protection Agency's (EPA) definition is frequently cited: "Environmental justice is the fair treatment and meaningful involvement of all people regardless of race, color, national origin, or income, with respect to the development, implementation, and enforcement of environmental laws, regulations, and policies" (U.S. EPA, 2020). As nurses caring for individuals, families, and populations, we advocate for a healthy environment while valuing diverse beliefs, cultures, and communities.

A final concept relevant to environmental and family health is the precautionary principle. The precautionary principle states that, in cases of serious or irreversible threats to the health of humans or ecosystems, acknowledged scientific uncertainty should not be used as a reason to postpone preventive measures (WHO, 2004). In 2004, the American Nurses Association developed the *Principles of Environmental Health for Nursing Practice* (see Table 6-1), which featured the precautionary principle as a guiding principle. In this document, ANA states: "Where an activity raises threats of harm to the environment or human health, precautionary measures should be taken even if some cause-and-effect relationships are not fully established scientifically" (ANA, 2007, p. 7). The principle was discussed as far back as 1998 at the Wingspread Conference on the Precautionary Principle (Science & Environmental Health Network, 2018) and is still important because it encourages nurses and other health care professionals to be proactive in reducing the environmental hazards affecting human health. Similarly, CNA also advocates for the precautionary principle and the role of nurses in environmental health in their *Nurses and Environmental Health* position paper (Table 6-2) (CNA, 2017).

Table 6-2	Canadian Nurses Association's Nurses and Environmental Health

The role of nurses in environmental health includes:

- assessing and communicating risks of environmental hazards to individuals, families, and communities
- educating patients, families, and communities about environmental health and how to address key environmental health issues
- showing leadership in personal practices that support and reduce harm to the environment
- collaborating with interdisciplinary colleagues to identify and mitigate environmental health risks in practice environments
- advocating for policies that protect health by preventing exposure to those hazards and promoting sustainability
- producing nursing science, including interdisciplinary research, related to environmental health issues
- promoting the development of natural and built environments that support health

Source: © Canadian Nurses Association. Reprinted with permission. Further reproduction prohibited.

Environmental Health and Family Health

As nurses, it is important that we understand the connection between the environment's health and the health of families. Chapter 1 in this textbook defined family health as an approach that considers all aspects of life affecting the family, and the environment is a variable influencing family health care. Environmental health is a critical factor throughout the human life span because the physical environment can contribute to maintaining health, causing illness, or exacerbating comorbid conditions. Children and babies are especially vulnerable because their immature body systems are less able to moderate the effects of air, soil, and water pollution or the effects from chemicals in water, food, and household products.

Nurses seek to advocate for a just and equitable health care system that provides health care services and resources equitably to all individuals, families, and communities. Many examples, however, demonstrate the negative health impacts on people of color or those living in poverty due to the influences of living or working in unhealthy environments. This topic will be covered in more depth later in this chapter.

Families are key units within society, and each has a significant impact on the health of its members. Families live within and are constantly interacting with their physical as well as social environments. It should also be recognized that families have some ability to have an impact on their own home and surrounding environment. Teaching families to develop safe indoor and outdoor areas around their home is another way that nurses can support the environmental health of families. The rest of this chapter will explore in more detail how aspects of environmental risks, hazards, policies, and literacy have an impact on and relate to family health.

ENVIRONMENTAL HEALTH RISKS

Overview

Families are connected to and interact with the environment throughout their lives. These short- and long-term interactions with the environment can have an impact on each family member's health and well-being. The health impact may occur soon after the exposure, or it may not appear for many years or decades. Environmental health risks affect families collectively and as individuals. Families often experience similar health risks because of their consistent exposures to environmental hazards in the home or local community. Even environmental exposures that occur to one family member in the workplace or school can affect other family members. For example, pesticides present on the clothing of a father working in an agriculture setting may also contaminate his child when he comes home and embraces his child. The exposures of a mother to workplace pollutants or chemicals may affect her fetus if she is pregnant. This section will introduce some of the major sources of environmental health risks and provide a case study to demonstrate the impact of environmental health risks on an indigenous First Nations population in Canada.

The distinction between environmental health risks and socially determined health risks is not always clear. As previously mentioned, SDOHs originate from factors or influences of society or culture. SDOHs, environmental influences, biological and genetic components, and personal lifestyle are factors that make up an ecological model of health. When considering the intersection of these factors with health care systems, we can think of families as being connected in a collaborative relationship with the health care ecosystem. For this chapter, we will focus on the health risks with predominantly environmental aspects and especially those that influence family health.

Environmental Health Risks

Environmental health risks may originate from a number of environmental factors. These may include air quality, water quality, soil and land quality, disease-carrying biological organisms, weather and climate, geological events, natural and human-created chemical toxins, and solar or ground (e.g., radon) radiation.

Air Pollution

The quality of the air is influenced by local as well as distant sources of pollution. Specific pollutants are generated depending on the source, and they may include ozone, nitrogen dioxide, carbon monoxide, sulfur dioxide, lead, mercury, and particulate matter. Local industries, vehicles, and home-cooking fuels can create anthropogenic sources of pollution that affect the health of families. For example, the rates of asthma and other respiratory diseases are found to increase when families live in close proximity to roadways, especially those with diesel vehicles. Coal-fired electricity-generating plants are significant contributors to local, regional, and global air pollution and produce toxic metals that can also contaminate water systems. In many parts of the world, families still use biofuels (e.g., wood, charcoal, coal) to cook and/or heat their homes. Many of these homes lack proper ventilation of the smoke from these sources, and the smoke has a significant impact on the health of the home dwellers, especially the mothers and children. According to WHO (2018), "close to 4 million people a year die prematurely from illness attributable to the household air pollution from inefficient cooking practices using polluting stoves paired with solid fuels and kerosene."

Air pollution and its associated health risks may also be attributed to natural sources. Wildland fires and volcanoes may produce very high levels of air pollutants that can affect large geographic areas. The health effects of air pollution from any source often have a disproportionate impact on lower socioeconomic groups, whose members often work outdoors or have limited resources for air-filtering systems in their homes. Young children and older adult family members with existing cardiovascular or respiratory diseases are especially susceptible to impacts from wildfire smoke pollutants and particulates. Climate change has resulted in increased periods of drought and changes in precipitation patterns that have created conditions for longer and more extensive wildfire seasons.

Water Pollution

Although water pollution may originate from natural sources, the predominant source is anthropogenic. Sources of water pollutants may include chemicals and toxic metals from industries, excess nutrients and animal wastes from agriculture, chemicals from homes and lawn products, and human waste from treatment plants. Even though most families get their home water from treated community water systems, these treatment systems do not address all potential waterborne health threats. Most water treatment systems focus on eliminating risks from biological contaminants, and water polluted with disease-causing microbes is still a significant health risk in developing countries. An often unknown health risk from polluted community water systems in developed countries is from chemical contamination. The impact of this type of water pollution is evident in the tragic environmental health consequences that affected the population of Flint, Michigan, around 2014. Although the new water source was considered safe from biological contaminants, its corrosive effects caused lead from aging water pipes to leach into the water and produce excessive lead levels in household water. Older homes, where the majority of the lower socioeconomic population resides, were more likely to have water lines susceptible to the corrosive effects of the new water and thus to the increased lead exposure. According to the National Resource Defense Council (NRDC, 2018), a local pediatrician stated, "Lead is one of the most damning things you can do to a child in their entire life-course trajectory." In Flint, nearly 9,000 children were supplied lead-contaminated water for 18 months (NRDC, 2018).

Soil and Land Pollution

The quality of the soil or land that a family is exposed to may also have short- or long-term impacts on health. The specific pollutants may be different in urban or rural areas, but nurses should understand the historical uses of the land within their community. Contaminants from previous uses (e.g., mining or ore processing and refineries) may linger in the soils for extended periods of time, long after the soil-polluting industries have ceased their operations. Recognizing a family member's location as a source of potential health risk may relate directly to, or have an impact on, a person's current health condition. Young children are especially susceptible to the effects of exposure to contaminated soil. Young children's physiological systems are not yet fully developed, and they also interact more directly with the soil through their crawling and active play activities in outdoor settings. Even if the family's home environment did not have historical exposure to soil contaminants, the use of lawn or garden pesticides or other chemicals can lead to elevated environmental exposures for children and pregnant women. Soil pollutant exposures to the adult members of a family may occur within the context of their employment. Agricultural workers may be expected to work in areas recently sprayed with pesticides or herbicides, but they may have minimal barrier protection from these chemicals. Workers in mining industries may be exposed to harmful substances (e.g., coal dust), or they may also be exposed to chemicals used in the processing of mining ores. Environmental justice issues are relevant considerations with soil or land pollutants because in many urban or suburban communities, the land available for low-income population housing may have been contaminated at one time by industries that no longer exist. When converted into housing developments, these lands are often located in less-desirable locations and become the affordable choice for those in lower socioeconomic brackets.

Biological Disease Agents

Disease-carrying biological organisms pose environmental health risks for family health. Some of these organisms may have global prevalence (e.g., influenza, COVID-19), or they may be more limited in their distribution (e.g., malaria, tuberculosis). The health, social, and economic burden of diseases from biological organisms is extensive. Although global life expectancy has increased, biological diseases still affect morbidity, personal productivity, and family health. When one member of a family becomes ill, other members may also be exposed and acquire the same illness. In addition, caring for ill family members creates additional burdens to the economic and functional aspects of a family.

Disease from these organisms may be acquired through direct contact with the infectious agent or through a vector (e.g., mosquito) that transmits the disease-causing agent to the human. The list of disease-causing organisms and vectors is extensive, but they can be grouped into the categories of bacteria, viruses, parasites, *rickettsia*, and prions. There are certainly larger organisms (e.g., snakes, rabid dogs) that may pose a health risk, but the numbers of people affected by these animals are significantly lower compared to those infected with microbial organisms. The risk of exposure to family members depends on the disease agent's mechanism for infection and environmental factors that support the organism's life cycle or availability of the vectors. Climate change, with extended warm seasons and overall warmer temperatures, has led to expanding ranges of certain disease-carrying mosquitoes. For example, with dengue fever, cool winter temperatures have historically limited the incidence of this disease in the continental United States. However, there has been an increase in the distribution of dengue outbreaks in the southern United States over the past decade that is believed to be associated with the warming climate of those areas (Butterworth et al., 2017).

Meteorological Risks

Weather and climate may cause environmental events that can pose health risks to families. Extreme heat, hurricanes/typhoons, tornadoes, and blizzards are examples of meteorological events that can directly alter the health and welfare of individuals, families, and populations. Global climate change is having a direct impact on weather patterns. One significant concern associated with climate change is the increased frequency and duration of extreme heat events. Older adults, children, and those with existing cardiovascular disease are especially vulnerable to the effects of extreme heat. Extreme heat events are also tied to environmental justice issues because many families with reduced socioeconomic status often lack protective measures such as insulated housing or air conditioning. These families often live in areas of a community where green spaces are also lacking, which exacerbates the local effects of high temperatures. Agricultural and construction workers are at higher risk to the effects of extreme heat events because their work is outdoors.

An increase in other extreme weather events, such as hurricanes, is linked to climate change. Greater numbers of and more intense hurricanes have been noted over the last decades, and hurricanes directly and indirectly increase mortality and lead to long-term increases in morbidity (Woodward & Samet, 2018). Families that live in flood-prone areas or in older or poorly constructed houses are more vulnerable to the impacts of hurricanes or major rain events. The disproportionate impact of Hurricane Katrina on certain populations in the United Sates offers an example of the injustices that families of color or poverty face due to environmental threats. When Hurricane Katrina struck New Orleans in 2005, communities of color made up a large majority of the flooded neighborhoods. Failures of the levee system and an incompetent governmental response raised the national consciousness regarding a legacy of systematic and structural racism of African Americans and the effects of many generations living at or below the poverty level (Allen, 2007).

Besides the environmental health risks already mentioned, climate change has additional impacts on food production, distribution, and consumption. These include declining global crop yields from extreme weather events, diminished fisheries from increased water temperatures and ocean acidification, and increased foodborne illness from pests or the chemical contamination of food to control such pests. Extreme weather events, which are increasing in number due to climate change, can significantly affect the growing and distribution of food. Damage from weather events to agricultural products is exacerbated because of the prevalence of monoculture forms of food production that have large areas of land dedicated to the production of just a few agricultural products. If crops are not yet mature, weather events can affect the harvesting and distribution of these products. The modern food system relies on an intact and consistent transportation system. Interruptions from flooding or severe storms can interrupt this supply chain across the country. Families who rely on access to fresh fruits and vegetables in their local store may see a loss of these products due to weather events in another part of the country.

Miscellaneous Environmental Health Risks

Radiation may pose an environmental health risk to certain family members and communities. Radiation exposure can be from a number of sources, but two of the most common include ultraviolet (UV) light from the sun and radon from ground or water sources. Radiation can significantly increase the risk of cancer for those exposed throughout their lifetime. Family members, especially those with light-colored skin, are at risk for multiple types of skin cancer due to UV exposure. Those who choose to sunbathe outdoors or in tanning beds, or who are employed in outdoor occupations, increase their risk of developing skin cancers with their excessive or long-term exposure to UV radiation.

Radon is a decay product of uranium, and it is an extremely toxic, colorless gas naturally found in soil and rock. A small percentage of radon exposure can come from communities that use deep water aquifers, although the major exposure is from the soil. Environmental radon is considered one of the largest sources of human exposure to ionizing radiation and is considered a leading cause of lung cancer (Friis, 2019). Tests are available to measure home radon levels, as are methods to mitigate excessive radon exposure. However, there is often a lack of knowledge about possible radon sources in communities, and even if these sources are known, homeowners may not choose to spend the money to measure their home's radon levels. If a homeowner has an unsafe amount, the cost of installing mitigation measures can be many thousands of dollars.

Noise is an environmental health risk and poses a risk for hearing loss. Although most noise pollution is anthropogenic, some natural sources (wind, thunder) may also have an impact on a person's hearing. Common sources of excessive human-produced noise occur in occupational settings (industry, agriculture, logging, mining), homes (loud music, lawnmowers, power tools), and transportation (trains, planes). Regardless of the source, short- or long-term exposure to high levels can lead to a loss of hearing acuity. The costs of hearing testing and hearing aids may be beyond a family's budget. A loss of hearing has a minimal direct impact on a person's health, but the social isolation and depression that can accompany hearing loss may create a profound impact on the quality of life of an individual and her or his family.

Environmental Health Risk: Canadian First Nations Peoples and Oil Tar Sands

This case study presents the environmental health impact of oil tar sands development on a First Nations family in the Peace River area of Alberta, Canada. The case provides a brief introduction of the Ducharme family and the health issues they believe are associated with environmental pollution from oil tar sands development near their home. The perspective of this case is from that of a home-health community nurse. The nurse uses a descriptive epidemiology approach to identify the health-related impacts on this family from environmental exposures to pollution connected to tar sands development (Figure 6-1). Epidemiology is the basic science used as a framework to investigate population health-related events and answers the what, who, when, where, and why questions of health-related events.

Here is a brief review of these categories as used in descriptive epidemiology:

- **What = Case Definition:** This clearly defines the acute illness, chronic disease, or health risk.
- **Who = Community Characteristics:** Identifies common inherent and acquired characteristics of the population with the acute illness, chronic disease, or health risk. Such characteristics include demographic factors (age, race, sex), marital status, socioeconomic status, common behaviors, cultural behaviors, and environmental exposures.
- **When = Time:** Identifies time-related aspects of the health risk (annual, seasonal, daily).

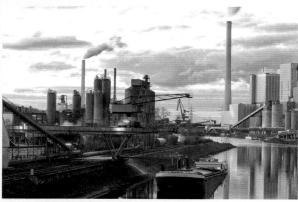

FIGURE 6-1 Example of a Processing Plant (Photo for Illustrative Purposes Only) *Source: © istock.com/Bim*

Environmental Health Risk: Canadian First Nations Peoples and Oil Tar Sands—cont'd

- **Where = Place:** Identifies the influences of geography and environment on the identified health risk. Are there geographic variations within the population that affect risk? Are there special positive or negative influences from locations such as home, worksites, or schools?
- **Why = Causes:** Identifies the causes or etiologies of the health risk to the population.

Background: The Family
The Ducharme family has five members. André, the father, is a 32-year-old male of Métis heritage. André was raised in Manitoba but moved to the Fort McMurray, Alberta, area 12 years ago to find work in the oil industry. He has worked as a truck driver for the past 10 years and married Nuna, whom he met when she worked in the cafeteria of the company cafeteria. Nuna, a 28-year-old female, is of First Nations Cree descent, has spent her entire life in the Fort McMurray area, and has many relatives that live close by. André and Nuna have been married nine years and soon after marrying, they moved to the Peace River area (northwest of Fort McMurray) because André was offered a better-paying position. Nuna has not worked outside the home since they moved to Peace River and dedicates herself to caring for her children and being active in local school and community events. Their children include Kitchi, an 8-year-old boy; André Jr., a 6-year-old boy; and Nuttah, a 2-year-old girl who was born premature at 30 weeks. They live in a three-bedroom mobile home on a rented lot within the Peace River city limits. The family has been concerned about André Jr.'s worsening asthma, and Nuttah's primary-care providers are concerned about her not meeting her childhood physical and mental developmental milestones.

Background: The Community
Within the Alberta province of Canada, and in the general vicinity of Fort McMurray (including Peace River), lies an enormous area of recoverable oil known as oil tar sands or just tar sands. The area of this resource is estimated to be larger than the state of Florida. Tar sands are a mixture of mostly sand; clay; water; and a thick, molasses-like substance called bitumen. The hydrocarbons that make up the bitumen are used to produce gasoline and other petroleum products. Historically, developing tar sands into fuels was cost-prohibitive because of the isolated location of tar sands areas, the extensive infrastructure needed to process tar sands, and the long distances to viable markets. The tar sands bitumen mined in the Alberta site is typically transported to distant refineries in the United States; thus, it poses additional health risks from spills during transport and noxious and dangerous emissions during refining.

On the recommendation of the Ducharme family's primary-care clinic, a community health nurse was contacted to look for possible environmental health risks that may be affecting this family. The nurse uses descriptive epidemiology to gather the assessment data, from which interventions may be planned and initiated to improve health. The information below provides an overview of the nurse's work.

What = Case Definition
Research into the health and social effects of tar sands mining and processing has demonstrated an increased incidence of leukemia, lymphomas, and other cancers and problems of acute nausea, headaches, skin rashes, and respiratory problems from emissions and odors (Lambert, 2011; NRDC, 2014). Other suspected health problems include reproductive impacts (e.g., birth defects) and decreased mental capabilities in children from the exposure to methylmercury. Social effects include impacts to traditional food-gathering activities from the pollution and infrastructure effects on traditional food (fish, caribou) sources (NRDC, 2014). The environmental exposures experienced by the Ducharme family and their health issues appear to be correlated, but the nurse knows a direct causation would be difficult to validate.

Who = Community Characteristics
The current population of the tar sands area in Alberta is a mixture of First Nations, Métis, and Caucasian peoples. The majority of the Caucasian population arrived in this area as part of the tar sands development. The Métis are considered an Aboriginal group of Canadians with a mixed European and Indigenous ancestry. The Chipewyan and Cree make up the majority of the First Nations peoples in this general area. The 2016 census showed a population of greater than 65,000, with a majority being Canadian citizens (approximately 88%) and in the 15 to 64 age range (77%), and origins identified as North American Aboriginal (approximately 10%), other North American (approximately 33%), and European (approximately 44%) (Statistics Canada, 2017).

(continued)

Environmental Health Risk: Canadian First Nations Peoples and Oil Tar Sands—cont'd

The First Nations tribes in the tar sands area represent a small percentage of the total population, but they also experience the greatest impact to their lives and health due to the tar sands development. Some Indigenous people do benefit from the opportunities for economic improvement through employment within the production facilities and associated infrastructures. However, these people are at risk for the greatest impact on their cultural way of life. There are also increased health risks to the Indigenous peoples due to traditional food-gathering aspects and their exposures to land, air, and water pollution.

When = Time
The time-related aspects of the tar sands health risks are both current and historical. Direct exposure to the environmental pollutants may create acute health conditions such as skin rashes and respiratory problems (e.g., asthma or chronic obstructive pulmonary disease [COPD] exacerbation). Cancers are typically a result of chronic exposure and may take years to decades to develop, which thus complicates the attribution of cause to a specific environmental factor.

Where = Place
The geography of the tar sands area is predominantly low-elevation boreal forest, with generally severe winters and mild to warm summers with a borderline subarctic climate. There are numerous lakes and rivers that fall with the Athabascan River Watershed. The rivers flow north, eventually connecting to the Arctic Ocean. The primary uses of land in northern Alberta have been forestry, oil and gas production, recreation, and grazing. The Ducharme family's mobile home residence is drafty, inadequately insulated, and cramped for an active family of five. The family's home lies within a few miles of the tar sands processing plant and sits along the highway where heavy truck traffic consistently transports materials to and from the plant.

Why = Causes
Directly connecting environmental health risks, such as those encountered with the tar sands development, to specific health outcomes is difficult. Disease such as cancer have many etiologies and are often the result of exposures over many years. Cancer and other diseases *may be* correlated with the exposure to increased toxic air pollutants from drilling and processing or water pollutants such as methylmercury and polycyclic aromatic hydrocarbons (PAHs), but a direct causation model is challenging to establish. Epidemiological studies may show changes over time for the incidence and rates of cancer to an exposed population. Many members of the Peace River community believe there have been significant health impacts from the increased air pollutants and noxious odors created by the excavation of tar sands (Nikiforuk, 2013). A true, randomly controlled trial to demonstrate cause and effect between environmental health risks and diseases is impossible to design and unethical to conduct. A polluter's role in causing disease is extremely difficult to demonstrate; therefore, the attestation of liability is rarely accomplished in cases of disease from environmental exposures.

Questions for reflection on the nursing care of the Ducharme family:

1. As the community health nurse, what could you do to assist the Ducharme family and other First Nations people in improving their health? What interventions would be your primary focus for reducing illness or improving the Ducharme family's health?
2. What could the community nurse do to assist the Ducharme family and First Nations people in reducing their environmental health risks in the Peace River community? What are the known and potential environmental health risks in this case?
3. Identify the environmental justice aspects of this case. Who are the victims?
4. What aspects of the Ducharme family and the First Nations people put them at risk for experiencing injustices?
5. How could local health care workers advocate for policy changes to reduce the impacts of the environmental health risks?

NATURAL DISASTERS, NURSING, AND FAMILIES

What Are Disasters?

There are several ways to define a disaster. One definition is that a disaster is an event that forces a group of people to seek help outside their usual set of resources. Using this definition, if an event takes place in a town that requires assistance from another city to respond effectively, the event is a disaster. Other definitions suggest that a disaster is an event that causes damage, kills, or hurts people. This definition often includes a monetary threshold, a definitive number of damaged buildings, or a definitive number of lives lost to determine which events qualify as disasters. In this chapter, a disaster is defined as any event that overwhelms a given group of people's capacity to meet their needs and forces them to seek outside assistance. This definition is useful because it can be scaled to fit a variety of situations. A disaster may affect a single family, a large family group, a neighborhood, or a city.

Environmental health and disasters are similar because both are the result of intricate, multifactor interactions in and between complex systems. Both are also the result of natural phenomena interacting with human lives. It is essential to recognize that a disaster is not the event but the consequences and effects of the event on people and social systems. Thus, an earthquake is a disaster when it causes a bridge over a river to collapse. The ruined bridge impedes the movement of people. It prevents people from evacuating the affected area, alters the flow of the river, disrupts transportation, restricts the delivery of medical supplies, and keeps adults from going to work and children from going to school. This example demonstrates how disasters result from an interaction between the built environment and an event that disrupts human activity.

The number of disasters worldwide is growing, and the consequences of those events are rapidly intensifying. Wildfires, hurricanes, floods, tornadoes, and droughts are examples of environmentally related disasters that affect increasing numbers of people every year. These events kill people directly and disrupt communities by hindering economic systems, interfering with the delivery of goods and service, and contributing to disease outbreaks. For these reasons, nurses should be ready to respond to disasters and, more important, take steps to prevent them from happening to minimize their effects.

Disasters and Environmental Health

The interaction between the natural and built environments is a critical component of understanding disasters and how they affect families. Although disasters result from events that may not be foreseeable or may not be avoidable, risk mitigation and effective planning can help minimize the adverse outcomes resulting from various events (Paton, 2003).

Environmental health is particularly essential when considering disasters because of the contributions the environment can make to a disaster event. The current understanding of hazards

and disaster phenomena links environmental issues to human risk; flooding, drought, and wildfires are excellent examples of disaster events that result from environmental conditions. Both human-caused and natural disasters result from numerous contributory factors, including environmental changes from natural processes or human contributions. Although natural events are powerful phenomena, the damages they inflict on people result from human planning and decision making. The risk that any event poses to human beings results from the relationships people have to their surroundings and from natural forces outside human control.

For example, when people are displaced by drought or human conflict, the displacement may cause quick population shifts that overcrowd cities and increase risks. Cities become overcrowded, and municipalities cannot keep up with their community's changing nature. Existing policies and the delivery of goods and services fall behind the demands of the growing population. Housing is often scarce, sanitation services become taxed, and health services may be overburdened. These factors increase the vulnerability of the community, steadily increasing its susceptibility to a trigger event. In collaboration with one another, these dynamics result in an ongoing elevated risk and increased consequences when a disaster event does occur. Growing evidence suggests that over the long term, human activity contributes to changes in the environment (e.g., climate change) at multiple levels and thus contributes to disastrous events.

Disasters, like environmental health, are the result of complex systems interacting with one another. Disasters are categorized as natural and human-made, suggesting that some disasters cannot be anticipated or planned for and others can. Regardless of the source, all disasters result from events unfolding in the physical world and interacting with human choices. Those choices include policy, land zoning, population movement, and political and governmental conflict (Burkle, 2020; Khorram-Manesh & Burkle, 2020).

Policy and decision making that have an impact on environmental health also affect the risks and potential threats to communities. For example, the placement of a water treatment facility or industrial waste storage facility may be appropriate under optimal conditions. However, if a geological event takes place (e.g., earthquake), the consequences of that event can be amplified by the contamination released from the damaged facility. Policy choices are also a critical component of human-caused disasters. Unlike natural disasters, human-caused disasters are the result of human activity, and the results from options chosen can be identified and recorded by examining policy and policy choices. A thorough discussion of how families are affected by health policy is included in Chapter 4.

Disasters and Families

Disasters are, by definition, disruptive. They interfere with the normal day-to-day operations of individuals, families, and communities. Disasters can diminish or eliminate the critical aspects of family functions. They lessen the ability of families to respond to existing and ongoing stressors. In addition, they create new, potentially life-threatening stress on families and family members.

Disasters damage and disrupt physical structures and the built environment. They may destroy homes, hospitals, emergency services, places of worship, and schools. Because these things are essential to families, they represent interference and disruption to a family's existing, predisaster support network. The physical disorder to transportation services may also change the delivery of goods and services that families depend on. Food and other household goods may become scarce. Child-care, elder-care, and health care services may close. Municipal services may also fail, and families may no longer have access to clean water or to electricity for heating and air conditioning, and garbage and sewage disposal systems may become inoperative.

The combined consequences of these factors increase risk for the spread of diseases. Poor hygiene from lack of clean water and disrupted sanitation services creates an optimal setting for the spread of communicable disease. These stressors create physical risks and functional challenges for families as they try to overcome and respond to disasters.

Children and older family members, because they are dependent on others, are more vulnerable to the effects of disasters. They rely on other members of the family and may have only a limited capacity to contribute to the family's needs during a disaster. They are also at greater risk of suffering from the mental health trauma associated with disaster events.

What Can Nurses Do?

Because nurses provide health care across the life span and in multiple areas, they are uniquely capable of playing a crucial role in disaster management. In their various professional capacities, nurses can focus on hazard identification, risk mitigation, and disaster preparedness and response. Nurses can also advocate on behalf of families and communities to develop policies that will make communities safer.

Nurses can work with individual families to help them identify the risks they face. These threats may be found in the surrounding area and could be natural or human-made hazards, or a combination of the two. Once risks have been identified, nurses can help families minimize the potential consequences of those dangers. This process builds on the dynamics of the family. The nurse works with the family to help family members understand their strengths and bolster their advantages and strengths. Mitigation is an essential step because it has the potential to moderate the impact of a disaster. Mitigation activities can reduce the severity of the consequences of a disaster event and lessen the impact on the family.

When total reduction of consequences cannot be achieved, nurses can strengthen the family to minimize adverse outcomes. The disaster management cycle (Figure 6-2) illustrates the phases in which nurses have an opportunity to act. The disaster management cycle is a continuous process and is comprised of at least four critical stages: risk mitigation, preparedness, response, and recovery. The

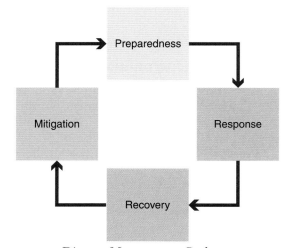

FIGURE 6-2 Disaster Management Cycle

disaster management cycle serves as a powerful tool to help families identify the steps to protect themselves. Essential ideas illustrated by the process show the need for ongoing assessment, planning, and preparedness, and the crucial importance of preparedness before and after an event takes place.

Discussing disasters may be upsetting for families. Nurses need to be sensitive to how families respond when discussing disaster-related threats such as injury to loved ones, separation from children and elders, and destruction of the home or possessions. Nurses need to promote engagement and a sense of personal interest among the family members to help them recognize their stake in the disaster preparation efforts.

Nurses can help families prepare and mitigate hazards, but they must also be sensitive to the limits on a family to make changes in their environment. The nurse may be better positioned to help families when they have well-established connections to the community. When nurses are trusted by the community, they can build on existing bonds and established trust when offering help.

Risk Awareness

Perception of risk is vital to the disaster planning process because it helps emergency planners determine if at-risk communities are aware of the threats they face. Risk perception also influences whether or not members of an at-risk community will make efforts to ready themselves for potential threats. Risk is a complex and dynamic concept determined by exposure to threats and the capacity to respond to an adverse event (Paton, 2003).

Vulnerability

Vulnerability is also a crucial aspect of understanding disasters. The International Federation of Red Cross and Red Crescent Societies (IFRC) defines vulnerability as "the diminished capacity of an individual or group to anticipate, cope with, resist and recover from the impact of a natural or man-made hazard" (IFRC, 2020). Vulnerability is one factor used to understand a person's or a community's risk. Exposure is often associated with poverty, but it is also a result of gender, social class, age, existing illness, mental health, previous trauma, housing status, and access to resources. As mentioned earlier, the disaster preparedness cycle

is an excellent tool for explaining to families how they can minimize their vulnerability and take steps to diminish the consequences of hazards.

The Disaster Management Cycle

Each phase of the disaster management cycle is critical to nurses working with families. It illustrates opportunities and responsibilities in each stage and can be shared with families to help them understand the outcomes needed in each phase of the cycle. Resources to help families in their disaster preparation can be found in Box 6-1. "The disaster management cycle illustrates the ongoing process by which governments, businesses, and civil society plan for and reduce the impact of disasters, react during and immediately following a disaster, and take steps to recover after a disaster has occurred" (Global Development Research Center, n.d.).

Mitigation

Mitigating known hazards is the single most important step that families can take in anticipation of disastrous events. Guided by the disaster management cycle, nurses should work collaboratively with families and communities to identify and understand the risks they face. Nurses working in this role must know that risk perception is a complex phenomenon that is influenced significantly by community perception of hazards and is guided by what community members feel is worth protecting.

BOX 6-1

Family-Focused Internet Resources for Disaster Preparedness

- "Ready" Build a Kit: An official website of the U.S. government https://www.ready.gov/kit
- "Be Prepared. Get Connected. Take Action": American Red Cross, Northern California, Coastal Region, Emergency Preparedness Guide https://www.redcross.org/content/dam/redcross/local/NCCR/148816preparednessguide_web.pdf
- U.S. Department of Agriculture (USDA): Disaster Resource Center https://www.usda.gov/topics/disaster
- "Get Ready": Government of Canada Disaster Preparation website https://www.getprepared.gc.ca/index-en.aspx

Once risks are identified, efforts to minimize them should be the next step. As much as possible, threats should be reduced at this phase before they become disasters. Often these threats cannot be addressed by individuals, families, or even entire communities. Municipalities, states, or federal entities generally have the responsibility and capacity to handle the identified community threats. Infrastructure problems, zoning issues, and lack of community resources are examples of factors beyond an individual family's control. Nurses working in at-risk communities can also play a role in community organization. They may amplify and ensure that the community's concerns are shared with the proper policymakers, act as subject matter experts when applicable, or serve as advocates by helping community members articulate their problems.

Preparedness

Preparedness offers families another opportunity to protect themselves. During the mitigation and preparation phases, families can eliminate potential threats and ready themselves appropriately for dangers they cannot entirely prevent. In this phase, families can gather supplies they may need during an event, develop and practice disaster plans, and organize themselves and their friends if a disaster event takes place.

Response

The response phase involves actions to protect life and support the physical needs of an affected population. This phase, which immediately follows an event, is marked by a sense of urgency, and the highest priority is to address physical health and lifesaving needs. Nurses may also be involved in patient transport, working in shelters, providing food, or finding new housing. The spotlight during response is meeting the basic needs of families and individuals. A crucial concern during this phase is family separation. Every effort should be made to keep families together.

Communities Affected by the Kīlauea and Lower Puna Eruption on Hawai'i Island

This case study explores the effects of the Kīlauea and Lower Puna eruptions on a family living outside Hilo on Hawai'i Island (Figure 6-3). The case will present a timeline of the event, describe the affected area, and illustrate the dynamic relationships between policy, culture, and a Hawaiian family's needs during the disaster.

Background

In May 2018, a series of eruptions began that would eventually open 24 volcanic fissures and cover more than 6,000 acres of land. The Lower Puna lava flows, part of the Kīlauea eruptions, was responsible for destroying more than 700 homes and over 1,600 acres of farmland. Recovery efforts forced the County of Hawai'i to ask for $800 million in recovery funds, a large amount of which came from the federal government. Much of the damage took place in areas where lava flowed during previous

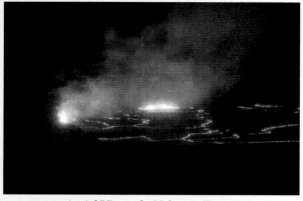

FIGURE 6-3 Aerial View of a Volcanic Eruption.
Source: © istock.com/JTSorrell

Communities Affected by the Kīlauea and Lower Puna Eruption on Hawai'i Island—cont'd

eruptions. The land was inexpensive in these areas, and building codes were lenient. This affordable land was attractive to many people who would otherwise have been unable to purchase land in Hawai'i.

The Lower Puna eruption began on May 3, 2018, and would become the most massive eruption of Kīlauea in recent history. More than 2,000 residents had to evacuate from affected areas; roads were closed; and the regional electrical provider, Puna Geothermal Ventures, had to close. The Lower Puna event was not a single eruption located in a single space. Instead, it consisted of many lava flows, lava fountains, and gas vents throughout the region. Volcanic activity also caused a series of ongoing earthquakes.

One of the largest earthquakes took place on May 4. The 6.9 magnitude event could be felt across the Puna district of Hawai'i Island. These earthquakes contributed to the closure of Puna Geothermal Ventures, which is responsible for a quarter of the island's electricity.

Lava flows were responsible for isolating neighborhoods and communities when roads were destroyed. In some cases, entire subdivisions were buried beneath large flows. The flows also destroyed landmarks and natural features in the area. Green Lake, the largest freshwater lake in Hawai'i, was evaporated when lava entered Kapoho Crater. Kapoho Bay was filled with lava, which destroyed recreational and culturally significant sites.

An examination of the events clarifies that much of the damage happened in areas where lava flows had been in the past, areas where land was inexpensive and easy to build on because it could not be insured. There was little effort to regulate development in those areas. Residents did an excellent job of responding to warnings, listening to disaster managers, and taking care of one another. However, they had put themselves at risk by living in these areas identified as high risk in previous risk assessments. These events illustrate the relationship between people, policies, and the natural environment, and how those components interact to form a disaster.

A Family Facing Disaster

The Nakamura family lived in Leilani Estates outside Pāhoa, 24 miles from Hilo. Russell Nakamura is a 51-year-old construction worker who grew up in Hilo. Russell is Japanese, Hawaiian, Filipino, and Okinawan. Russell's wife Kalei grew up on Maui. Kalei is Hawaiian, Korean, Irish, and Portuguese. She is 48 years old and works at Hilo Airport. Russell and Kalei have three children: Hoku, who is 16, attends school on O'ahu; Jasmine, 13, and Keone, 10, live with their parents. Russell's father Daichi was living with the family when the eruptions started. Russell has two sisters and a brother living on the Big Island, as well as many cousins. Kalei also has family on the Big Island, although they live on the island's Kona side, more than 2 hours away.

The Nakamuras were able to evacuate their home ahead of many of their neighbors. Russell, Kalei, and the two younger children moved in with one of Russell's sisters in Hilo. Daichi moved in with Russell's brother. Russell was laid off from work because the homes he was working on were affected by the eruption. Although the family's home was not destroyed, they spent several months with Russell's sister. Because they acted early, they moved all of their belongings out and stored them with various friends and family until they could return home.

The family received considerable help from their family and were able to relocate. Despite the opportunity to move in with family and the support they received, they encountered challenges. Two weeks after moving away from their home, Russell and Kalei were informed that Hoku was performing poorly in school. She reported to her school's health clinic and told the school nurse she could not sleep and was "always worried about her family." Russell could not return to work for six months, and when he did, his commute time doubled. Two months after the eruptions started, Keone, the family's youngest, was diagnosed with asthma. Because several of Kalei's coworkers had to ask for time away from work to respond to issues caused by the eruptions, Kalei's hours increased to more than 60 hours per week.

Hawaiian History

Native Hawaiians, kānaka maoli, or kānaka ōiwi, are the indigenous people of Hawai'i. The Hawaiian way of life was profoundly disrupted by Western contact starting in 1778. The foundational values of health, land use, and social structure were irreversibly changed when people coming to the islands brought with them new diseases, new religions, and capitalism. The end of the Hawaiian Kingdom began in 1893 after a group of American plantation owners, with the help of the U.S. Marines, initiated a

(continued)

Communities Affected by the Kīlauea and Lower Puna Eruption on Hawai'i Island—cont'd

coup. Queen Lili'uokalani, the last reigning monarch of Hawai'i, was removed from power, and Hawai'i was eventually annexed in 1898. These events are part of a long process that contributed to Hawaiians losing their land and the death of nearly 90% of kānaka ōiwi. Today, kānaka maoli continue to endure significant challenges, including disproportionate negative health statistics, overrepresentation in the prison system, and lower income status than other ethnic groups in Hawai'i.

Questions for reflection on the nursing care of the Nakamura family:

1. What are the known and potential risks posed by the volcanoes in this case? How did the previously identified risks threaten families before the eruptions? Did these same risks also benefit the people living in the region?
2. Identify the environmental justice aspects of this case. How did the building codes work in favor of families looking to own land and build homes on Hawai'i Island? Do community health nurses have a responsibility to question zoning or building codes?
3. What historical issues put Native Hawaiians at risk for experiencing injustices? How does that history connect to the Nakamura family?
4. Do the risks faced by Native Hawaiians differ from those faced by other residents of the area? How might those risks be experienced and/or expressed in a family as ethnically diverse as the Nakamuras?
5. What could a community health nurse do to assist residents in the area avoid future risks?
6. How could a community health nurse advocate for policy changes to reduce the impacts of disaster risks?
7. What were the Nakamura family's immediate needs? Do you believe they are currently at risk? What risks might they face over the next year after the eruptions subside?
8. How does the unique geography of Hawai'i play a role in the challenges that the Nakamuras face? How does the issue of distance and the complications of traveling between islands change your assessment of this family's needs?

Recovery

The recovery phase provides an opportunity to help families return to a state at least as stable as they were in before the disaster. Individual families recover in collaboration with their community as a whole. Nurses need to appreciate that various plans should be integrated and occur in concert with each other. The goods and services that communities rely on will return to optimal functioning in relationship to one another, but this process takes time and requires significant interoperational effort.

Communities are often frustrated during the recovery phase because of the time required and the realization that things may not be the same as they were before the disaster. People become aware of the limits of the available assistance, and some communities may feel abandoned. Some parts of the community may recover quicker than others, meaning some individuals may return to work and school while others do not. Assistance may not be equally available or may require substantial bureaucratic involvement. This period can last for months or years and may cause substantial stress and trauma to families and communities.

Nurses must play a role in this phase. They can take care of patients and may be the first to recognize changes in people's health. They can advocate for policy and funding requirements by bringing the conditions of the communities they care for to the attention of lawmakers and other officials. Nurses can also act as subject matter experts and offer their expertise to community members to communicate their needs.

ENVIRONMENTAL HAZARDS AND FOOD SAFETY

Healthy food provides the necessary nutrients and calories for a healthy body. Food also serves as the center for family interactions, celebrations, and cultural experiences. In this chapter, the focus has been mostly on health risks encountered by families from the physical environment. Food can be obtained from both natural environments (e.g., oceans) and from anthropogenic sources (e.g., agricultural lands), and this section will focus on how biological, physical, and chemical food hazards may affect food safety and family health.

Chemical Hazards

Chemical hazards in food may come from naturally occurring toxins, but they are due more frequently to contaminants introduced during the production, storage, or packaging of food. Natural toxins may accumulate in marine foods (e.g., shellfish) due to algal blooms, or they may be present in wild foods such mushrooms. Families that gather or harvest these sources of food may be unintentionally poisoned, with outcomes ranging from mild illness to death. Appropriate and timely community education may reduce the risk of these natural sources of food poisoning.

Anthropogenic sources of chemical hazards in food may be related to the presence of heavy metals, pesticides, or additives. Heavy metals, such as lead, arsenic, and mercury, may contaminate food. These heavy metals may find their way into the food through irrigation systems, polluted water bodies, livestock feed, or leaching from metal cans. Acute exposures to an excessive amount of foodborne heavy metals are very unusual, but the long-term effects of low-level exposure are unknown. The developing fetus may be especially susceptible to the impact of heavy metal ingestion, even though the mother may not experience negative health symptoms.

Pesticides are used extensively in modern agricultural practices to prevent damage from insects or other pests and to boost harvest yields. These chemicals may directly contaminate food sources or produce polluted water systems during runoff from the fields. Most consumers are exposed to pesticides from dietary sources, but the risks may be significantly reduced through appropriate washing or peeling of the produce. Unfortunately, the potential risks of long-term exposure to low levels of pesticide residue on foods are unknown due to the lack of adequate longitudinal studies. Safe levels established by governments are often based on short-term exposure in adults, and the impact to infants or those with compromising health conditions is not adequately understood. In a landmark study in the mid-1990s, low levels of multiple pesticides were found in baby foods. In response, the U.S. federal government passed the Food Quality Protection Act. In the 20 years since its passage, many of the harmful pesticides have been banned, and testing has confirmed that amounts of pesticide residue in baby food have dramatically decreased (Lunder, 2016). Outbreaks of pesticide poisonings from food sources do still occur, and appropriate health department surveillance is important to minimize the spread of these outbreaks. Because of the distance food may travel from its source to points of consumption, tracing the location and cause of contamination can be challenging for health officials.

Physical Hazards

Food safety may be affected by physical hazards. Examples include items from the land such as pieces of wood, bones, seeds, shells, and stones or other items such as glass or metal that were incorporated into the food during growing, harvesting, processing, or storage. Physical objects may also be unwittingly introduced in the home during food preparation. Compared to chemical and bacterial hazards, physical objects rarely cause significant health risks for most families, and the majority of these objects pass through the gastrointestinal system without causing harm. With sharp physical objects, however, there are risks of laceration, puncture, or infection requiring medical care; with solid objects, there is a risk of dental fractures.

Biological Hazards

Microbial organisms are probably the most common and well-known agents affecting food safety. Microbes of concern may include bacteria, viruses, parasites, worms, fungi, and prions. Table 6-3 identifies some of the most common microbial agents associated with illnesses from consumption of tainted fresh produce.

In this text, discussing the unique illnesses from exposures to the multitude of disease-causing microbes is not practical, but a general overview is warranted. With food contamination, most bacteria and viruses produce localized infections that affect the gastrointestinal system and produce symptoms of abdominal pain, nausea, vomiting, and/or diarrhea. With some exposures, the microbe's toxin (e.g., botulism) is responsible for the symptoms and health outcomes. Especially with bacterial toxins, the illnesses may disseminate to other body systems with fever, headaches, kidney damage, and neurological impairments.

Giardia, a protozoal organism, may be transmitted by food or water and produces giardiasis, with the typical gastrointestinal effects of diarrhea. Worms, such as *Trichinella* and tapeworms, are

Table 6-3	**Common Microbes Associated with Illnesses from Fresh Produce**		
BACTERIA	**VIRUSES**	**PARASITES**	**FUNGI**
Salmonella spp.	Hepatitis A virus	*Cyclospora*	*Alternaria* sp.
Escherichia coli	Rotavirus	*Cryptosporidium parvum*	*Fusarium* sp.
Campylobacter spp.	Norovirus	*Giardia* sp.	*Aspergillus niger*
Vibrio spp.	Norwalk and Norwalk-like	*Trichinella* spp.	

Source: Alegbeleye et al., 2018.

foodborne hazards generally transmitted through meat products, especially if they are improperly cooked. Infections can range from the person being asymptomatic to mild gastrointestinal distress, to life-threatening effects from invasion of the heart and central nervous system.

Food safety is especially important for maintaining family health and may be significantly affected by food-related disease organisms. Families often share meals, and thus multiple family members may become ill from the same contaminated food source. Many gastrointestinal diseases may also be spread among family members through unintended ingestion of fecal matter from an infected individual. Improper handwashing of one individual preparing the family's food may spread the illness-causing microbe to others. Children and older adults are especially vulnerable to foodborne hazards, and they often experience more serious consequences from the loss of fluids and electrolytes associated with diarrhea and/or vomiting. In addressing the biological hazards associated with food, nurses can assist families in reducing their exposures by advocating for immunizations, proper hygiene practices, and appropriate food preparation.

ENVIRONMENTAL JUSTICE ISSUES

Environmental justice calls people to action to advocate for fair treatment and equitable involvement of all people regardless of ethnic background, race, national origin, or income status and concerning the development, execution, and enforcement of laws, policies, and regulations that govern and shape the relationship between people and the surrounding environment (U.S. EPA, 2020). The environmental justice movement began with individuals, mainly people of color, from communities most affected by pollution and other environmental threats. Those people, motivated by the situations they saw in their communities, sought to address the reality that people who live, work, and play in the most polluted environment are commonly people of color and people who have lower incomes. Environmental justice advocates have demonstrated that the excessive exposure among these communities was deliberate and did not happen accidentally (NRDC, 2020).

The goal of environmental justice is to provide equal protection to all people and possibly nonhuman entities such as animals and aspects of the environment. Environmental justice means that all people enjoy the same degree of protection from environmental threats and have equal access to the decision-making mechanisms that guide policy to create the healthiest environment to live, work, and play in (U.S. EPA, 2020). Equitable and just treatment of all communities means that no population would be forced to bear the consequences of environmental exposures resulting from industrial, municipal, and commercial operations more than any other. Ensuring this reality often means all community members are involved in creating or revising federal, state, and local laws, regulations, and policies. Meaningful participation among all communities depends on equitable access to decision-making procedures and the capacity to communicate with governing bodies and decision makers. Communities also depend on access to and the ability to share accurate, up-to-date information with the intent of informing community members of possible threats (U.S. Department of Energy, n.d.).

Environmental Health Burden on Unempowered Members of Society

Unempowered members of society are at particular risk for the consequences of environmental health risks, for several reasons. The unempowered are those members of society who are the least able to influence the mechanisms of decision making and the creation of laws, policies, and regulations, and who have the least economic resources available to them. Within the larger society, people without acknowledged power may have no other choice but to endure environmental threats without recourse to make changes. They may be segregated to parts of the city or town closest to various threats, such as contaminated water, air, or soil. Members of these communities may have to work in high-risk environments and face significant exposures both at home and at work.

These communities typically do not have the resources to move or to take steps to mitigate their risk exposures. Disempowered members of the community cannot ask for or demand policy change. They may not have the money, time, or capacity to speak on their own behalf, or they may not have access to the legal or regulatory systems.

Their risk exposure makes them more susceptible to the burden of diseases caused by environmental threats. If community members are already sick, the efforts to care for ill family members further consumes the community's limited resources. Environmental threats attributed to environmental injustice practices may cause asthma, immune deficiencies, cancers, and cognitive problems such as dementia. These pathologies result in tremendous burdens to families caring for their sick relatives.

Environmental Health Risks to Migrant and Undocumented Workers

Migrant and undocumented workers are victims of environmental injustices. They are at particular risk for environmental exposures because of their work settings and inability to access the legal systems in the countries where they are employed. The inability to seek legal protection is arguably the most significant challenge faced by migrant workers. They may find themselves unable to leave jobs that put them at risk and with no alternative to challenge employers' unhealthy work environments.

Undocumented workers live with the constant threat of being discovered and facing deportation, which may mean separation from their families. When undocumented workers try to escape hardships and possible threats of violence in their home countries, deportation may be a life-threatening situation. The threat of being sent away may supersede the threat they feel from environmental exposures. Migrant workers often work in jobs that put them at significant risk. Agricultural, construction, and fisheries work, with jobs often held by migrant workers, is risky and often exposes workers to environmental hazards, chemicals, toxins, and poor working conditions. Extreme temperatures, pesticides, chemicals, and poor working conditions pose unique risks to immigrant workers (Moyce & Schenker, 2018).

Environmental Health Risks and Poverty

People living in poverty are at greater risk of exposure because they have fewer resources available to protect themselves from potential threats and little capacity to respond when facing hazards. Poverty creates a dynamic situation that forces people to make choices in the short term with little regard for long-term consequences. Low-wage workers may be forced to endure workplace hardships that put them at significant risk due to toxins, chemical exposures, temperature extremes, and long working hours. These threats are similar to the hazards faced by migrant workers because both groups have few choices and limited power for creating change. Poverty, by its very nature, limits options. These limitations are not confined to the work available to people. Poverty may also restrict where people can live, how much they eat, and the recreational activities available to the family.

The Urban/Rural Divide

Rural communities may be challenged because of their socioeconomic status as a whole. Rural community members may have few resources to support them when they are challenged, and there may be limited opportunity for advocacy within the community. Rural communities often have limited employment opportunities, and challenging a large employer because of work-related environmental risks may come with significant consequences.

The tyranny of distance also challenges many rural communities. The resources and support a community needs may be several hours away, or they may require travel by airplane or boat only when the weather conditions permit. These factors create profound barriers to exchanging information, meeting deadlines, attending meetings, and filing required documents, as is often required when working in or trying to change bureaucratic decision-making systems.

Native and First Nations Communities

Environmental health is particularly important to Native American and First Nations communities because of their unique history and relationship with the land. Native and First Nations people may connect and understand their relationship to the land and the familial and spiritual way a person is tied to the land. Native American and First Nations people may see themselves as descendants of the land and may conceptualize their relationship to the land the way that they conceptualize responsibility to a living relative. With these beliefs, community members may feel a significant responsibility to care for and protect the land. When these dynamics are present, it is imperative to be culturally respectful of the community member's beliefs.

Indigenous people often express their identity through activities rooted to, with, or on the land. These expressions of self often require access to land and activities undertaken in the natural environment. Cultural activities may include eating food gathered from the land or animals raised on the land and could increase their health risks if they contain toxins or contaminants (see the case study titled Communities Affected by the Kilauea and Lower Puna Eruption on Hawai'i Island).

These activities with increased exposure to potential environmental health threats should be carefully considered. The complicated nature of relationships between community members, the land, and the land's resources may pose a significant challenge to nurses working with Native and First Nations peoples. Asking community members to limit their access to the resources of the natural environment, or their cultural sources of identity, may be as spiritually and emotionally damaging as the physical threats posed by toxins and other hazards.

With the presence of other social challenges faced by Native and First Nations communities, these environmental stressors exacerbate the risks

to families. Parents may feel they have failed to teach children their culture. The children may feel disappointed with their parents and grandparents, whose approval and acknowledgment are critical to their identities within the broader community.

Globalization and Health

Globalization contributes to the ongoing issues of environmental health largely because globalization is motivated predominantly by economic factors. The factors that put people who have lower incomes at risk and that put profits above the people, animals, and the natural world are largely the motivators for globalization. The trade- and market-driven agendas of globalization, by definition, cross national boundaries and make environmental regulation and legislation complicated.

Seeking environmentally sustainable globalization creates a dilemma. Despite research suggesting that unchecked industry depletes and damages natural resources, puts humans at risk, and accelerates global warming, advancing environmental protections is not without its own costs. Nations that institute meaningful environmental protections inevitably face disadvantages in the global marketplace due to increased production costs or reduced products. This forces nations and workers to decide if they value their market advantage or their environmental protections more. Nurses may be challenged with having to help families and communities make choices between protection from potential environmental threats and a robust economy.

ENVIRONMENTAL HEALTH RISKS: THE BUILT AND COMMUNITY ENVIRONMENT

Nurses working with families must recognize that environmental health threats can be found in many places where family members work, play, and live. These locations may share risk factors, or the threats may be precisely located in one site and not another. Nurses need to consider the amount of time different family members spend in these different settings to determine the extent to which each person may be exposed. Some of the risks mentioned in this section have been addressed in other sections of this chapter.

Home

Home environmental health concerns include indoor air quality, lead paint, carbon monoxide, radon, pesticides, molds, and chemical exposures. These are examples of threats within the house itself. Other threats may come from the surrounding area but are of equal importance.

Proximity to broad thoroughfares and freeways where pollutants are consistently higher, noise pollution, industrial or agricultural exposures, surface and groundwater contaminants, and toxic waste management are examples of threats posed within the local geographic area in which families may live. Poor air quality has been identified as a contributing factor in premature death, increased cancer rates, respiratory and cardiovascular damage, and increased asthma in children.

Indoor air pollution in some communities ranks among the highest risk factors faced by families. In communities where solid fuels are used for cooking and cleaning, indoor air pollution contributes to pneumonia, chronic respiratory issues, and lung cancer. Although the evidence is less clear, some data suggest that indoor air pollution is associated with asthma; tuberculosis; cataracts; and issues during pregnancy, including low birthweight, heart disease, and cancer (WHO, 2016, 2018).

All family members do not equally share the burden of these threats. Women, children, and older relatives may be at higher risk because they have greater exposure to indoor pollutants. Children and older adults may not have the physiological resiliency to protect themselves and may be more prone to getting sick after minimal exposure.

Work

As mentioned previously, a person's workplace can pose a significant health risk. The nature of the work, particularly for those with limited options, often forces people to take risks to their health that they may not otherwise. The working environment exposes people to toxins, biological agents, heat, the sun, pesticides, and other harmful chemicals.

Workers are often dependent on policy and legal standards to protect them in the working environment. Regulations arguably serve the single most significant protective force in the work environment. Regulation and a means of enforcing policies ensure that employers adhere to practices that minimize risk and protect workers. Unfortunately, policies may be difficult to enforce in isolated rural areas and especially with undocumented workers.

School

Like the home, schools pose several threats associated with indoor environmental hazards. Examples of school-bound risks include lead paint, radon, water and air quality, asbestos, proximity to roads and thoroughfares, and possible chemical exposures.

Schools differ from the home environment because families have less control over potential environmental hazards associated with the school buildings and grounds. Local policy may dictate attendance, but it may not offer families control over where their children go to school, the buildings' conditions, and the risks within the surrounding neighborhoods. Parents may have limited awareness of the dangers that their children are exposed to and may learn of ongoing threats only after considerable exposure periods.

Public Spaces

Public spaces are essential to families because they offer recreation, participation in sports, and community involvement. Public spaces may be outdoors, such as parks or water recreation areas, or indoors, such as shopping malls, theaters, religious services buildings, and sports venues. These spaces are crucial not only for individual families but also for communities as a whole. They provide neighborhood members a chance to meet with one another and to create and nurture social ties.

Public spaces, like schools and the workplace, may hide several environmental threats. Air and water quality, pollutants associated with roads and highways, industrial and agricultural pollutants, and toxins in the built environment are some of the threats that families may face in their community spaces. Public spaces should bring people together; support prosocial behavior; and provide unique opportunities for entertainment, relaxation, and exercise. However, the presence of environmental hazards may reduce community members' desire to spend time in these spaces.

The Nurse's Role

Understanding these risks helps nurses assess potential exposures and prepare families to mitigate hazards or advocate for safety measures. Nurses need to be prepared to take an epidemiological approach, consider each family member's exposure potential, and plan accordingly. Interventions may include making changes in and around a family's home, helping the family to make changes where their behavior may reduce threats, or advocating for broader changes such as requiring lead paint or asbestos to be removed from housing.

Nurses may find themselves having to do home inspections or facilitating in the process to gather sample specimens to identify threats such as lead in water and paint, mold, radon in the air, or contaminants in soil. Nurses may also be the first to recognize symptoms of exposure in their patients and should report their findings appropriately. Nurses can take advantage of screening and assessment tools made available by city, county, regional, and federal entities.

Nurses may play a critical role in communicating risks to threatened communities and families. Nurses are often responsible for explaining to their clients the potential hazards they may encounter. To familiarize themselves with home-related risks, nurses may wish to review the National Center for Environment Health's *Healthy Housing Inspection Manual* (Centers for Disease Control and Prevention [CDC] & U.S. Department of Housing and Urban Development [DHUD], 2008). The goal of risk communication is to motivate change in people by making them aware of the negative outcomes that various threats pose. Nurses should be sensitive to their clients' needs and circumstances when explaining risks because some clients will have limited opportunity to change their circumstances or alter their exposure to threats. Nurses working in community settings have to advocate tirelessly for families, minimize threats, and nurture community-based strengths within community members.

ENVIRONMENTAL HEALTH POLICIES

As the risks posed by environmental threats have become better recognized, protection from environmental hazards is increasingly seen as a human right. One of the primary goals of environmental health policy is eliminating health disparities and the uneven burden that vulnerable populations feel from adverse outcomes. The goal of policy formation is to leverage organizational power to create systemic frameworks of influence that regulate or guide other entities' behavior within a determined space of action (Neira et al., 2017). Public policy ensures that the needs of affected communities are appropriately met according to the members of those communities. The enormous burden placed on low- and middle-income communities by environmental health issues such as air pollution, sanitation, and hygiene cannot be overstated.

Policymakers seek to create strategies that ensure community members, businesses, and public services interact with one another equitably. Well-designed policy sustains a framework that provides for the safety and longevity of communities, businesses, and resource groups by delineating how those entities interact with one another.

One of the central objectives of environmental health policies is to provide systemic laws, regulations, and procedures that protect people using structural procedures to improve environmental conditions. Ideally, policies are put into place in all environments where risks are identified to minimize or eliminate those risks. The challenge of implementing environmental health policies is in recognizing the risks before significant consequences have affected communities.

Environmental policy formation must be sensitive to the interconnectedness of environmental issues; a holistic approach that appreciates the complex interactions of multiple systems and subsystems is essential to creating effective policy. Policy formation should consider scientific, economic, and cultural issues. It is also imperative that policy be responsive to changes in the people's demands and the current understanding of issues. The expectations of business entities place their own demands on the broader environmental landscape, which may be at odds with emerging scientific information.

Several ideological principles can be used to guide policy formation. The focus of these various philosophies is to protect the environment, wildlife, and human health. Different approaches focus their efforts on various factors, but all share the desire to offer protection to more than just people.

Policy grounded in environmental justice advocates for the idea that all people, regardless of their background, socioeconomic status, gender, age, ethnicity, or religion, be equally safe from hazards and environmental threats. Proponents of environmental justice recognize that threats may result from power inequalities that leave some people more vulnerable than others.

Precautionary policy stems from the idea that prevention of harm should be one of the most important motivating factors in policy formation (see Table 6.1 and Table 6.2). Policy should anticipate risks and be structured in a way that minimizes those risks before adverse outcomes occur. Advocates of precautionary policy may champion rules that offer protections before evidence of adverse outcomes is established. In cases where existing science suggests a negative outcome may be possible, precautionary policy will err on the side of caution rather than wait to see what would happen to the people, animals, or other entities they seek to protect (Friis, 2019).

Policy Formation

Policy formation is often a prescriptive, iterative process that involves sequential steps, analysis, and improvement. In the first phase of the process, policymakers define the issue they want to address. During this step, participants work to ensure that they have adequately determined the issue they hope their policy will address. The issue has to be a recognized concern, and there has to be evidence that realistic steps can be taken to eliminate or reduce the adverse outcomes of the problem.

Policymakers set an agenda and establish a timeline and priority list to determine how they want to approach the problem and in what order. Budgetary constraints and resource limits pose significant barriers to developing policies effectively. Planners have to look for procedures that consider various obstacles while remaining responsive to the complexity of environmental issues.

Policy establishment is the selection of policies or procedures that will be put into place to protect people, animals, or the environment from the recognized threats. In this phase, the guidelines are instituted and made available for application.

Policy implementation happens when the established policies are put to use and begin to change how things happen in the real world. To see change, established policies have to be put to use over time so that outcomes can be measured, and the value of the policies can be accurately assessed. When policies change quickly, it will be challenging to determine if they have produced the desired outcomes that policymakers sought during the formation phase.

Risk Assessment and Risk Management

Two of the most critical aspects of policy formation are risk assessment and risk mitigation. These issues play different roles in the policy process, guiding the creation and need for policy as well as serving as benchmarks for desired outcomes of policy implementation.

Risk assessment is a profoundly complex process that involves an analysis of data and evaluation of known threats. Despite efforts to be thorough, policymakers can rarely account for every possible hazard, nor do they have access to all the information they need. There will always be unknown factors influencing outcomes and potentially causing harm.

Policymakers have to weigh the cost benefits of implementing any plan, recognize the costs of implementation, and weigh those costs against the benefits the policy seeks to create. In some situations, the risk of an identified hazard may be so minimal that implementing a policy is not worth the return on investment. The more complex the environmental concern, the more difficult it may be to determine the cost-benefit ratio.

Environmental policies ideally reduce risks and minimize hazards. Policies should put into place procedures and safeguards that protect the identified entities from known hazards or prevent adverse outcomes. Successful policy implementation ideally protects groups of people by eliminating risks on a large enough scale to have the broadest effects.

Policy and Nurses

One of the most effective ways of developing appropriate policies is to involve community members and as many stakeholders as possible. Policymakers should seek input from as many people as possible to ensure that no perspective is being minimized in the earliest phases of policy formation. This is a task particularly well suited to nurses who have extensive experience listening to clients, helping them amplify their concerns, and advocating as needed. Nurses can take part in this process as policy informer, policymaker, and community supporter.

ENVIRONMENTAL HEALTH LITERACY

Environmental literacy, also known as ecological literacy or ecoliteracy, is an awareness about the environment, environmental problems, and the knowledge or methods to address those problems. Environmental health literacy has generally been embedded in the literature of the biological and health sciences, but the jargon and language of these sciences is often too technical or specialized for people to understand and act upon. For the purposes of this chapter, the more appropriate concept of environmental health literacy comes from the Society for Public Health Education (SOPHE, n.d.) and states,

> environmental health literacy integrates concepts from both environmental literacy and health literacy to develop the wide range of skills and competencies that people need in order to seek out, comprehend, evaluate, and use environmental health information to make informed choices, reduce health risks, improve quality of life and protect the environment.

With the increasing and deleterious impact of environmental health problems (e.g., global climate change, air and water pollution), nurses and other health care professionals must address the need for an enhanced environmental awareness into their practice. Finding ways to integrate environmental health literacy into health activities of clients can provide families with the skills and knowledge to reduce impacts on their health from environmental sources. As health care professionals, nurses share a sacred connection with their clients. Nurses and other health care professionals have an obligation to promote environmental health literacy among our colleagues and our communities.

One example of supporting the work of health care providers in advancing environmental health literacy is the Collaborative on Health and the Environment (CHE). This organization has created a multimedia e-book, *A Story of Health*, to promote health and prevent disease (CHE, 2019).

This award-winning resource is an interactive document with multiple chapters that feature embedded information, links to online resources and videos, graphics, and in-depth information for clinicians. The stories are accessible to an educated lay public. The e-book connects health and the environment in a series of stories using fictional people and their families and communities to enable readers to explore the risk factors for disease as well as how to prevent disease and promote health and resilience (CHE, 2019).

Nurses support a holistic view of human health, and they must extend this view beyond the bedside and recognize the connections between the environment and health. They need to inform and work with families and communities to see the environment–health connections and find ways to improve both. Promoting environmental literacy and praxis in which nurses learn to think globally as they practice locally will be good for the profession, good for the people, and good for the earth (Laustsen, 2006).

SUMMARY

Family health is affected by the health of the environment. This is particularly important within the scope of community and public health nursing; however, knowledge of environmental health issues is valuable for nurses working with families in any setting and in all communities. Nurses working with individual families or at the community or population level have a responsibility to develop and implement interventions that reduce environmental health risks and improve the environmental health literacy of families.

- The ecological model of population health views human health as the center of multiple intersecting influences such as behavior; social, family, and community networks; living and working conditions; and the broader influences of national or global factors.
- Families may suffer health effects associated with environmental health risks and hazards that come from air, water, soil, and land quality; disease-carrying organisms; weather and climate; geological events; and natural and human-created chemical toxins and biological hazards.

- Environmental health has a disproportionate impact on certain families and population groups. Health policy should be designed to eliminate and reduce disparity and the burden on vulnerable families.
- Environmental health risks associated with the built and community environment predispose families to health threats where family members work, play, and live.

Nurses across all settings need to integrate an awareness of exposure risks in their assessments of individuals and families.

- Nurses have the opportunity to advance environmental health literacy in individuals and families. This includes an awareness about the environment, environmental problems, and the knowledge or methods to address those problems.

Families Across the Health Continuum

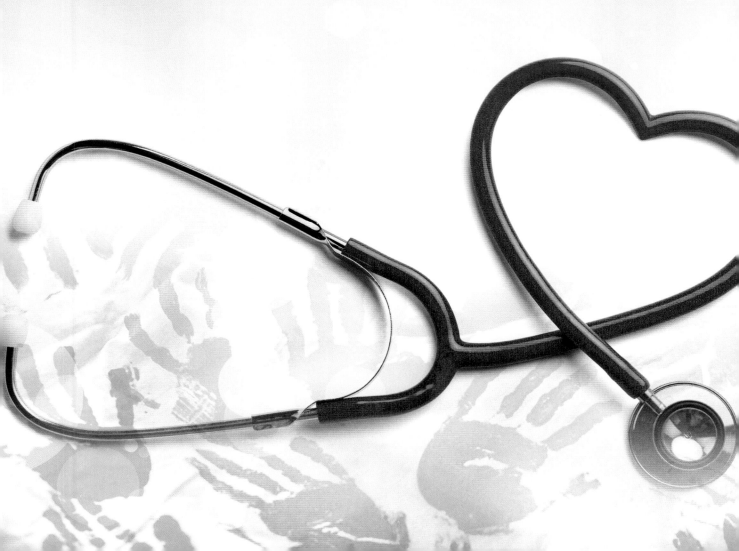

chapter 7

Family Health Promotion

Annette Bailey, PhD, RN

Josephine Pui-Hing Wong, PhD, RN

Mandana Vahabi, PhD, RN

Michèle Parent-Bergeron, PhD, RN

Critical Concepts

- *Family* is commonly defined as the basic social unit of the community and society that consists of people connected either by blood, marriage, adoption, or cohabitation. In this textbook, the definition for *family* also includes the following: the family is who the members say it is.

- The health and well-being of families are influenced by the social, economic, and environmental conditions in which they are born, live, and work; therefore, family health promotion is embedded in community and population health promotion.

- Families define, value, and experience health, health promotion, and disease prevention differently. It is important for nurses to conceptualize and assess the health status of families based on sociopolitical determinants of health.

- Family health promotion is not merely techniques and behavioral activities; it is a way of thinking and acting to strengthen the quality of family life and the health of family members.

- Family health promotion focuses on family interactions shaped by internal family processes and external factors that are structural (i.e., factors that are beyond one's control, such as race, class, income).

- Family health promotion occurs within the dynamics of social, historical, and political structures, so understanding these structures is an essential part of nursing care.

- Health equity in family health promotion is best advanced through culminating and intersecting efforts of policy, research, and practice.

- Nurses have an ethical and social responsibility to care for families in empowering ways, which means strengthening all aspects of families that are necessary for their social adjustments, safety, and growth.

- The role of nurses is to plan, provide, and evaluate nursing services to achieve the highest level of health and well-being possible for families.

INTRODUCTION

Families of all sizes and compositions form the basic units of communities and serve as the fundamental promoters of individual and community health (Hanson et al., 2019). Communities are woven together by family units, and the distinctive nature of each family unit serves in the overall strength and uniqueness of communities. As a unit, families play a significant role in promoting the overall well-being of family members across the life course through resource sharing, supporting decision making, supporting varied family transitions, and fostering connections and a sense of belonging (Carroll & Vickers, 2014; Thomas et al., 2017). However, the contributions of families go beyond the boundary of the immediate family to supporting the stability and vibrancy of community and social infrastructures. The relationship between families and communities is a reciprocal transaction; consequently, family health promotion should not be conceptualized simply by compartmentalizing different aspects and functions of families. A more collective perspective of family health promotion considers the varied and complex dynamics that families exist in, and particularly how historical and systemic issues determine the health experiences of different families.

The sociopolitical conditions that families experience are complex. Many families in the United States are navigating poverty, food insecurity, social injustice, racial discrimination, community violence, and legacies of colonization. These societal issues impinge on families' functionality, their growth, and their well-being (Anderson, 2019; McCalman et al., 2018). Therefore, family health promotion is not merely a set of techniques and activities focused on helping families change patterns of health behaviors. Family health promotion is a way of *thinking* about the dynamics of historical social, economic, and political structures and the effects on family health, and *acting* on factors that impede and promote family relationships, growth, and their ability to thrive as a unit. Thus, a major task of family health promotion is the engagement of critical frameworks in practice that compel nurses and other health care professionals to understand the unique needs and perspectives of families and intentionally engage with families in empowering ways.

The purpose of this chapter is to demonstrate a critical understanding of family health and family health promotion from the perspective of health equity. We begin by contextualizing the definition of family through an equity lens. We then discuss the application of theoretical frameworks in nursing care for diverse families with attention to social determinants of health. We also elaborate on strategies for promoting family health while demonstrating how nurses can assess families and promote their health through empowerment.

DEFINING FAMILY AND FAMILY HEALTH

Family is commonly defined as the basic social unit of the community and society that consists of people connected either by blood, marriage, adoption, or cohabitation. In Chapter 1, the term *family* is defined in many ways, but the most salient definition is the following: the family is who the members say it is. In Western societies, many people think about "family" in terms of biological and/or legal relatedness, maternal and/or paternal functions, living structure and arrangement, and normative relationship patterns. Historically, the dominant image of the family is a traditional two-parent household; however, this has changed. In the United States, the number of two-parent households is on the decline, while divorce, remarriage, and cohabitation are on the rise; the number of single-parent households is growing, and Americans are having fewer children (Pew Research Center, 2021). In Canada, demographic shifts mean that more children are living in their parents' households longer, and, as the number of older adults in Canada has increased, more are living with their adult children (IES, 2021). It is important to note that contemporary families are diverse and dynamic units of social relationships, and they continue to evolve and transform over time based on changing social and political contexts of society. As individuals interact with social systems, their meaning of socially constructed identities (race, gender, class, age, and sexuality) are reconstituted, and their responses to traditional views shift (Battle & Ashley, 2008). A traditional, Eurocentric model of family, therefore, does not adequately account for all family types, especially as social norms about family and cultures continue to change.

Definitions of *family health* have evolved from anthropological, biopsychosocial, developmental, family science, cultural, and nursing paradigms. Family scientists have defined healthy families as resilient and as possessing a balance of cohesion and adaptability that is facilitated by good communication (Walsh, 2016b). Other definitions of family health focus on the totality of the family's existence and include the internal and external environment of the family. This perspective is rooted in general systems theory and the ecological systems theory (Novilla, 2011). A holistic definition of family health encompasses all aspects of family life, including interaction and health care function. For the purposes of this chapter, *family health* is a holistic, dynamic, and complex state. Family health is more than the absence of disease in an individual family member or the absence of dysfunction in family dynamics. Rather, it is the complex process of negotiating and solving day-to-day family life events and crises, and providing a quality life for its members (Novilla, 2011). Today, the notion of family has to be understood in the contexts of social identities, power relations, and the dynamic interactions between families and society. It is important for nurses to understand that the health and well-being of individuals and families is influenced by social and historical inequities.

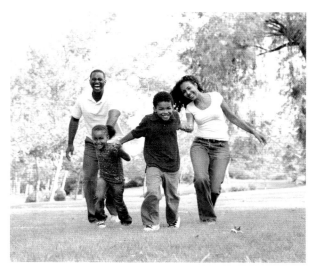

© *Monkey Business Images/Monkey Business/Thinkstock.*

FAMILIES AND POPULATION HEALTH EQUITY

Scientific advancements in the 20th century have improved human life expectancy significantly. However, increasing evidence shows that not all populations benefit equally from access to technology or key resources that support economic development. For example, in developing countries where technology is restricted, income-generating activities, innovation, and opportunities to reduce poverty are limited (Mirza et al., 2019). Individuals and families that lack access to health care have inherent risks, and socioeconomic status may have the most significant impact on health. Socioeconomic status consists of the lifelong evolving status of a person's financial situation, educational attainment, and employment status (McMaughan et al., 2020). While access to care is necessary for the protection and promotion of health, Woolf (2019) suggested that it is just one of the critical domains necessary for health, which include (1) health care, (2) health behaviors, (3) the physical and social environment, (4) socioeconomic status, and (5) public policy—"all of which have complex interrelationships" (p. 196).

Social Determinants of Health

The social determinants of health (SDHs) influence families and health equity significantly. The SDHs are the conditions in which people are born, grow, work, live, and age and the broader systems that shape living conditions (World Health Organization [WHO], 2021b). The systems include economic policies, health agendas, social policies, and political systems. At all levels of income, health and illness are consistent with social status and most responsible for health inequities; the lower one's economic position, the poorer one's health (WHO, 2021b). Examples of SDHs that influence health equity in positive and negative ways include income, employment, education, access to food, work and life conditions, social support, relationships in the community, and access to health care.

The U.S. Department of Health and Human Services (2021) developed the place-based framework, *Healthy People 2030*, to identify five key areas of SDHs:

1. Health care access and quality: The connection between access to health services and health (e.g., access to primary care, health insurance, health literacy)

2. Education access and quality: The connection of education to health and well-being (e.g., graduation rates, higher education, language and literacy, early childhood services)

3. Social and community context: The connection between where people live, work, and play and their health and well-being (e.g., community and civic engagement, workplace relationships, discrimination, incarceration)

4. Economic stability: The connection between financial resources and socioeconomic status and one's health (e.g., income, cost of living, poverty, food security)

5. Neighborhood and built environment: The connection to where people live and their health and well-being (e.g., housing, neighborhood, and environment)

The framework supports understanding the health of vulnerable populations in the context of their circumstances and daily lives. This can help nurses develop interventions that promote the health of families and advocate for health and social policies that reduce vulnerability. Populations at risk for marginalized social status are more vulnerable to health disparities. For example, the Affordable Care Act (ACA) helped to ensure health care coverage for millions of Americans. After the law was implemented, the uninsured rate among Black Americans actually declined despite 2.8 million Black Americans obtaining coverage through the ACA. By 2018, the uninsured rate was 9.7 percent, while the uninsured rate for White Americans was just 5.4 percent (U.S. Census Bureau, 2019b).

In addition to social marginalization, income insecurity and low socioeconomic status have enormous influence on health outcomes of families. Family household income, level of education, and the type of jobs that family members hold all contribute to family health status (Marmot, 2015; Woolf, 2019). Specifically, family members' health practice, physical and mental health, early child development issues, relationships, and family functioning are implicated in overall health status. The development of children within families is a strong indicator of how families are

economically and socially positioned. Children in higher-income families tend to flourish and score higher on all development measures (Marmot, 2015), while limited access to educational and other resources often diminishes the emotional and psychological health of children in low-income families (Guhn et al., 2020; Hodgkinson et al., 2017).

It is important to note that social and economic disparities are not natural occurrences or coincidences. Challenges to the quality of life and flourishing of families have their roots in social inequalities, social policies, political decisions, and oppressive histories. It is critical to recognize that income and health disparities are associated with and are reinforced by preexisting structural violence of racism, sexism, and classism (Shumway, 2017; Kirton, 2018).

When racial and gender inequality are combined with poverty, significantly more detrimental health and social consequences are seen for children in low-income families (Livingstone & Weinfeld, 2015). Beyond child development, research demonstrates that poverty is disruptive to all dimensions of family functioning. Poverty negatively affects interactions and relationships between family members, resulting in diminished interest in family activities, conflict in parental roles, and compromised parent-child relationships (Banovcinova et al., 2014). Like other health inequities, poverty operates from intersecting social and structural nuances; however, the effects are felt and maneuvered at the family level, creating challenges in family health and functioning.

Nursing care that recognizes the lived experiences of families, which is a tapestry of intertwining and complex factors and circumstances, can instill empathy and humanity into the gaps in health promotion that exist for families that are marginalized and at risk for experiencing health inequities. The following sections present a few examples of the sociopolitical contexts of challenges faced by marginalized families. It is beyond the scope of this chapter to describe families from all contexts. We focus on families of Indigenous people in Canada, Black families in the United States, and LGBTQ+ communities to illustrate the complex dynamics and impact of vulnerability and health and social inequities. The use of the term *Indigenous people* in this chapter refers to First Nations, Inuit, and Métis Peoples in Canada collectively and is used to reflect Indigenous experiences in health care. It is important to recognize this distinction, when appropriate, considering that the term *Indigenous* has recently replaced the term *Aboriginal*, which is still acceptable and widely used (The Indigenous Health Writing Group of the Royal College, 2019).

Indigenous Families in Canada

Indigenous communities have unique collective cultural values, beliefs, and practices. Colonization has disrupted the cultural experiences and practices of Indigenous families everywhere and continues to shape their lives and livelihood (Palmater, 2017). Colonization is not simply the misappropriation of Indigenous land. It is a form of structural violence legitimated by racist public policies and laws to displace Indigenous families from their ancestral and granted Territories, and to justify the legalized kidnapping and stealing of Indigenous children from their families, both in the residential school era and in the present-day so-called child protection systems. In Canada, residential schools were government-sponsored religious schools developed to assimilate Indigenous children into Euro-Canadian culture, which led to cultural genocide and destruction of Indigenous families (Wilk et al., 2017). Cultural genocide included separating and isolating Indigenous children from their families and cultures and forced assimilation into the dominant European culture without granting them similar rights and dignity. Residential schools not only inflicted trauma and abuse on Indigenous children; they also systematically eroded and undermined all aspects of well-being for Indigenous families and communities through disruption of the structure, cohesion, and quality of family life (Aguiar & Halseth, 2015). Indigenous children forcibly taken from their families and placed in residential schools were stripped of their language and culture, their names were changed, siblings were separated, and parent visits were discouraged and controlled. Disruption of family life (i.e., parent-child(ren) bonding, intimacy, extended family relationships) contributed greatly to alienation, estrangement, and negative coping. When Indigenous children, especially those abused in residential schools or foster homes, returned to their families, many were unable to form trusting relationships or positive connections with their parents or families. Reintegration into family and community proved challenging for many because of a loss of identity. They were too far removed from their own Indigenous roots. A loss of individual and cultural identity and broken family bonds continued for generations (Truth and Reconciliation Commission of Canada, 2015). After decades of investigating reports of mistreatment, neglect, malnutrition, physical and sexual abuse, and efforts to ban Indigenous languages in residential schools, the Truth and Reconciliation Commission of Canada concluded that the policy of forcible removal of Indigenous children was "cultural genocide" (Fontaine et al., 2015). In the same report, the Commission estimated that more than 150,000 children attended the residential schools and more than 6,000 died, never returning home. Recently, the community of Tk'emlúps te Secwépemc, which was the location of the largest school in the Indian Affairs residential school system, Kamloops Indian Residential School, reported finding a mass grave holding the remains of 215 children, including some as young as three years old (Kamloops, 2021). The physical health outcomes linked to residential schooling included poorer general health, increased rates of chronic and infectious disease, and poor self-rated health (Wilk et al., 2017). The devastating impact of colonization also manifested in disproportionately high levels of mental health disparities in the form of abuse, addictions, violence, and suicide within Indigenous families (Bourassa et al., 2015; Wilk et al., 2017). At the same time, colonialism has worked in tandem with structural racism to produce discriminatory legislation such as the Indian Act in Canada. Anti-Indigenous colonial racism produces and perpetuates all forms of systemic discrimination and barriers embedded in the policies and procedures of organizational structures affecting the daily life and well-being of Indigenous families (Richmond & Cook, 2016). For example, Indigenous communities in Canada continue to experience disproportionately high rates of infant mortality (Richmond & Cook, 2016). For many years, and still now, Indigenous pregnant women living in rural or remote reserves have been removed from their families and support networks between the gestational age of 36 and 38 weeks and transferred to birthing services in urban centers for delivery. This transfer can occur sooner if a pregnancy is considered to be at high risk (Lawford et al., 2018). Known as Health Canada's birth evacuation or maternal evacuation policy, the evacuation of women from rural and remote communities to give birth in hospitals located in southern urban centers was intended to reduce infant mortality rates, especially for Indigenous women who are often considered at greatest risk (Olson & Couchie, 2013). However, this evacuation practice negates the holistic needs of Indigenous women. Traveling away from traditional and ancestral homelands to give birth is contrary to traditional birthing practices and ontologies for many Indigenous women (Lawford et al., 2018). Yet this policy of forced birth travel is still in effect. Indigenous leader Dr. Pamela Palmater argued that pregnant Indigenous women, like other Canadian women, should have the option with support to give birth in their communities. In 2017, the federal government tried to remedy this situation by offering to pay for Indigenous women to bring a buddy with them to urban birthing centers. However, the buddy system cannot replace the cultural and spiritual practice of birthing within one's family and community. As a result of the policy, Indigenous women continue to experience high levels of stress, isolation and loneliness, a lack of choice, weight loss and physical suffering, financial stress, fear and worry, and even shame for having a family, which further exacerbates risks for optimal maternal and infant health (Lawford et al., 2019). Indigenous people are resilient, and many of their communities have flourished; however, "the impact of colonialism continues to have profound health effects for Indigenous peoples [families] in Canada and internationally" (Browne et al., 2016, p. 1). Defining Indigenous families, therefore, cannot be done in the absence of colonial context, and their health, resistance, and resilience, cannot be fully understood outside their social experiences.

In the United States, American Indian and Alaska Native women also experience health inequities and are vulnerable to poor health outcomes. In addition to higher rates of preterm birth, infant mortality rates for babies born to American Indian women are higher than for babies born to White women (Centers for Disease Control & Prevention [CDC], 2018). Contrary to Indigenous women in Canada, some American Indian and Alaska Native women tend to have better access to prenatal care due to greater access to Indian Health Services within some local communities. American Indian and Alaska Native women who have moved to urban communities, away from tribal reservations and rural communities, may experience more barriers to accessing health care (Raglan et al., 2016). Overall, American Indian and Alaska Native women are two to three times more likely to die from pregnancy-related complications than White women (CDC, 2018). There is strong evidence to suggest that lifetime chronic experiences of stress, racial discrimination, and economic marginalization contribute to these health disparities (Gupta & Froeb, 2020).

Racism in the Black Community

Slavery has contributed to systemic racism, structural barriers, and widespread social oppression that results in an overall lack of access to equitable socioeconomic and political resources for many Black families and communities. This has perpetuated a cycle of poverty for them and has created significant vulnerability for health risks. Challenges that Black families experience, produced through multigenerational traumas of slavery, are often overlooked or denied because of a lack of value and acknowledgment of their experiences. It is important to note that the perpetual oppressions against Black families and communities are not limited to material marginalization. Dehumanization, brutality, and mistreatment are significant elements of slavery that have permeated the experiences of Black families for generations. Racism, in the form of stereotypes and discrimination and originally derived to justify the enslavement of Black people, is an epidemic. Racist stereotypes function as symbolic violence, especially against Black men, who are constructed as primitive, animalistic, and dangerous. This perception has resulted in police brutality, high rates of homicide, and overincarceration of Black men (Alang et al., 2017). While Black men's experience with police brutality and incarceration stretch back for many years, media coverage of the recent social justice protest sparked by the public killing of George Floyd by a White police officer and subsequent conviction, helped to shed light on the severity of this problem for Black families.

The COVID-19 pandemic has revealed inequities in the U.S. health care system by the shockingly disproportionate death rates among Blacks, who represent a third of hospitalized patients with COVID-19 yet make up only 13% of the U.S. population. At one point during the pandemic, Black Americans living in Chicago made up 43% of the cases and 56% of the deaths from the virus (City of Chicago, 2021). A recent study from the United Kingdom demonstrated that Black participants had a four times higher risk of being hospitalized due to COVID-19 complications, even after controlling for economic and physiological risk factors (Lassale et al., 2020). Several possible biological explanations are under investigation that are specific to COVID-19 that increase the risk for Black individuals and families; however, perhaps the most critical risk factors are related to well-known health inequities. Black individuals are disproportionately affected by greater than 45% of vascular-related diseases and are 37% more likely to develop lung cancer than White Americans, despite lower exposure to cigarette smoke (Ajilore & Thames, 2020), which predisposes individuals to the complications of COVID-19. The social determinants of health that most significantly affect poorer health outcomes, such as socioeconomic instability, education, and environment, have a direct impact on access to regular health care and the quality of health care (WHO, 2021b). In addition, evidence suggests that there is medical bias in testing and treatment of Black people with COVID-19 (Infectious Disease Insights, 2020). It is difficult to believe that social inequities such as these continue to persist despite the evidence of consistently poor effects on health. Structural forms of racism and discrimination are critical to understanding the context for health care experiences and health outcomes.

Structural barriers and racism can create intense trauma among Black families, with negative outcomes stemming from the involvement, injury, and death of Black members of the community in gun violence (Bailey et al., 2015; Bailey & Velasco, 2014).

The loss of Black men due to violence and incarceration has left a gap in Black families, resulting in an increasing number of Black women parenting Black households (Livingstone & Weinfeld, 2015). Although Black mothers have continued to raise strong, resilient Black children, their efforts are continually threatened by pervasive systemic racism that forces them into poverty and other social suffering. Racial stratification and pay inequity—specifically income inequality for Black female-led homes—also present social and economic challenges for Black families (Livingstone & Weinfeld, 2015). Multigenerational poverty caused by slavery has influenced the migration of Black families across diverse national contexts, resulting in prolonged separation of families. The migration of African and Caribbean Blacks to countries such as Canada, the United States, and the United Kingdom is driven by the need to obtain a better life for themselves and social, educational, and economic progress for their children and families (Taylor et al., 2017). Black immigrants' decision to migrate is involuntary; it is born not of choice but of displacement (James & Davis, 2012). The historic and material conditions that have shaped Blacks' migration are remnants of slavery and colonialism manifested in the 21st century. In defining Black families, it is critical to understand that Black family structures are often constructed and re-created in response to the social and economic impacts of racism, sexism, and classism.

Stigma-Discrimination Matters: Impact on LGBTQ+ Families

Heterosexism, homophobia, and discrimination have a negative impact on the lives and well-being of LGBTQ+ individuals and their families. Before 1995, same-sex parents were not allowed to apply jointly for an adoption. It was not until 2005, when the Civil Marriage Act passed, that same-sex parents were granted the same rights as heterosexual parents (Government of Canada, 2021). In the United States, activism to obtain equal rights for same-sex marriage started in the 1970s. In 2015, the U.S. Supreme Court finally made same-sex marriages legal in all 50 states (Wootton et al., 2019). According to the U.S. Census Bureau (2019b), there are approximately

543,000 same-sex married-couple households and 469,000 households with same-sex unmarried partners living together. There are also about 191,000 children living with same-sex parents.

Although some countries, including Canada and the United States, have legalized same-sex marriages, LGBTQ+ persons and their families are vulnerable to discrimination based on sexual orientation and gender identity. Equitable access to resources that support family functioning and relationships, including steady and meaningful employment, access to high-quality health care, access to fair and affordable housing, and more, are all socioeconomic vulnerabilities that can have a negative impact on physical and psychological health.

Whether in communities, health care, or the workplace, LGBTQ+ families experience higher levels of discrimination and microaggression because they do not reflect the normative form and structure of family (Haines et al., 2018). Due to homophobia and stigma, LGBTQ+ children and youth are sometimes rejected by their parents and families, putting them at increased risk of social isolation, diminished self-concepts, negative coping, mental illness, substance use, suicide, and HIV vulnerabilities (McCann & Brown, 2019). Fighting against stigma and discrimination, the social movement organization Parents, Friends and Family of Lesbians and Gays (PFLAG) was formed in the 1990s, first in the United States and Canada and subsequently around the world. PFLAG plays an important role in changing societal attitudes and advocating for equitable policy change (Broad, 2011). Many LGBTQ+ people have also established a cutting-edge strategy of forming so-called families of choice to promote their personal and collective resilience (Hull & Ortyl, 2019). Chosen or created families are sources of strength for LGBTQ+ individuals who are rejected; these families function as a buffer to reduce the impact of homophobic violence, abuse, and microaggression experienced by LGBTQ+ individuals and to improve their resilience (Hailey et al., 2020; Haines et al., 2018). However, systemic discrimination continues to affect LGBTQ+ families negatively. Black LGBTQ+ persons and their families, in particular, are also vulnerable to experiences of racism and homophobia and are more likely to be pathologized for not fitting with the dominant ideas of family (Battle & Ashley, 2008). Defining LGBTQ+ families should be integrated and connected within the context of social identity and intersecting social politics. LGBTQ+ family health and nursing care is discussed in greater detail in Chapter 8.

The three family scenarios discussed reinforce the idea that the relationship between families and communities is a reciprocal transaction. When the definition of family is not understood based on its unique form and structure, its collective roles and functions in the historical, social, and political life of the community may be overlooked. Emphasis on the background and context of the individual and family experience can provide nurses with opportunities for health promotion that are equitable and family-centered.

THEORETICAL PERSPECTIVES FOR FAMILY HEALTH PROMOTION

Families are microcosms of communities and societies that engage in complex processes of negotiating resources, solving day-to-day life events and crises, and helping its members thrive (Novilla, 2011). Social and community resources are not simply external factors; they are generated and sustained by public policies and politics and are therefore a central part of the dynamic and complex relationship between families and local and global communities. Families are best understood as entities within a wide and complex spectrum of interactions, and *family health* is best understood as a holistic, dynamic, and multifaceted state.

Ecological Perspective

An ecological perspective emphasizes the intricate dynamics between families and environmental factors that influence health. From this perspective, health care providers can advance their understanding of all aspects of family life, including the varied and complex dynamics that families exist in, their interactions, and overall family health care functions (Kokorelias et al., 2019; Novilla, 2011).

In an ecological perspective, the family is conceptualized as being part of something much larger yet at the center of a complex social system that includes the individuals, family, community, and society (Novilla, 2011). The individuals and family interact with the components of the system as they develop their values, family-level beliefs, and behaviors. In using an ecological model, nursing researchers are able to study how physical, social, economic, and political factors interact to shape the health of families and communities, and they can work across relevant disciplines to identify effective strategies that promote health equity at multiple levels, as illustrated in Figure 7-1.

The figure provides an ecological view of families within society. As shown, the family is nestled in circular, connected relationships that go beyond their immediate household to the broader community and society. The figure shows the complex interconnections and relationships that shape the health of families. While families are

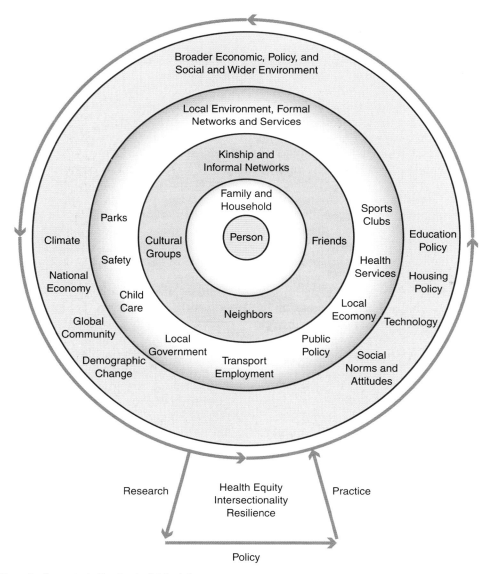

FIGURE 7-1 Bronfenbrenner's Ecological Model   *Source: Diagram by Joel Gibbs, based on Bronfenbrenner's (1979) Ecological Model (Scott, Laing, & Park, 2016, p. 7).*

an entity on their own, with unique cultures, interactions, and dynamics, the boundaries of family dynamics are permeable to the influences of community and societal issues. As the center to all surrounding circles, families can exert influences beyond their immediate households. This is demonstrated by the lines for each concentric circle. The interaction between families and each aspect of their environment is a necessity to meet their social, emotional, and economic determinants of health. Interactions with informal networks like friends and cultural groups foster connectivity, social support, and informal resources. Local environments serve in the provision of recreation, health service access, employment and educational opportunities, and safety. The broader economic and social environment sets the tone for national economies, family and health policy, societal and cultural norms, and environmental effects. Chapter 2 discussed how the bioecological perspective includes both *nature* (biological) and *nurture* (environmental contexts) of growth and development for members of the family, and the family as a whole, *over time*.

Families are as healthy as the environments around them. The complexities of a family's experiences are often realized in their interactions within local and broader communities. Systemic barriers, limited equity policies, and prejudicial influences can mean poor health and well-being outcomes for families with multigenerational effects. As a result, family health promotion is embedded in community and population health promotion, and the intersection between research, policy, and practices is foundational to family health promotion.

The intersection of research, policy, and practice is constructed at the base of the ecological model to indicate that family health should move beyond simply understanding a family's interactions with the broader society to taking actions through research, policy, and practice that address interactions that hamper the progression of all families. Such actions should be grounded in principles of equity, intersectionality, and family resilience.

In family health promotion, nurses focus on the health and well-being of individual family members as well as on families as holistic units that make up communities. Because families are diverse, nurses are likely to work with families of different cultural backgrounds, compositions, and health practices. Nurses have an ethical and social responsibility to care for all families in empowering ways, that is, with cultural humility and structural competency. Cultural humility is an active process of continuous critical self-reflection about how nurses' worldviews and biases affect their professional practice and negatively affect the experiences and health outcomes of the families they work with (Hughes et al., 2020). Structural competence refers to nurses' ability to recognize that the health of individuals and communities is determined by myriad structural factors that require upstream solutions (Hansen & Metzl, 2016). Strengthening families; preserving family culture and customs; and promoting social adjustments, safety, and growth for families is achievable through actions focused at critical points of influence between families, community, and society.

Whether at the bedside or in community settings, nurses come into practice with power—power to empower or oppress. Nurses have an ethical and social responsibility to provide nursing services for families in culturally safe ways. In the context of health equity, this responsibility requires nurses to address both personal biases that have an impact on their care and the structural oppression that has an impact on a family's health. The concept of cultural safety speaks to the work of nurses at the structural level to promote family health. In addressing inequities in health outcomes, especially for Indigenous people, nurses are encouraged to attend to the concept of cultural safety, which "prompts nurses to reflect on the structures, discourses, and assumptions that frame the delivery of health care and what can be done to counteract power differentials in health care" (Pauly et al., 2015, p. 131). Cultural safety is necessary to mitigate impacts of discrimination, stigma, and historical trauma by addressing the policies and practices that marginalize the power of families accessing health care. Strengthening families; preserving family culture and customs; and promoting social adjustments, safety, and growth for families is achievable through actions focused at critical points of influence between families, community, and society. However, this requires an active process of continuous critical self-reflection about how nurses' worldviews and biases affect their professional practice and negatively affect the experiences and health outcomes of the families they work with (Hughes et al., 2020).

An ecological model provides nurses with a broad understanding of the multilevel influences on the health of families. Combining this model with other theoretical perspectives can help nurses design and implement relevant family research and translate evidence into practice to achieve family-centered health promotion.

Health Equity Perspective

Health equity means that every person has a fair and just opportunity to access the resources that they need to be as healthy as possible (Braveman, 2014). Health equity gaps are responsible for the downward spiraling of health among families at the lowest extreme of health and wealth—these are the poorest and most disadvantaged families in our society. For families experiencing inequity, multiple stressors unfold across multiple aspects of their social and political surroundings. Health equity for families is achieved through identifying and removing systemic barriers that determine their access to economic, social, political, and environmental resources for health.

Caring for families at all stages of illness and wellness requires understanding and consideration of their unique experiences in society, and especially how these experiences affect their wellness process. An understanding of the uniqueness of a family's experiences can help nurses plan and deliver care in a family-centered manner. For example, from an ecological perspective, nurses working with Indigenous families understand that their interactions are infused with systemic and structural nuances that are interdependent and relational with a family's history, their culture, and their environment. Indigenous children and families require equitable access to high-quality and culturally respectful health services to address disparities and transform their health (Greenwood et al., 2018).

In regard to understanding the impact of structural social factors on Indigenous families, Gerlach et al. (2018) found that working with Indigenous children and families from a health equity perspective includes learning from them, rather than about them; understanding how family's well-being is influenced by trauma, adversity, and multifaceted social determinants; and being responsive to a family's experiences of raising children in social isolation influenced by the broader sociohistorical context. Using a health equity lens, nurses can better recognize the uniqueness of families and approach their care with an openness to understand their needs. They can also intentionally engage with families with less judgment in their attitude and demeanor. When nurses do this, they can advocate on behalf of families with greater authenticity.

Intersectionality Lens

Intersectionality is a concept defined as:

a theoretical framework that posits that multiple social categories (e.g., race, ethnicity, gender, sexual orientation, socioeconomic status) intersect at the micro level of individual experience to reflect multiple interlocking systems of privilege and oppression at the macro, social-structural level (e.g., racism, sexism, heterosexism) (Bowleg, 2012, p. 1).

In other words, the intersectionality framework enables nurses to analyze how a myriad of social factors interact on multiple levels to understand how health outcomes are revealed across diverse population groups and geographical contexts (Kapilashrami & Hankivsky, 2018).

Figure 7-1 demonstrates how families are embedded in interconnected and relational networks at the community, institutional, and structural levels. It is not enough to understand that differences in opportunities have an impact on families' differential experiences with health. Understanding the intricate ways in which certain factors unique to race, class, gender, and sexuality intersect and operate together at different levels of power in families' vulnerability is necessary to promote health equity and social justice for families (Collins & Bilge, 2016). For example, we know that gender inequality affects women economically and socially. However, Black women's experiences with inequities are further complicated by race; thus, they have fewer and lesser opportunities than White women. When sexuality is added in the mix, then the intersecting identities of transgender women of color expose them to added discrimination, more inferior health care experiences, and poorer overall health outcomes (Howard et al., 2019). This shows that a single factor cannot account for the health outcome of families. The health of families is a result of the intersection of multiple factors—personal, environmental, social, and political factors—that are mutually influencing. The intersecting effects of these factors are strengthened by systems of power relations in society that work to produce different lived experiences and access to opportunities for children and families who are marginalized. An intersectionality lens helps us understand the complexities of family life, decisions, actions, and interactions within the domains of power and intersecting systems of oppression. When used in combination with a health equity lens, an intersectionality lens sheds light on how family interactions at different levels of the ecological model—for example, the institutional (e.g., policies) and structural (e.g., racism)—shape inequities for families (Kapilashrami & Hankivsky, 2018).

To better understand how families' unique identities and structural position in a system of power influence their differential experiences, López and Gadsden (2016) suggest that practitioners, researchers, and educators adapt an *intersectionality health equity lens*, which illuminates the subtleties of race and class systems of oppression in shaping health and well-being for children and families in communities that are marginalized by systemic oppression. An intersectionality health equity lens enables nurses to engage in *critical reflection* to become aware of the ways that oppression operates to reinforce and magnify health inequities. When nurses understand these intertwining systems of oppression, they can take actions to address health disparities and discrimination experienced by these families in the health care system and beyond. For example, thinking from an intersectionality and health equity lens, nurses working with Black families affected by violence (e.g., police brutality) would consider its connection to racism and generational trauma, as well as its overall impact on the success and health of Black families. From this perspective, nursing actions would attend to positive changes at the macro level (political representation, public policies, institutions), meso level (organizations), and micro level (programs/service). Intersectoral collaboration and coordinated efforts that engage families as partners may

shift and reduce the impact of traumatic experiences (Heberle et al., 2020).

Resilience Perspective

Many families grapple with multiple, cumulative, and persistent challenges that may affect all members within the family unit and the family as a whole. These challenges may include chronic illnesses, community violence, death of family members, grief and loss, discrimination, complex trauma, poverty, job loss, prolonged unemployment, and relationship breakups. When members of families are overwhelmed with these acute or chronic stressors, their health and well-being are compromised.

At the same time, many families can overcome these challenges and survive. What makes some individuals and families recover and others break down? Regardless of the level of stressors families face, it is important for nurses to apply a family resilience perspective to identify protective factors that keep families resilient. Research has shown that it is important to support families to access their inner capacities and external resources that enable them to bounce back and continue to achieve their health goals (Walsh, 2016a, 2016b; Burnette et al., 2020).

Family resilience is the ability of the family to cope with adversity and to overcome life challenges. When families move through a crisis by adapting to stressors and maintaining a positive level of function, they often grow stronger and more resourceful (Walsh, 2016a). The family's ability to grow and thrive despite adversity is often intrinsically motivated, but it can also be externally reinforced or fractured. From an ecological perspective, the interactions between individual, family, peer group, community, and larger system variables play a role in perpetuating stressors, as well as serving as protective factors for nurturing and building resilience during hard times. Therefore, efforts toward promoting family resilience have to be embedded as transactional processes between families, their social and community networks, access to resources, and ability to navigate barriers in their complex environments (Breitkreuz et al., 2014; Ungar, 2011). Nurses working with families need to acquire a critical understanding of resilience-building actions and support needed in the extended family and community (Piel et al.,

2017) that can activate and sustain family recovery and growth.

What do these perspectives, or lenses, mean to you as students? How do these fit into the construction of your identities? We come in relation to each other from a point of differences—different experiences, different backgrounds, different cultures. These differences, however unique, shape our perspectives and our view of the world and each other. Our view of the world determines what we do. These lenses compel us to appreciate differences in coming to an understanding of how our humanity connects us. From this perspective, nurses care for diverse families with the intention to strengthen a family's ability to promote their health and connect to their broader community.

FAMILY HEALTH PROMOTION ADDRESSING DETERMINANTS OF HEALTH

In addressing family health at all of its levels of complexity, nurses should understand the relationship between social determinants of health at different dimensions of health and how these determinants serve as barriers in addressing vulnerabilities in diverse families. Reading and Wein (2009, 2013) proposed a framework called the *Integrated Life Course and Social Determinants Model of Aboriginal Health* to provide deeper understanding of the link between determinants of health and health equities for Indigenous individuals and families at the proximal, intermediate, and distal levels. The model builds on what has been described in this chapter as the social determinants of health (WHO, 2021b).

While the framework is focused on health promotion for Indigenous families, it is versatile and applicable to other families, particularly when nurses seek to develop ways to promote the health of individuals and families based on their unique circumstances. Proximal determinants of health are conditions that directly affect the physical, mental, and spiritual health of families. These determinants contribute to stressors and influence behavioral change at the family level. Income, education, food insecurity, and the neighborhood where families live are all considered proximal determinants because they influence family instability, violence, poor parenting, the risk of injuries, chronic illnesses, and mental health issues for families. Intermediate determinants of health can be thought of as directly arising from proximal determinants. For example, low income and living in disadvantaged neighborhoods are results of inequitable educational access or limited community infrastructure. These, along with a lack of environmental support and cultural cohesion, have fostered inequitable access to opportunities for families at the community level. Distal determinants of health have the most detrimental influence on family health because they are rooted in social, political, and economic structures that construct both proximal and intermediate determinants of health.

Understanding the complex intersections among these three levels can help nurses explore opportunities to address vulnerabilities within families. Nurses can focus on understanding the extent to which different levels (proximal, intermediate, distal) are associated with poor health outcomes for families, and they can also begin to identify strengths in the family that can be utilized to build resilience and capacity for health promotion. To better conceptualize these levels of intersecting health determinants, we illustrate them as the crown (proximal), trunk (intermediate), and root (distal) of a tree in Figure 7-2.

Nurses may believe it is easier to focus on the proximal level (crown) when dealing with complex issues; however, it is important to understand that interventions and resources targeted at the distal level (root) can make long-term differences for families at all levels by exposing, interrupting, and eliminating barriers faced by families. Therefore, understanding how the health of families fits within the context of the broader society is critical in truly addressing health equity (Gerlach et al., 2018). For example, nurses working with families experiencing crisis and loss related to gun violence in their community should consider how the family may have been affected by historical, economic, and sociopolitical factors in their community. In this situation, the role of the nurse when working with the family would include demonstrating respect for their humanity, creating a culturally safe environment for care, maintaining sensitivity for their experiences, and advocating for equitable opportunities for them to access high-quality care that is grounded in social justice principles.

For example, having access to care that recognizes that people have a right to self-determination can be fundamental to creating conditions for equal access to health and health care (Richmond & Cook, 2016).

On a broader level, nurses have the opportunity to demonstrate leadership in advocating for policy that supports equity within the health care system and community. Discrimination can exist within the health care system (intermediate/ trunk), and nurses that are mindful of the risks of implicit bias have the opportunity to reduce the

effects on health for all families, including Indigenous families (Allan & Smylie, 2015). In a study that assessed discrimination within health care, Wylie and McConkey (2019) found that implicit bias was so normalized that many health care professionals were unaware that it was a problem. Addressing discrimination and bias within health care organizations can improve interactions and relationships with all families, which is critical within family health promotion. Equity policies to inform distribution of health resources and govern accountable and respectful interactions at the

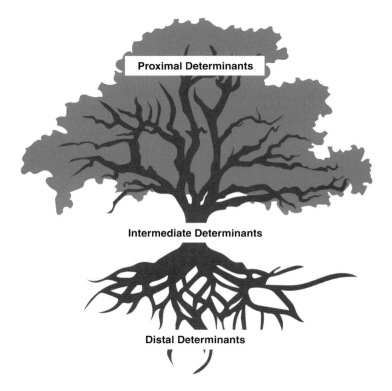

Proximal (The Crown)
- Health behavior
- Physical environments/ neighborhood
- Employment/income
- Education
- Food insecurity

- Trauma/mental health
- Self-esteem
- Chronic illness
- Violence
- Addictions
- Homelessness

Intermediate (The Trunk)
- Health care systems
- Educational systems
- Social environment
- Community infrastructures, resources, and capacities
- Cultural continuity/respect

Distal (The Root)
- Colonialism/Indian Act
- Slavery
- Racism and social exclusion
- Self-determination
- Policies/politics

FIGURE 7-2 Intersecting Levels of Determinants of Health: Proximal, Intermediate, and Distal *Source: © Charlotte Loppie.*

organizational and systems level are necessary for promoting safety for families in the health care process. Health equity in family health promotion at all levels can be advanced by connecting efforts of policy, research, and practice, as shown in Figure 7-1.

Family Health Promotion and Nursing Practice

Empowering nursing practice is concerned with uplifting humanity, without bias, judgment, or blame. An equity lens that considers the lived experiences of families can lead to the empowerment of families and enhance policy, research, and practice in nursing. Family health promotion is a way of thinking and acting that is informed by social, economic, and political issues and by social justice principles and ethics in nursing. In addition to their roles as health care professionals and leaders in the community, nurses are engaged citizens who see how social and economic inequities contribute to health vulnerabilities, compound illness severity, and place the success and well-being of individual and families at risk. In the next section, we discuss three examples of issues affecting families today, including the societal impact, and the role of the nurse in assisting families.

Gun Violence Loss

The United States has a higher rate of community gun violence than any developed country (Wang et al., 2020). Black males living in disadvantaged neighborhoods in the United States and Canada are disproportionately affected by gun violence injury and death (Butters et al., 2011; Kalesan et al., 2018). According to a recent analysis by the Violence Policy Center (VPC) (2020), the state of Missouri had the highest homicide victimization rate among Black Americans for the fourth year in a row, with a rate of 57.30 per 100,000 and nearly 11 times the overall homicide rate. In 2017, the national homicide victimization rate for White Americans was 3.06 per 100,000 (VPC, 2020). Black males also disproportionately bear the burden of disenfranchised grief and trauma from losing multiple friends and family members to gun violence (Smith & Patton, 2016). Due to the untimely and tragic nature of these deaths, Black families suffer prolonged grief and trauma that affect family

function and stability. This is particularly devastating for Black parents because of the racially stigmatizing discourses that occur when children are lost to gun violence, police brutality, and other types of violence (Bailey et al., 2013; Wamser-Nanney et al., 2019). Because of the stigma of gun violence in the community, Black families have increased risks due to decreased access to victim services, diminished social support, and decreased social empathy for their grief (Bailey et al., 2015; Hannays-King et al., 2015).

Nurses working to promote the health of Black families affected by the loss of family members to gun violence should consider how environmental-context stressors exacerbate their experience, including to increase their grief and contribute to physical and mental health risks. This first requires nurses to understand how the history of racism and oppression (*distal determinants of health*) influence their experience with gun violence loss and their access to psychological resources for their grief. It is crucial to explore conditions such as poverty and neighborhood context (*proximal determinants of health*) that make Black families vulnerable to intense trauma experiences. Skilled broad assessments of trauma experiences of individuals and the family overall, as well as the situation, can be critical to providing support that is unique to the needs of the family. Implementing and advocating for trauma-informed approaches to care in the community can be an effective tool for family nursing.

The Nurse Family Partnership (NFP) is an example of a home-visiting program implemented by registered nurses before and after women give birth and continuing for two years after delivery. The program is designed to improve prenatal care, care coordination, and healthy pregnancy behaviors and to support the infant-maternal bond (Morsy & Rothstein, 2019). Home visits that support and promote baby and toddler development, as well as provide guidance to mothers on self-care and stress management, family planning and parenting, and employment support, reduce the child's exposure to maltreatment and to risks for developing toxic stress responses, and enhance the child's environment with better maternal health (Morsy & Rothstein, 2019). Nurses can work directly with parents and families to strengthen their environment and build resilience that can protect them from the effects of stress and trauma. Nurses can also engage in community-level interventions that support trauma-informed approaches, including the following:

- Support family involvement in parenting programs that mitigate toxic stress exposure for parents and children.
- Practice collaboratively across interdisciplinary teams in health care and in the community in order to refer families to professionals and programs that support healing and build resilience, including social services, grief counseling, and trauma specialists.
- Support teachers, preschools, and schools with education about the short- and long-term effects of toxic stress, the importance of developing positive coping skills, and the value of trauma-informed approaches.
- Advocate for inclusive, safe, and culturally sensitive environments for children and families in the community.
- Prioritize psychological and physical safety for individuals, families, staff members, and communities (Morsy & Rothstein, 2019; Isobel & Edwards, 2017).

This list of trauma-informed approaches is not exhaustive; there are many ways that nurses can contribute to safer, healthier, and more resilient communities. To assist the reader with the process of integrating and applying nursing knowledge to the care of families, the following case study about the Martin family is presented. Refer to Chapter 12 for additional information.

Food Insecurity

Individual and household food insecurity remains an important public health issue and is a key social determinant of health for families. Food insecurity is defined as the disruption of food intake or eating patterns due to a lack of income or resources (U.S. Department of Health and Human Services, 2021). In 2017 and 2018, over 1.2 million children in Canada lived in food-insecure households, which means that they lived in homes where they lacked access to adequate, nutritious, and culturally acceptable food to support a healthy and active lifestyle (Dietitians of Canada, 2021). Food insecurity affects about 11% of households in the United States, including one out of every eight adults, and one out of every six children; they live in households that are food insecure based on not being able to afford

Case Study: Family Affected by Gun Violence Injury

Thomas Martin, a 22-year-old Black male, married, with four children, was brought to the emergency room of a large urban hospital late one night in life-threatening condition after being shot multiple times. The bullets punctured some of his major organs and damaged his spinal cord. He lost a significant amount of blood and was resuscitated twice during emergency surgery. Although Thomas survived 22 hours of surgery to remove bullets from his body, he lost a kidney and was paralyzed from the waist down. Upon transfer to the general surgery unit of the hospital, the nurses learned that he was shot by a rival gang member during a drug deal. Health care personnel could be heard referring to Thomas as the "nocturnal pharmacist." Over several months of his hospitalization, police guarded the room. Family members were devastated and anxious. They spoke about the shame they felt as a result of his shooting and their experience of being disregarded by health care professionals. The family visited frequently and offered prayers around the clock. Thomas's recovery transpired into a long and arduous journey, with several subsequent and complex surgeries. During this time, Thomas's wife divorced him. She received sole custody of the four children. Thomas became depressed, angry, and confrontational. See Figure 7-3 for a detailed Martin family ecomap.

As you think about the case, reflect and document your response to the following questions:

1. How might Thomas's situation affect his family?
2. What are the challenges and opportunities in health promotion for this family?
3. Describe the key determinants of health related to Thomas's experience with gun violence injuries.
4. How can the health care team's views on health inequity influence their actions to facilitate recovery for Thomas and his family?

Case Study: Family Affected by Gun Violence Injury—cont'd

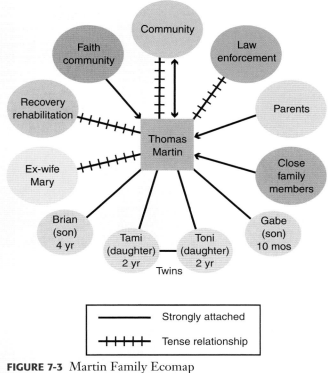

FIGURE 7-3 Martin Family Ecomap

balanced meals or worrying that they will run out of food before they can buy more (Frongillo et al., 2019). Research reveals a clear association between household food insecurity and negative physical and psychosocial health outcomes, demonstrating that adults and children in food-insecure households are prone to poorer overall health; decreased physical functioning; poorer cognitive, academic, and psychosocial development; increased maternal depression; and poorer-quality parent-child interaction (Hodgkinson et al., 2017). More specifically, researchers have found that the most common chronic conditions for adults facing food insecurity were diabetes, hypertension, and arthritis (Basu et al., 2017; Garcia et al., 2018).

Food insecurity also has the potential of adversely affecting family relationships and well-being. People living in food-insecure households appear to be more vulnerable to feelings of anxiety, powerlessness, worthlessness, family dysfunction, and psychological impairment such as depression and suicide/suicidal thoughts. Such problems are believed to stem from a preoccupation with obtaining food or having to access food through socially stigmatized means, such as using food banks, selling belongings, or stealing (Seivwright et al., 2020; Vahabi & Damba, 2013).

Population subgroups that experience an elevated rate of poverty, including single-parent households, older adults, recent immigrant families and communities, and Indigenous communities, are at risk for food insecurity. Nurses working with families need to recognize that food insecurity, as a proximal determinant, is connected to other competing proximal determinants such as income and lack of affordable housing (National Academies of Sciences, Engineering, and Medicine, 2017; Vahabi et al., 2013) that have to be addressed concurrently to improve families' well-being.

Nurses have a vital role in reducing food insecurity. Nurses have the ability to assess the

Table 7-1	Levels of Food Security	
FOOD SECURITY	**KEY INDICATORS EVIDENCE**	**POSSIBLE IMPACT ON THE HOUSEHOLD/ HEALTH OF THE FAMILY WITH VARYING LEVELS OF FOOD SECURITY**
High	High food security. No reported or observed indications of challenges with access to healthy food. Individuals and the family have the ability to access food on a regular basis, demonstrate choice of foods, and make accommodations based on desires and needs.	Individuals and families have the ability to adapt food choices to a healthy lifestyle. Healthy food choices can enhance energy, improve learning, and support job performance. Opportunities for food-related activity in family celebrations, cultural events, and community activities. Increased opportunity for health promotion activities in the family to promote health and prevent disease.
Moderate	Moderate food security. Occasional reported or observed indications of challenges with access to healthy food (e.g., insufficient food supply on an intermittent basis). May not show signs of nutritional challenges.	
Low	Low food security. May experience low food quality, variety, or choice of foods. May lack the resources (e.g., income, community services) to support a desired diet or optimal nutrition. May or may not be experiencing hunger on a regular basis. May or may not show signs of a reduced food or nutritional intake.	Families may be making choices between food and medicine, or between food and health care. Individuals may miss work or school due to interrupted sleep patterns or feelings of hunger, stress, or worry. Moderate to high levels of stress, anxiety, with an impact on behavior. Feelings of frustration, powerlessness, guilt, or shame. Stressors related to access to food consume thoughts, taking time and energy away from other activities.
Very Low	Very low food security; food insecurity. Individuals and/or the family may experience hunger due to a lack of access to food or a delayed or intermittent access to food over the course of the day or month. Parents and caregivers may report inability to feed children in the home. Abnormal or inconsistent eating patterns. May demonstrate a preoccupation with food. May report periods of fasting that cycles with periods of bingeing. Physical signs or symptoms of food insecurity, malnutrition (e.g., underweight, obesity, anxiety, exacerbation of chronic conditions, cognitive or behavioral challenges).	Situation may be complicated by other factors (e.g., lack of housing, transportation). Inconsistent work or school performance due to hunger or inability to concentrate. Increased risk for crime-related activity in order to eat or feed family. Increased risk of chronic health conditions (e.g., anemia, arthritis, cognitive challenges, mental health conditions). More frequent hospitalizations due to the related impact on certain conditions such as diabetes as a result of hypoglycemic events (Basu et al., 2017).

individual's and the family's level of food security during care interactions. Levels of food security are described in Table 7-1. When a need is identified, nurses can intervene swiftly to refer people to local food-based programs such as community kitchens, community gardens, senior centers, and food banks. Nurses can also connect people to federally funded food programs that can serve as a first-line of defense against hunger and food insecurity (Altarum Healthcare Value

Hub, 2020). Offered on a sliding scale basis, the Supplemental Nutrition Assistance Program (SNAP), formerly known as food stamps, has been shown to reduce food insecurity by up to 30% (Keith-Jennings et al., 2019). The Special Supplemental Nutrition Program for Women, Infants, and Children (WIC) is a public health nutrition program providing nutrition education, breastfeeding support, and access to nutritious food for pregnant women and mothers of small children experiencing low or reduced income. Another program available to students in public schools, based on the income level of their household, is the National School Lunch Program (NSLP), which provides one or two nutritious meals a day. By advocating for an assessment of food security during all health care encounters, nurses can engage other members of the health care team in interventions that support food security. While screening for food insecurity does not eradicate the underlying problems, it enables nurses and other health care professionals to expand their plan of care to other priorities affecting family health that result from socioeconomic issues, such as experiencing temporary or consistent unemployment, experiencing housing instability, and being exposed to stress or violence.

Stigma Reduction for Family Health

As described in previous sections, the effects of intersecting stigma and discrimination (homophobia, transphobia, heterosexism, racism, sexism) are devastating to family functioning and the health and well-being of family members. Children and youth who self-identify as LGBTQ+ experience a disproportionate burden of bullying and victimization at school (Espelage et al., 2018), in the community (Elipe et al., 2018), and even at home (McDermott et al., 2019), resulting in social isolation and mental health challenges, including anxiety, depression, self-rejection, and suicide risks. Youth who are rejected by their families often become homeless (Rhoades et al., 2018).

It is important to note that the harm of stigma and prejudice is not limited to youth who self-identify as LGBTQ+. Stigma can also affect children and youth whose parents or family members are LGBTQ+. While research has shown that there are few differences in psychosocial, emotional, and social development between children of sexually underrepresented parents and children with heterosexual parents (Reczek et al., 2016), some studies show that children with lesbian mothers reported more bullying related to their own sexuality and family structure (Goldberg & Garcia, 2020). Other youth with same-sex parents reported experiences of both direct and indirect stigmatization as well as structural stigma embedded in government policies (e.g., law on same-sex

marriage), schools, faith organizations, mass media, and other institutions. These different forms of stigma and discrimination contributed to anxiety and fear among these youth, and many coped by being defiant or detaching from these experiences (Kuvalanka et al., 2014).

Despite evidence that child development and children's well-being are not determined solely by the structures of families, misinformation and biases continue to stigmatize families of LGBTQ+ communities. Two recent studies demonstrated that the determinants of child health and well-being are similar between families with heterosexual parents and families with same-sex parents. In 2014, Crouch et al. studied 500 children from 315 same-sex families to find that parental gender, surrogacy, and donor status had little impact on the overall health and well-being of children of same-sex parental families. They found that the stronger predictor of better child health outcomes was living in a stable family environment with a higher household income. Similarly, a study that drew on population health data of over 20,000 households in the United States also found that, similar to households with heterosexual parents, the health of children with same-sex parents is determined by family socioeconomic status rather than by diverse family forms (Cenegy et al., 2018). The researchers also highlighted the heterogeneity among same-sex couple families in terms of ethnoracial and socioeconomic diversity and the need to consider the systemic disadvantages in terms of income and education faced by families.

Based on existing evidence, family health promotion in LGBTQ+ communities is best achieved using an ecological approach to reduce stigma and systemic discrimination. Nurses need to keep in mind how racism, sexism, homophobia, and transphobia intersect to produce vulnerabilities and inequities among LGBTQ+ families. At the macro level, nurses can advocate for equitable access to determinants through public policies (e.g., employment equity, housing, income, access to health care). At the meso level, programs and services designed to reduce stigma and discrimination are critical. Unbiased education and social marketing campaigns that engage stakeholders in all settings—schools, workplaces, faith organizations—can lead to community-wide attitude change (Hull et al., 2017). Community education programs that engage parents in safe, open, and nonjudgmental discussions about sexuality and social justice have been found to be effective in addressing homophobia and sexual stigma (Katz-Wise et al., 2016; Narushima et al., 2014 Wong & Poon, 2013). These efforts enable children, youth, and adults to speak out against stigma and discrimination against LGBTQ+ youth and families, as demonstrated by the growing movement of gay-straight alliances at school and in the community (Day et al., 2020). At the micro level, access to culturally safe and structurally inclusive programs and services is needed to address the psychosocial needs of and promote resilience among LGBTQ+ children, youth, and families.

CONSIDERATIONS FOR PROMOTING FAMILY HEALTH

Nurses interact with families in clinical and community settings, and they witness the complex social burdens on families that foster anxiety and stress. Nurses are placed in a position of authority and leadership to address the consequences for patients and families. In community settings, nurses often work with entire families in health promotion programs, whether in maternal-child health promotion, community development, or mental health promotion programs, or communicable disease management. In these situations, nursing actions focus on addressing key determinants of health, facilitating access to resources, family resilience building, and advocacy efforts. Regardless of the setting, nurses and families converge and plan interventions that promote the health of the individuals in the family and the family as a whole. Health promotion is often aimed at one or more of the social determinants of health and is essential to achieving health equity and optimal health outcomes.

Up to this point, we have discussed family health promotion from the perspective of health equity. Next, we provide consideration for nurses that involves considering ideologies, attitudes, and actions in preparation for working with and engaging with families within health equity frameworks.

Shifting Mainstream Ideologies

Like other professionals, nurses are products of their environments and their education. Through processes of environmental or educational socialization, we acquire ideologies on how to think, interact, and react. When these ways of being are not congruent with providing high-quality health care that is free of racism and discrimination, nurses have an important responsibility to address potential bias and cultivate new ways of learning and acting, which can be challenging. When faced with unfamiliar circumstances, the practice of nursing can be thought provoking, or even morally and ethically difficult. This requires a willingness for nurses to demonstrate humility and curiosity that will help them acquire new perspectives and grow in their understanding for their practice caring for patients and families.

Nursing practice in any form or setting is meant to intervene at the point of vulnerability and illness through equitable and ethical care. Horrill et al. (2018) challenge nurses to practice in ways that create physical and emotional safety and disrupt discourses that perpetuate socioeconomic and racial barriers in health care settings. Nurses are also urged to improve access to health care for diverse individuals and families, challenge their assumptions, and practice using lenses of cultural safety and health equity (Browne et al., 2016). Nurses can do this by assessing the skills they bring to engaging with diverse families, challenging their own beliefs and assumptions about families, and modeling behaviors that interrupt racism and discrimination in the health care setting.

Personalizing Determinants of Health

A variety of social determinants of health combine to create unique configurations of varying degrees of health outcomes for families (Barnes et al., 2020). We often think of the impact of determinants of health broadly. However, determinants of health are not equal in their impacts on families, even with recognition of the intersecting burden of co-occurring determinants. For example, the impact of racism on Black communities carries a heavy weight because of its consequences for access to opportunities, the barriers to advancement for individuals, and the impact on mental and physical health of families. Yet the experiences that lead to these outcomes are quite varied. Because experience matters, nurses need to conceptualize the health status of diverse families based on skilled assessment of the pertinent determinants of health and plan care that is high quality and free of discrimination and racism. While nurses must focus on the intersection of race, racialization, and oppression in implicating health and access to care, they must also consider how social and structural determinants of health affect all people who are vulnerable. By knowing this, nurses can assess each family effectively in order to identify their relevant needs, engage them in health promotion programs, promote resilience building and well-being, and work to change systems that deny the basic human rights to families (Barnes et al., 2020). In consideration of health promotion specifically for Indigenous families, the Truth and Reconciliation Commission of Canada (2015) provides a set of actions for nurses in health promotion to redress the legacy of residential schools and advance the process of Canadian reconciliation. This includes completing training in anti-Indigenous racism and discrimination, such as the San'yas program (Provincial Health Services Authority, 2021). We also suggest the following resources to assist with this training:

1. *Evidence Brief: Wise Practices for Indigenous-Specific Cultural Safety Training Programs* (Churchill et al., 2017)
2. *Indigenous Allyship Toolkit: A Guide to Honouring Culture, Authentic Collaboration and Addressing Discrimination* (Hamilton Niagara Haldimand Brant Local Health Integration Network, 2019)

SUMMARY

In this chapter we discussed family health and family health promotion from the perspective of health equity.

- Individuals and families do not exist in isolation; they are uniquely positioned within their community and within multilevel social systems.
- Family health cannot be understood sufficiently outside the intersection of social, political, historical, and economic factors: conditions that affect families differently. For example, health interactions and health outcomes for Indigenous and Black families include an experience that is informed by historical issues, structural conditions, and familial circumstances.
- An ecological perspective, in combination with other critical lenses, can provide nurses with a broad understanding of the complex dynamics between health outcomes and the social determinants of health.
- Strengthening families and promoting the development of resilience can be done through the use of relevant research, programs and services, and policies that support family-centered health promotion.
- Nurses are well prepared to advocate for improved access to quality health care for all families, including those that are vulnerable and underserved, by challenging their assumptions and delivering care that is culturally safe, ethical, and equitable.

chapter 8

Nursing Care of LGBTQ+ Families

Paul S. Smith, PhD, RN, CNE

Patrick Robinson, PhD, RN, ACRN, CNE, ANEF, FAAN

Kiki Fornero, MSN, RN

Critical Concepts

- Nurses care for families with members who have unique gender identities, sexual orientations, and family structures in a variety of settings and circumstances with increasing visibility and frequency.

- Historical, political, sociocultural, religious, and economic contexts influence the meaning of gender, gender identities, and gender expressions.

- Gender and sexuality are socially constructed concepts that vary across place and time.

- Gender, gender identity, and sexual orientation diversity are evident across ethnicities, cultures, age groups, and socioeconomic classes.

- Lesbian, gay, bisexual, transgender, and queer (LGBTQ+) persons experience family through a variety of biological and social structures that include kinship ties and chosen family.

- As minorities with a historically marginalized and stigmatized population, LGBTQ+ individuals and families experience significant life-span barriers to health and well-being, as well as barriers to legal and social protections under the law that lead to health disparities.

- Heteronormativity, racism, sexism, ageism, and other powerful social identities often intersect with gender diversity and result in increased barriers to care and thus increased health risks among the LGBTQ+ population. Nurses often care for families experiencing challenges at these intersections of diversity.

- Language and social ideas about gender are always evolving. Many cultures do not share the same language or social constructs related to gender identity, sexuality, and gender expression. Effective family nurses embrace this developing language and seek to create safe and respectful dialogue from the position of the learner when caring for LGBTQ+ individuals and their families.

- Families with LGBTQ+ members are working to achieve the same socially prescribed functions of all families: to rear responsible and independent children, provide emotional and instrumental support to one another, and provide family member health care across the life span.

(continued)

Critical Concepts—cont'd

- Effective family nurses examine their own understandings and biases of gender, sexuality, and families and reflectively seek to serve LGBTQ+ families with efficacy and compassion.

- Nursing care of LGBTQ+ families is an act of social justice, especially when focused on health promotion and removing barriers to health care that result in health disparities in the population.

INTRODUCTION

Until 1961, same-sex behavior was illegal in every U.S. state, and not until 2003 were antisodomy laws struck down by the Supreme Court; at that time, 14 states still considered same-sex behavior criminal (Baker, 2019). After multiple failed attempts, sexual orientation was added to the Canadian Human Rights act in 1996 (CBC News, 2015). Homosexuality was considered a sociopathic personality disorder in the first edition of the *Diagnostic and Statistical Manual* (*DSM*) published in 1952 and remained in the second edition until its removal in 1973 (Drescher, 2015). While nowhere close to the start of the fight for LGBTQ+ civil rights, the watershed events in the movement in the United States (the Stonewall Inn riots) and Canada (raids at four gay bathhouses in Toronto) occurred in 1969 and 1981, respectively (History.com Editors, 2021; CBC News, 2015). Marriage equality did not come to either country until the 21st century, with the U.S. Supreme Court decision in *Obergefell v. Hodges* in 2015 and by passage of the Civil Marriage Act in Canada in 2005 (History.com Editors, 2021; CBC News, 2015).

This chapter begins with these historical events to demonstrate how very recent the societal understanding and movement toward acceptance of sexual and gender diversity has been in the United States and Canada. In less than two generations, illegal activity is now sanctioned by marriage. As such, phenomena related to LGBTQ+ identities and families continue to evolve rapidly. Like any phenomenon, language must be used to describe it. The language used in this chapter should be considered a best attempt to use appropriate and affirming language. However, language comes down to choices, and the language chosen herein may not necessarily represent all members of the LGBTQ+ community's perspective.

LGBTQ+: PEOPLE AND A COMMUNITY

The term *LGBTQ+* is an acronym (lesbian, gay, bisexual, transgender, queer and the + encompasses a list of other identities that fall under the queer umbrella). It attempts to be inclusive by listing different types of identities and more recently the name of a community that includes people with these identities and others. Sometimes the term includes the letters *I* to include those who are intersex and *A*, which stands for "ally." Allies don't necessarily identify with one of the identities represented by the other letters but wish to identify as a member of the community. A plus sign (+), as used within this chapter, sometimes follows the term to indicate that any attempt at categorizing the community by individual letters would fall short. It is estimated that 4.5% of the U.S. population identifies as LGBTQ+ (Conron & Goldberg, 2020), which equates to 11,343,000 people. An estimated 1.7% of the Canadian population (aged 18 to 59) identifies as gay or lesbian, and 1.3% identify as bisexual, for a total of 1,096,200 people (Statistics Canada, 2017).

Sexual and gender diversity are complex phenomena that are not necessarily related. For example, a particular sexual orientation does not suggest a particular gender identity, or vice versa. Attempts to define terms relevant to discussions of the LGBTQ+ community are fraught with difficulties because there are multiple perspectives on definitions and meaning, and use continues to evolve. Thus, the terms discussed in the following sections are only one set of conceptualizations; others exist.

Sexual Orientation

Sexual orientation is an inherent or immutable enduring emotional, romantic, or sexual attraction to other people (Human Rights Campaign [HRC], n.d.). A person may be attracted predominantly to people of one gender, both binary genders, transgender or genderqueer people, or those who may identify as nonbinary or agender. Most commonly, people are **heterosexual** and are attracted to people of the opposite gender in a binary male/female model. Heterosexuals are widely referred to as straight and the term heterosexual often means "being straight." **Homosexual** people, most commonly identifying as gay (males or females) or lesbian (female), are attracted to those of the same sex. People with a **bisexual** orientation are attracted to others of either binary sex. Some persons find their sexual orientation is somewhat fluid across the life span, or it is more person-dependent than it is concrete or static. Using data from the daily Gallup Tracking Survey, 10,338,000 adults in the United States are estimated to identify as LGBTQ+ (Conron & Goldberg, 2020).

The concept of sexual orientation continues to evolve. Growing numbers of people identify as pansexual (not limited in sexual choice with regard to biological sex, gender, or gender identity) and omnisexual (involving, related to, or characterized by a diverse sexual propensity) (Lacey, n.d.). In addition, some people identify as demisexual, meaning sexual attraction only when an emotional bond has developed, regardless of gender (Ferguson, 2019). Some people identify as asexual (not experiencing sexual attraction) and greysexual (rare or limited sexual attraction) (Asexual Visibility and Education Network, 2020). Such identities demonstrate the increasingly complex nature of sexual orientations with which people identify.

Evidence suggests that sexual orientation is biologically determined (Roselli, 2018). It is a normal expression of human sexuality and not a preference over which one may exercise self-agency. Therapeutic efforts to change sexual orientation (i.e., conversion therapy, reparative therapy) have been denounced in policy statements by a majority of mainstream medical and mental health organizations (e.g., American Counseling Association, American Academy of Pediatrics, American Psychiatric Association) (Human Rights Campaign, n.d.b.). Indeed, it is widely held that such practices may result in the reinforcement of social stigma as well as psychological, social, and family relationship damage (Human Rights Campaign, n.d.c.).

The identity of queer is pertinent to the discussion of sexual orientation. Originally a pejorative, the term *queer* has emerged as a preferred identity for many, with emerging evidence that the identity is distinct from those who identify as gay or lesbian (Goldberg et al., 2020). The term *queer* will also be discussed subsequently with gender identity.

Biological Sex

Sex is related to the X and Y chromosomes, with XX defined as female and XY as male. Chromosomes drive sex determination and differentiation, which initiate pathways that lead to primary (genital) and secondary (body) characteristics mediated through various hormonal pathways in utero and throughout life. However, there are also cases of people born with single sex chromosomes and three or more chromosomes, so there is a range of chromosome complements, hormone balances, and phenotypic variations that determine sex (World Health Organization [WHO], n.d.). Sex is typically assigned to a person at or increasingly before birth based on external genitalia.

While sex is commonly thought of as male or female, there are individuals born intersex or who discover that they are intersex at some point in their lives. *Intersex* is a nonspecific term that means a person has a sexual or reproductive anatomy that does not fit with what is typically considered either male or female (InterACT, 2020b). For example, a person may have a vulva or vulva-like structure and internal testes. There are also people with mature ovarian and testicular tissue (World Health Organization, n.d.). The term *intersex* may cover many anatomical, genetic, and physiological variations. It is estimated that one in 1,000 to one in 2,000 children are born each year with clear indications of intersex status. More subtle presentations are also known to exist.

Gender Identity

Gender identity is one's innermost concept of self as male, female, a blend of both, or neither. It is how individuals perceive themselves and what they call themselves (Human Rights Campaign, n.d.f.). People whose gender identity is different from their biological sex or that assigned to them at birth may identify as **transgender**. A much more recent addition to the English lexicon is the term **cisgender,** which denotes those whose gender identity is the same as their biological sex. An estimated 1,397,150 people identify as transgender in the United States (Conron & Goldberg, 2020). There is no one way for people who consider themselves part of the transgender community to identify. Some individuals may choose to identify as a transman or a transwoman. Others may not use the *trans-* prefix. Similarly, there is no one way to be transgender. For some, gender-affirming therapies such feminizing or masculinizing hormones and genital surgery to achieve alignment with gender identity are critical components of transitions. Others may choose hormones, but not surgery, or they may opt for other types of surgery that bring the appearance of their body in alignment with their gender identity, such as mastectomy or breast augmentation. Box 8-1 contains a summary of the most common gender-affirming therapies.

Another common gender identity is nonbinary, meaning the person does not identify as a man or woman but rather as something other than the socially constructed meaning of those terms. The binary myth of sexual and gender diversity is discussed in the next section. Other terms related to this identity include *genderqueer, agender,* and *bigender,* although definitions of all those terms may differ across contexts and speakers (National Center for Transgender Equality, 2018). Related is the idea of a gender-fluid identity, where a person does not identify with a fixed notion of gender. Some nonbinary people identify as members of the transgender community, while others do not.

As with sexual orientation, the identity of queer is claimed by people with diverse gender identities. As such, queer has emerged as an identity used by the LGBTQ+ community to communicate broadly that they do not identify or conform in some way to the dominant cultural definitions related to sex, gender, or sexuality.

The way people refer to themselves and want to be referred to is not always clear from how people look or choose to present themselves (see the next section on gender expression). Along with gender identity comes the use of pronouns that may or may not fit others' expectations. Box 8-2 provides information about pronouns that are often used by people who are transgender or nonbinary. Use of correct pronouns is a critical area for building trusting and productive relationships with patients.

BOX 8-1
Gender-Affirming Therapies

Feminizing

Hormones: Goal is development of female secondary sex characteristics and suppression/minimization of male secondary sex characteristics.

- Estrogens: 17-beta estradiol (bioidentical to that from the human ovary)

Antiandrogens: Goal is development of female secondary sex characteristics and suppression/minimization of male secondary sex characteristics.

- Spironolactone (direct antiandrogen receptor activity and suppressive effect on testosterone production)
- 5-alpha reductase inhibitors (block conversion of testosterone to dihydrotestosterone)

Augmentation mammaplasty: Goal is defined breasts.

- Silicon or saline implants under the breast tissue or pectoralis muscle

Vaginoplasty: Goal is creation of vulvovaginal structure.

- Penile inversion where vaginal lining is created from penile skin. Clitoris is created from a portion of the glans penis
- Orchiectomy is performed. Labia are created from scrotal skin

Masculinizing

Hormones: Goal is development of male secondary sex characteristics and suppression/minimization of female secondary sex characteristics.

- Testosterone (all available preparations are bioidentical)

Masculinizing chest surgery: Goal is sculpture of a masculine-appearing chest.

- Subcutaneous mastectomy via a periareola incision
- Inframammary mastectomy with free nipple grafting

Phalloplasty: Goal is creation of penis.

- Free flap (radial forearm) or pedicled flap (anterior lateral thigh)
- Performed after hysterectomy and vaginectomy (or vaginal mucosal ablation)
- Scrotoplasty with or without testicular implants
- Erectile implant to allow rigidity for penetration

Metoidioplasty: Goal is to create a phallus from local tissue

- Testosterone causes growth of clitoris
- Scrotoplasty, hysterectomy, and vaginectomy may be similar as with phalloplasty

Source: Deutsch, M. B. (2016). *Guidelines for the Primary and Gender-Affirming Care of Transgender and Gender Nonbinary People* (2nd ed.). https://transcare.ucsf.edu/guidelines

BOX 8-2

Gender Pronouns

People use the pronouns that fit their identity. The correct pronoun is not always discernible from how a person chooses to express their gender. The correct pronoun is often revealed in conversation. However, misgendering (making assumptions about gender identity and verbalizing it through the use of the wrong pronoun or name) is a microaggression that stigmatizes and erodes trust. It is critical to simply ask people what pronouns they use if you are unclear.

Many transgender people use the common binary pronouns (he/him/his or she/her/hers). However, many members of the transgender, genderqueer, and nonbinary community choose to use gender-neutral pronouns such as the following:

They*	Them*	Theirs*
Ze (zhee)	Hir (here)	Hirs (heres)
Ze (zhee)	Zir (zhere)	Zirs (zheres)
Xe (zhee)	Xem (zhem)	Xyrs (zheres)

Note that these are used as singular pronouns.

Most electronic health records do not assist in providing readily visible pronouns that people use.

Without formal documentation, health care providers may make assumptions and misgender a patient. Misgendering occurs when a person uses language that wrongly identifies the gender identity of another. While using the wrong pronoun (referring to someone as he when the person uses the pronoun *she*) is a prime example of misgendering, using the wrong name is common in health care settings. Not all transgender people legally change their name from the one assigned at birth. For some, it is undesirable, while for others, it is too costly or not safe due to social circumstances. Electronic health records are challenging because the legal name is often the only name that appears, and it appears with great frequency. For some transgender people who have claimed a new name, the name assigned at birth is called the deadname. Using the birth name (for example, when a nurse first meets a patient) is referred to as deadnaming, which can be a painful form of misgendering.

It is important to note that specific gender identities do not correlate directly with specific sexual orientations. For example, most people, including those who are transgender, are heterosexual and identify as straight (Conron & Goldberg, 2020). However, transgender people also identify as gay, lesbian, and bisexual. For example, a person who was assigned female at birth may grow up identifying as straight. At some point, the person comes to identify as a man; however, his sexual interests and attractions remain the same, so he identifies as a gay man.

Gender Expression

Gender is usually expressed through appearance (hairstyle, clothing, facial hair, makeup, etc.), voice, and behavior (Human Rights Campaign, n.d.f.). Gender expression can be classified as conforming and nonconforming. The reference is to societal expectations of what is considered to be masculine or feminine. Often there is congruency between gender identity and gender expression. For example, a cisgender woman chooses to wear dresses, heels, and makeup. However, another cisgender woman may choose men's clothing and short-cropped hair. This person may be referred to as tomboyish, or within the lesbian community, she may refer to herself as a butch.

THE BINARY MYTH

In Western cultures, sexual orientation and gender are seen as essentially fixed binary concepts. The exception is that there is common understanding of bisexuality, but even in this case, the concept is categorical, and a person is one thing or another. However, both research evidence and the lived experiences of people suggest that the concepts are more accurately characterized in terms of spectrums, with various possibilities across a life span (Matsuno & Budge, 2017; Savin-Williams, 2016).

A useful way to think about a person's sexual and gender diversity is to conceptualize it as a unique intersection of multiple spectrums. Figure 8-1 displays this conceptualization using lines representing the spectrums of sexual orientation, gender identity, and gender expression. These spectrums are anchored on the ends with the common binary terms related to these concepts. The lower portion of Figure 8-1 demonstrates that spectrums intersect at any given point to create

There are multiple dimensions of sexual and gender diversity. Each dimension is a spectrum of identities anchored on each end by binary concepts. People identify somewhere along each spectrum. The dimensions represented here are meant to be illustrative and not exhaustive.

A useful way to think about the complex individual sexual and gender-related identity of a person is to picture it as a unique intersection of spectrums. The top figure suggests an identity such as cisgender, straight man; whereas the lower figure may represent a person who identifies as nonbinary and pansexual.

Cis ———————————— Trans
Gender identity

Conforming ———————————— Nonconforming
Gender expression

Straight ———————————— Gay
Sexual orientation

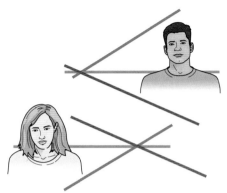

FIGURE 8-1 Multiple Spectrums of Sexual and Gender Diversity

a unique individual. Some intersections are far more common than others; for example, a cisgender, masculine-conforming gay man is common. Location on each spectrum among individuals is independent of location on the other spectrums, so infinite, unique possibilities exist.

THE LENS OF CULTURAL HUMILITY

Frameworks are useful in organizing thinking in general, but they can be particularly helpful in understanding unfamiliar phenomena. Cultural humility is a process of self-reflection and discovery to understand yourself and others to build trust (Hughes et al., 2020). It was initially conceived as a model for developing productive, authentic, and therapeutic relationships between health care providers and patients. It acknowledges the shortcomings of the desire for cultural competency, which in the context of this chapter would assume a cisgender heterosexual norm and a willingness to understand variances from this. Instead, cultural humility focuses on a commitment to continuous learning about oneself and others (Hughes et al., 2020). This approach allows health care providers not only to address their implicit biases but also to improve patient-provider interactions as providers become aware of their

own shortcomings, thus creating a more equal power dynamic (Sprik & Gentile, 2020).

It is a useful framework in working with LGBTQ+ people and their families because every person has a sexual and gender identity. The ability to cocreate a caring, trusting relationship with members of the LGBTQ+ community begins with understanding one's own identity, along with biases, preconceptions, and prejudices. Such reflections lead to comfort in asking questions of patients and seeking meaning. One can never be competent in another person's sexual and gender identity. Instead, one can be humble and open to continued and evolving understanding. This is true for all nurses, including those who are themselves members of the LGBTQ+ community.

For health care providers, two online resources that include valuable information when providing care for LGBTQ+ individuals and that would enhance a provider's self-reflection are Fenway Health (https://fenwayhealth.org) and Lavender Health (https://lavenderhealth.org). These sites highlight education and policies as well as available services for the LGBTQ+ community. Lavender Health includes a workplace climate scale that allows for discussion related to creating an inclusive and affirming workplace climate for LGBTQ+ nurses (Lavender Health, 2016).

For nurses or other health care providers who identify as LGBTQ+, there is a need to maintain objectivity when providing care for LGBTQ+ patients and families. Nurses who identify as LGBTQ+ may need to reflect on their own issues around disclosure because they may internalize societal intolerance and carry an unconscious shame about their sexual identities as well as a fear of what may happen when people know they are LGBTQ+ (Yingling, 2019). While there is much ongoing discourse on improving LGBTQ+ health and patient outcomes, little attention has been given to exploring experiences of LGBTQ+ health care professionals (Lim et al., 2019). LGBTQ+ nurses may experience stress as a result of a hostile or homophobic work environment that may lead to burnout, work dissatisfaction, increased turnover, and difficulty being authentic in the workplace (Silva & Warren, 2009; Yingling, 2019).

Eliason et al. (2018) analyzed qualitative data from 277 health care professionals who identified as LGBTQ+. Identified sources of stress for these providers included religiously and politically conservative coworkers, coworker/patient lack of knowledge, stresses of being closeted, and concerns about coming out to patients (Eliason et al., 2018). In addition, the consequences of being "out" at work were identified as including lack of promotions, gossip, and anti-LGBTQ+ comments and behaviors in the workplace (Eliason et al., 2018). Of the participants, 18% reported having negative coping strategies, which highlights the extra burden of stress often experienced by LGBTQ+ health care providers (Eliason et al., 2018).

While there is little literature on the topic of LGBTQ+ providers, one resource that an LGBTQ+ health care professional may utilize is the GLMA (previously known as the Gay & Lesbian Medical Association) *Health Professionals Advancing LGBTQ+*. GLMA was founded in 1981 as the American Association of Physicians for Human Rights, with the mission of ensuring equality in health care for LGBTQ+ individuals and health care professionals (GLMA, 2020). In 2002, GLMA expanded its mission to include health professionals of all kinds because previous membership was open only to physicians, residents, and medical students (GLMA, 2020). In 2013, the first GLMA Nursing Summit was held to form a nursing entity focusing on LGBTQ+ health and on LGBTQ+ nurses and allies to engage on improving LGBTQ+ issues in nursing.

HEALTH DISPARITIES AND LGBTQ+ PEOPLE

While LGBTQ+ people have made significant gains in the United States and Canada in terms of legal and civil rights, bias and social stigma are still prevalent for many members of the community. Minority stress describes the adverse effects of social stigma and prejudice on mental health (Meyer, 2003). Such stress contributes to higher levels of substance use disorders among LGBTQ+ people than their heterosexual or cisgender counterparts (Institute of Medicine [U.S.] Committee on Lesbian, Gay, Bisexual, and Transgender Health Issues, 2011). Also, LGBT smoking rates are 68% higher than the general population (King et al., 2012). Such health behaviors lead to increased risk of morbidity and mortality, including those attributable to cardiovascular disease.

In addition, LGBTQ+ people are disproportionately affected by mood and anxiety disorders, which have significant health consequences and lead to higher levels of suicide than the general population (Cochran et al., 2003). Transgender and other gender nonconforming people are at particularly high risk from death by suicide, with family rejection, discrimination, and denial of even basic accommodations (access to bathrooms, housing, etc.) being contributing factors (Narang et al., 2018).

Access to quality, appropriate health care services is an additional driving factor in LGBTQ+ health disparities. LGBTQ+ people often find that health care providers are ignorant about or dismissive of their unique health needs and concerns. Worse, providers are sometimes seen as unwelcoming and discriminatory. In a review of 17 published reports of nurses' attitudes toward LGBTQ+ patients, Dorsen (2012) found that all studies revealed evidence of negative attitudes. Patients who perceive health care providers as being uncomfortable with them may be reluctant to reveal their sexual orientation or gender identity or to seek health care at all (Eliason & Schope, 2001). Such a lack of trust can prevent early detection or misdiagnosis of multiple conditions. Lack of access to health care and social services is exacerbated by poverty; 22% of LGBTQ+ people living in the United States live in poverty compared to 16% of their cisgender straight counterparts (Badgett et al., 2019).

While great strides have been made in combating the global HIV pandemic over the past four decades, transmission continues at alarming rates among specific populations. Men who have sex with men are still at the highest risk of HIV infection. The estimated number of new U.S. HIV infections in 2018 was 36,400, with 67% among men who have sex with men (Centers for Disease Control and Prevention [CDC], 2020b). In Canada, 2,165 new cases of HIV were identified in 2016, with 52% attributable to male-to-male sexual contact (Public Health Agency of Canada, 2018). A recent meta-analysis suggests that 14% of transgender women in the United States are living with HIV (Becasen et al., 2019).

LGBTQ+ FAMILY STRUCTURES

The definition of family has evolved significantly over the 20th and 21st centuries. Only approximately 46% of children in the United States under 18 years of age live in a home with two married heterosexual parents in their first marriage (Pew Research Trust, 2015). Family structures for LGBTQ+ people are increasingly diverse, with family members across various sexual and gender identities. Using the definition of *family* as two or more individuals who depend on one another for emotional, physical, and economic support, members of LGBTQ+ families are often self-defined.

Evolving societal norms, including marriage equality in both the United States and Canada, have contributed to the changing landscape of LGBTQ+ family structures. The LGBTQ+-family-affirming legal and societal trends are in stark contrast to the norms as late as 20 years ago when even in emergencies or end-of-life care, gay and lesbian couples were not legally allowed to participate in decision making, have access to information, or have the right to hospital visitation in many cases.

Estimates from the U.S. National Health Interview Survey (Gates, 2014) suggest that there are 690,000 same-sex couples in the United States, 18% of whom reported that they were married. An estimated 19% of same-sex couples and lesbian, gay, and bisexual individuals who were not in a couple were raising children under the age of 18 in the home, which means that an estimated 30,000 children under age 18 have married same-sex parents, while 170,000 have unmarried same-sex parents (Gates, 2014). According to the 2016 Canadian Census, there were 72,880 same-sex couples, representing 0.9% of all couples (Statistics Canada, 2017). One-third of these couples were married, and 12% had children living with them. Half of all same-sex couples in Canada lived in four of the country's five largest census metropolitan areas: Toronto, Montréal, Vancouver, and Ottawa–Gatineau (Statistics Canada, 2017).

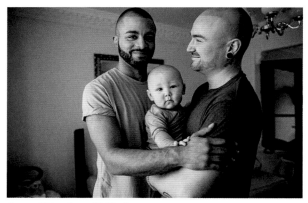

Source: © *istock.com/SolStock*

In the not-too-distant past, same-sex families were denied access to health care options that could support reproduction and were not permitted to be named parents of children in families they created. This, along with societal expectations for marriage and childbearing as well as stigma, led to a one-family structure specific to LGBTQ+ families in North America: a family founded through a mixed-orientation marriage (MOM). A MOM is typically one in which one partner identifies as heterosexual of one sex (e.g., straight female), and the other partner is a homosexual or bisexual of the opposite sex (e.g., gay male). Early research of MOMs estimated that 20% of gay men married women in their lifetimes (Janus & Janus, 1993). Such marriages often occur among social groups with more generally conservative social and religious viewpoints that forbid same-sex relationships (Hernandez et al., 2011). LGBTQ+ individuals desiring to remain part of the community and experience "family" may enter into heterosexual marriages to participate fully in this experience.

Another type of family structure sometimes seen in the LGBTQ+ community would be considered "living apart together." An example of this would be when a gay man is the sperm donor for a lesbian couple. The gay man does not live in the household but is clearly family because he is involved to various degrees in parenting and different roles in that family. Other family structures could include older LGBT community members assuming a parental, mentoring, or protective role with LBGT youth (Levitt et al., 2015) and community members forming intimate nonsexual bonds akin to siblings or cousins. Health care providers cannot make assumptions about who might comprise one's family of choice. Nurses need to ask about friends and family members and their respective roles. Nurses can advocate for assessment forms and organizational policies that support processes that affirm as relevant key members of individuals' families.

NURSING OF PARENTS AND CHILDREN

Birth of an Intersex Infant

The gender binary is socially reinforced during pregnancy and immediately after the birth of a newborn. Questions regarding a developing fetus or newborn's biological sex are a persistent topic of conversation and typically include only recognition of male and female categories. For these reasons, parents may experience stress when uncertainty exists regarding the biological sex assignment of their new baby. Parents face difficult decisions regarding the selection of potential treatment options and may feel pressured to decide on a socially prescribed gender category by which to rear the baby. Nurses have a unique opportunity to provide support and education to new parents to ease any stress and mark the experience of welcoming their child with joy.

Culture drives perceptions of people with intersex conditions and guides treatment during infancy. Over the last 70 years, and within the context of the biomedical model, birth of an intersex infant was treated as a medical emergency, and surgical intervention was initiated shortly after birth (Ovadia, 2013). While surgical intervention may be necessary to address urological emergencies in intersex newborns, surgical correction of reproductive anatomy is controversial. The practice of prompt surgical intervention of reproductive anatomy was grounded in gender psychology that assumed that infants are gender neutral at birth but should be conditioned in accordance with their assigned sex (Lev, 2006). Medical treatment of intersex youth

has also included hormonal therapy based on the sex assigned at birth to manipulate expression of physical characteristics. Past medical treatment of intersex infants prioritized normalizing appearance of anatomy over functionality or satisfaction and relied on heteronormative assumptions regarding gender identity and sexual expression (Lev, 2006). In some cases, individuals were unaware that they were born intersex or that they received surgery during infancy until well into adulthood. These individuals also faced difficulty in accessing medical records that detailed their surgical history because the records had been closed (InterACT, 2020b). With increased awareness of issues surrounding biological sex and its relatedness to gender identity and expression, approaches to care and the medical treatment of intersex infants have evolved.

Contemporary approaches are informed by emerging understanding of the harms done by interventions that intersex individuals did not have the opportunity to consent to. Examples of lasting harms stemming from unconsented treatment include psychological trauma, damaged familial bonds, decreased sensation and sexual satisfaction, impaired reproductive ability, and the need for ongoing surgeries due to complications or to repair procedures that do not match the individual's gender identity (Lev, 2006). Care of the intersex infant includes an interprofessional team with various specialists, including neonatologists, surgeons, urologists, and endocrinologists specializing in pediatrics; nurses; case managers; geneticists; ethicists; psychologists; and psychiatrists (Callejas-Agius et al., 2012; Ovadia, 2013). In light of the ethical issues surrounding the birth of an intersex infant, it is acceptable to defer any treatment not deemed medically emergent until the parents and child give informed consent.

Advocacy organizations such as InterACT take the position that no surgical intervention should take place until the child is old enough to articulate her or his gender identity and assent or consent to treatment (InterACT, 2020b). This position recognizes the rights of intersex individuals to self-determination and body autonomy. Parents may struggle to delay treatment if they believe that early intervention will enhance their child's psychosocial adjustment or allow them to avoid stigma later in life (Gardner & Sandberg, 2018). The American Academy of Pediatrics holds the position that the treatment plan for intersex individuals should remain

BOX 8-3

The Nurse's Role in Caring for Families with an Intersex Child

- Advocate at the health care organization to include nondiscrimination policies for intersex people.
- Respect privacy by avoiding disclosure of intersex status to members outside the care team, and avoid unnecessary physical examination of the intersex individual.
- Suggest that parents delay filing the birth certificate or selecting a name until they feel ready to do so.
- Advocate that the interprofessional team include a mental health specialist experienced in working with intersex individuals.
- Assess the parents' concerns and value systems.
- Maintain empathy and engage in active listening.
- Avoid the urge to offer information until the parents signal readiness.
- Educate the parents about the difference between biological sex and gender as well as the possibility of the child expressing gender uncertainty as time passes.
- Encourage parents to keep a journal documenting their feelings through the decision-making process to share with their child later.

flexible and be guided by the needs and beliefs of the child and family (Gardner & Sandberg, 2018). The nurse holds an important role in addressing the questions and concerns of the parents of an intersex newborn as well as advocating for the family. The scope of the nurse's role in advocating for the family with an intersex child are outlined in Box 8-3.

PREGNANCY WITH GENDER AND SEXUAL MINORITIES

As with other diverse populations, nurses should adapt practices that center on the unique needs of gender and sexual minorities during pregnancy. To support expectant parents, nurses must make an effort to be well-informed about the patient's family structure. People define family in a myriad of ways. Families can be comprised of members who are biologically or legally bound, but neither is required when forming or defining a family. It is not uncommon for lesbian, gay, and transgender parents to have children from previous relationships with a different-sex or same-sex partner, and members of the

health care team should approach their understanding of familial bonds with openness and without judgment. As is the case with different-sex parents, expectant same-sex or transgender parents may be members of a unique family structure that will guide the nurse's assessment, planning, and interventions.

Pursuing Pregnancy

When the decision to pursue parenthood is made, LGBTQ+ singles and couples have a range of options to consider. For example, if there is a desire to conceive a child rather than adopt, couples might discuss who will become pregnant and how the partner will participate in pregnancy, labor and delivery, and care of the infant after birth (Bushe & Romero, 2017). Single individuals must also decide how they will conceive, construct family, and foster community for support during pregnancy and after the birth of the child. The nurse might offer a single patient or couple interested in conceiving an overview of options for assisted reproduction or answer questions to support decision making.

Assisted reproduction can be a costly undertaking, so providing information to individuals and couples early in the planning process is a priority. The nurse should keep in mind that individuals seeking to conceive a child may have tried unsuccessfully to become pregnant outside a health care setting due to social stigma and cost barriers (Kim et al., 2020). The first step for transgender patients who desire to pursue pregnancy is to discontinue hormone therapy (Garcia-Acosta et al., 2019). Individuals seeking to conceive may choose to use the sperm of someone known to them or opt for an anonymous donor. Considerations for deciding on a donor include the type of involvement the family wants from the donor, as well as the donor's genetic makeup. Lesbian couples also have the option of implanting one partner's fertilized egg in the partner who will bear the pregnancy (Bushe & Romero, 2017). In conjunction with intrauterine insemination or embryo transfer, hormonal therapy may be used to improve the likelihood of successful implantation. In this case, the nurse educates the patient and partner on how to administer injections and store fertility-enhancing medication as well as providing emotional support throughout the process.

When a patient or couple experiences difficulty in achieving pregnancy, the nurse holds an important role in assessing emotional health, coping strategies, and physical health status. The patient or couple experiencing impaired fertility often go through a grieving process. The relationship dynamics of a couple may change as a result of impaired fertility, although these changes can be both positive and negative (Riederer et al., 2019). Gender and sexual minorities may experience stigma in the health care setting when dealing with infertility. Research aimed at exploring fertility issues in self-identified lesbians is limited, and findings remain inconclusive due to small sample sizes or flawed methodologic grounding (Kim et al., 2020). The nurse can be instrumental in educating fellow members of the health care team about the risk of implicit bias regarding impaired fertility in individuals who identify as lesbian.

Considerations for the Perinatal Period

Once a pregnancy is viable, different needs emerge to ensure that gender and sexual minorities receive personalized care. Staging an inclusive environment in obstetric clinics and labor and delivery units requires intentionality. A first step might be to ensure that reading and education materials reflect gender and sexual minorities and diverse family structures (Bushe & Romero, 2017). Health care team members should ask the patient or couple for their pronouns and preferred terms to describe parenting relationships. Because gender exists on a spectrum, a same-sex couple may ask to be referred to as "parents" rather than "moms" or "dads" (Bushe & Romero, 2017). On the other hand, another couple may distinguish their titles as "mama" and "mommy." The nurse must maintain a sense of cultural humility as the preferences, identities, and roles of the developing family are learned.

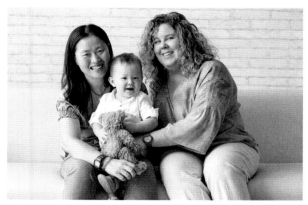

Source: © istock.com/DragonImages

After establishing rapport with the family, the nurse obtains a comprehensive health history. Forms should include a variety of familial relationships and expansive gender identities, including offering open-ended response options. The health history and intake assessment guides the development of the plan of care, so it may be necessary to extend questions to the pregnant patient's partner, when applicable. For example, the nurse may ask for the partner's medical history if their egg was implanted in the partner carrying the baby, or ask for information about how the baby was conceived as it relates to diagnostic testing and risk mitigation (Bushe & Romero, 2017). Questions may seem intrusive to the patient and family, so the nurse should take care in offering explanation about the relevancy of questions to avoid making the family feel marginalized.

A common societal idea equates pregnancy with femininity and assumes that pregnancy is experienced only by people who identify as female. The health care team should keep in mind that the experience of pregnancy is not limited to individuals who identify as a woman or female and offer education to support choices during labor, delivery, and the postpartum period. The perinatal period includes many physiologic changes that may be unsettling to gender-expansive individuals. For example, transgender men who become pregnant discontinue hormones well in advance of conception and notice changes to their physical features that make them appear more feminine (Garcia-Acosta et al., 2019). The nurse sensitized to these experiences is better positioned to provide emotional support. During labor and delivery, nurses should ask the patient how they refer to their anatomy and consistently gain consent before performing physical assessment (Garcia-Acosta et al., 2019). The nurse can advocate for offering hospital gowns, equipment, and décor in a variety of colors instead of limiting the color palette to pink.

Nurses and providers should have a good understanding of the patient's plan for nourishing and bonding with their newborn. Another opportunity to implement inclusive language is to describe lactation and feeding as chestfeeding rather than as breastfeeding if the terminology resonates with the patient (Garcia-Acosta et al., 2019). Hormonal therapy may be introduced or discontinued if one or both parents express a desire to breastfeed or chestfeed their newborn (Bushe & Romero, 2017;

Garcia-Acosta et al., 2019). The parent who carries the baby during pregnancy may be uncomfortable with the idea of breastfeeding or chestfeeding due to physical changes that occur when lactating. The nurse can remain supportive of the patient's decision to cease milk production by offering alternatives such as bottle feeding with donor milk or formula, or using an apparatus where milk flows through a prosthetic breast that the parent wears on their chest (Bushe & Romero, 2017). Parents might be willing to explore alternatives if the nurse explains that breastfeeding or chestfeeding not only provides nourishment but also facilitates bonding with the newborn.

Establishing the Birth Certificate

The nurse or registered nurse case manager may play a role in helping new parents understand the legal implications of being listed on the newborn's birth certificate. Due to the complexity of filing and legally asserting parental rights, as well as the excitement and fatigue experienced after a birth, the family should discuss the birth certificate before the baby is born. Although the individual who gave birth is listed on the birth certificate automatically, some states fail to uphold the legal rights of the nonbirth parent for gender and sexual minority couples. In states where the nonbirth parent's rights are challenged, they may be unable to consent to medical treatment, travel with their child, or enroll them in school and other programs (National Center for Lesbian Rights [NCLR], 2019). If a known sperm donor is used to conceive a child and the family expresses the desire to include them on the birth certificate, all parties should be counseled about the legal ramifications of doing so. Families might consider reinforcing the nonbiological parent's legal status through formal adoption (NCLR, 2019). In addition to offering support and education as new parents establish who will be listed on the birth certificate, nurses can advocate to policymakers to amend the birth certificate form to include gender and sexual minority relationships, such as listing parent one and parent two rather than mother and father.

Through pregnancy, and as decisions about formal/legal and informal titles are reached, the parent who did not give birth might feel less visible or detached from the process because attention is focused on the pregnant partner. It is important to note the expectant couple's relationship dynamics and intentionally involve the parent who is not pregnant so that they feel included in the process (Bushe & Romero, 2017). Couples may still be working to establish familial roles as they answer questions from extended family and friends about how they define their roles. To ease parents' worry or frustration, the nurse can reinforce the idea that familial roles are dynamic and will likely shift over time.

Surrogacy

Laws: Adoption is challenging for single people and same-sex couples in the United States and abroad. Another path to parenthood might be surrogacy to avoid barriers to adoption or because of a desire to be biologically linked to the child (Fantus & Newman, 2019). Surrogacy is another form of assisted reproduction wherein a person with female reproductive anatomy carries a pregnancy for another person or couple. Similar to intrauterine insemination, a range of options exists when considering parenthood through surrogacy. First, a surrogate or gestational carrier should be selected. The surrogate or gestational carrier may be a family member, close personal friend, or acquaintance, or the person can be anonymous. The surrogate may donate an egg to be fertilized or, when a gestational carrier is used, the egg can come from a known or anonymous donor and implanted in a person who will not be biologically linked to the child (Tsai et al., 2020). Same-sex couples with male reproductive anatomy must decide if one or both partners will provide sperm for fertilization and plan for situations in which an embryo becomes unviable (Fantus & Newman, 2019). The decision of whose genetic material is used is guided by desire for a biologic link to the child.

Laws guiding surrogacy arrangements have been contentiously debated for decades. For this reason, the role of the surrogate in child rearing should be established early in the planning process. While it is customary for the intended parents to cover the surrogates' medical expenses, variability exists across the United States and abroad regarding laws recognizing surrogacy contracts as well as the allowance for financial compensation of the surrogate (Tsai et al., 2020). In some parts of the United States and Canada, financial compensation is prohibited in an effort to protect women from coercion or being treated as a commodity (Fantus & Newman, 2019). Similarly, laws governing who will be listed on the newborn's birth certificate vary across the United States, while Canada allows for both parents to be listed on the birth certificate and for second parent adoption, and some provinces legally recognize three-parent families (Fantus & Newman, 2019). The nurse or case manager is tasked with knowing parenting laws in their state and supporting the surrogate and intended parents as they navigate the process.

Supporting Fathers Through Birthing and Discharge: The nurse plays a significant role in educating new parents about the care for their newborn in an effort to start the family on a good trajectory. Men pursuing parenthood through surrogacy require special care and consideration to ensure that education is effective and well received. Specific considerations guiding nursing care of fathers using a surrogate/gestational carrier is included in Box 8-4. During pregnancy, the nurse is professionally, legally, and ethically obligated to protect the confidentiality of the surrogate or gestational carrier (Tsai et al., 2020). However, details about the progress of the pregnancy can be disclosed to the intended parents if the surrogate/gestational carrier authorizes consent. Given that the intended parents are not experiencing the pregnancy firsthand, they may require more time or explanation about the progress of the pregnancy during clinic visits.

The confidentiality of the surrogate/gestational carrier must also be protected during labor and delivery. When possible, and if the surrogate agrees, the intended parents are included in the labor and birth of the newborn. The health care team should look for opportunities to include the intended parents in education and the delivery experience. After delivery, the focus of education should shift to equipping new fathers with the skills needed to care for the newborn. As with any new parent, the new father(s) should be taught how to feed, bathe, position, and change diapers for the newborn. New father(s) will need to decide whether to acquire breast milk from the surrogate/gestational carrier or donor or whether they will use formula (Tsai et al., 2020). They will also need to decide on whether to vaccinate the newborn. Given variability in paternity leave, the nursing team may have to repeat education if one parent misses information due to a need to continue working (Logan, 2020). Strong collaboration among the nursing team, including passing on information about the newborn's family structure during handoff report, eases the intended parent's transition to fatherhood.

BOX 8-4

Considerations for Working With Surrogates and Intended Fathers

- Prior to conception:
  - Discussions about who will be present at appointments; maintenance of health habits during pregnancy, such as avoiding caffeine or restricted foods; and posting to social media about the pregnancy
  - Disclosure of the surrogacy arrangement to the child
  - Planning for complications
- During pregnancy, labor, and delivery
  - Create an environment inclusive of fathers.
  - Be understanding of variable paternity leave and reinforce education, when necessary.
  - Pass along information about the parenting arrangement during handoff report.
  - Inquire about how each parent wants to be addressed.
  - Act as a liaison between the parents and health care team.
  - Identify both parents on the newborn's ID card.
  - Create and update binders about state laws regarding parental leave and parental rights.

Adoption

Many professional organizations endorse same-sex couples adopting children (HRC, n.d.d.), yet LGBTQ+ people still face challenges when pursuing parenthood through adoption. Many same-sex couples experience discrimination and may have been denied rights to adoption in the past. Once an adoption is granted in the United States and Canada, same-sex couples must navigate claiming parental rights of an adopted child differently than mixed-sex couples. For example, some states recognize only one legal parent in a same-sex couple, leaving the second parent to claim parental rights through second-parent adoption or through coparenting or custody agreement (HRC, n.d.e.). The health care team should maintain awareness that

LGBTQ+ families may experience financial, mental, and emotional strain due to legal challenges and discrimination through the adoption process.

Prospective adoptive parents should visit the pediatrician with the child's medical record before the adoption is formally completed to establish a comprehensive health plan (Jones & Schulte, 2019). The preadoption health visit also offers the opportunity to reconcile the new parents' vaccination history, administer vaccinations when indicated, and address potential environmental challenges to ensure a smooth transition once the child is brought home (Jones & Schulte, 2019). If a preadoption visit is not possible, the new family's first encounter with a nurse may be a well-child visit. Depending on the circumstances leading to a child being placed for adoption, the child may be malnourished or may have been exposed to substance use, violence, or other trauma (Jones & Schulte, 2019). The first well-child visit should include a thorough review of vaccination records, medical and social history, a complete physical assessment, assessment of developmental milestones, relevant diagnostic tests, and discussion about emotional well-being and psychosocial adjustment of the child and family (Jones & Schulte, 2019). The nurse can remain a supportive figure for the new family by supporting each member as they adjust to changes and by developing a collaborative, family-centered plan for managing holistic health concerns.

A Child Identifies

Coming Out: When a child or adolescent realizes their attraction to people of the same sex, they will likely seek information about what their attraction means and contemplate coming out to family and friends. *Coming out* refers to a process where a person makes their sexual orientation or gender identity known to others (American Academy of Pediatrics [AAP], 2012). A child or adolescent may first approach a trusted friend, school official, or member of the health care team for support and guidance on how to come out to their parents. It is important to remind the youth that the timing of coming out depends on their safety and comfort level so that they avoid feeling rushed.

When the youth decides that the time is right to come out, the nurse will extend support to the family. The nurse's support should focus on facilitating the family's acceptance of their child. The level of family acceptance carries significant implications for the long-term physical and mental health trajectory of the child (Newcomb et al., 2019; Substance Abuse and Mental Health Services Administration [SAMHSA], 2014). Family rejection of LGBT+ youth may lead to high-risk behaviors, incarceration, mental health distress such as depression and suicide, or placement in foster care (Newcomb et al., 2019; SAMHSA, 2014). The nurse's role in supporting the child and family through the coming-out process is to facilitate family acceptance. Connecting parents with organizations such as Parents, Families, and Friends of Lesbians and Gays (PFLAG) may have a positive impact on the child's experience with coming out because parents will be able to access information and connect with other families who share similar experiences.

The Family Acceptance Project offers guiding principles for clinical care and support of the family when a child identifies as LGBTQ+. Hallmarks of the Family Acceptance Project include recognizing that parents may struggle to accept their LGBTQ+ child due to concerns that the child will be bullied or victimized (SAMHSA, 2014). It is the responsibility of health care providers to meet parents where they are, provide resources and information, and address concerns (SAMHSA, 2014). Care providers should maintain awareness that acceptance is not a linear process, and acceptance and rejection may coexist. Parents may have questions about conversion therapy, which aims to change the sexual orientation or gender identity of LGBTQ+ individuals. Providers should offer insight into the lack of scientific grounding for conversion therapy and the enduring harmful effects that these programs perpetuate. Organizations, including the American Psychological Association, advise that conversion therapy should be avoided, and in some states the practice has been made illegal (Mallory et al., 2019). The nurse should aim to offer a nonjudgmental space for families to express their progress on acceptance.

LGBTQ+ youth are at higher-risk of being bullied in person or online than their heterosexual or cisgender peers (U.S. Department of Health and Human Services [USDHHS], 2017). Bullying not only threatens the physical safety of the youth experiencing it but also has a negative impact on their mental health and performance at school. As with any school-aged child or adolescent, the nurse should incorporate assessment questions to discern if bullying is occurring, from whom, and in what form. The nurse should also assess overall emotional well-being and complete focused psychological screening, if indicated (Fish, 2020). When necessary, the nurse completes focused mental health assessments including depression, anxiety, or suicide-risk surveys. Care must be taken when approaching sensitive questions regarding mental health and emotional well-being. The nurse should explain that each assessment is commonly completed with people in the same age category and not guided solely based on gender identity or sexual orientation. Normalizing mental health assessments for all patients, regardless of gender identity or sexual orientation, and reiterating the emphasis on maintaining confidentiality and physical and psychological safety help to reduce feelings of being othered.

The majority of schools that offer sexual education programs fail to teach about LGBTQ+ sexual health, and some states ban the inclusion of any information (HRC, n.d.a.). During clinical encounters with any youth, a comprehensive health assessment includes discussion and education about sexual health. A focus on LGBTQ+ sexual health prevents the spread of misinformation, promotes safety, mitigates risk, and supports the family's knowledge development. When providing LGBTQ+ inclusive sexual health education, the nurse should highlight LGBTQ+ relationships in a positive light and use gender-neutral terms to describe anatomy or when referring to partners (HRC, n.d.a.). The nurse should also avoid assuming the type of sexual partners the youth might have and convey that pregnancy or sexually transmitted infections are not limited to heterosexual sexual encounters (HRC, n.d.a.). LGBTQ+ inclusive sexual health education can offer the opportunity to answer questions and open communication about sexual safety and risk prevention if the youth has come out to their family and is comfortable involving their parent(s) during the visit. Parents can be empowered to advocate for inclusion of LGBTQ+ sexual health education in their child's school (HRC, n.d.a.). The nurse should also provide encouragement to parents to continue open discussions about sexual health with their child.

Coming Out as Transgender: Evidence suggests that children as young as eight can recognize that their gender is not aligned with the sex assigned to them at birth (Olson et al., 2015). Families access the health care system as they navigate their reactions, feelings, and questions regarding transgender identity. Many factors, including social stigma and fear of rejection, influence the mental health of transgender youth, who are at higher risk of anxiety, depression, eating disorders, self-harm, substance use, and suicide than their cisgender peers (Rafferty, 2018; Fish 2020). Interactions with the health care team can influence how the family and child adjust to emerging gender identity.

The clinical environment can signal whether the health care team are open and equipped to provide sensitive care to transgender patients. Signage and resources featuring people of diverse gender identities can create an opening for youth to approach the conversation about coming out as transgender with the health care team. In addition, offering a gender-neutral bathroom helps patients feel more comfortable during clinic visits (Rafferty, 2018). Normalizing asking for each patient's pronouns and having staff members display their pronouns on their name badge also open the door for conversations about gender identity. Pronouns and the name designated by the patient should be documented in the patient's medical record and used during interactions with the health care team (Rafferty, 2018). An inclusive environment also creates the opportunity for patients who are not questioning their gender identity to learn and ask questions.

The American Academy of Pediatrics endorses a gender-affirmative approach to care. The gender-affirmative approach recognizes that (1) gender identity forms in response to interrelated factors, including biology, socialization, development, and culture; (2) gender identity occurs on a spectrum; (3) transgender identity does not constitute a mental disorder; and (4) when mental health issues exist, they are the result of stigma or negative experiences (Rafferty, 2018). Parents benefit from learning about the gender-affirmative approach from the nurse as a way to demonstrate support for their child, validate their desire to protect their child from harassment, and begin to process their own feelings. In turn, transgender youth can benefit from having supportive and well-informed parents as they make decisions about gender expression and explore treatment options. Research demonstrates that strong communication, even as disagreement occurs, can improve outcomes for families with transgender children (Rafferty, 2018). Therefore, in cases where parents are struggling to accept their child's gender identity, the nurse can have a role in facilitating communication within the family.

Coming out as transgender is a multistage process (Rafferty, 2018). The first stage is social affirmation, in which an individual begins telling people about transitioning their gender identity and altering the way they express gender through clothes, hairstyles, and so on. The second stage is legal affirmation, in which state and federal documents are changed to reflect the transition. The third stage is medical affirmation. During this stage, children and adolescents may begin taking cross-sex hormones to suppress the start of puberty, with the support of their parents. The last stage is surgical affirmation, in which the individual has their body surgically altered so that it aligns with their gender identity. These procedures include removing breasts, ovaries, the uterus, or testes and reconstructing genitalia. Some features may be added, such as breast implants or other reconstruction, to enhance masculine or feminine features (Rafferty, 2018). The health care team should only inquire about the patient's surgical history as it relates to gender transition when it directly relates to care or treatment decisions. This approach demonstrates respect for privacy. Surgical intervention is typically reserved for adult patients, although sometimes adolescents undergo these procedures. The family requires mental health support through all phases of the child's transition. Nurses have a responsibility to assess how the family is functioning and coping as well as to offer supportive resources.

HEALTH CHALLENGES AND DISPARITIES IN EARLY AND MIDDLE ADULTHOOD

On balance, sexual and gender minorities face the same health concerns found in the population at large. There are notable disparities, however, in several specific domains (Institute of Medicine Committee on Lesbian, Gay, Bisexual and Transgender Health Issues and Research Gaps and Opportunities, 2011) for members of the LGBTQ+ community, who report poorer overall well-being than those in the mainstream population. They report a higher number of acute physical symptoms

and chronic conditions and indicate, at a higher rate than their heterosexual peers, that their health precludes them from participating in everyday physical activities (Institute of Medicine Committee on Lesbian, Gay, Bisexual and Transgender Health Issues and Research Gaps and Opportunities, 2011).

Patterns of risk and relative wellness differ by sex. Fewer lesbians and bisexual women report excellent or very good health when compared with heterosexual women, whereas there is no difference in health status reporting by sexual orientation among men (Institute of Medicine Committee on Lesbian, Gay, Bisexual and Transgender Health Issues and Research Gaps and Opportunities, 2011). Lesbians are more likely to be overweight or obese (Simoni et al., 2017). Gay men have been found to have a significantly lower body mass index (BMI) and participate in more physical activity compared to their heterosexual counterparts, who tend to participate in less physical activity and have a higher BMI (Fricke & Sironi, 2020). According to data obtained from the 2016 Behavioral Risk Factor Surveillance System, bisexual persons had lower rates of breast cancer screening adherence, and lesbian and gay persons had decreased likelihood of cervical cancer screening adherence (Charkhchi et al., 2019). Lesbian, gay, and bisexual persons have higher rates of tobacco, alcohol, and drug use (Simoni et al., 2017). Gay and bisexual men account for more than half of those living with HIV or AIDS; they are at an increased risk for anal cancer and some sexually transmitted infections (STIs) (e.g., syphilis) (Institute of Medicine Committee on Lesbian, Gay, Bisexual and Transgender Health Issues and Research Gaps and Opportunities, 2011). HIV occurs in about 28% of transgender women, and it is reported that most are unaware they are infected (Kates et al., 2016).

It is important to note that very little methodologically sound research has been conducted on physical health status and health disparities among transgender individuals. To date, the primary focus of research has been on the effects and side effects of hormone therapy. This research provides some evidence that transgender women are at greater risk of venous thromboembolic disease and elevated levels of prolactin associated with feminizing hormone therapy (Weinand & Safer, 2015).

Transgender men may experience elevations in liver enzymes, loss of bone mineral density, and increased risk for ovarian cancer associated with masculinizing hormone therapy (Braun et al., 2017; Institute of Medicine Committee on Lesbian, Gay, Bisexual and Transgender Health Issues and Research Gaps and Opportunities, 2011). In 2011, the Committee on Health Care for Underserved Women reported that more than half of those who identify as transgender have obtained injected hormones outside a traditional medical setting. Yet recent research supports that gender-affirming hormone therapy has positive psychological effects, reducing symptoms of anxiety and depression, lowering perceived social distress, and improving the quality of life and self-esteem effects in both transgender adolescents and adults (Nguyen et al., 2018). Ultimately, the lack of access to quality health care for transgender care and associated health issues stands as the largest health risk. In relation to sexual health, LGBTQ+ persons face similar health care and education as the rest of the population. STI prevention is a high priority, as is pregnancy risk for those who possess female reproductive organs (regardless of their gender identity and sexual orientation) and typical screenings for reproductive cancers regardless of sex or gender identity.

Health Challenges and Disparities in Late Adulthood

As is the case for earlier phases of development, the health concerns of LGBTQ+ adults are not distinct from those of heterosexuals, and available research is minimal. It appears that lesbians and bisexual women in late adulthood have slightly higher rates of breast cancer than heterosexual women.

HIV remains a significant risk factor, particularly for men and transgender women. In 2018, 17% of new HIV diagnoses were in individuals older than age 50 (CDC, 2020b). This is a particularly salient finding for family nurses because most HIV prevention campaigns are not directed toward older adults (Institute of Medicine Committee on Lesbian, Gay, Bisexual and Transgender Health Issues and Research Gaps and Opportunities, 2011). Older LGBTQ+ people living with HIV are another such group, which is especially relevant to aging men and transgender women, who have unique needs (Institute of Medicine Committee on Lesbian, Gay, Bisexual and Transgender Health Issues and Research Gaps and Opportunities, 2011). Worldwide, about 20% of transgender people are

living with HIV; this number increases to 27% for transgender women who are sex workers (Poteat et al., 2015). Although LGBTQ+ people comprise a subgroup of older HIV-positive individuals, a small Canadian qualitative study of persons living with HIV who are age 50 and living in Quebec (Wallach & Brotman, 2012) identified concerns that include employment and living conditions, premature aging, shrinking social networks, and challenges to maintaining intergenerational relationships or finding acceptance in older peer networks. Disclosure to family, peers, and providers that results in nonaffirming responses can exacerbate experiences of stigma, social isolation, and mental health issues (Daley et al., 2016a, 2017).

Many LGBTQ+ adults believe that their status as sexual and gender minorities helped them to prepare for older age. Although they are twice as likely as their heterosexual peers to be single and living alone, they report having developed greater resilience and better support networks.

Access to and utilization of health care for older LGBTQ+ adults is particularly troubling. A large percentage (40%) report that they have not disclosed their sexual orientation to their primary care provider (Espinoza, 2014). They fear that they will not be treated fairly or will be denied care. In fact, 65% of transgender adults fear that they will have limited access to adequate health care as they get older (Espinoza, 2014). In addition, prior or present discrimination among chronically ill LGBTQ+ older adults is positively correlated with an increase in physical and emotional symptoms for them and for their caregivers (Institute of Medicine Committee on Lesbian, Gay, Bisexual and Transgender Health Issues and Research Gaps and Opportunities, 2011). This highlights the need for nurses to consider even unrelated caregivers within the context of LGBTQ+ family care.

A groundbreaking and award-winning American documentary released in 2011, *Gen Silent* (Maddox, 2011), pointed to the importance of understanding the particular concerns, including isolation, stigma, and discrimination, that are part of the lives of six older single and partnered LGBTQ+ people and caregivers. In that film, the lives of an older gay couple, a single transgender woman, and an older lesbian couple are profiled in light of their health and social care needs, including their chosen families and the need for LGBTQ+-affirmative community. A key focus of that movie highlighted the resilience and resistance in LGBTQ+ communities. As Espinoza (2011) indicated, although LGBTQ+ older adults have often experienced years of invisibility and discrimination, they have also been witnesses to LGBTQ+ activism during their lifetimes and have seen incredible movement in social acceptance and policy development for LGBTQ+ people in the United States, Canada, and many other countries. Individual LGBTQ+ people and allies across diverse communities and geographic areas are spearheading health policy change at the federal level for LGBTQ+ people through collectives such as the Diverse Elders Coalition (Espinoza, 2011) in the United States, which includes communities of Southeast Asians, Hispanics, Native Americans, and Asian Pacific people. Similarly, in Canada, Rainbow Health Ontario (Travers, 2015) and seniors-specific networks such as the Senior Pride Network (n.d.) in Toronto, along with nursing and other health provider networks, have been active in advocating for program and policy change to support LGBTQ+ older people locally and provincially.

Although LGBTQ+-specific supports, including social groups for older people or welcoming LGBTQ+ seniors groups, are now becoming available to some extent in large cities in North America, the vast majority of social or health supports for older people assume that older people are heterosexual and cisgendered. Even though LGBTQ+ people are diverse with respect to age, culture, ethnicity, and language, organizations and providers who create seniors-focused programs and services geared to specific language or cultural groups are unlikely to have considered the relevance of LGBTQ+ diversity in the communities they serve. Seniors-focused services, whether they are faith-based or provided through other social agencies, must consider that their diverse communities across ethnicity and language include lesbians, gay men, bisexuals, and transgender people (Brotman et al., 2007; Daley et al., 2017). LGBTQ+ seniors-focused social and recreational networks are emerging more frequently in the United States and Canada, and such resources for older people are becoming aware of the value of undertaking needs assessments and policy change to create welcoming environments and relevant programs to meet the needs of the often-hidden LGBTQ+ groups they serve (Services and Advocacy for GLBT Elders and National Center for Transgender Equality, 2012; Tang, 2015).

As health issues surface for older people that require them to engage with health and social services, seniors-focused programs, or condition-specific programming, they may be more likely to use home-care services and may be anticipating the need for some sort of congregate care, such as assisted living or long-term care for themselves or their partners. Most older LGBTQ+ people have established care providers and, to varying extents, support networks and prefer to age in place, even if safety is relative. To move to another place entails coming out again and learning the perils of that new environment. With few exceptions, however, LGBTQ+ people are invisible in long-term care, residential, and congregate facilities, and it is with trepidation that most LGBTQ+ people plan for the possibility of institutional care (Daley et al., 2017). Fear and anxiety mark thoughts of planning for long-term care for many older LGBTQ+ people, a life transition that is often difficult for many individuals and families in any context (Stein et al., 2010). Health care providers, families, and others providing support in planning for long-term care may not be aware of the individuals' LGBTQ+ identities. LGBTQ+ people worry that, because care providers may lack knowledge or understanding about older LGBTQ+ people, they will neglect them or express overt disapproval or more subtle hostility, and that this may result in being neglected, excluded, or ridiculed (Tang, 2015). Since few long-term care or residential facilities are openly LGBTQ+-positive in terms of the material provided to prospective patients and families, and assessment forms are unlikely to have categories to ask about sexual orientation or gender identity, older LGBTQ+ individuals—even those who have been open in many aspects of their lives—may go back into the closet (Daley et al., 2017). McIntyre and McDonald (2012) described environments that LGBTQ+ people face in residential and long-term care institutional facilities where "the place of home as the private domain is replaced with an 'intimate public space' rife with heteronormative assumptions" (p. 132). In addition, sexuality is often assumed to be irrelevant to older people, and sexual orientation and gender identity may be assumed to be narrowly associated with one's sexuality rather than relevant to the holistic health and well-being of LGBTQ+ people. Health care providers; staff, including volunteers; families; and other residents often lack knowledge and understanding about LGBTQ+ people and are unaware of the needs of LGBTQ+-identified older people and the importance of being able to create an environment that reflects their personal priorities, as well as one that can include partners and visible markers of LGBTQ+ community. Given such dynamics in residential care facilities where individuals may be increasingly dependent on care providers for physical, social, and spiritual support in relation to complex personal care needs, palliative care, and dementia care, the importance of LGBTQ+-affirming providers and organizations cannot be underestimated (Institute of Medicine Committee on Lesbian, Gay, Bisexual and Transgender Health Issues and Research Gaps and Opportunities, 2011; McGovern, 2014; Tang, 2015). Although currently no LGBTQ+-specific long-term care facilities are available in Canada, advocacy initiatives are underway to develop these in the future (Tang, 2015).

Recent Canadian research on LGBTQ+ home care in Ontario, Canada, showed that home-care providers were unlikely to have received training in the home-care environment explicitly on LGBTQ+-focused health issues and that the curriculum in their professional programs lacked LGBTQ+-focused content, with the result that providers and patients identified concerning gaps in LGBTQ+-affirming home care. However, when care providers and home-care agencies were made aware of the specific health issues that are important to LGBTQ+ people, they were often receptive to making policy changes and promoting service provider education to enhance the LGBTQ+-affirmative environments (Daley et al., 2016a). LGBTQ+ communities stress that building health care provider and organizational LGBTQ+ cultural competence is essential. LGBTQ+-identified individuals are otherwise bearing the burden of constantly teaching providers about LGBTQ+ health issues and affirming environments, adding to the everyday minority stress that affects their lives (Institute of Medicine Committee on Lesbian, Gay, Bisexual and Transgender Health Issues and Research Gaps and Opportunities, 2011).

Aging, Older Adults, and LGBTQ+ Families

LGBTQ+ seniors comprise anywhere from 2 to 7 million people of the total U.S. population and more than 335,000 Canadians (Fredriksen-Goldsen, 2011; Lim & Bernstein, 2012). However, older LGBTQ+ families have often been invisible in communities of older people as well as to health and social service providers and to the policymakers and decision makers whose focus is to enhance the health and well-being of older populations. Similar to other subgroups of LGBTQ+ populations, there is very limited health and health service research on older LGBTQ+ people and their families, but it is needed to inform responsive and relevant health and social care. Nurses and interdisciplinary health care providers interact with older LGBTQ+ people and their families in all health care settings, from primary care to long-term care.

Most older LGBTQ+ people dwell in the community and, similar to other older people, many hope to age in place, often having established a level of comfort and familiarity in what they call home. Several factors shape the aging experience for LGBTQ+ people. First, the historical context of LGBTQ+ people in society is relevant. Because they have grown up in eras where sexual orientation was considered a pathology and same-sex sexual activities were criminalized, older LGBTQ+ people, especially those older than 75 years, are unlikely to have come out, whereas those who are somewhat younger may be more likely to disclose their sexual orientation, although many still remain in the closet in some aspect of their lives. For many, there is an ongoing need to manage disclosure because they fear discrimination or victimization (Fredriksen-Goldsen, 2011). Second, because they grew up at a time when traditional family structures prevailed and same-sex marriage was not an option, they are less likely to have a spouse or children and thus face isolation. Older transgender people are particularly invisible (Daley et al., 2017).

Older LGBTQ+ people are diverse in many ways, including ethnicity, language, and socioeconomic status; as the Institute of Medicine Committee on Lesbian, Gay, Bisexual and Transgender Health Issues and Research Gaps and Opportunities (2011) has indicated, however, research is very limited in this regard. Ageism is a reality in our social worlds, and for LGBTQ+ people, sexuality and gender interact with other social dynamics such as racism to affect the availability of social support, housing, and experiences of stigma that diverse groups of older LGBTQ+ people may face

(Institute of Medicine Committee on Lesbian, Gay, Bisexual and Transgender Health Issues and Research Gaps and Opportunities, 2011). Thus, although older LGBTQ+ people are often seeking care for chronic diseases such as cancer, diabetes, and heart disease, they may also be dealing with social determinants such as discrimination, housing, and social support, which influence the possibility of achieving good mental well-being (Institute of Medicine Committee on Lesbian, Gay, Bisexual and Transgender Health Issues and Research Gaps and Opportunities, 2011; Kertzner et al., 2011). In contrast with the general population, in which older women are more likely to live alone, older gay and bisexual men, more than older lesbian or bisexual women, are more likely to live alone, which has implications for their mental and emotional well-being (Fredriksen-Goldsen et al., 2015). Older women in general often face financial vulnerability, and older lesbian women, who worked at a time when employment for women was less likely to provide them with pensions and benefits, may face particular financial challenges (Daley et al., 2017). Similarly, older adults of color, many of whom have often faced poverty or who have had and continue to have precarious work in low-income sectors, live with economic insecurity, which can affect their access to health care as well as their health outcomes (Espinoza, 2011). The experiences of aging for ethnic and racial LGBTQ+ minorities, such as African Americans, Two-Spirit First Nation and Native Americans, or Aboriginal transgender people seeking housing or health care, can reflect multiple dynamics of discrimination based on race, sexuality, and gender (Brotman & Ryan, 2004; Institute of Medicine Committee on Lesbian, Gay, Bisexual and Transgender Health Issues and Research Gaps and Opportunities, 2011). LGBTQ+ older adults may have experienced discrimination when accessing elder-care services, employment, and housing opportunities (Center for American Progress, 2020), which can lead to social isolation relevant to their income security and their mental health as well as their ability to thrive independently and in the community.

Older transgender people, either those who transitioned years before or the increasing number who are transitioning in their older years, often face health care systems and networks for older people that are not prepared to meet their needs. Concerns about being able to access meaningful care from a health care provider who is nonjudgmental and knowledgeable about trans-specific clinical care, networks, and resources for social support and other strategies that can enhance their mental health and well-being is crucial for transgender people to thrive as they age. This can be particularly important because transgender people can be disenfranchised on many levels, such as being alienated from families of origin, including their children and grandchildren (Finkenauer et al., 2012).

Family Caregiving for Older Adults

There are virtually no empirical reports on disability within the LGBTQ+ community, although loss of independence with aging or illness is a concern for sexual and gender minorities just as it is for members of the heterosexual community (Institute of Medicine Committee on Lesbian, Gay, Bisexual and Transgender Health Issues and Research Gaps and Opportunities, 2011). Many older LGBTQ+ people are themselves caregivers for partners, friends, and family of all ages (Brotman et al., 2007).

Twenty percent of LGBTQ+ persons between the ages of 40 and 61 report that they do not know who would take care of them if they became ill or disabled; this number increases to more than one-third for those who do not have a partner or a spouse (MetLife Mature Market Institute, 2010). LGBTQ+ individuals are three to four times less likely to have children than heterosexuals (Espinoza, 2014). Indeed, among those who serve as caregivers, more heterosexual individuals report caring for family members (65%) when compared with their LGBTQ+ counterparts (53%). This underscores the importance of close relationships with friends and families of choice and should be noted by nurses who are involved in planning or coordinating in-home care or who are communicating with care providers. Genograms and ecomaps are useful to home-care nurses to develop the client story and visualize the resources and challenges of LGBTQ+ families (see the case study about the Boyle family).

It is important for nurses and other health care providers to understand that the structure of caregiving appears to be different within sexual and gender minority populations. For example, half of LGBTQ+ caregivers are men, whereas 75% of heterosexual caregivers are women (Institute on Aging, n.d.). Gay men also report spending more time in caregiving tasks. They spend an average of 41 hours per week; their lesbian counterparts spend 26 (MetLife Mature Market Institute, 2010). The sensitivity of nurses to what may seem to be small or insubstantial differences in caregiving goes a long way in reducing perceived bias for patients, thereby making experiences of care more satisfying. An effective means of empowering LGBTQ+ caregivers is the completion of advance directives, including medical proxy or power of attorney forms to delineate each family member's role clearly, especially in states where there are no other forms of legal protection or acknowledgment of family relations and responsibilities.

Certainly, beginning with the need to support HIV-positive members of the LGBTQ+ community when no services existed, LGBTQ+ communities often developed circles of care to offer the health care and personal support that individuals required (Brotman et al., 2007; Maddox, 2011). LGBTQ+ older adults have distinct networks of support from peers, who are often older themselves. As Fredriksen-Goldsen (2011) has noted, "Despite the fact that their support systems differ and they often lack legal protection for their loved ones, an alarming 30 percent do not have a will and 36 percent do not have a durable power of attorney for healthcare" (p. 6). As indicated in one Canadian study, given barriers to home-care services, families, friends, and communities are often relegated to providing postsurgical support for transgender people, for instance (Daley et al., 2016a).

In Canada, health care providers and LGBTQ+ communities have collaborated to create tools for interdisciplinary service providers. In 2008, Toronto collaborated with LGBTQ+ seniors and care facilities to develop the LGBT Long Term Tool Kit (City of Toronto, 2008), which offers health care providers and organizations a systematic approach to creating positive space in long-term care facilities. In a home-care context, researchers created two tools for provider organizations based on Ontario-wide research (Daley et al., 2017) with home-care providers and LGBTQ+ home-care users. The LGBTQ+ Access and Equity Framework (Daley et al., 2016a) is a user-friendly tool that offers home-care organizations a way to assess systematically and comprehensively their organizations and strategies to work toward providing LGBTQ+-affirmative care. Both tools emphasize the need for engaging leadership across the organization and for developing partnerships with LGBTQ+ communities in meaningful ways in order to develop and evaluate programs that serve sexual and gender minorities by building LGBTQ+ community capacity.

A second resource, *Queering Home Care* (Daley et al., 2016b), is a one-page tool created when home-care findings were mapped onto an existing home-care patient values statement. To support the development of welcoming health care environments for LGBTQ+ people, each section of the original patient values statement was revised to illustrate the unique concerns of LGBTQ+ people in order to align with high-quality care. Sections include a focus on high-quality care, partnering in decision making, being respected in the health care encounter, and having the necessary information. For instance, in the section on Being Respected, the following phrase was added to the *Queering Home Care* version:

To receive care that respects cultural, ethnic, spiritual, linguistic and regional preferences . . . having your home including chosen art work and photos and partner(s) and friends respected and having your chosen language including pronouns for yourself and your chosen supports respected. (p. 1)

Strategies to move LGBTQ+ family care forward in a context of aging include:

- building nurses' knowledge and understanding of LGBTQ+ health issues for diverse groups of older people and LGBTQ+ histories of oppression and resilience
- building LGBTQ+-affirming cultural competency that includes the use of affirmative language; opportunities to examine attitudes and values, including how ageism and racism intersect with heterosexism, biphobia, and transphobia; and holistic clinical assessments that take a strengths-based approach to high-quality care
- engaging with LGBTQ+ communities in needs assessments to support responsive LGBTQ+-focused programs and services, as well as LGBTQ+-affirmative programs and services to serve broader populations
- developing LGBTQ+-aging-focused curriculum in nursing education and training opportunities such as professional

orientations and in-services in long-term care facilities

■ advocating for LGBTQ+-affirmative policies and programs in health and social care and broader communities

The following case study about the Boyle family will assist the reader with the process of integrating and applying nursing knowledge to the care of LGBTQ+ families.

Case Study: Boyle Family

An Older Woman in Transition

Robin Boyle was raised as a biological female who, at the age of 48, began exploring gender identity and the process of transitioning to a transgender man. During this time, Robin challenged many traditional notions of family to support *their* (Robin's chosen pronoun) care during the transition process. Nurses providing care to families with transgender members must first identify the pronouns preferred by the transgender members by simply asking. Often, transgender people identify and introduce themselves as John (he, him, his) or Chris (they, them, their) when in social situations.

Today, Robin Boyle (they, them, their) is a 53-year-old Asian transgender man. Robin was raised in a closely knit family in a rural area of Texas. Robin's parents came to the United States as refugees at the end of the Vietnam War and came to live in Texas through a sponsorship by the Southern Baptist Church. Robin was the younger of the family's two daughters. At age 22, Robin married a heterosexual African American man, David, and had two children through this marriage: a son named Jonathan and a daughter named Alexandra. Robin and David were high school sweethearts in Texas and moved to Southern California after they married to escape the conservative beliefs back home. They believed that Southern California would allow their children to live a life filled with diversity and support for their mixed-race family. For the first 10 years of this marriage, Robin was a stay-at-home mother and was very active in their children's lives. Robin and David were active members of the United Church of Christ in their hometown because of its open and affirming doctrine. They participated in numerous rallies throughout California to show their support for same-sex marriage for their fellow church members. As Robin became more active in the LGBTQ+ community, they became close friends with Tony, a transgender man who was very open with Robin about his struggles in transition. During the next few years, Robin began counseling with a social worker who had several clients in the LGBTQ+ community and had been recommended by Tony as someone that Robin could trust. Robin began to reflect on the many different experiences of childhood and youth, and began envisioning life without the fear and repression that had been routine in Texas. At the age of 48, Robin began exploring their gender identity and sought support from their primary health care providers for hormones in the process of transitioning.

At the time of the transition, Robin's daughter Alexandra, now 24, was pregnant with her first child. She was overwhelmed by her mother's announcement of her transition and struggled to know how to explain things to her in-laws. During an argument with Robin, Alexandra told them that this was an attempt to refocus attention away from what should be Robin's support for Alexandra's pregnancy. Alexandra was angry and stated: "I wanted my mother to be with me during my delivery, not some man I don't know!" Robin is a trained doula and had planned to provide direct support during Alexandra's delivery but now feels unwelcome. Alexandra's husband, Chris, has been very supportive of Robin's transition because many of his classmates from Stanford self-identified as members of the LGBTQ+ community, including his best friend. Chris believes Robin should be Alexandra's doula, which is leading to friction and conflict in their relationship.

Robin's son Jonathan, now 26, is pursuing his master's degree in nursing to become a family nurse practitioner and has been very supportive of his parent's transition but continues to use "Mom" when talking about Robin. He was fortunate enough to have several classes in his primary-care course that focused on issues of LGBTQ+ health but never expected to have to apply this information to his own family. Jonathan has been living at home with his 2-year-old son Iggy since the death of his partner during childbirth. Robin has been helping Jonathan raise their grandchild, providing day care while Jonathan is at school. Robin, Jonathan, and Iggy have been living with David in a three-bedroom home. When gender transition began, Robin moved into Alexandra's empty bedroom because David did not identify as being gay and felt this is what he would have to be to remain intimate with Robin. Robin and David had individual and joint sessions with Robin's counselor for the past year. Although these sessions helped them to live together amicably, David felt strongly that their relationship cannot continue through Robin's transition and filed for a divorce. Robin had insurance through David's company but will not be covered once the divorce is finalized. Currently, testosterone injections are covered by David's insurance; after the divorce, however, Robin will need to apply for Medicaid (called

Case Study: Boyle Family—cont'd

Medi-Cal in California) because of their limited income (see the Boyle family genogram and ecomap in Figures 8-2 and 8-3, respectively).

Robin's friend Tony has helped with resources about Medi-Cal and the process that must be completed to receive coverage for testosterone injections and gender-affirming surgery. Medi-Cal will cover the hormones and surgery, but coverage is decided on a case-by-case basis, and there is no guarantee that Robin's medical needs will be covered. Robin needs to file a treatment authorization request (TAR), explaining why their hormones and surgery are medically necessary. It can take several months for this application to be considered; if denied, the appeal will entail legal expenses and further time. When Medi-Cal expanded its Medicaid coverage with the Patient Protection and Affordable Care Act, many more services for the transgender population became available. Like many of their friends in the LGBTQ+ community, Robin considered moving to Ontario, Canada, where there is access to universal health care that covers all physician and hospital services except elective surgery. If Robin moves to Canada, the concern becomes that they will no longer be able to have a nurse practitioner as their primary-care provider because testosterone is considered a controlled substance that must be prescribed by a physician. In addition, Robin will need to get support from their providers to show that this surgery is medically necessary.

Robin has decided to have top surgery only—that is, a double mastectomy—and has begun the process of applying for Medi-Cal. Unfortunately, as long as Robin is living with David, David's income is considered part of the household income, and they are over the limit by $1,000 monthly for Robin to qualify for assistance. David's insurance company stated they will terminate Robin's coverage as soon as the divorce is final, no matter the living arrangements. Robin estimates they will be uninsured for at least 6 months before qualifying for state assistance. Robin wanted to arrange for as much of the transition as possible to happen during summer vacation from school, as they had arranged a transfer to a new school where fewer explanations would have to be made about Ms. Boyle becoming Mr. Boyle. Robin knows faculty are not exempt from bullying, teasing, and transphobic remarks from students and others at high school. Fortunately, there is a gender-neutral bathroom available at the new high school and the administration has encouraged its use. At the current place of employment, all the bathrooms are labeled male or female for faculty or staff members and for students. Robin has continued to use the women's restroom but feels increasingly out of place.

Robin's church and its members remain very supportive during the transition, but there are a few friends who have begun to take sides as they learned of the impending divorce between Robin and David. Some of these friends expressed concern for the

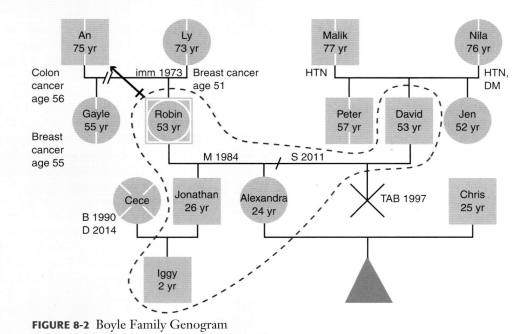

FIGURE 8-2 Boyle Family Genogram

(continued)

Case Study: Boyle Family—cont'd

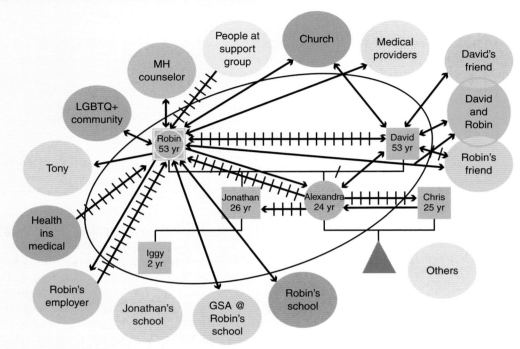

FIGURE 8-3 Boyle Family Ecomap

confusion that Iggy may feel, which Robin sees as a projection of how these friends are feeling. Iggy used to call Robin "Nana," but recently has switched to "Bobin." Overall, Iggy just seems content to have his favorite playmate around the house baking cookies.

Robin has begun taking testosterone during the last 2 years. Since undergoing the transition and beginning testosterone, Robin has been growing more body hair, their voice deepened, and their relationship with their female body parts has become strained. Robin has been using binders since beginning the transition to minimize their large breasts but developed an ongoing problem with candidiasis, often with chafed, raw, intertriginous areas that sometimes have a foul odor. The daily routine of binding their breasts, the fear of an embarrassing odor, and the pain led to Robin's decision for a double mastectomy. Robin's primary-care provider scheduled a mammogram, but Robin has been cancelling and rescheduling these appointments. Robin hoped the mastectomy would eliminate the need for mammograms but recently learned this will not be the case. Although the procedure will reduce the risk by 90% to 95%, Robin carries the *BRCA1* gene and will need ongoing surveillance (Ochaney et al., 2019). Robin is beginning to understand the psychological term *gender dysphoria* in a very personal sense. Although Robin has been using this diagnosis as they were preparing the TAR, it was not until these body changes that Robin felt any unease with transitioning. Robin knows this transition is essential to their psychological well-being to become the man they have known to be inside, but deciding how much surgery to have or not based on financial concerns has worn Robin down. Robin has not had a Pap smear in more than 10 years, with the last one being slightly abnormal. Even with a strong family history of colon cancer, Robin was trying to avoid a colonoscopy. The thought of going to an outpatient procedure center, filling out the registration forms with male identification, and then having to answer questions from the nurses and doctors before and after the procedure explaining the transition was overwhelming for Robin. With Robin's insurance situation in limbo, limited income, and family demands, these routine health maintenance procedures seemed low priority.

Robin began mourning the loss of the relationship with David and feels isolated. At the transgender support group, a woman began to show an interest in Robin but the advances were deftly deflected. Robin has been reading a lot online, chatting with others, and is considering living an asexual lifestyle. Robin learned over time that intimacy does not need to include sex and does not feel safe exploring their sexuality until the transition is complete.

Case Study: Boyle Family—cont'd

Questions for reflection on the nursing care of the Boyle family:

- What are your own biases that may affect the way you provide care for Robin?
- What are the stressors and barriers for the Boyle family?
- What are the strengths and facilitators for this family?
- What practices and nursing interventions would you prioritize in caring for this family if you were to be caring for Robin as a nurse on an inpatient surgical unit at the time of the double mastectomy?
- What practices and nursing interventions would you prioritize for this family if you were caring for Robin in a primary-care setting when doing an intake and history to establish care?
- How would you find resources for LGBTQ+ families in your community?
- How would you, as Robin's nurse, either in the United States or Canada, be able to act as an advocate for transgender health rights affecting the experience of the Boyle family?

SUMMARY

Nurses provide direct care to LGBTQ+ families in a variety of health care and community settings. In order to be most effective providing care that meets the specific needs and concerns of LGBTQ+ families across the life span, nurses must:

- Begin with the close examination of their own belief systems and biases.
- Apply an attitude of openness and develop an appropriate vocabulary, consulting with the families they care for from the position of learner.

- Recognize that LGBTQ+ families are at increased risk for several health and health-related problems that range from physical and psychological illnesses to social, political, and health care access barriers.
- Provide direct, compassionate, and competent care to the LGBTQ+ family population by engaging in and developing practice to meet the specific needs of the community.

chapter 9

Genomics and Family Nursing Across the Life Span

Louise Fleming, PhD, MSN-ED, RN

Marcia Van Riper, PhD, RN, FAAN

Critical Concepts

- Genomics refers to the study of all genes in the entire genome, whereas genetics refers to the study of a particular gene.

- Genomic medicine (also called genomic health care) is an emerging discipline that involves using genomic information about an individual as part of that person's clinical care and the health outcomes and political implications of that clinical use.

- Advances in genomics and technology have dramatically altered the landscape of health care by providing the tools needed to determine the hereditary component of many diseases and conditions, as well as to improve our ability to predict susceptibility to genetic conditions, onset and progression of genetic conditions, and responses to medications.

- Biological members of a family may share the risk for disease because of genetic factors.

- Families respond to genetic discoveries in their own unique way; even within the same family, members react differently.

- When a genetic risk is identified in a family, the two major nursing responsibilities are to help family members understand that the genetic risk is present and to make sure decisions about testing, management, and surveillance are well-informed and fit with individual and family beliefs, desires, values, and circumstances.

- Results of genetic tests are considered private and thus should not be disclosed to other family members without the tested individual's consent.

- Nurses play a critical role in helping individuals and families find accurate information and access resources when they have concerns about genetic and genomic health risks.

- All nurses, regardless of their areas of practice, need to be able to apply an understanding of the effects of genetic risk factors when conducting assessments, planning, and evaluating nursing interventions; ideally, a family perspective should be used.

Some illnesses run in families, and people commonly wonder if they or their children will develop a disease or condition that is present in their parents or grandparents. This is especially true now that stories about advances in genomics and the experience of living with genetic conditions appear in the popular media on a regular basis (Angier, 2017; Grady, 2020; Heidt, 2020; Zimmer, 2020). Nurses are likely to be among the first health care providers that individuals and families go to with questions about genomics and health because nurses are typically viewed as trusted health care providers with a long history of providing holistic family-focused care (Van Riper, 2020). Nurses have traditionally shown expertise in bridging gaps among health care providers, individuals, families, and communities (Lee et al., 2017). Therefore, the ability to apply an understanding of genetics and genomics in the clinical setting needs to be a priority for all nurses because it helps to ensure that individuals and families that might benefit from genetic services receive appropriate education and referral (Boyd et al., 2017).

During the past two decades, there has been growing recognition around the world that genomic knowledge and skills need to be incorporated into nursing education and training. Because of this, there have been ongoing efforts to provide genomic education and resources to nurses in educational and clinical settings (Calzone et al., 2018; Dewell et al., 2020; Lee et al., 2017; Limoges & Carlsson, 2020). In addition, in some countries, there have been national efforts to require basic competencies in genetics and genomics for all nurses (Boyd et al., 2017; Tonkin et al., 2020).

In the United States, an independent panel of nurse leaders from clinical, research, and academic settings developed a set of guidelines called the *Essential Nursing Competencies and Curricula Guidelines for Genetics and Genomics*. These guidelines were originally endorsed in 2009 and updated in 2011 by nearly 50 organizations in the United States. All nurses need to have minimal competencies in genetics and genomics regardless of their academic preparation, practice setting, or specialty (Van Riper, 2020). Nurses in all areas of practice are expected to participate in genetic risk assessment, play a pivotal role in explaining genetic risk and genetic testing to patients and families, and support informed health decisions and opportunities for early intervention (Lee et al., 2017). Essential

genetic and genomic competencies for nurses with graduate degrees were developed by a consensus panel in 2011 and published shortly thereafter. The advanced competencies are based on the assumption that nurses with graduate degrees have already achieved the core essential competencies.

A recent scan of nursing curriculum, regulatory documents, and practice standards in Canada revealed a very limited amount of genetic and genomic content (Limoges & Carlsson, 2020). There is evidence, however, that Canadian nurses, especially community health and pediatric nurses, have been incorporating genetic knowledge into practice for decades. In 2006, Bottorff and colleagues (2006) published findings from a qualitative study describing nurses' roles in providing clinical genetic services related to adult-onset hereditary disease and factors that influence genetic nursing practice in Canada. Semi-structured interviews were conducted with 22 nurses from five Canadian provinces (Bottorff et al., 2006). Factors identified as supporting genetic nursing roles included their nursing background, being part of a multidisciplinary team, and receiving mentorships. Challenges to establishing roles in genetic nursing included role ambiguity, lack of recognition of nursing expertise, limited availability, isolation, and instability of nursing positions. More recently, an initiative, supported by the Canadian Nurses Association and Ontario Genomics, was developed to engage nurses in all domains of practice to develop a framework to guide nursing strategies toward genomic literacy (Limoges & Carlsson, 2020).

Genetic conditions are often described as family diseases or conditions, and genetic testing is often considered to be a family experience. Until recently, however, much of what was known about the experience of being tested for or living with a genetic condition focused on the individual (Lewitt-Mendes et al., 2018; Long et al., 2018; von der Lippe et al., 2017). Fortunately, this is changing. More and more researchers are recognizing the need to illuminate the family experience of being tested for or living with a genetic condition (Boardman, 2020; Mendes et al., 2019; Myllyaho et al., 2019; Pruniski et al., 2018; Van Riper et al., 2020).

It is important for nurses to be aware of the effect of genetics and genomics on families because biological family members share genetic risk factors. In addition, families function as systems with shared health risks that affect the whole family, and family processes mediate how individual family members and the family as a whole respond to these health risks. Family members inevitably have an effect on each other's lives and, in many cases, they support each other in seeking and maintaining healthy growth and development, regardless of their biological kinship. All nurses, regardless of their areas of practice, must be able to apply an understanding of the effects of genetic risk factors when conducting assessments, planning, and evaluating nursing interventions; ideally, a family perspective should be used.

This chapter describes nursing responsibilities for families of persons who have or who are at risk for having genetic conditions. These responsibilities are described for nurses working with individuals and families across the life span. Genetic conditions are lifelong, so families living with genetic conditions need ongoing care and support. The goal of the chapter is to describe the relevance of genetic information within families when there is a question about genetic aspects of health or disease for members of the family. Family nursing knowledge is incomplete without an understanding of how families influence and are influenced by the way in which individual family members adapt to the experience of being tested for or living with a genetic condition.

GENETICS AND GENOMICS

Advances in genomics and technology have dramatically altered the landscape of health care and nursing practice by providing the tools needed to determine the hereditary component of many diseases and conditions, as well as to improve our ability to predict susceptibility to genetic conditions, onset and progression of genetic conditions, and responses to medications (Doble et al., 2017; Gibbs, 2020; Henderson & Mudd-Martin, 2018). *Genomics* refers to the study of all the genes in the entire genome, whereas *genetics* refers to the study of a particular gene. *Epigenetics* is the study of changes in gene function that are heritable and that are not attributed to alterations in DNA sequences. For these and other definitions of genetic terms, refer to the *Talking Glossary of Genetic Terms* (National Human Genome Research Institute [NHGRI], n.d.). Genomic medicine (also known

as genomic health care) is an emerging discipline that involves using genomic information about an individual as part of their clinical care and the health outcomes and political implications of that clinical use (NHGRI, n.d.).

The human genome consists of approximately 3 billion bases of DNA sequence, and more than 99% of these bases are the same in all individuals (National Institutes of Health, 2017), making individuals more genetically similar than different. Individuals inherit genetic material from their parents and pass it on to their children. Some conditions result from a change or mutation in a DNA sequence of a gene. A *gene* is defined as the basic physical and functional unit of heredity (National Institutes of Health, 2017). For example, Huntington's disease results from a specific change within the DNA sequence in a particular gene. It is an example of a condition traditionally referred to as a Mendelian or single-gene disorder, and it follows an identified pattern of traditional inheritance in families—in this case, autosomal dominant inheritance. Persons who are biologically related may have inherited many of the same DNA sequences in addition to having shared common environments with other family members; this combination ultimately increases risks for having similar specific illnesses.

Researchers also identify common genetic variations known as single-nucleotide polymorphisms. These variations may not cause an actual disruption in the DNA coding but can often be used as tools that help scientists and clinicians recognize DNA variations that may be associated with disease. These conditions include common disorders, such as diabetes, that are observed to occur more frequently in families but do not follow a traditional pattern of inheritance.

A core competency for nurses is to maintain knowledge of the relationships of genetic and genomic factors to the health of individuals and their families. Cancer provides an example of the relationships between genes, environment, and health. The development of a malignant tumor is the result of a complex series of changes at the cellular level. Several genes protect against cancer by regulating cell division (during mitosis); mutations in those genes can occur during the course of a person's lifetime and thus affect one's predisposition to cancer. A person may be at increased risk of developing cancer if an inherited mutation occurs in one of those genes or if they are exposed to environmental factors that influence genetic mutations. For example, tumor suppressor genes help protect against the development of breast cancer. If a woman inherits a mutation in a tumor suppressor gene (such as the *BRCA1* gene), she has lost some of her protection against breast cancer from birth, but she will not necessarily develop cancer unless other cellular changes (some of which are influenced by factors such as her reproductive history) occur during her lifetime. Others in her family may also have inherited the same mutation and are similarly at risk. If she subsequently becomes a smoker, she has an additional increased risk for lung cancer because of the environmental influence of smoking on cell division in her lungs. In families where smoking is the norm, there may be a perceived familial condition because of the shared environmental and genetic influences on several members of the family. Box 9-1 lists inherited and multifactor inherited genetic conditions.

BOX 9-1

Examples of Inherited and Multifactor Inherited Genetic Conditions

Inherited Genetic Conditions

- Huntington's disease
- Cystic fibrosis
- Sickle cell anemia
- Familial hypercholesterolemia
- Congenital adrenal hyperplasia

Multifactor Conditions—Combination of Genetics and Environment

- Heart disease
- Diabetes
- Most cancers
- Alzheimer's disease
- Neural tube defects

GENETIC TESTING

Types of Genetic Testing

Genetic testing can be performed for several purposes, including prenatal diagnosis, diagnosis of a genetic condition in a newborn, detection of carrier status, confirmation of a genetic diagnosis, predictive testing for familial disorders, and pre-symptomatic testing. See Table 9-1 for types of genetic tests. In addition, NHGRI has a webpage designed to address frequently asked questions about genetic testing. Prenatal testing is offered during pregnancy to help identify fetuses that have certain genetic conditions. The most common

Table 9-1	Types of Genetic Tests
Diagnostic	Performed when signs and/or symptoms of a genetic condition are present. Confirms whether or not an individual has the suspected condition.
Carrier	Detects whether a person is a carrier of either an autosomal recessive or an X-linked disorder.
	A carrier of an autosomal recessive condition usually has no signs of the condition and will be at risk for having an affected child if the other parent is also a carrier. He has one normal copy of the gene in question and one mutated copy.
	A female carrier of an X-linked condition has one normal copy of the gene on the X chromosome and one mutated copy of the gene on the other X chromosome, and generally has no signs or very mild signs of the condition. Her sons have a 50% chance of having the condition, and her daughters have a 50% chance of being carriers.
Predictive or presymptomatic	Performed on healthy individuals. Detects whether they inherited a mutation in a gene and therefore whether they will or may develop a condition in the future.
Prenatal diagnosis	Genetic test performed on the fetus. Indicates whether the fetus has inherited the gene mutation that causes a specific condition and therefore whether the child will develop that condition.
Pharmacogenetic (PGx) testing	Analyzes a person's genes to understand how drugs may move through the body and be broken down. The purpose of PGx testing is to help select drug treatments that are best suited for each person.
DTC genetic testing	DTC genetic tests are marketed directly to the general public, usually via the internet. DTC genetic testing provides access to an individual's genetic information, usually without involving a health care provider.

conditions tested for prenatally are neural tube defects (NTDs), Down's syndrome, trisomy 13, and trisomy 18. Carrier testing can tell people if they have (carry) a gene alteration for a particular kind of inherited disorder called an autosomal recessive genetic disorder, such as cystic fibrosis, sickle cell anemia, or congenital adrenal hyperplasia (CAH). Predictive testing can identify individuals who have a higher chance of getting a disease before the symptoms appear. Predictive testing is available for inherited genetic risk factors that make it more likely for someone to develop certain cancers, such as colon or breast cancer. Presymptomatic genetic testing can indicate which family members are at risk for a certain genetic condition that is already known to be present in their family. This type of testing is performed for people who have not yet shown symptoms of a disease, such as Huntington's disease.

In an effort to bridge the transition from the development of a genetic test to diagnostics and treatment, the National Institutes of Health launched the Genetic Testing Registry (GTR), a free online tool that can be used to obtain a comprehensive list of available genetic tests. The GTR webpage includes links to a variety of clinical resources such as GeneReviews, MedGen, Online Mendelian Inheritance in Man (OMIM), and Orphanet, as well as links to consumer resources, including Genetics Home Reference. GeneReviews is a collection of peer-reviewed, expert-authored descriptions of genetic conditions presented in a standardized format. The reviews provide clinically relevant and medically actionable information regarding diagnosis, management, and genetic counseling. MedGen is a webpage where users can search for specific genetic conditions, related genes, and clinical features. It also includes practice guidelines. OMIM is an online catalog of human genes and genetic disorders. Orphanet is a portal for rare diseases and orphan drugs. The consumer resources provide consumer-friendly information about genetic conditions and links to support organizations.

The National Comprehensive Cancer Network continually updates guidelines that specify what kind of screening is indicated for a person who has a gene mutation that increases the chances of cancer developing. For example, family members may seek testing if they are at greater risk for familial colon cancer. In some cases, clinical practice guideline criteria recommend that genetic testing be done to determine whether a person is at risk.

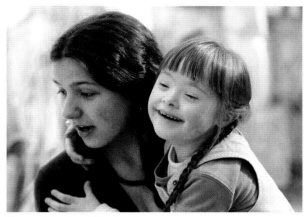

Source: © *istock.com/Denkuvaiev*

Another type of genetic testing that is rapidly being integrated into clinical practice is pharmacogenetic (PGx) testing (Cheek & Howington, 2018; Hippman & Nislow, 2019; Rollinson et al., 2020). PGx testing is performed to examine an individual's genes and thus determine how medications are absorbed, move through the body, and are metabolized by the body. The purpose of PGx testing is to allow health care providers to tailor individualized drug treatments that are specific to each person. For example, before starting a patient on warfarin (one of the most commonly prescribed drugs in the United States and many other countries), PGx testing can be done to figure out what starting dose would work best for the patient. Adjusting the dose based on the patient's genotype can help avoid toxicity and improve efficiency.

Certain gene mutations can affect how an individual's body metabolizes some medications. For instance, patients can be tested to see if they are ultrarapid metabolizers (1% to 10% of the population), extensive metabolizers (majority of the population), intermediate metabolizers, or poor metabolizers. Ultrarapid metabolizers may need a higher dose of a medication because they metabolize drugs so quickly that they may never reach a therapeutic concentration. Intermediate and poor metabolizers may require a lower-than-normal dose.

Information about drug labeling that includes pharmacogenomics information can be found on websites such as Drugs@FDA: FDA Approved Drugs. The U.S. Food and Drug Administration

(USFDA) also has a webpage titled Table of Pharmacogenomics Biomarkers in Drug Labeling that is a useful tool for the community. Herceptin (trastuzumab) is an example of a drug for which obligatory genetic testing has been developed. The purpose of obligatory testing is to identify a subset of women with breast cancer who overexpress HER2/neu, because these women are likely to be the only patients with breast cancer who will benefit from taking Herceptin. Nurses need to understand PGx testing so they can provide comprehensive care, especially at the time of discharge. Nurses who have a good understanding of PGx testing can play a critical role in making sure that drug doses are optimized and drug reactions are avoided.

Direct-to-Consumer Genetic Testing

Traditionally, the only way a person could undergo genetic testing was to go through health care providers such as physicians, nurse practitioners, and genetic specialists. However, it is now possible to undergo genetic testing in one's home. Direct-to-consumer (DTC) genetic testing is a type of genetic testing that is marketed directly to consumers via television, the internet, or print media (National Institutes of Health, 2017). Once the genetic test is ordered by the consumer, a test kit is mailed directly to the person's home. The test kit typically includes instructions for how the DNA sample is to be collected (often by swabbing the inside of the cheek) and a return envelope. Consumers are notified of their results either by mail or by phone, or the results are posted online. With some DTC companies, a genetic specialist or other health care provider is available to discuss the results by phone.

Several companies offer DTC testing, with one of the most well-known being 23andMe. Currently, 23andMe offers consumers three options: (1) ancestry testing plus traits, (2) health plus ancestry service, and (3) VIP health plus ancestry services. The third option, which costs almost four times as much as the second option, is for consumers who want premium customer support and priority testing. Some DTC tests are evaluated by the USFDA but not all. Generally, DTC tests for nonmedical and basic wellness purposes are not reviewed by the USFDA before they are offered. DTC tests for moderate to high-risk medical purposes, which may directly affect medical care, are more likely

to be reviewed by the USFDA to determine the validity of test claims.

When reviewing tests, the USFDA assesses:

- whether a test can accurately and reliably measure what it claims to
- whether the measurement is predictive of a certain state of health
- what a company says about its test and how well it works

The USFDA also examines whether the test offers accurate information that can be readily understood by a consumer without the involvement of a health care provider (USFDA, 2019).

It is important for nurses to be aware of DTC genetic testing so that they can advise their patients who are interested in DTC testing to meet with a health care provider or a genetic specialist to learn more about this type of testing and its accuracy and applicability to health care. Nurses and other health care providers should also be aware of the reliability (or unreliability) of DTC genetic testing. The main concern with DTC genetic testing is that, without guidance from a health care provider or genetic specialist, the individual may make significant decisions about prevention or a particular treatment that is based on incomplete or inaccurate information (USFDA, 2019; NHGRI, 2020). Studies have demonstrated that DTC testing is not always done in a uniform manner, which leads to results that are unreliable and inaccurate (Tandy-Connor et al., 2018). There have also been reports indicating that, if an individual submits his or her DNA sample to multiple companies, the results may be contradictory. For example, one DTC company might say that the person is at increased risk for developing prostate cancer, whereas another DTC company says that the person is at moderate risk, and a third DTC company says that the person is at low risk. Obviously, these results would be difficult for even a genetic specialist to interpret. Many individuals who undergo DTC testing also seek genetic counseling to understand their findings (Marzulla et al., 2020).

Potential Advantages and Disadvantages of Genetic Testing

Nurses should understand the differences in the types of genetic tests that families may consider and the potential advantages and disadvantages of

BOX 9-2
Potential Advantages and Disadvantages of Genetic Testing

Potential advantages of testing include:

- Opportunity to learn whether one has an increased likelihood of developing an inherited disease; in those who prefer certainty, this can help resolve feelings of discomfort, even if the result shows the person has inherited the condition
- Relief from worry about future health risks for a specific disease if the test is negative
- Information that can be used for making reproductive decisions
- Information to inform lifestyle choices (e.g., food choices, smoking, alcohol use, contraceptive choice)
- Information to guide clinical surveillance or management of the condition
- Information for other family members about their own status

- Confirmation of a diagnosis that has been suspected (e.g., that early or nonspecific signs and symptoms are caused by a specific condition)

Potential disadvantages are that the test results may provide:

- A source of increased anxiety about the future
- If the result is negative, guilt at having survived when others in the family are affected (so-called survivor's guilt)
- Concern about potential discrimination based on genetic test results
- Regret about past life decisions (such as not having children)
- Changes in family attitudes toward the person who has been tested (such as less reliance on them for support)

---

genetic testing, which are summarized in Box 9-2. Nurses who participate in discussions about genetic testing must maintain current knowledge about these tests as well as about new technology for testing and interpretations of results.

Genetic tests have limitations that vary according to the specific test. For some tests, not all persons who want the test may qualify, which occurs when their family history does not suggest that the disease has a major genetic component or when the genetic mutation that causes the disease has not been identified. For some tests, it is possible that a result may be difficult to interpret. For some conditions, genetic mutations have been discovered that are associated with the disease in that family. Because many genes may be associated with one condition, or several different mutations may be possible in a gene, it is often necessary to test an affected family member first to try to identify which gene is involved and which type of mutation is causing the condition in that family. A sample is taken from the affected person to determine whether a genetic mutation can be identified that is associated with that condition. This may not be possible if the affected person in the family has passed away or if the affected person refuses to undergo the genetic testing to help other family members.

Another limitation of genetic testing is that the results may not be definitive. This is especially true with any type of genetic screening such as prenatal and newborn screening. For example, a mother who undergoes prenatal screening may be told that she is at increased risk for having a child with Down's syndrome. Or new parents may be informed that their infant's test results from newborn screening for cystic fibrosis are in the positive range for that screening test. A positive result of a screening test simply means, however, that a diagnostic test is required to determine if the results of the screening are correct (e.g., the fetus has Down's syndrome or the newborn baby has cystic fibrosis). It is important for parents to understand that, in some infants who test positive, a diagnostic test result can indicate that the infant has a genetic condition and will need further evaluation and treatment; in other cases, however, subsequent tests will be normal. When an infant undergoes further evaluation and is found not to have the condition, the first test result is sometimes referred to as a false positive, or an out-of-range result that requires further testing.

In many cases, families first learn of an abnormal screening result either by phone or during a follow-up visit. Families often respond with fear and distress to the news, and many turn to the internet for information about the genetic test or condition (USFDA, 2019; Pappas, 2018). Nurses can help guide parents to credible websites concerning condition management and help them review information obtained online (Brockow & Nennstiel, 2019; Sjöström et. al, 2019).

DISCLOSURE OF GENETIC INFORMATION TO FAMILIES

Down's Syndrome

Much has been written about parental satisfaction with family/provider interactions surrounding the diagnosis of Down's syndrome, and there have been ongoing efforts to help health care providers become more prepared to share positive results from prenatal screening and diagnostic testing (Crombag et al., 2020). However, reports of parental dissatisfaction with the informing process continue to appear in the popular literature. There continue to be reports of health care providers giving families inaccurate, out-of-date information about what life is like for individuals with Down's syndrome and their families. Nurses need to be well informed about types of prenatal testing being offered, and they need to know the difference between prenatal screening and diagnostic testing. In addition, they need to be prepared to give expectant parents more than just technical information about the genetic test. Nurses need to provide information about choices that will have to be made by expectant parents following a positive test result, resources for families who receive a positive result, and up-to-date information about life with Down's syndrome in the 21st century (Van Riper et al., 2016). Findings from an ongoing cross-cultural study about adaptation and resilience in families of individuals with Down's syndrome (Van Riper et al., 2016) revealed that parental preference concerning the informing process match fairly well with the guidelines recommended by the National Society of Genetic Counselors (Sheets et al., 2011). Therefore, nurses are encouraged to become familiar with these guidelines. Recommendations include informing parents early in the process, even when a suspected diagnosis has not been confirmed; delivering the news in private and when the parent(s) or support persons are available; using their preferred language; and supporting the family with accurate information and resources (Sheets et al., 2011).

Results of Genetic Testing and Communication Between Nurses and Caregivers

Studies have been conducted examining parents' reactions to newborn screening and recommendations for improving communication (Brochow &

Nennstiel, 2019; Seddon et al., 2020: McCarthy, 2020). Reactions from the parents after hearing their child had a genetic condition ranged from "very scary" to "not concerned." Common emotions reported by parents include shock, panic, and worry. In addition, some parents reported feeling guilty. Concerning recommendations for improving communication, seven main themes were identified:

- *Provider characteristics:* The provider should be knowledgeable, known to the family, and an effective communicator.
- *Provider approach:* The provider should be calm and reassuring, answer questions, be honest, not downplay results, be sensitive, use simple language, speak to both parents, take their time, and address the parents' questions.
- *Timing of the notification:* Inform the parents as soon as possible, but not on a Friday afternoon. Some parents specified that they would have preferred not to be notified until the diagnosis was confirmed, not suspected.
- *Communication channel:* Parents desired to be told in person rather than on the telephone and that providers not leave a message on the answering machine or in voice mail.
- *Care coordination:* Parents preferred being referred to an appropriate specialist as soon as possible and that there was direct communication between the primary-care provider and the specialist.
- *Information:* Parents wanted written materials and a follow-up process in place if additional questions arose in the first few weeks following being told about the diagnosis.
- *Family support:* Parents wanted access to other families having a child with the condition, adults with the condition, and support groups to hear life experiences.

Certain genetic conditions, such as salt-wasting CAH, are life threatening without proper treatment. Families learning of their child's CAH diagnosis in the first few weeks following birth may become overwhelmed because not only are they learning their child has an inherited, genetic condition, but also that their failure to treat the CAH adequately can result in the death of their child (Fleming et al., 2017a; Fleming, 2016; Boyse et al., 2014). CAH requires parents to administer oral steroids, typically hydrocortisone, up to three times daily to affected children. In addition, parents must supplement maintenance steroid doses with oral "stress dosing" during times of illness and an emergency intramuscular (IM) injection of hydrocortisone when a child is unable to tolerate oral medications and/or if signs of adrenal crisis are present. This need for stress dosing, either orally or by injection, related to simple viral and bacterial childhood illnesses is frequent and unpredictable, often requiring parents to make complex treatment decisions (Fleming et al., 2017a). Girls born with CAH often experience virilization, which results in atypical genitalia at birth caused by elevated testosterone related to adrenal dysfunction (boys born with CAH have typically appearing male genitalia) (Fleming et al., 2017b). Nurses and other health care providers must be sensitive to families during this challenging time and be willing to provide needed support. This support may include repeating management instructions, putting families in touch with local and national support groups, and referring families to pediatric endocrinologists and pediatric urologists in a timely and clear manner.

FAMILY DISCLOSURE OF GENETIC INFORMATION

Access to genetic information gained from genetic testing as well as from family history raises a host of questions for the family regarding confidentiality that includes the following: who to tell, what and when to tell them, and how much to share. Nurses must maintain the confidentiality of each family member's genetic testing information. It is completely up to the individual to determine whether or not to reveal information about genetic risks, testing, disease, or management. Results of genetic tests are private, so they should not be disclosed to other family members without the tested person's consent. In the United States, the Health Insurance Portability and Accountability Act (HIPAA) permits disclosures of health information if there is an immediate and serious threat to the person and if the disclosure could reasonably lessen or prevent the threat (U.S. Department of Health and Human Services [USDHHS], 2017). In most cases, however, the choice of disclosure of genetic information is an individual decision that is made in the context of the family.

Family members may prefer to maintain privacy regarding their decision to undergo testing, even within the family. This decision may reflect an attempt to avoid disagreements within the family, to protect others in the family from sadness or worry, or to prevent discrimination or bias. For example, people who have predictive Huntington's disease testing may be reluctant to share this information with their primary-care provider. The reluctance may be because they fear that any notation in their medical record may be accessed by an employer or insurance provider, which may lead to loss of employment or insurance. Although there are laws that prohibit insurance or employment discrimination based on a person's genotype, some individuals may remain concerned that revealing their genetic information may place them at risk for future discrimination.

When one person in a family has a condition that is caused by an alteration in a single gene, such as a gene associated with hereditary breast or ovarian cancer, the person with the mutation is asked to notify others in the family that they too may have this same DNA mutation. In general, the family members themselves pass on this information, but occasionally, with the consent of all concerned, direct conversations can occur between the nurse and other family members. It is up to the individual family members and the family as a whole about how, when, and with whom to share their genetic information. Concerning hereditary breast cancer, mothers report anxiety about upsetting their children and causing unnecessary worry with disclosure; however, avoiding disclosure has profound effects on their children, including children developing blasé and conflicting attitudes toward breast reconstruction surgery as well as misunderstandings of the full implications of risk management decision making (Rowland et al., 2016).

Both individual and family relationship factors can influence communication among family members. Therefore, nurses should have a good understanding of their patient's personal beliefs about sharing genetic risk information with family members. Typically, close relatives are told of the new diagnosis shortly after it has been made; however, sometimes a longer period of time is needed so that the affected person can make sense of the genetic test result for themselves. Nurses should be patient, empathetic, and caring during conversations with the family as disclosure decisions are made. Box 9-3 depicts an example of family communication about genetic information.

BOX 9-3
Family Communication of Genetic Information

Brian, a 46-year-old man, is the oldest of three siblings. He is married but has no biological children. Brian was aware that his mother died of bowel cancer at the age of 38 years, and although this worried him, he hid his anxiety from both friends and relatives. He never discussed his mother's death with his wife or siblings. Brian had been experiencing abdominal pain for some months when he collapsed at work one day and was taken to his local hospital emergency department. He was found to be anemic and suffering a bowel obstruction. A tumor located near the hepatic flexure of the large colon was removed successfully. Brian was informed that his family and medical history indicated that it was likely he had inherited a mutation in an oncogene that predisposed him to bowel cancer. He was advised to share this finding with his siblings and recommend that they seek advice and screening for themselves. Brian was reluctant to discuss the issue with his siblings but did tell his wife. Brian chose not to disclose this information to his siblings. Several months later, at the encouragement of his wife, they met with the cancer nurse to discuss the situation. The cancer nurse helped Brian decide what information to share with his siblings. They created a plan for how and when to share the information. Subsequently, both Brian's sister and brother had genetic testing. Brian's sister was found to carry the mutation. She was screened, and she worked with the nurse to devise a plan to tell her children about their possible risk when they reached 18 years of age.

Parents: To Tell or Not to Tell

Parents form views about how and when to tell their children early after a diagnosis and typically feel responsible to communicate this information to their children themselves. Parents of a child with a genetic disorder take into consideration what to tell their children about the condition based on the developmental level of the child and the child's extent of interest in knowing about the genetic condition. Parents who are unsure about informing their children may feel that it would be better coming directly from a health professional. Parents of children with genetic conditions may choose not to share information because they have concerns about school issues, obtaining health care

for their children, and insurability or employability of their children. Nurses have a significant role in helping parents decide what information to share with their children about their genetic condition based on their developmental level. Family nurses also help parents determine how much information to share with outside sources, such as schools, day care, or employers, about their child's genetic condition.

Concealing Information: Family Secrets

Families choose to keep genetic information quiet for a variety of reasons. Sometimes information is kept a secret out of a desire to protect other family members. Some keep it secret because they feel shame. Still other families may choose to keep information confidential because the exploration of genetic inheritance may reveal other personal information. For example, consider a family with four sisters who want health advice because their father has a form of familial colon cancer. In the course of obtaining the family history, the mother confides to the nurse that her husband is not the biological parent of the oldest daughter and that others in the family do not know this history. In this situation, the nurse recognizes that the oldest daughter does not share the same risk for this disease as her sisters, but the nurse would not be permitted to reveal that information to any family member without the mother's permission. This family secret can create conflict for the nurse because the lack of disclosure might mean the eldest daughter is exposed to unnecessary procedures, such as a colonoscopy (which carries a risk for morbidity). The nurse would discuss the issue of risks for procedures with the mother so that she can consider all the information in deciding to tell her daughter the family secret. The mother would have to decide if the benefits of disclosure outweigh the distress the daughter may experience by learning about her parentage.

Family Reactions to Disclosure of Genetic Information

Families are unique and respond to genetic discoveries differently. Even within the same family, the responses of family members may vary. Some members may seek predictive testing to determine whether they have inherited the genetic condition. Others choose not to seek testing. Some members react to genetic discoveries with grief, loss, and denial. The nurse's role is to support all family members in their reactions and ultimate choices.

Children, regardless of age, may wonder if they will have the same condition as their parent. For example, this may be the case for teens who have a parent or grandparent with Huntington's disease, an autosomal dominant condition. Guidelines do not recommend predictive testing until a teen is old enough to provide informed consent. However, delayed disclosure to children can lead to increased family tension that can result in misunderstanding, blame, and secrecy. Teenagers should be given the opportunity to discuss concerns about genetic testing, but parents should be involved in and support their child's final decision. Nurses should offer the opportunity for them to ask questions and discuss their concerns, including offering to facilitate a family discussion. Box 9-4 depicts a family working with an adolescent about genetic testing.

Older adults may have varied experiences with genetic conditions that they have seen in their families over the years and can serve as a valuable source of information regarding family history of genetic conditions. Advances in genomics will make susceptibility testing for common diseases of middle and old age (such as coronary artery disease or cancer) more common.

Family members possess beliefs about their own risks and who in the family will develop a genetic condition, and these beliefs are often based on the family's previous experience. For example, if only male relatives have been affected by an autosomal dominant condition that could affect either sex, female members in the family may believe they are not at risk. Sometimes preselection beliefs are based on the fact that the person thought to have inherited the condition physically resembles the affected parent or shares a physical characteristic (such as hair color) with other affected relatives. A preselection belief may influence the person's self-image and overall functioning. For example, those who believe they will develop a condition may make different career choices, avoid long-term relationships, or decide not to have children. Box 9-5 depicts a case study that demonstrates preselection beliefs.

BOX 9-4
Working With an Adolescent About Genetic Testing

Susan is a 17-year-old young woman whose mother developed breast cancer at age 42 and had to have a double mastectomy. Susan's mother is now recovering from her surgery and doing well. Susan's maternal grandmother and one of her maternal aunts died from breast cancer in their forties. Susan's mother chose to have genetic testing to learn about the possible genetic cause of her breast cancer. The test results revealed that she has a *BRCA1* gene mutation, which significantly increases a woman's lifetime risk of developing breast cancer. At her annual health care appointment, Susan tells the nurse about her family history of breast cancer and that her mother has a *BRCA1* gene mutation. Susan says that she would like to know what her risk is for inheriting this gene and that she would like to have genetic testing to find out if she carries the same *BRCA1* gene as her mother. She says that she is worried about her younger sister, too. Susan tells the nurse that she does not want to worry her mother or family by talking with them about her concerns. The nurse informs Susan that she is free to express her concerns with her and her physician and that they can talk with her about how best to discuss the issue with her mother and express her concerns. The nurse also lets Susan know that when she is 18 years old, she will be old enough to provide informed consent to have genetic testing for the *BRCA1* mutation that her mother has. The nurse recommends that when Susan is 18, she consider genetic counseling with a genetic specialist to learn more about her risk and the *BRCA1* genetic testing.

DECISION TO HAVE GENETIC TESTING

In some circumstances, family members may want to know the likelihood that they will develop a condition in the future, which is referred to as either *predictive* or *presymptomatic* testing. Typically, the physical risk for undergoing genetic testing is minimal, but not so for the emotional risk. The test results may have a significant effect on a person emotionally, influence medical decisions, and result in discrimination. Undergoing genetic predictive testing requires nurses to work with clients so that they make this decision in a way that meets

BOX 9-5
Preselection Beliefs

John is a 21-year-old man who has recently graduated from college and is trying to decide what career he wants to pursue. John has a family history of Huntington's disease (HD) on his mother's side. His mother's brother and her father have both passed away from HD. His mother, age 45, is currently in good health. John is very worried that he will develop HD because it is in his mother's family. John makes an appointment to talk to his health care provider about his concerns. As the nurse is taking his vital signs, John tells them about his concerns that he will develop HD. He says that he doesn't know if his mother has it, and he is worried because it seems to occur in the males of the family, and he resembles his uncle who died from HD. John says that he would like to go to medical school, but he is scared that he will develop HD when he is young and it will greatly affect his career. He also tells the nurse that he has a girlfriend to whom he is very attached, but he is afraid to consider getting married because he does not want to put her through the experience of losing him to HD. He says that he has not even told her about his family history. The nurse tells John that she understands his concerns and encourages John to talk with his doctor about how he can learn more about his risk for HD. The nurse encourages him to consider having genetic counseling to talk further about his risks and available genetic testing for HD to learn more. John thanked the nurse for their support and suggestions and says that he will surely talk with his medical provider further about his concerns and options.

their specific needs while staying alert to the non-physical risks. Nurses involved with these families should be able to identify the sources of emotional distress and offer effective strategies to help mediate distress, help patients make informed decisions about medical interventions, and help them handle possible discrimination.

Emotional Health

Family members seek or avoid genetic testing for a variety of reasons. Some elect to know whether or not they carry a mutation so they can reduce their fear of the unknown or make life choices, such as having children. Some people decide not to have predictive testing because they believe

this knowledge would increase their level of anxiety and would prompt a constant watch for developing symptoms (Anderson et al., 2019). Test results mean different things in different situations, which makes these decisions to undergo testing even more complex and multifaceted. For example, a positive test for a *BRCA1* or *BRCA2* breast cancer mutation does not mean the individual has a 100% chance of developing breast cancer, so taking precautionary measures requires weighing costs and benefits. In other situations, such as in the case of Huntington's disease, if an individual carries the autosomal dominant condition, he will develop the disease. Some choose not to be tested for fear that they would lose hope.

Even adjustment to a negative result—meaning that a person does not have the genetic pattern of the disease—can be difficult. Some people who find that they are not at risk of developing a genetic condition experience so-called survivor guilt, which can be described as a sense of self-blame or remorse felt by a person who, in this case, will not develop a condition that others in the family will develop.

Medical Decisions

Physicians and nurse practitioners are in an excellent position to work closely with individuals and families in making well-informed decisions about their health based on genetic and genomic information. These health care providers have the ability to refine and personalize medical care that is based on the client's genetic makeup. For example, there is an increased probability that treatment outcomes will result in fewer adverse effects from medications, such as pain management being determined on the basis of whether a client is a known fast metabolizer or is slow to metabolize certain kinds of drugs. But just because there are many tests available does not mean that the best option is for the individual to have genetic testing done. Advanced practice nurses need to work closely with the individual and family in deciding to conduct genetic testing; they should explain what the test would show and how specific the results might or might not be, and explore what options are possible based on the outcome of the testing.

After conferring with the health care provider, some individuals may choose not to have genetic testing at that time. Instead, these individuals may elect to undergo regular checkups and screenings, such as more frequent mammograms. In contrast, when a person has genetic testing and tests positive for a specific disease, a cascade of decisions then befalls that person, including preventive or prophylactic treatments, degrees of treatment, risks of treatment, and benefits of treatment. For example, a woman may decide to undergo surgery, such as sterilization, to avoid passing on to offspring a condition such as cystic fibrosis or sickle cell anemia, or someone with positive results for the *BRCA1* breast cancer mutation may elect to have a bilateral mastectomy.

Discrimination

Many individuals choose not to undergo genetic testing because they fear discrimination. For example, a person may be concerned that she may be bypassed for promotion if it was known that she tested positive for a medical condition. In the United States, the Genetic Information Nondiscrimination Act (GINA) of 2008 protects individuals from discrimination initiated by an employer or health insurance company (Genetic Discrimination, 2020). Under GINA, insurers may not use genetic information to set or adjust premiums, deny coverage, or impose penalties for preexisting conditions, and they may not require any genetic testing. Unfortunately, the GINA law does not apply to employers with fewer than 15 employees, and it does not include protection against discrimination when an individual seeks to obtain life insurance, short-term disability insurance, or long-term care insurance. GINA does not protect members of the military, veterans, federal employees, or the Indian Health Service. Each of these sectors of society is protected against discrimination by other laws and statutes.

Under GINA, an employer may not make any decisions about hiring, firing, promoting, pay, or assignment based on any genetic information. The Patient Protection and Affordable Care Act of 2010 also prohibits denial of insurance coverage based on genetic information. GINA is significantly more stringent and specific in preventing discrimination by employers and health care insurance agencies (Genetic Discrimination, 2020), however, because it defines genetic information as including medical history.

ROLES OF THE NURSE

When a genetic risk is identified in a family, nurses, together with others on the health care team, have two major responsibilities: (1) help family members understand that the genetic risk is present and (2) make sure decisions about testing, management, and surveillance are well-informed decisions that fit with individual and family beliefs, desires, values, and circumstances.

This section suggests ways that nurses should review their own beliefs and values when working with families. It covers how to conduct a risk assessment and genetic family history, the importance of working with a couple in preconception education, and the role of nurses as genetic information managers.

Personal Values: A Potential Conflict

Nurses must become aware of cultural values that differ from their own family cultural values. Cultural awareness allows nurses to tailor their practices to meet the needs of the family. Box 9-6

BOX 9-6

Cultural Awareness for Working With Families

Kate is a genetic nurse working in a pediatric clinic for children with inherited metabolic conditions. She was scheduled to see a family whose son had a rare inherited metabolic disorder to discuss the parents' future reproductive options, including prenatal diagnosis. When the family entered the room, she noted with surprise that the parents and the child were accompanied by both sets of grandparents. She quickly arranged for more chairs to be brought into the room. Kate was quite disconcerted to find that the paternal grandfather repeatedly answered questions that were directed to the parents, and she continued to address the parents. Eventually, the child's father explained that, according to his culture, the oldest male relative on the father's side was responsible for making the decision that would affect the family; therefore, it was critical that the grandfather be fully involved in all discussions. While reflecting with her mentor, Kate realized that, in the future, she would ask the family at the beginning of the family conference to share any specific cultural needs she should know about in order to help meet their family needs.

demonstrates how a nurse who does not understand a family's cultural values could contribute to a poor outcome.

It is a difficult emotional situation when nurses' personal values conflict with those of families. One example of this type of conflict occurs when the nurse personally does not agree with the family decisions relative to the potential risks of having a child who is genetically predisposed to having a terminal disease. It is unethical, however, for nurses to try to influence the decisions of the family or family members because of their own personal views.

Another type of conflict occurs when opinions within the family vary. In this type of situation, the role of the nurse is to facilitate family members expressing their views. In clinical genetics, more than one family member may be involved in decision making, and nurses should respect each person's autonomy.

Conducting a Genetic Family History

As described in Chapter 5, a genogram collects useful information about family structure and relationships. Nurses can use a three-generation family pedigree to provide information about a potential genetic inheritance pattern and recurrence risks. The genetic risk assessment enables nurses to identify those family members who may be at risk for disorders with a genetic component so that they can be provided appropriate lifestyle advice, screening recommendations, and possibly reproductive options. Information on standardized pedigree symbols and the construction of a genetic family pedigree is available to the public through the Centers for Disease Control and Prevention (CDC) webpage called Family Health History: Genomics and Precision Health.

The purpose of drawing the family tree using a genetic family pedigree is to enable medical information to be presented in the context of the family structure. Obtaining a genetic family history in this systematic manner helps ensure inclusion of all critical information in the analysis. The process of obtaining a detailed health history and causes of family deaths is as follows:

- Start with the client.
- Next, include the client's immediate family members.

- Continue with the client's mother's side of the family.
- Then add the client's father's side of the family.
- End with relatives who have died, including their cause of death.

Relatives who are not biologically related, such as those joining the family through adoption or marriage, should also be noted with the appropriate pedigree symbol. The reason that relatives who are not biologically related are noted in a pedigree with a special symbol is to identify them as family members who are not at risk for passing on or inheriting harmful genes from the family they have joined.

Obtaining a family genetic history is a nursing skill that requires technical expertise and knowledge of what should be asked, as well as sensitivity to personal or distressing topics and an awareness of the ethical issues involved. Box 9-7 outlines the components of a genetic nursing assessment. Information given by patients is considered part of their personal health record and should be treated as personal and private information.

Drawing the genetic family pedigree or family tree for at least three generations often provides important data about the potential inheritance pattern. When a condition affects both male and female

---

BOX 9-7

Components of a Genetic/Genomic Nursing Assessment

A genetic nursing assessment includes the following information:

- Three-generation pedigree using standardized symbols
- Health history of each family member
- Reproductive history
- Ethnic background of family members (as described by the family)
- Documentation of variations in growth and development of family members
- Individual member and family understanding of causes of health problems that occur in more than one family member
- Identification of questions family members have about potential genetic risk factors in the family
- Identification of communication preferences for genetic health information within the family

members and is present in more than one generation, a *dominant condition* is suspected (Figure 9-1). Conditions that affect mainly male relatives, with no evidence of male-to-male transmission, increase suspicion of an *X-linked recessive condition* (Figure 9-2). When more than one child is affected of only one set of parents, it may be evidence of an *autosomal recessive condition* (Figure 9-3).

Nurses should not assume that a condition is genetic merely because more than one family member has it. Family members who are subject to similar environmental influences may have similar conditions without a genetic basis. One such example is a family with a strong history of lung cancer. For example, Bob, a 62-year-old man, was affected by lung cancer. His two brothers and father all died of lung cancer. Bob expressed deep concern about having a genetic predisposition that he could pass on to his sons. The family history revealed that Bob's father and every male member of his family worked underground as coal miners from the age of 14 years. In addition, they all smoked at least 20 cigarettes a day starting when they were teenagers. None of the women smoked, nor did they work in the mines, and none developed lung cancer. In this family, the cancer could likely be attributed to environmental rather than inherited causes.

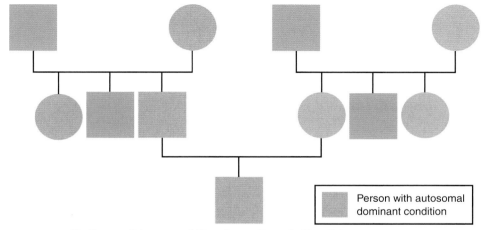

Person with autosomal dominant condition

FIGURE 9-1 Pedigree of Autosomal Dominant Genetic Condition

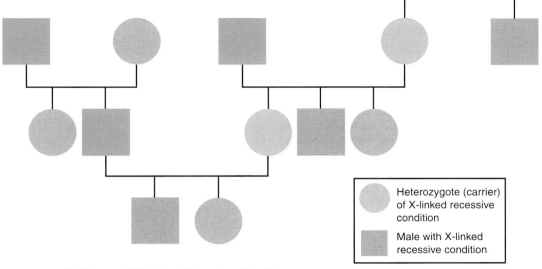

Heterozygote (carrier) of X-linked recessive condition

Male with X-linked recessive condition

FIGURE 9-2 Pedigree of X-Linked Recessive Condition

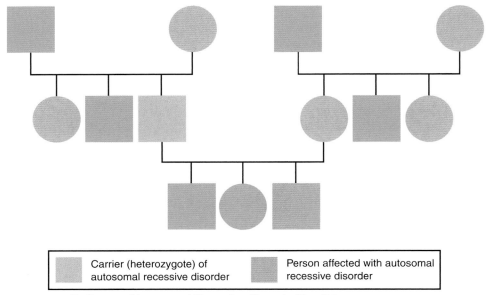

FIGURE 9-3 Pedigree of Autosomal Recessive Genetic Condition

Preconception Assessment and Education

Preconception counseling is an intervention that includes providing information and support to individuals before a pregnancy to promote health and reduce risks. It is ideal when a family has the opportunity to discuss difficult genetic decisions before a pregnancy. During a pregnancy, the emotional ties to the existing fetus may complicate the decision-making process for the parents. Preconception counseling enables a couple to explore options without time pressures.

One aspect of preconception education is conducting a health risk profile that includes family history; prescription drug use; ethnic background; occupational and household exposures; diet; specific genetic disorders; and habits such as smoking, alcohol, or street drug use. When nurses identify information that may present a health risk in future offspring, they should explore whether the individual or family wants a more extensive evaluation from a genetic specialist. Box 9-8 provides an example of preconception education for a couple concerned about genetic risks for offspring.

In addition to identifying inherited conditions, preconception counseling includes education regarding other risk factors that could change the outcome of a pregnancy. During preconception counseling, for instance, family nurses explain the importance of taking an adequate amount of folic acid, one of the B vitamins, which is known to decrease the number of babies born with NTDs (CDC, 2020). Box 9-9 provides more information about NTDs.

BOX 9-8
Preconception Education

Jay and Sara are college students who are planning to be married. Both are of Ashkenazi Jewish ancestry. Although both have heard about Tay-Sachs disease and the availability of carrier testing, neither has had the carrier test. When Sara visited the student health office, she talked with the nurse about her fears that she may not be able to have healthy babies. She knew that Tay-Sachs disease, a degenerative neurological condition, is more common in Ashkenazi Jewish families and that no treatment will alter the course of the disease. Sara was interested in learning more about the carrier test. The nurse offered to refer Sara to a genetics specialist who would help the couple explore the following childbearing options:

- Decide to have or not have biological children
- Have a pregnancy with no form of genetic testing
- Have a preimplantation genetic diagnosis
- Have a pregnancy and have a prenatal genetic diagnosis with an option to terminate an affected fetus
- Have a pregnancy using a donor gamete from a noncarrier donor
- Adopt a child

Risk Assessment in Adult-Onset Diseases

Genetic history taking is important in the adult population to assess for risk factors that are pertinent to common diseases, such as cancer and coronary heart disease. The risk assessment is based on the genetic family pedigree, but additional genetic or biochemical testing may be used to clarify the potential risk to each individual. To ensure privacy, health care providers must obtain consent from all living relatives before accessing their medical records and confirming relevant medical history. Family members who are seeking information are advised of their risks and options for clinical screening and follow-up. One example is the assessment of risk for cancer when there is a strong history of cancer in the family. Nurses must explore feelings of grief and anxiety about the future as well as beliefs about the inheritance pattern. Providing explanations enables families to understand the information and helps them learn possible options to reduce the risk for cancer in their family members.

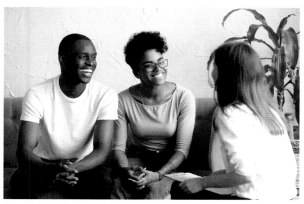

Source: © istock.com/fizkes

Increasingly, women with a family history of breast or ovarian cancer or both are seeking to reduce their risks for these conditions. All women have a risk for breast cancer (13% of women in the general population) and may be offered mammography screening according to the standards of care or regional health policy. For women with a genetic family history that is consistent with familial breast and ovarian cancer, genetic and familial cancer specialists should discuss earlier and more frequent screening. The challenge of decision making with hereditary breast cancer is demonstrated in the complicated process of weighing risks and benefits.

With appropriate treatment, some health problems with a major genetic component may improve or at least remain stable. But many genetic conditions lead to increasing loss of health and function throughout the person's life span. These genetic conditions require more and more complex care from both health care providers and the family. In the chronic phase of a genetic condition, individuals and family members not only come to terms with the permanent changes that come with the onset of illness symptoms but also must adapt their family routines and roles, and locate needed resources to meet changing health care needs.

Providing Information and Resources

An essential nursing competency includes the ability to identify resources that are useful, informative, and reliable for patients and families. It is the role of nurses to ensure that recommended websites include relevant and evidence-based information. Patients and families need psychosocial and medical information about genetics; therefore, any information that is prepared for distribution should include material on both types of needs.

Evaluation of Genomic and Genetic Nursing Interventions

Genomics and genetics are relatively new fields in nursing, but some work has assessed the value of genetic services, including nursing input, for patients and their families. Nurses must expand their assessment skills to include detailed family histories, understand the elements of genetic testing, and facilitate care coordination for genetic and genomic conditions and therapies (Boyd et al., 2017). Nurses should aim not only to be knowledgeable

Case Study: Evaluation of Nursing Intervention

Fiona is a 5-year-old kindergartener. Her teacher is concerned that she does not appear to be progressing as well as expected and asks the school nurse, John, to check her hearing. John arranges for Fiona's parents to bring her for a hearing test. He asks Fiona's mother about Fiona's medical history; the mother says that she has always been a well child and has not had any ear infections but has developed some "funny patches" on her skin. They have not caused a problem, but the mother has wondered what they are and if they could turn cancerous. John checked her skin and noted that they seem to be café-au-lait patches—small, pale brown pigmented areas of the skin. He reassures the parents that the café-au-lait patches are not harmful but could indicate an underlying cause for Fiona's slight learning problems. He drew a genetic family pedigree or family tree (Figure 9-4) and noted that Fiona's father and his mother (Fiona's paternal grandmother) had unusual skin lumps but no other medical problems.

When the pediatrician sees the family, she measures Fiona's head circumference and examines her skin. She confirms that the skin marks are café-au-lait patches and that Fiona has eight of them. Fiona's head circumference is larger than average, on the 97th percentile for her age. A diagnosis of neurofibromatosis type 1 is made. The pediatrician explains that this is a genetic condition but that it could have arisen for the first time in Fiona or may have been inherited from one of her parents. Neither parent is aware of the condition in the family. The pediatrician examines both parents and finds that Fiona's father has a large head circumference and has several raised lumps on the skin, called *neurofibromas*. He tells the pediatrician he needed extra help with math at school, but he finished college and works teaching French. He has never been concerned about the lumps because his own mother had dozens of them, and apart from having one removed because her shoe was rubbing against it, they did not cause her a problem.

The pediatrician is aware that children with this condition may have learning problems. She recommends that Fiona be evaluated to identify whether Fiona would benefit from extra help at school. Because high blood pressure and malignancies can be a result of the condition, she also plans for Fiona and her father to have an annual checkup. Fiona's brother, James (9 years old), is also examined but has no signs of the condition and does not require any further assessment.

When John is informed of the diagnosis, he helps the family identify reliable sources of information on the internet and provides Fiona's parents with information about neurofibromatosis organizations.

Questions for reflection on the nursing care of Fiona and her family:

1. What are the primary roles for nurses related to genomics and working with families?
2. What strategies can nurses implement to support the family's understanding of using internet resources to support their learning?
3. How can nurses use professional reflection when working with families to address genetics?

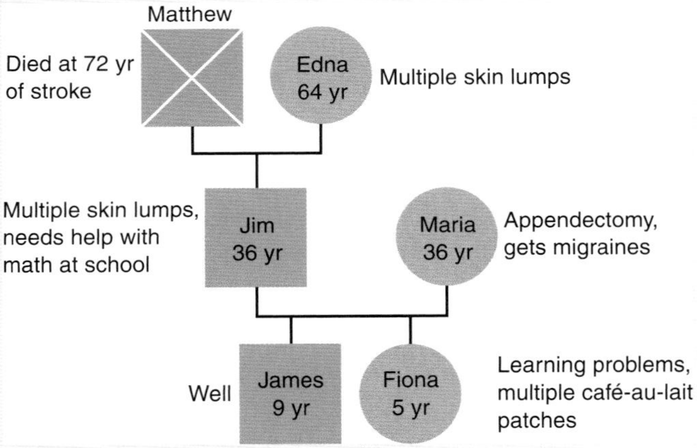

FIGURE 9-4 Genetic Pedigree: Fiona's Family Tree

about genomics but also to provide individualized care and to address the needs and specific agendas of each family. Case Study: Evaluation of Nursing Intervention, provides an example of a nurse's evaluation of interventions with a family whose child has a genetic condition.

Although it is not possible for health care providers to have current knowledge about every condition, nurses exhibit competence in this area by having an awareness of their limitations, being open to discussion, finding appropriate resources, and referring to specialists when required. It is essential that nurses working in all types of settings be prepared with an adequate knowledge foundation to explain the basis and implications of genetics and genomics.

SUMMARY

The following major concepts were discussed in this chapter:

- Families share both social and biological ties. Identifying biological risk factors is an essential component of professional nursing practice, and a nursing assessment is incomplete without identifying biological factors that may place individuals or their offspring at risk for genetic conditions.
- Nurses providing care to families across all health care settings and throughout the life span must maintain current knowledge of genomic aspects of health and risks for illness to assist families in obtaining information and further evaluation if needed.
- Nurses work with families on assessment, identification of issues influencing family members' health, facilitating appropriate referrals, and evaluating the effect of these activities on the family's health and well-being.
- Family values, beliefs, and patterns of communication are integral components of how families cope with and respond to family members with medical conditions that have a genetic component.

chapter 10

Families Living With Chronic Illness

Kimberly E. Kintz, DNP, ANP-BC, RN

Mindy B. Zeitzer, PhD, MBE, RN

Critical Concepts

- Chronic illness is a global phenomenon with the potential to worsen the overall health of a nation's people and limit the individual's capacity to live well.

- Healthy lifestyle behaviors and early detection or screening may prevent some forms of chronic disease.

- Chronic illnesses that occur at birth or early childhood are most likely to be genetic and require special attention during developmental changes and across the life span.

- Nurses must use evidence-based knowledge to empower families with the information, skills, and abilities to manage chronic diseases over the life course and prevent complications and comorbidities.

- Family-focused care is important for prevention and management of chronic illness when it occurs; this type of care involves intentional nursing action that meets both the individual's and family's needs.

- Knowledge about disease self-management and adherence to a therapeutic medical regimen is essential for individuals and their family members if they are going to prevent additional complications.

- Nurses use various actions (e.g., teach, coach, demonstrate, counsel) to assist individuals and their family members to cope with the stress of uncertainty, powerlessness, and anticipatory and ambiguous losses that accompany chronic illnesses.

All members of the family are affected when one of its members has a chronic illness. When an individual is diagnosed with a chronic illness, it becomes necessary for the individual and the family to learn to manage the disease or disorder while living a quality life. Individuals with a chronic condition often battle to stay healthy, live active lives, retain a high quality of life, and prevent complications. This battle is waged primarily within the confines of the family. When an individual is diagnosed with a chronic illness, whatever it might be, family members must incorporate unexpected changes into their roles and daily processes, manage disabilities imposed, and identify ways to do it with the resources they have available and within a context of uncertainty. Managing uncertainty is a significant concern for individuals and families living with chronic illness (Brown et al., 2020; Hummel, 2019b). Family members are challenged to balance the needs of the ill family member with their own needs and the needs of the family as a whole.

Chronic illnesses often require complex care, and many people have more than a single condition. People with chronic illnesses can experience complications or comorbidities that make situations even more difficult. For example, a person diagnosed with type 2 diabetes may also have hypertension, hyperlipidemia, and neuropathy. A person with Parkinson's disease may also have a serious sleep disorder, constipation, chronic pain, and Lewy body dementia. Individuals with a chronic illness often require care from multiple health care providers. Nurses are crucial in helping families coordinate care from by multiple providers and access to potential resources. The complex needs can create havoc for families, especially those with limited access to care and resources, as they attempt to manage many thorny situations daily. The holistic approach of nurses is crucial to the individual and family adaptation and management of living with chronic illnesses across the life span. Chronic illnesses have an impact on the lives of infants, children, adolescents, young adults, older adults, and persons 65 years and older. Chronic illnesses affect the physical, emotional, intellectual, social, vocational, and spiritual functioning of the person with the condition as well as the family members. Wide variations exist in the ways different chronic illnesses and conditions affect individuals and the family's physical, mental, and spiritual health; employment; social life; and longevity.

Differences in the ways families accommodate a chronic illness exist and are influenced not only by the level of disability and associated symptoms but also by individual, family, and systemic factors. Families differ in their perceptions of disability, their backgrounds, cultural and spiritual beliefs, and access to needed resources. Care responses differ depending on whether the symptoms are constant (cerebral palsy), episodic (migraine headaches), relapsing (sickle cell anemia), worsening or progressive (diabetes, Parkinson's disease, or certain types of cancer), or degenerative (Alzheimer's disease or Rett syndrome). Details of the unique individual situation vary with the age of the individual, previous family experiences, level of disease complexity, individual's motivation or ease in managing the illness, unique family member relationships, and distinct personalities and values. Regardless of the type of chronic illness experienced, one thing remains the same: Various family members are likely to be involved at several levels.

Because family members are the most enduring care providers, they might be viewed as the biggest resource for individual care over time. Family members generally offer the constancy and continuity of care needed for the most optimal health outcome. Most health care providers come and go in the lives of individuals with chronic conditions, offering medical management, education, and counseling for brief times. But it is generally family members that provide the needed ongoing and persistent care across time.

The purpose and focus of this chapter are to describe ways for nurses to think about the impact of chronic illness on families and to consider strategies for helping families manage chronic illness. The first part of this chapter briefly outlines the global statistics of chronic illness, the economic burden of chronic diseases, and three theoretical perspectives for working with families living with chronic illness. The chapter begins with the importance of integrating ethnoculture in family health care and the impact of chronic illness on family life. Four theoretical approaches are introduced for assisting nurses to think about the best way to assist the family living with chronic illness. The rest of the chapter captures a variety of possible nursing actions to assist these families. Two case studies are presented in this chapter: one family who has a member living with type 1 diabetes and another family helping an older parent and grandparent manage Parkinson's disease. Although each family experience with illness is completely individual, many of the challenges that these two families demonstrate are universal to other families supporting members living with different chronic illnesses.

WHAT IS CHRONIC ILLNESS?

Definitions for what constitutes chronic diseases vary widely, although most definitions seem to address duration and limitations in function and may include mental health conditions. Whether the condition is a physical or a mental health condition, there is a need for ongoing treatment and management of the condition (Raghupathi & Raghupathi, 2018). Different approaches used to measure the prevalence and consequences of chronic diseases and health conditions in children contribute to the lack of uniformity and acceptance of a definition. The terms *chronic disease* and *chronic illness* are often used interchangeably by health care providers and researchers. Larsen (2019) differentiates between *condition* and *illness* as follows: "*condition* refers to the pathophysiology of a disease" whereas *illness* is referred to as "the human experience of a disease and refers to how the disease is perceived, lived with, and responded to by individuals, their families and health care professionals" (p. 4). This chapter will utilize the term *chronic illness* as much as possible.

The term *chronos* is the root word for "chronic" and refers to time; however, the term *chronicity* has various definitions. Chronic illnesses have been defined as conditions that last or are expected to last more than 3 to 12 months and result in functional limitations and/or need ongoing medical care (Raghupathi & Raghupathi, 2018). Another definition describes a chronic illness as a health condition that requires long-term coordination of health care that is comprehensive and includes continuity of care (Reynolds et al., 2018). The World Health Organization (WHO) uses the term *noncommunicable diseases* (NCDs) interchangeably with chronic diseases that are not passed from person to person, generally have a slow progression, but have a long duration. WHO (2018c) describes four main types of NCDs: cardiovascular diseases (such as heart attacks and stroke), cancers, chronic respiratory diseases (such as chronic obstructive pulmonary disease and asthma), and diabetes.

INTEGRATING ETHNOCULTURE IN FAMILY NURSING

With the rapidly changing world today, nursing care must be understood not only in the local context but also with a global (international) vision as nurses strive to meet the needs and demands of individuals and families experiencing chronic illnesses. Both Canada and the United States are experiencing demographic shifts because of growing multicultural and multilingual communities. The rapidly changing population patterns require nurses who can assess and meet the needs of diverse family groups that are living longer with complex chronic health conditions.

Nursing: Addressing Health Needs of a Multicultural Society

The increasing migration between and within nations suggests that health care providers may experience both benefits and challenges in today's health care arena. For many, life in the United States is an international experience. For nursing, what this means is that, in order to meet the health needs of diverse communities, nurses must be not only qualified but also culturally knowledgeable and ready to adapt to the changing needs of a rapidly diversifying population with multiple languages and cultural health beliefs and health needs. Beliefs and self-management are a combination of cultural beliefs and traditions. Patients and their families are best served when nurses focus not only on the differences but also on the similarities within and among various cultural groups. Family nursing focuses on the strengths of individuals, families, and their communities. Global population shifts require that nursing meet the needs of diverse communities. Ethnocultural frameworks assist nurses with making client-centered assessments and inclusive management plans:

- Nurses achieve cultural knowledge by first desiring the knowledge and by actively engaging in cultural encounters with patients from diverse backgrounds.
- Nurses must self-reflect and acknowledge biases and discriminatory practices that prevent meaningful communication and interactions with unfamiliar community members.
- When working with individuals and their families, nurses must consider the client's worldview, environmental context, values, beliefs, religious patterns, and health practices.
- When developing plans of care, nurses assess and include long-standing, culture-bound traditional beliefs and practices.
- Nurses must be knowledgeable about biocultural variations, disease incidences, and health inequities in the populations they are serving.
- Nurses must become familiar with the historical, political, economic, and public policies that affect chronic illness management.

Addressing the needs of diverse communities is not a new phenomenon, but it has become a focal point for nurses and other health care providers. Examining the integration of diversity in health care is timely and warranted, especially because the nursing profession in the United States, as in other nations, is limited in the number of nurses from different racial and ethnic backgrounds with the skills to navigate health matters in diverse environments. In the United States today, 80% of nurses self-identify as White (American Association of Colleges of Nursing, 2019). What this means is that the percentage of U.S. nurses of underrepresented backgrounds is at odds with the increasing national and global demographic shifts.

The Canadian Nurses Association (2013) expressed the need to describe the diversity profile of nurses in order to help human resources planning. In 2019, Canadian men represented 9% (396,085) of the total employed registered nurses (Canadian Nurses Association, 2020). The National League of Nursing (NLN) suggests that a lack of racial, ethnic, and gender diversity in the health professions limits our ability to provide appropriate care for families in a changing environment. The lack of diversity in the health profession perpetuates health care inequities, societal biases, and stereotyping (NLN, 2016).

CHRONIC ILLNESS: A GLOBAL CONCERN

Chronic illness is a global issue and is one of the leading causes of mortality and disability in the world. From 1999 to 2014, four of the five leading causes of death in the United States were from chronic diseases, two of which (heart disease and cancer) accounted for approximately 52% of all deaths (WHO, 2018c). Canada has very similar statistics, with cancer being the leading cause of death and accounting for 30% of all deaths (Government of Canada, 2019b). Worldwide chronic conditions such as cardiovascular diseases, cancer, chronic respiratory disease, and diabetes are responsible for 80% of these deaths (WHO, 2018c). These four prominent chronic diseases are linked by common and preventable biological risk factors, notably high blood pressure, high blood cholesterol, and excess weight, and by related major behavioral risk factors, such as unhealthy diet, physical inactivity, and tobacco use (Chen et al., 2018; WHO, 2018a).

Various factors, such as a growing older population; an increasing life expectancy related to advances in public health and clinical medicine; and lifestyle-associated modifiable behaviors such as tobacco use, excessive alcohol use, insufficient physical activity, and poor nutritional habits, have all contributed to the increase in chronic illnesses (Hajata & Stein, 2018; Waters & Graf, 2018; WHO, 2018c).

WHO (2018c) estimated that out of the 41 million people who died from chronic disease, 15 million were under the age of 69 years and 85% of those premature deaths occurred in low- and middle-income countries. Projections are that the percentage of people worldwide older than the age of 60 years and living with chronic illness will increase between 2015 and 2050 from 12% to 22%. Common chronic conditions associated with aging include diabetes, hypertension, chronic obstructive pulmonary disease, hyperlipidemia, depression, cancer, and osteoarthritis. Many older individuals live with multiple chronic illnesses and complex conditions. As individuals get older and experience more chronic illnesses, they are at risk for geriatric syndrome. Geriatric syndrome is not a chronic illness or specific disease diagnosis but a cluster of five clinical symptoms: incontinence, pain, malnutrition, cognitive impairment, and frailty. Geriatric syndrome is associated with a higher mortality rate when present in older adults (Schiltz et al., 2019; WHO, 2018a). Cardiovascular disease is the number one cause of death around the world and accounts for 31% of all global deaths (WHO, 2017). Cardiovascular disease morbidity and mortality could be reduced by addressing risk factors such as tobacco use, unhealthy diet, obesity, physical inactivity, high blood pressure, diabetes, and elevated lipids (WHO, 2017). Worldwide, obesity has tripled since 1975. In 2016, approximately 39% of adults 18 years or older were overweight, and 13% were obese. In 2019, the number of obese and overweight children under the age of 5 years was estimated to be over 38 million. Obesity in children, once considered a problem in high-income countries, is rising in low- and middle-income countries (WHO, 2020a).

Cancer is the second leading cause of death around the world and accounted for approximately

9.6 million deaths in 2018 (WHO, 2018b). The most common cancer deaths are cancers of the lung, colorectal region, stomach, liver, and breast (WHO, 2018b). According to WHO, tobacco use is the most important risk factor for cancer because it is estimated to cause 22% of global cancer deaths (WHO, 2020b). In addition, tobacco use is the primary cause of chronic obstructive disease, such as emphysema and asthma, worldwide.

In 2014, about 422 million adults worldwide were living with diabetes, an increase from 108 million in 1980, with the majority affected by type 2 diabetes (WHO, 2020c). When diabetes is not well managed, it leads to complications that include heart attack, stroke, kidney failure, limb amputation, vision loss, and nerve damage. In 2016, diabetes caused approximately 1.6 million deaths, with many of these deaths (43%) occurring in those under the age of 70 (WHO, 2020c).

When pain becomes a comorbidity, the challenges to individuals and their family increase tremendously. Many chronic conditions involve chronic nonmalignant pain (Palylyk-Colwell & Wright, 2019). Chronic nonmalignant pain is one of the most prevalent and costly health care problems addressed in primary health care settings and affects about 100 million American adults, which is more than the total number affected by heart disease, cancer, and diabetes combined (McCann, 2018).

The United States and Canada are experiencing increased racial, ethnic, language, cultural, and family system changes. Combined with the increase in life expectancy, rising health care costs, a greater number of individuals living longer with chronic diseases, and the increasing need for family health support, nurses experience unprecedented challenges in providing care to families.

Family Health: Why Diversity Matters

It is well recognized that racial and ethnic underrepresented populations suffer disproportionally from not only chronic debilitating conditions but also from preventable acute ailments and social conditions associated with poor health outcomes. According to the Office of Minority Health (2019), Hispanics/Latinx suffer disproportionately from obesity, asthma, liver disease, diabetes, and related complications. Diabetes is a major concern among subgroups of Hispanics because of

visual and renal impairment, higher rates of amputations, and premature death. Among African American populations, heart disease, strokes, cancer, asthma, diabetes, lung diseases, HIV/AIDS, and homicide are of greater concern at younger ages. Among Native American/Alaska Natives, the leading causes of death are diabetes, heart disease, cancer accidents, strokes, and infant death. Asian Americans share health risks similar to those for other underrepresented groups, including cancer, heart disease, strokes, and accidents. Although the risk factors, morbidity, and mortality rates vary among and within these underserved populations, a concern is the paucity of health data available on the health of underrepresented groups. For nurses, it is imperative that evidence-based measures be increasingly available to assist individuals and their families and communities managing disabling chronic conditions. Without adequate data and tools for improving health care, nurses may not be able to assist the growing number of individuals and families from diverse backgrounds and all citizens living with and managing chronic debilitating conditions.

Surveillance of Chronic Illness

How do we know how many people have chronic illness and whether the problem is getting better or worse? In public health, one approach is the availability of surveillance data that are systematically collected over time. This information is used to analyze a problem and help identify trends of change over time. The following are examples of some of the surveys and surveillance systems that are used in the United States:

- Behaviorial Risk Factor Surveillance System (BRFSS)
- National Ambulatory Medical Care Survey (NAMCS)
- National Healthcare Safety Network (NHSN)
- National Health Interview Survey (NHIS)
- National HIV Surveillance System
- National Hospital Discharge Survey (NHDS)
- National Notifiable Disease Surveillance System (NNDSS)
- National Vital Statistics System (NVSS)
- Youth Risk Behavior Surveillance System (YRBSS)

In the United States and Canada, the Behavioral Risk Factor Surveillance System (BRFSS) is a survey used by the Centers for Disease Control and Prevention (CDC) to collect national information regularly. This is a state-based or province-based system of health surveys conducted via phone. The survey tracks health risk factors and uses the findings to improve the health of the nation's people who are 18 years of age and older. For example, when asked, "Have you ever been told by a doctor that you have diabetes?" participants from southern states such as Arkansas, Louisiana, Mississippi, Alabama, South Carolina, Tennessee, Kentucky, and West Virginia had the highest prevalence of yes responses, with an average of 12.4% to 16.7%, compared with 10% as the national average (CDC, 2020b). These types of statistics assist health care providers in developing target population-specific programming. In 2019, more than 59% of the U.S. adult population drank alcohol in the past 30 days, with approximately 18.3% reporting binge drinking and 7.6% reporting heavy drinking (CDC, 2020b). The CDC (2019) defines *binge drinking* as a pattern of drinking that brings a person's blood alcohol concentration (BAC) to 0.08 grams% or above. This typically happens when men consume five or more drinks, or when women consume four or more drinks, in about 2 hours. Binge drinking is common in young adults 18 to 34 years of age. However, adults 35 years and older account for more than half of the binge drinking. Binge drinking has serious unintended consequences such as motor vehicle accidents, falls, burns, and alcohol poisoning. Alcohol poisoning accounts for roughly 2,200 unintentional deaths a year in the United States (CDC, 2019).

Another survey instrument used to collect information about chronic illness risks is the National Health and Nutrition Examination Survey (NHANES) (2020) in the United States and the Food and Nutrition Surveillance in Canada. The National Cardiovascular Data Registry is a database used to capture information about particular individuals. The National Program of Cancer Registries in the United States and the Canadian Cancer Registry are both surveillance organizations that focus on collecting, monitoring, and interpreting trends in cancer risks among a variety of populations. Large cohort studies, such as the Framingham Heart Study (2017), provide retrospective information about groups of people that

share similar experiences. The Canadian Tobacco Use Monitoring Survey (CTUMS) (2019) describes the smoking trends in Canada from 1999 to 2017. Other data regarding chronic diseases are identified through individual records, from insurance companies, and via reviews of death certificates.

Surveys have revealed that internationally the burden of chronic disease in adults and children is increasing in low- and middle-income countries, and despite increasing awareness and commitment to address chronic illness, global actions to implement cost-effective interventions are inadequate (Chen et al., 2018; Hajat & Stein, 2018; WHO, 2018d). The cause of the increase of chronic diseases in these countries is not easy to pinpoint. Most of the research on chronic illness factors has been conducted in developed countries.

Economic Burden of Chronic Illness

Chronic diseases are not only common; they are also costly for families and society. By 2030, it is estimated that 83.4 million people in the United States will be living with three or more chronic diseases. In 2016, the total direct costs for chronic disease health care were $1.1 trillion (Waters & Graf, 2018). Between 2015 and 2050, the total estimated economic burden for cancer medical costs is estimated to be $10.4 trillion (Chen et al., 2018). The economic burden of chronic disease in the United States by 2050 is estimated to be $94.9 trillion. The global cost of chronic disease in 2030 is estimated to be $47 trillion by 2030 (Chen et al., 2018); cardiovascular disease cost is estimated to be $863 billion and to rise to $7 trillion by 2050 (Chen et al., 2018). Diabetes costs are projected to cost the global economy $2.1 trillion by 2030 (Bommer et al., 2018).

The national economic burden of Parkinson's disease is estimated at $51.9 billion, with approximately 1 million individuals being diagnosed in 2017 (Yang et al., 2020). The total estimated economic burden includes an estimated direct medical cost of $25.4 billion and an indirect/nonmedical cost of $26.5 billion, which includes (1) $14.2 billion for individuals with Parkinson's disease and caregiver burden combined, (2) $7.5 billion for nonmedical costs, and (3) $4.8 billion due to disability income received for those individuals with Parkinson's disease (Yang et al., 2020). When chronic illness is considered, it is useful to recognize that, in addition to the associated dollar costs of various chronic diseases, there is also a loss in productivity and wages because of absenteeism.

In Canada, chronic disease costs are estimated at $190 billion annually, with an additional $122 billion associated with indirect income and productivity losses (Chronic Disease Prevention Alliance of Canada, 2017). In 2019, the economic burden of diabetes in Canada was about $30 billion, which is a significant increase from $14 billion in 2008 (Diabetes Canada, 2019). In 2010, the three major chronic lung diseases (cancer, asthma, and chronic obstructive pulmonary disease) had an economic burden in Canada of $12 billion, with projections of this number doubling by 2030 (Theriault et al., 2012).

In 2019, 14% of Canadians aged 15 and older (roughly 4.3 million people) smoked (Government of Canada, 2019a). However, this is a decrease from 2014, when roughly 18.1% of Canadians aged 12 and older smoked (Statistics Canada, 2020). Tobacco use causes nearly 8 million deaths per year worldwide, with 1.2 million of the deaths occurring in nonsmokers exposed to secondhand smoke (WHO, 2020b). In the United States, more than 480,000 deaths occur annually from cigarette smoking and from secondhand smoke (CDC, 2020d). The total economic burden of smoking is estimated to be more than $300 billion a year. Indirect costs, including loss of productivity when an ill person cannot work and the loss of productivity in the workplace when family leave is taken, was estimated to be $156 billion (CDC, 2020d). Economic costs for chronic illnesses such as diabetes are continuing to increase. The global economic costs are estimated to increase significantly from $1.3 trillion in 2015 to $2.1 trillion in 2030 (Bommer et al., 2018). In Canada, the economic cost of diabetes was approximately $30 billion in 2019, which accounts for about 3.5% of public health care spending in Canada (Diabetes Canada, 2019). In 2020, diabetes was reported to cost Americans $327 billion. Direct medical costs were $237 billion and indirect costs, such as disability, work loss, and premature death, were $90 billion (CDC, 2020c). Financial costs for this disease are even greater when the family pays for additional health care needs, such as over-the-counter medication and medical supplies, additional visits to optometrists or dentists, health complications that occur

before the diabetes is diagnosed, lost productivity at work for the individual and family members, and costs for informal caregiving. Because of continued emphasis on treatment of disease and related complications rather than prevention, the cost of diabetes continues to climb.

- At the current rate, a 42% increase in cases of the seven chronic diseases is predicted by 2023, with $4.2 trillion in treatment costs and lost economic output.
- Modest improvements in preventing and treating diseases could avoid 40 million cases of chronic disease by 2023, with the economic effect of chronic illness decreased by 27%, or $1.1 trillion annually from the current cost.
- Decreased obesity rates, a large risk factor linked with chronic illness, could result in productivity gains of $254 billion and avoid $60 billion in annual treatment expenditures.

Many with chronic illnesses fear they will be unable to afford needed medical care, a fear not unfounded because medical costs for those with chronic illness tend to be higher. Families with a child or an adult member with a chronic condition often face economic challenges. For example, in diabetes management, although medical insurance may cover the costs of medications and supplies such as syringes and glucose testing strips, other health-promoting activities might require out-of-pocket expenses. A person with diabetes needs to eat a balanced diet, which requires the purchase of foods high in nutritional value—food that might be more expensive than less healthy foods.

Lay caregivers, although posing far less of an economic burden on the health care system, come with their own set of costs. Still, the cost of funding caregiver services and support is small compared with the value of their contributions. Policy recommendations that can make these relatively less costly unpaid caregivers' services (Family Caregiver Alliance, 2018) less burdensome to families include the following:

- Implement family-friendly workplace policies (e.g., flextime, telecommuting).
- Expand the Family and Medical Leave Act (FMLA) and include the definition of eligible employees under FMLA beyond

the care of immediate family members to include care for siblings, in-laws, and grandparents.

- Provide adequate funding for the Lifespan Respite Care Program. This program coordinated systems of accessible, community-based respite-care services for family caregivers of children and adults of all ages with special needs (Administration for Community Living, 2019).
- Provide a tax credit for caregiving.
- Permit payment of family caregivers through consumer-directed models in publicly funded programs (e.g., Medicaid home, community-based services waivers).
- Assess family caregivers' own needs through publicly funded home and community-based service programs and referral to supportive services.

Costs Associated With Children and Youth With Special Health Care Needs

In addition to the health care provided in clinical settings, children and youth with special health care needs (CYSHCN) often require illness management and health maintenance in the home (Mattson & Kuo, 2019). The increased time and care demands of CYSHCN can make it difficult for family caregivers to be employed fully, and emotional stress and financial burdens can result. It is estimated that family caregivers provide 1.5 billion hours of care annually for the 5.6 million CYSHCN (Romley et al., 2017). A child might need special therapy such as physical, speech, or occupational assistance. In addition, these families may have to pay more for everyday living expenses, such as water, heating, or special clothes or equipment, that are not included in their health plan. Parents of CYSHCN may lose pay if they need to take days off from work to care for their child (Mattson & Kuo, 2019; Romley et al., 2017).

Parents working in low-income jobs often do not receive adequate health insurance benefits. Some families earn too much money to qualify for public subsidies but not enough money to cover the health care expenses of raising CYSHCN. Compared with children in higher-income (and also lowest-income) households, children living in such lower-income families are more likely to have gaps in insurance coverage and more likely to be uninsured (Romley et al., 2017).

Ethical Considerations in Chronic Illness

Within health care ethics, four primary principles are often discussed: autonomy, beneficence, nonmaleficence, and justice. When it comes to chronic illness, these principles are not regularly considered, and little research exists examining the ethics involved with chronic illness and chronic care. Health care professionals including nurses, patients, and their families, however, potentially encounter several ethical problems.

Because much of the management of a chronic illness is provided by the patient or the family at home rather than a health care professional, many ethical issues are overlooked (Walker, 2019). For example, privacy in chronic care goes beyond just protecting patient data; chronic illness can have an impact on self-perception and self-confidence resulting from altered appearance and stigma, making privacy issues reach beyond the walls of the health facility (Mahmoud, 2018). In addition, informed consent goes beyond just consenting for a specific procedure; rather, it is an ongoing process for care and management that is ever changing (Walker, 2019). Baskin (2020) describes how patients seek care in the emergency department for chronic conditions that cannot be controlled adequately at home and how providers often feel a negative bias toward the patients seeking this type of care in an emergency setting. These patients, however, are subsequently sent back to their home environments without adequate resources and where they continue to be uncontrolled (Baskin, 2020). These situations just described are only a few examples of ethical problems with justice and resource distribution as well as with autonomy and self-determination.

How do nurses make sense of the inequality of health care resource distribution that leads to inequitable health outcomes? This is one example of an ethical problem that falls under the principle of justice. Justice is defined as "fair, equitable, and appropriate distribution of benefits and burdens" (Beauchamp & Childress, 2019, p. 268). As noted earlier, large amounts of resources are spent around the world on the management of chronic conditions. Hallway conversations and small-group discussions often involve nurses discussing the inequality of care and available resources for patients. When it comes to chronic illness, several problems contribute to this inequality. Many of these problems have been discussed previously and include health disparities and bias, socioeconomic status, and social determinants of health. These issues are out of the nurse's control, but they can weigh heavily on a nurse, particularly when a patient has poor outcomes. Much of the care and management needed for chronic illness is provided at home by the patient or the patient's family. Nurses can provide education, but if patients lack means (e.g., financial, insurance, cognitive, physical, etc.), they may not be able to obtain the care they need at home to ensure positive outcomes and maintain their desired quality of life. There remains an inequity gap between the care nurses and other health care professionals are able to provide in a health care facility and the varying degrees of care that patients are able to receive at home on an ongoing basis. The evidence shows that justice concerns—that is, decreased resources and access to care—correlate with patients having worse outcomes (Khullar & Chokshi, 2018). This can ultimately leave nurses feeling distressed about poor outcomes for their patients.

Autonomy and the right to self-determination is another problem area in chronic illness. This is an important principle because it also integrates respecting the patient and the patient's sense of self-worth. When health care professionals discuss autonomy and self-determination, the topic typically centers around consent/informed consent in an acute setting, such as for a particular procedure. In patients with chronic illness, consent is not a one-time occurrence for a particular action or procedure. Because patients experience chronic illness over a long period of time, self-determination is an ongoing process, one that has the potential to change frequently. Nurses often find it difficult to accept a patient's or family's choice not to adhere to proposed management plans. Nurses should understand that patients and families deal with these illnesses on an ongoing, daily basis, not on a short-term, one-time-only basis, and that they often experience suffering that can change the

perspective and goals of the patient. Often, patients use different decision-making processes for different stages of their illness that takes into account a variety of changing factors. The ability to care for oneself, the resources involved and the difficulty in accessing those resources, the emotional and mental effort, stigma, level of control, and suffering often weigh heavily and have an impact on the decisions and actions of the patient. It is important for the nurse to honor patients' desires to control their lives and their care because this ultimately shows respect for the patient and the patient's sense of worth and self-determination.

The Nurse's Role

While ethical issues can be difficult to think about, knowing that the role of the nurse is to support and advocate for the patient helps define the role in these difficult circumstances. Protecting the patient's right to self-determination points to the need for nurses to assess patients' choices at the present time and discuss those choices with them while knowing that patients' choices and actions change over time. Taking the time to gain a better understanding of the patient's experience and avoiding stereotyping and labeling helps to provide the support the patient needs. Also, having a better understanding for the suffering of the patient helps to inform the patient's decisions and the nurse's understanding of those decisions (Baskin, 2020). Ultimately, the goal is to support and advocate for patient's choices with both family members and the other health care professionals, which will help protect the patient's right to autonomy and self-determination. Justice-related concerns are often a broader issue, but using the nurse's role of advocacy to help connect patients to needed resources within the community can be helpful. Examples of such resources include support groups, free clinics, educational material, transportation resources, and so on. This can also help the patient achieve the best outcomes.

Ethics related to chronic illness is not discussed frequently in the literature, and more research is needed. It is important for nurses to understand, however, that ethical issues do arise in chronic care. Discussing these issues helps to bring them to the forefront so problems can be addressed, and better care can be provided.

THEORETICAL PERSPECTIVES: WAYS TO UNDERSTAND CHRONIC ILLNESS

Family health care within a frame of chronic illness works best when it moves beyond merely the individual or cultural focus and toward considering the family as a whole plus its individual parts (Rolland, 2019). Understanding illness beliefs on a family level enhances the nurse's ability to work with family members to develop a plan of care that works for the entire family. Few ethnocultural models address the application of transcultural assessment when working with families dealing with a chronic illness. Nursing is well positioned to use transcultural models that integrate multiple worldviews, with a greater emphasis on the strengths of individuals managing chronic conditions and the nurses who assist in their care.

By using an ethnocultural model as an overarching perspective of working with families, nurses strengthen their ability to establish relationships with families in context as they apply chronic illness models in their practice. The Ethno-Cultural Gerontological Nursing Model (ECGNM) (Phillips et al., 2015), is one of the few transcultural models that include family care. By using multiple theoretical perspectives, nurses have more flexibility to offer options to families in the management of their chronic illness. Three additional models specific to living with chronic illness are briefly explained: Rolland's Chronic Illness and the Life Cycle: A Conceptual Framework (1987), the Family Management Style Framework (FMSF) (Knafl & Deatrick, 1990, 2003; Knafl et al., 2012), and the Family Health Model (FHM) (Denham, 2003). These models provide unique perspectives on assessment, goal planning, nursing actions, and outcome evaluation using a family-focused point of view in chronic illness.

ECGNM

ECGNM lays the groundwork for focusing on diversity with an aging population (Phillips et al., 2015); however, it is also applicable to other populations. A central principle of this model is that patients are best served when nurses focus not only on the differences but also on the similarities within and among cultural groups, with particular focus on the strengths of individuals, families, and generational cohorts in the communities in which they live. By assessing various macrosocial and microsocial forces, family nurses working with individuals and families dealing with a chronic illness are better able to assess the needs and resources available to families.

A review of ECGNM demonstrates the interrelationship between macro- and microsocial influences, thus assisting nurses to assess how various forces intersect and influence individual, family, and ethnocultural groups' interpretation of health, illness, and life events in various phases of their lives (see Figure 10-1). The top and lower frames of the model list various macrosocial factors, including historical, political, economic, and public policy factors, as well as the environmental climate and stereotypes. On the lower frame, group influences are outlined, including discrimination, health and self-care, traditions, how gender and cohort influences interact with historical events, and the meaning ascribed to these elements by individuals and family. Running across the center of the model are microsocial (personal) dimensions such as health, biological and generic variations, individual and family experiences, modes of communication, resources, and sociocultural factors that in turn influence the interpretation, responses, and ultimately health experiences and health outcomes. In an analysis of the utility of ECGNM for working with diverse Latino populations, Ruiz et al. (2016) demonstrated how health, culture, language, and aging intersect and contribute to health outcomes for this population. The model has been used successfully to analyze various family beliefs, knowledge, confidence, and experiences from various cultural backgrounds and experiences of health across the continuum (Crist et al., 2017; Crist, Montgomery, et al., 2018; Crist, Ortiz-Dowling, et al., 2018).

As proposed, ECGNM offers nurses an expanded framework for conducting a more comprehensive assessment of individuals and families. For nurses, the model provides an expanded framework for gaining insight into the strengths of a family as well as exploring a wider net of creative resources that may be utilized by families living with a chronic illness or other challenging life event.

Historical Period Events

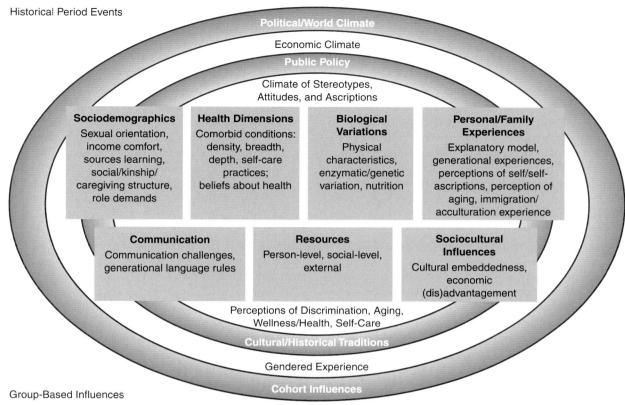

FIGURE 10-1 Ethno-Cultural Gerontological Nursing Model (ECGNM) *Source: Reprinted with permission from Phillips, L., et al. [2015]. Developing and proposing the Ethno-cultural Gerontological Nursing Model.* Journal of Transcultural Nursing, *26(2), 121.*

Rolland's Chronic Illness and the Life Cycle: A Conceptual Framework

Chronic illnesses can be categorized by their traits, as outlined in Rolland's (1987, 2018) Chronic Illness and the Life Cycle: A Conceptual Framework. This framework outlines how the following three aspects come together in families and explains how families with similar illness stories adapt differently:

- *Illness type:* Illness type encompasses several components, including onset of the illness (acute or gradual), course of the illness (constant, progressive, episodic/relapsing), outcome of the illness (fatal, unpredictable, nonfatal), level of disability resulting from the conditions (capacitating or incapacitating), and uncertainty.
- *Time phases:* Time phases of the chronic illness include diagnosis/initial crisis, mid-illness/chronic, or terminal phase.

- *Components of family function:* Family function components include organization and structural patterns, communication processes, belief and belief systems, and development such as multigenerational patterns. (See Figure 10-2.)

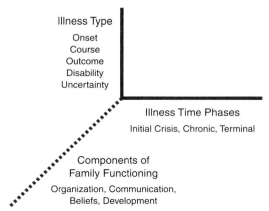

FIGURE 10-2 Family System Illness (FSI) Model: Three Dimensions *Source: Reprinted with permission of Guilford Press.*

In Rolland's framework, the preceding elements of chronic illness affect family functioning, strengths, and vulnerabilities. Rolland's framework recognizes several influences on the illness, disability, and loss that occurs. These influences include the family and the individual's life course, family patterns, and belief systems (culture, ethnicity, race, spirituality, gender, and socioeconomic status). For example, although some chronic conditions involve primary disabilities, such as those occurring from birth anomalies, other conditions, such as strokes, myocardial infarctions, secondary blindness, or kidney failure, are acquired disabilities resulting from lifestyle patterns or delayed or ineffective treatment of other conditions. The reactions and adaptations of the individual and family to a chronic condition differ according to whether the disability is considered on-time and expected versus off-time and unexpected. Although some people with chronic conditions have lives fraught with pain, depression, and mental or physical difficulties, others experience satisfying lives with only minimal difficulties. The family processes, development, and beliefs influence the experience of the patient and family with the illness.

FMSF

FMSF was designed to help nurses understand how families who have a child with a chronic condition integrate management of the chronic illness for the child into the everyday living needs and routines of the family as a whole. The original work on the development of FMSF was conducted by Knafl and Deatrick in 1990. This original work has been refined over time to be one of the most significant longitudinal studies of a family assessment instrument. The assessment instrument Family Management Measure (FaMM) (Knafl et al., 2011, 2007) helps nurses understand the needs of families who have children with specific chronic conditions, such as brain tumors (Deatrick et al., 2006), children undergoing palliative care at home (Bousso et al., 2012), and adolescents who have spina bifida (Wollenhaupt et al., 2011). With updates over time, the framework has become more applicable to a broader range of families managing childhood chronic illness (Knafl et al., 2012) and now incorporates contextual influences on the experience. This framework has also been used to increase understanding of challenges for families who have an older adult with dementia (Beeber & Zimmerman, 2012). More recently, the framework has been adapted to include children (Beacham & Deatrick, 2019) as well as to understand familial response to parental advanced cancer (Park et al., 2019). Figure 10-3 depicts the revised FMSF model (Knafl et al., 2012).

Understanding the family's responses to a chronic condition provides ways for family nurses

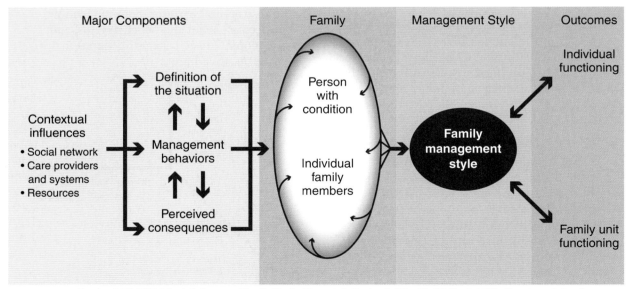

FIGURE 10-3 Revised FMSF Model *Source: Knafl, K. A., Deatrick, J. A., & Havill, N. L. (2012). Continued development of the Family Management Style Framework.* Journal of Family Nursing, *18(1), 11–24.*

to offer effective interventions to meet the needs of both the individual and the family. This framework includes five family management styles: thriving, accommodating, enduring, struggling, and floundering. The management style a family adopts is based on how the family members define the situation, manage the situation, and perceive the consequences of the situation. In FMSF, the parents each define what the child's chronic condition means for them individually and their family. Included in this definition is how the parents view the child. Does the parent view the child as a child who has a health issue that can be managed, or does the parent focus on the condition before the child and see the management of the health condition as tragic and difficult to manage? Influencing the definition are the parents' personal beliefs about the cause, seriousness, predictability, and course of the condition. Another component in defining the illness is how disparate or similar the two parents' perceptions are on how they view their child, the condition, parenting philosophy, and overall approach to management. Table 10-1 briefly outlines the five family management styles.

Managing the child's condition is another piece of the process of establishing a family's management style. To manage illness, parents combine their philosophy of parenting with their beliefs about their ability to parent a child with a chronic condition. One management approach may be that of being confident in their ability to parent and manage a chronic health condition. A second management approach may be when the parent views the child and situation as burdensome. A third approach is when parents feel they are inadequate in their abilities to parent a child with a chronic condition.

Another element of management concentrates on how the parent balances the ability to manage the chronic health condition with other aspects of family life. Parental management behaviors linked with chronic illness are often aligned with the parents' ability to establish consistent and effective treatment routines. Parents may not be well prepared to handle the caregiving responsibilities shortly after receiving a chronic illness diagnosis; they might require some coaching (Sullivan-Bolyai et al., 2004). Stable routines that allow for balance or equilibrium in daily life are essential for optimal disease management over time and change throughout the life course. For example, if the

chronic illness requires dietary changes, family members must learn ways to balance personal food preferences and prior eating patterns with the medical needs of the ill family member. Although specific management or routine activities may vary, a predictable and consistent routine is beneficial.

Finally, the ways parents focus attention on and perceive consequences of a chronic illness are an important consideration in determining the family's management style. Chronic illness can be viewed as a central feature of the family, an organizing focus, or a life aspect balanced with other responsibilities.

FMSF not only identifies cognitive and behavioral family aspects but also points to factors that may be predictive of family strengths or problems (Knafl & Deatrick, 1990, 2003; Knafl et al., 2012). Nurses using this framework are urged to consider the unique needs of individuals within the family, those of family members or member dyads, and the family as a whole. Family nurses should use this model as a guideline that outlines ways to think about how a family is responding to having a child with a chronic illness. Nurses can use this framework to help think of interventions that may help a family in the management of the situation and adaptation to living with a chronic condition. Nurses need to understand member dynamics and family processes as they assess care needs, provide education, and offer counseling.

FHM

Connections between chronic illness and families are tied to ideas suggested within FHM (Denham, 2003). This ecological model provides a lens to consider the multiple traits, interactive processes, and life experiences that influence the health and illness of interacting and developing persons. Families and individual members have infinite ways to define themselves as they interact and exchange information with larger societal systems and institutions. The family household is the hub of action where members depart and return as individual members are nurtured and socialized. FHM identifies member connections to each other and those beyond the household boundaries that have relevance to chronic illness. FHM uses three domains—contextual, functional, and structural—in which nurses perform assessments, plan care, provide nursing actions, and evaluate outcomes.

| Table 10-1 | **Family Management Style Framework** | | | |

View of the Child

THRIVING	ACCOMMODATING	ENDURING	STRUGGLING	FLOUNDERING
Parents view child from the lens of normalcy. They see the child as just as capable as other children. Their child has a chronic health condition that is incorporated into the everyday life of the child and the family as a whole.	Parents usually see their child from the lens of normalcy and being capable of living everyday life.	Parents fluctuate in their view of the child between that of normalcy and tragic. Sometimes see their child as capable and other times focus on the child's vulnerabilities.	Parents are inconsistent in how they view the child relative to normalcy capabilities and vulnerabilities.	Parents have primarily a negative view of their child and see the situation as tragic. They see the child as not capable and as vulnerable.
Parents view life as normal and incorporate the management of the health condition into the everyday life of the child and family.	Parents tend to view life as normal and caring for the child with a chronic condition, and the chronic condition as part of life.	Parents vary on how they view life: between normal or focused on the management of the health condition.	Parents are variable in how they view everyday life, but they see it primarily from a negative lens and management of the chronic condition overtakes their everyday life as a family.	Parents view the situation as a burden and have a sense of hatefulness about having to manage their child's chronic health condition.
Parents mutually agree in their viewpoints and definition of the child and their management approach.	Parents usually share the same viewpoints, definition, and management choices.	Parents usually share the same viewpoints, definition, and management choices.	Parents do not share the same viewpoints and definition and do not agree on management approaches, which creates much conflict between the parents.	Parents differ significantly on how they view the child, how they define the situation, and the management plan.

Management Behaviors

THRIVING	ACCOMMODATING	ENDURING	STRUGGLING	FLOUNDERING
Parents are confident in their management abilities and incorporate the management regimen into the life of the family. They are proactive in their problem-solving approach.	Mothers are confident in their abilities to manage the chronic condition. Fathers are not as confident as the mothers in their abilities to manage the illness. They are usually proactive in problem solving, but they are sometimes are reactive.	Parents are confident in their abilities, but they view the management regimen as burdensome. They are usually proactive in problem solving, but sometimes they are reactive.	Parental conflict is the overriding theme. Mothers see the management regimen as burdensome. Fathers express more confidence in their ability to manage the chronic condition. Neither parent anticipates problems that are routine; therefore, they are reactive to problems.	Parents view the management regimen as burdensome. They feel inadequate and overwhelmed. They are reactive to problems and are often overwhelmed or put into crisis mode when a problem occurs.

Perceived Consequences

THRIVING	ACCOMMODATING	ENDURING	STRUGGLING	FLOUNDERING
Parents view the child in the foreground and see the stress and hassles of the chronic health condition in the background. Parents have a positive outlook and create a new sense of "normal" for the family as a whole.	Parents usually place the child in the foreground and the stress and strains of the chronic condition in the background. In general, the parents have a positive outlook for the family as a whole.	Parents fluctuate in how they perceive the outcome and the stress and strains of the chronic condition on the child and the family.	Mothers typically have a negative view of the situation and future outlook for the child. Fathers tend to be more positive in their view of the future for the child.	Parents have a negative outlook and view of the future. They worry that their future as parents will be less happy and limited.

This model encourages nurses to consider ecological factors relevant to the family members and their household. Factors such as the neighborhood, community resources, community demographics, political milieu, and social environment also influence families' responses to chronic illness and disease management and affect outcomes.

Operational definitions suggest ways to describe the complex relationships among the biophysical and holistic aspects of a chronic illness and how these aspects affect family, health, and family health. In FHM, health is defined as an adaptive state experienced by family members as they seek to optimize their well-being and wrestle with liabilities found within self, family, households, and the various environments where they interact throughout the life course (Denham, 2003). This definition guides nursing practice roles useful for family care when a member has a chronic illness. Even when one has a chronic illness, health can still be possible, and well-being can be maximized.

Family health suggests that member transactions occur through system and subsystem interactions, relationships, and processes that have the potential to maximize processes of becoming, enhance well-being, and capitalize on the household production of health. Families strive to achieve a state where members are content with themselves and one another. That is, family health includes the complex interactions of individuals, family subsystems, family, and the various contexts experienced over the life course. The household becomes the pivotal point for coping with health and family health needs.

Contextual Domain

Family health is depicted with contextual, functional, and structural dimensions (Figure 10-4). The *contextual domain* includes all the environments where family members interact or have potential to be acted on, but it also includes the characteristics or traits of the family (e.g., socioeconomic

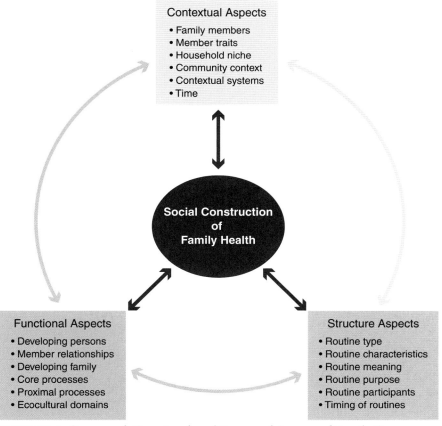

FIGURE 10-4 Contextual, Functional, and Structural Aspects of Family Care

status, educational attainment, extended kin relationships). The contextual domain is affected by the internal household environment (e.g., membership traits and qualities, culture, traditions, values) and external household environment (e.g., neighborhood, community, safety, larger society, historical period, political context). An ecological model helps nurses understand that nested life aspects can challenge or strengthen one's abilities to discern causes and outcomes. Over time, it is difficult to decipher the many powerful influencers; they overlap, intersect, and potentiate or negate important health factors.

The family household is a key family environment or context. The *household* refers to the physical structure(s), immediate neighborhood surroundings, material and nonmaterial goods, and tangible and intangible family resources of the members that live together. As people age, they often reflect back on many households where they lived and the various influences impressed upon self from those settings. The family context pervades all life aspects and affects personal interactions, values, attitudes, access to medical resources, and availability of support systems, and influences individual and family health routines. For example, a family living in poverty or lacking adequate health care insurance is unlikely to have the same access to medical care as a more affluent family. A rural family with a long tradition of cultural values about health or illness might minimize physical symptoms and be slower to seek medical care than an urban family with great confidence in science and the abilities of health care providers.

Functional Domain

The *functional domain* refers to the individual and cooperative processes that family members use as they interact with and engage one another during the life course. This domain includes individual factors (e.g., values, perceptions, personality, coping, spirituality, motivation, roles), family process factors (e.g., cohesiveness, resilience, individuation, boundaries), and member or family processes (e.g., communication, coordination, caregiving, control). These dynamic factors mediate the actions of individuals, family subsystems, and families as a whole as they seek to attain, sustain, maintain, and regain health. The core family functions of caregiving, celebration, change, communication, connectedness, and coordination alter as families face

health and illness; these are areas where nurses can assess, plan nursing actions, and collaborate with family members to improve chronic illness outcomes (Denham, 2003).

The experiences linked with chronic illness can test and burden the functional capacities of the family and its members. In some families, individual and group strengths can be rallied to address pressing concerns, whereas other families might have member conflicts that threaten the capacities of effective disease management.

Structural Domain

The contextual and functional domains are the situational and behavioral antecedents that family members use to construct family habits or patterns linked with health and illness outcomes. The third aspect of FHM is referred to as the *structural domain;* it is composed of six categories of family health routines: self-care, safety and precautions, mental health behaviors, family care, illness care, and member caretaking. Each routine category is comprised of complex multimember habitual actions that form interactive patterns that describe the lived health and illness experiences of family households (Denham, 2003). Family health routines are relatively stable but still dynamic actions or habitual patterns that can be recalled, described, and discussed from individual and family perspectives. What might initially appear as random or chaotic patterns to an outsider may represent to family members regularity, purpose, and value of individual routines.

Although routines have unique qualities and involve all household members, some aspects of them change and evolve over time. This evolution can be a voluntary and intentional act, or it can be a consequence of other events in the family's life. Family members tend to maintain the integrity of routines as long as they are viewed as meaningful. New life situations can cause some adaptations to occur, however. Health routines tend toward steadfastness, but the diagnosis of a chronic condition that demands medical management and the availability of new or different support or resources (i.e., contextual factors) can challenge prior valued routines. If the family uses effective modes of communication, can share roles, and is comprised of resilient personalities, it might be more capable of handling the changes during a chronic condition than those families lacking these qualities. Family members might be able to cooperate and deconstruct ineffective routines and reconstruct new ones better than a disorganized family or one where member conflict rules. Health and illness routines are ways family members can support or thwart the management of a chronic illness. Family-focused nurses who partner with individuals and families can collaborate with them to plan care, strategize ways to implement changes, and evaluate outcomes. The creation and stability of healthy family routines and lifestyles can be strengthened through cooperative efforts. Family health routines depend on the human and material resources needed for the individual and family to make needed changes. Functional perspectives give insight into ways families optimize health potentials and use resources to balance diverse and conflicting needs.

Well-Being

Family-focused nurses strive to assist individuals and families make the most of available resources to achieve health and well-being. *Well-being*, in the Family Health Care Model (Denham, 2003), is defined as a health state with actualized opportunities, minimized liabilities, and maximized resources. Well-being includes many dimensions, including biophysical, psychological, emotional, social, spiritual, and vocational. Well-being is achieved through accomplishment of family goals such as risk reduction, disease prevention, health maintenance, and self-actualization. Nurses aim to provide holistic care that enhances well-being and to partner with families to empower them when chronic illness is the concern. Nurses who provide family-focused care aid individuals and families to achieve their health goals. They also empower members to devise plans and identify ways to implement strategies, and evaluate whether goals are met. Nursing encounters become a means to target the household production of health or holistically address related or potentially related health attributes or threats.

In chronic illness, family-focused care assists multiple family members to adapt, accommodate, and use household resources to achieve well-being for the entire family. Based on FHM, family-focused nurses can use what are identified as core processes to consider family aspects relevant to chronic disease management and identify ways to empower individuals and families to meet care goals (Table 10-2). FHM suggests a variety of ways to understand what happens when a member has a chronic illness from contextual, functional, and structural perspectives (Denham, 2003). Table 10-3 identifies several areas that a family nurse might assess using this conceptual model.

PREVENTION OF CHRONIC ILLNESS THROUGH HEALTH PROMOTION

Many chronic conditions are preventable. Others, though not preventable, may be able to be delayed, thus ensuring more quality years of life. Prevention is an important factor to consider when understanding chronic illnesses. In fact, prevention has been a focus to reduce disease and improve health both within specific countries and worldwide. For example, WHO (2013) has implemented a Global Action Plan (2013-2020) with an initiative of 25% reduction of noncommunicable diseases such as cardiovascular disease, cancer, diabetes, and chronic respiratory disease by 2025. Because many preventable chronic diseases have common modifiable risk factors (tobacco use, unhealthy diet/poor nutrition, physical inactivity, and harmful use of alcohol), programs are often aimed at behavior change related to these. The Global Action Plan includes myriad policies and programs that can be adopted and implemented to aid health promotion and disease prevention (WHO, 2013).

Various prevention programs exist at the local, national, and federal levels. For example, the CDC's National Center for Chronic Disease Prevention and Health Promotion (NCCDPHP) (CDC, 2020a) has a budget of $1.2 billion (fiscal year [FY] 2020) to conduct research on the effects of chronic conditions and interventions, provide funding, and offer guidance on how to reduce common risk factors for chronic diseases, especially in groups affected by health disparities. Canada also has myriad programs, initiatives, and strategies to promote health and prevent chronic disease (Public Health Agency of Canada, 2019), including the Canadian Diabetes Strategy, Healthy Living Fund, and Integrated Strategy for Healthy Living and Chronic Disease (Public Health Agency of Canada, 2019). A program funded by the CDC, Communities Putting Prevention to Work (CPPW),

Table 10-2 Core Family Processes and Chronic Illness

CORE PROCESSES	DEFINITION	AREAS OF CONCERN	
Caregiving	Concern generated from close intimate family relationships and member affections that result in watchful attention, thoughtfulness, and actions linked to members' developmental, health, and illness needs.	Health maintenance Disease prevention Risk reduction Health promotion	Illness care Rehabilitation Acute episodic needs Chronic concerns
Cathexis	Emotional bonds between individuals and family that result in members' emotional and psychic energy investments into needs of the loved one.	Attachment Commitment Affiliation Loss	Grief and mourning Normative processes Complicated processes
Celebration	Tangible forms of shared meanings that occur through family celebrations, family traditions, and leisure time that might be used to commemorate special times, days, and events. These times are often used to distinguish usual daily routines from special ones, and they often occur across the life course and have special roles, responsibilities, and expectations.	Culture Family fun Traditions Rituals	Religion Hobbies Shared activities
Change	A dynamic nonlinear process that demands an altered form, direction, and/or outcome of an expected identity, role, activity, or desired future.	Control Meet expressed needs Meanings of change Contextual influences	Compare and contrast Similarities/differences Diversity
Communication	The primary ways that children are socialized and family members interact over the life course about health beliefs, values, attitudes, and behaviors, and incorporate or apply health information and knowledge for illness and health concerns.	Language Symbolic interactions Information access Coaching Cheerleading	Knowledge and skills Emotional needs Affective care Spiritual needs
Connectedness	The ways that systems beyond the family household are linked with multiple family members through family, educational, cultural, spiritual, political, social, professional, legal, economic, or commercial interests.	Partner relationships Kin networks Household labor Cooperation Member roles	Family rules Boundaries Tolerance for ambiguity Marginalization
Coordination	Cooperative sharing of resources, skills, abilities, and information within the family household, among members of extended kin networks, and larger contextual environments to optimize individual's health potentials, enhance the household production of health, maintain family integrity or wellness, and achieve family goals.	Family tasks Problem solving Decision making Valuing Coping Resilience	Respect Reconciliation Forgiveness Cohesiveness System integrity Stress management

Source: Modified from Denham, S. A. (2003). *Family health: A framework for nursing.* Philadelphia, PA: F. A. Davis, with permission.

Table 10-3 Assessment Using the Family Health Model	
CATEGORIES TO ASSESS	**SPECIFIC AREAS WITHIN EACH CATEGORY**
Contextual	• Developmental stage
	• Family traits
	• Availability of health insurance
	• Access to care
	• Demographics (age, education, sex, employment)
	• Social support
	• Culture and ethnicity
	• Political, historical, and environmental factors
Functional	• Stressors
	• Coping skills
	• Family roles
	• Member responsibilities
	• Communication patterns
Structural	• Illness characteristics
	• Family organization or chaos
	• Routines established
	• Ability and willingness to alter routines

was implemented in 50 communities and showed that, for less than $5 per person, 84% to 89% of health promotion and disease prevention programs can be covered, particularly tobacco, nutrition, and physical activity interventions and services (Honeycutt et al., 2016).

Nurses play an important role in advocating for health promotion and policy change related to helping societies improve health. Evidence shows that policy-based strategies and larger scale planning are often more effective at creating positive behavior change than individually based interventions (Leong et al., 2017). For example, in areas where policies have been implemented related to tobacco use, including increasing cost, decreasing availability, and adjusting marketing, the policies significantly reduced tobacco use rates (Rosen et al., 2010). Urban and neighborhood planning that included more walkable destinations, closer grocery stores, and fewer or further fast-food establishments correlates with less obesity (Boehmer et al., 2007; Durand et al., 2011; Garfinkel-Castro et al., 2017; Librett et al., 2006; Sallis et al., 2012).

While health promotion improves quality of life and helps prevent disease, some evidence shows it helps decrease costs as well. The 2010–2012 CDC CPPW program allocated $403 million to communities to reduce obesity, tobacco use, and exposure to secondhand smoke and saved $2.4 billion in direct medical costs (Soler et al., 2016). For example, a 35% tax on sugar-sweetened drinks ($0.45 per drink) led to a 26% decline in sales, with the conclusion that a 20% tax on these drinks would reduce obesity levels by 3.5% in U.S. adults (Mytton et al., 2012). Workplace programs instituted to improve the health of employees have shown a 25% savings each on health care costs, worker's compensation, absenteeism, and disability management claims costs (Chapman, 2005). On an individual level, smoking cessation saves $5 per pack; for an individual who smokes one pack per day, this can save $1,825 per year (CDC, 2015). In addition, many insurance companies provide lower insurance premiums for nonsmokers, thus creating additional savings (CDC, 2015).

In looking at gaps of current data collection systems, the Institute of Medicine (IOM) (2011) suggests that individual and collective data are needed that help understand the continuum of prevention, disease progression, treatment options, and their outcomes. Joseph et al. (2017) also explain the need for improved monitoring of progress and health information to better guide health policy development and implementation. A troubling aspect of all surveillance efforts is that we have little to no information about family roles, inputs, or outcomes in the prevention or management of chronic illness.

Nonetheless, chronic illness is often linked to behavioral and environmental risk factors that could be effectively addressed through prevention programs. For example, the increasing rates of obesity, leading to several chronic complications, could be prevented with changes in dietary and exercise behaviors and changes in our environment that encourage exercise. A 2017 Prevention and Wellness Trust Fund (PWTF) report highlights what was accomplished when Massachusetts lawmakers created PWTF to direct health care funding into disease prevention programs (Massachusetts Public Health Association, n.d.). Hypertension screening increased from 58% to 62%, with a projected 5-year, $2 to $3 million health care cost averted. In the 0- to 9-year-old population, asthma rates decreased from 13% to 10% in communities that instituted PWTF school-based education programs (Zotter, 2017). These changes could reduce climbing chronic illness rates and reduce related complications through preventive care.

IOM (2012) suggests taking a "health in all policies" approach to federal regulations, legislation, and policies that improve opportunity for health and physical function for those living with chronic illness. This report also recommends that community-based services available for persons with chronic disease align with health care services and insurance reform legislation. If such an approach were to be taken, legislators and those involved in policy writing would be more conscious of health risks and the ultimate costs resulting from legislative decisions. The U.S. Department of Health and Human Services (USDHHS) has done just this. For the past four decades, the department has published *Healthy People* every 10 years. *Healthy People* is a 10-year national initiative to improve the health of Americans (USDHHS, 2020). *Healthy People 2030* includes directives that delineate the need for evaluation of past and current health indicator sets and adds the importance of objectives related to disease and disease prevention such as social determinants of health, health-related quality of life, and LGBTQ+ health; reducing calorie intake from solid fats and sugars; increasing the proportion of the population who meet physical activity guidelines; and more (USDHHS, 2020). To curb the chronic illness epidemic, it is critical that innovative local, national, and global approaches continue to be developed and implemented to aid in disease prevention and management.

HELPING FAMILIES LIVE WITH CHRONIC ILLNESS

Family-focused nurses understand that when individuals have a chronic illness, whether they are young or old, their family is always involved in the care. Family members influence decision making, engage in family planning, and play roles that positively and negatively influence disease management.

Some people manage their chronic illness without much difficulty or help from others, whereas others require a great amount of assistance and significant family involvement. Many need little medical care, but others require extensive medical services that may include care from special health care providers, regular treatments or testing, multiple medicines, or intense therapies. Life can be completely disrupted when confronting long-term or chronic illnesses that affect physical abilities, appearance, and independence. Diminished endurance capacities; continual discomfort in physical, emotional, and social realms; and financial problems are just a few of the challenges that families face. New medical procedures, diagnostic tests, screening, and pharmacologic therapies have improved health and the ability to live with chronic conditions and have helped to increase the life span, so families are living longer with chronic illness.

IOM (2012) considered what it takes to live well with chronic illness and determined that it requires more than medical care and pharmacologic therapies. IOM suggests that a variety of health determinants affect the life course (i.e., biology, genes, behavior, coping responses, physical environment, sociocultural context, peers, and family). Some of these aspects are linked with learned behaviors, family households, and the communities where families live. One might classify persons as healthy, at risk, chronically ill, functionally limited, disabled, or nearing the end of life. These health outcomes are influenced by several factors; some are intrinsic or controlled by the individual, and some are beyond the individual and originate in the larger society (e.g., environmental risks, public policy, population surveillance, media, public health, community organizations, health care, social values). This section focuses on how to work with families to support the person with the chronic illness to participate in his or her own self-management and ways to help families adapt to living with a chronic illness and working with the family care provider.

Helping to Support Self-Management

Self-management is a crucial aspect to quality living and successful management of a chronic illness. Self-management includes self-efficacy, self-monitoring of illness, and symptom management that is conducted by oneself or by others as directed by the patient (Richard & Shea, 2011). Self-management is both a process and an outcome of family nursing care. The *Self-Management Support for Canadians With Chronic Health Conditions* report (Health Council of Canada, 2012, p. 7) outlines the following four recommendations to help the Canadian health care system support people living with chronic illness in a more systematic way. These recommendations should be applied to those living with chronic illness regardless of country:

- Create an integrated, systemwide approach to self-management support.
- Enable primary health care providers to deliver self-management support as a routine part of care.
- Broaden and deepen efforts to reach more Canadians who need self-management supports.
- Engage patients and informal caregivers as key parts of any systematic approach.

Family nurses work with the individual and family to support self-management of the illness. For example, adolescents and young adults who engage in self-management at the time they transition from pediatric to adult medical care are known to have improved health outcomes (Varty & Popejoy, 2019; Henry & Schor, 2015).

Diabetes is a clear illustration. Diabetes self-management, similar to self-management for any chronic illness, entails adhering to a prescribed medical regimen and making lifestyle behavior changes. Most of these actions largely occur outside nurses' and other health care providers' observation. Self-management calls for integration of prescribed treatments into the daily experience, and it requires highly motivated individuals to follow medically prescribed treatments and protocols that may not be understood fully. This means that the individuals must have some confidence that their health care providers know what they are doing and trust that following these directions will improve their quality of life.

The last several decades have produced a large body of research findings that suggest that self-efficacy is an important factor linked with a willingness to participate in specific behavior (Richard & Shea, 2011). Persons with higher self-efficacy are more likely to engage in more challenging tasks, set higher goals, and achieve them (Bandura, 1977). Individuals with the chronic illness and their family members have different levels of self-efficacy and may differ in their level of readiness for change. Nurses who understand self-efficacy and readiness to change can use these concepts as they collaborate with families to set goals and plan strategies for meeting them. Nurses assess families on their perceptions and abilities to make the changes and then assist them as they agree on what changes they can make together. Nurses can explore family members' desires and confidence in their ability to alter lifestyle habits that might support their family member with a chronic illness to adhere to lifestyle changes, such as diet. A nurse-led family conference might be a way for the nurse to share more information about why changes are needed, benefits that might be realized, and risks if no changes are made. Some agreement might arise on trying a few things differently each week and moving toward the goals by using small steps. Nurses should not be simply telling the family what needs to be done; they should be asking them what they need, identifying their concerns, and helping them set up a plan they are willing to achieve together.

Self-Management in the Older Adult Population

Although many older adults are able to manage their chronic illnesses without additional family or external support, some older adults have difficulty with self-management of their care and require additional support. One of the major aspects of nursing is to assist patients in self-management ability. Self-management of care is not disease management but rather the ability of an individual to direct and maintain control over his or her chronic illness (Richard & Shea, 2011). A metasynthesis of the literature identified five factors affecting self-management of care: (1) personal/lifestyle characteristics, (2) health status, (3) resources, (4) environmental characteristics, and (5) health care system (Schulman-Green et al., 2016). See Table 10-4 for a list of barriers and facilitators that affect self-management.

Personal/Lifestyle Characteristics

Personal/lifestyle characteristics are influenced by knowledge, beliefs, motivation, and life patterns. Individuals who successfully self-manage their care are knowledgeable about their medications and treatment plan and are able to apply that knowledge successfully to their daily lives (Richard & Shea, 2011; Schulman-Green et al., 2016). Nurses who use motivational interviewing assist patients in their self-care.

In order for individuals to self-manage their care successfully, they need knowledge about their disease, medications, and treatment, and how to apply that knowledge to their own care. When there is a lack of understanding and social support about their chronic illness, medications, or treatment, their self-management is impeded, and individuals are less likely to be successful with self-management (Lemstra et al., 2018; Warner et al., 2019; Griva et al., 2013).

Motivation and self-efficacy are intertwined and influenced by an individual's self-discipline or control over his or her personal choices. Stigma was identified as a motivating factor for individuals to take care of themselves so that they could avoid additional health care services and accommodations (Audulv et al., 2009; Ploughman et al., 2012; Warner et al., 2019).

Life patterns and the ability to establish a routine influence an individual's ability to self-manage successfully (Savoca & Miler, 2001). The ability to establish positive self-management routines is correlated with prior positive self-management experiences and subsequent positive health outcomes (Griva et al., 2013). Establishing daily routines is

associated with improved self-management behaviors such as eating healthy and exercising. Conversely, unstructured or disrupted routines negatively affect self-management and the ability of individuals to establish routines (Griva et al., 2013). In addition, aging is associated with impaired self-management primarily because of cognitive impairment and forgetting to take medication (Song et al., 2010).

Health Status

Health status and comorbidities influence self-management. Self-management is hampered by multiple factors, including severity of symptoms; length of illness; adverse effects from treatment, including medication; complex treatment and/or medication regimens; and cognitive function (Saunders, 2019; Schulman-Green et al., 2016). When combined with physical comorbidities, effective self-management is hampered (Griva et al., 2013; Ploughman et al., 2012). A family ecomap is an excellent instrument to help patients and families manage multiple illnesses.

Resources

Resources that influence self-management are financial resources, equipment, and psychosocial support (Lundberg & Thrakul, 2011; Newcomb et al., 2010; Saunders, 2019). Limited financial resources impair an individual's ability to self-manage. Many individuals experiencing chronic illness frequently have multiple medications they need to take daily (polypharmacy). Older adults and the chronically ill are often on a limited, fixed income and are forced to choose between refilling their medications or paying for housing, electricity, food, and transportation (Newcomb et al., 2010; Vest et al., 2013).

Equipment, specifically the internet, is both a barrier and a facilitator in self-management. The internet provides a wealth of information to individuals and can connect them with peer support and information about health conditions (Brand et al., 2010; Wellard et al., 2008). Conversely, the internet provides an overwhelming amount of health information that may not be from reliable and credible sources, causing the patient undue stress (Balfe, 2009). Older adults may experience technology challenges and find the internet too difficult to navigate or understand its content (Aponte &

Table 10-4	**Barriers and Facilitators to Self-Management**	
SELF-MANAGEMENT BEHAVIOR	**BARRIERS**	**FACILITATORS**
Personal and Lifestyle Characteristics	Lack of knowledge about:	Knowledge about: medication/treatment and chronic disease
	medication/treatment and chronic disease	
	Unstructured routine	Stigma as a motivator to improve health
	Disrupted routine	Motivation and self-efficacy
		Self-discipline
		Personal choices (self-determination)
		Establishing a routine
Health Status	Aging and associated cognitive impairment resulting in forgetting medication	
	Symptom severity	
	Length of illness	
	Adverse effects from treatment including medication	
	Complex treatment regimens	
	Complex medication regimens (e.g., frequent dosing or medication changes or complex regimen such as with warfarin), polypharmacy	
	Multiple comorbidities	
Resources		
Financial	Lack of insurance,	Financial support from family and friends
	underinsured, or limited insurance coverage	
	Limited financial resources	Political systems that do not discriminate
	High cost of medication	
	High cost of healthy foods	
	Cost of supplies	
	Loss of employment	
Equipment	Internet	Internet
	Inability to obtain assistive devices such as glucometers and pill boxes either because of cost or lack of awareness	
	Inability to obtain equipment	
Psychosocial	Lack of support (family, parental, peer)	Perceived positive support (family, parental, peer)
	Isolation	Access/participation in support groups
Environmental Characteristics		
Home	• Different dietary preferences among family members	
	• Conflict among family members over food served in the home	
	• Competing demands of family members experiencing chronic illness	

(continued)

Table 10-4 Barriers and Facilitators to Self-Management—cont'd

SELF-MANAGEMENT BEHAVIOR	BARRIERS	FACILITATORS
Work	• Time and schedule constraints impairing ability to self-manage diet, exercise, and medication • Food environment while at work (short lunch break, limited access to healthy foods)	
Community	• Lack of transportation to medical appointments or to the gym • Unhealthy food choices when dining out at restaurants	
Health Care System Access	Lack of access to: • Specialists • Nursing care • Self-management programs • Alternative therapy	Access to: • Specialists, nursing care, self-management programs, alternative therapy • Educational resources outside health care system (information from books, radio, brochures)
Navigating system/continuity of care	• Long wait lines for appointments • Unreturned phone messages • Confusing communication with clinic staff • Multiple health care specialists • Seeing different providers at every appointment hampers obtaining prescriptions • Inconsistent advice from providers	
Relationships with providers	• Avoiding conflict by not being honest • Limiting communication with provider • Language barriers (not speaking or reading English)	• Positive patient-provider relationship where the patient has time to share concerns with provider • Patient trusts provider • Patient feels supported by provider • Empathy from the provider • Collaborative approach where patient and provider problem-solve together • Shared goals • Adequate time to discuss changes in plan of care • Adequate time for patient to ask questions and obtain feedback • Confidence in provider's competence important when following provider recommendation • Good communication by provider and avoiding use of medical jargon or technical language • Regularly scheduled visits • Provider recommending culturally sensitive self-management strategies

Source: Adapted from Schulman-Green, D., Jaser, S., Park, C., & Whittemore, R. (2016). A metasynthesis of factors affecting self-management of chronic illness. *Journal of Advanced Nursing, 72*(7), 1469–1489.

Nokes, 2017). It is the role of the nurse to help patients and families use credible websites in their search for current information.

Psychosocial support can be perceived as a barrier and facilitator in self-management. Psychosocial support was perceived as positive and influential in self-management when received from peers or partners (Brand et al., 2010; Henriques et al., 2012). A lack of partner support was perceived as a barrier to self-management, especially with regard to new dietary changes. Social isolation (lack of support) is also a barrier to self-management (De Brito-Ashurst et al., 2011). Support groups with members experiencing the same health condition was a facilitator to self-management and provided opportunities for individuals to connect with communities and resources (Lowe & McBride-Henry, 2012; Rasmussen et al., 2011). Many families connect with support groups online, especially when the family caregiver finds it difficult to get out of the home. Nurses have an important role in connecting patients and family members with support groups to attend in person or online.

Environmental Characteristics

Environmental characteristics of the home, work, and community influence self-management. Barriers affecting self-management in the home include different dietary preferences among family members, differences in personal preferences among family members over food served in the home, and competing demands of family members experiencing health problems (Orzech et al., 2013; Wu et al., 2011). Work barriers include time and schedule constraints that impair the ability to self-manage diet, exercise, and medication (Lundberg & Thrakul, 2011; Oftedal et al., 2010). Community barriers to self-management are complex and multifaceted. Lack of transportation to medical appointments or to the gym was identified as a barrier, as was limited or unhealthy food choices served at restaurants and convenience stores (Lundberg & Thrakul, 2011; Pascucci et al., 2010). One technique used by family nurses is to help patients and families conduct a needs assessment.

Health Care Systems

Health care system factors that influence self-management include access to health care,

ability to navigate the health system, continuity of care, and relationship with providers. Access (or lack of access) to specialists, nursing care, self-management programs, and alternative therapies was perceived as an essential element of self-management (Brand et al., 2010; Lundberg & Thrakul, 2011; Lemstra et al., 2018; Ploughman et al., 2012). Educational resources outside the health care system (information from books, radio, brochures) were facilitators (Brand et al., 2010; Lundberg & Thrakul, 2011). If at all possible, the nurse working with the family should connect the patient and the family with a nurse navigator (see Chapter 1), whose role is to assist families that have multiple health care providers.

Barriers for individuals experiencing chronic illness include navigating a complex health care system and continuity of care. Long wait lines/times for appointments, unreturned phone messages, and confusing communication with clinic staff were also identified as barriers to effective self-management (Brand et al., 2010; Newcomb et al., 2010). Inconsistent continuity of care with multiple providers and/or specialists, inconsistent recommendations from providers, and difficulty obtaining prescriptions from different providers was identified as a barrier to care and self-management (Brand et al., 2010; Newcomb et al., 2010).

Collaboration and communication between the individual/family support and the health care professional is a critical component to improve adherence to medications and recommended treatment. Recommendations to improve adherence include medication and goals of treatment counseling, assessing patient's social support, and scheduling follow-up routinely with the same provider (Lemstra et al., 2018).

Relationships with health care providers and the influence on self-management are shown in Box 10-1. Too often, persons with chronic conditions see numerous clinicians who order treatments without considering how they might affect the whole family. Individuals and families benefit from coordinated care, which means providing treatments and medical visits in ways that integrate services and relevant communication among those providing care. Goals of coordinated care include improving health outcomes, identifying risks or problems early, avoiding crises, and ensuring cost-effectiveness of service delivery. Poorly

BOX 10-1

How Health Care Providers Influence Self-Care Management for Chronic Conditions

Positive Influences*

- Positive patient-provider relationship
- Patient trusts the provider
- Patient feels supported by the provider
- Provider expresses empathy
- Collaborative approach to care and shared goals and decision making
- Adequate time for the patient to ask questions and obtain feedback
- Confidence in a provider's competence when following provider recommendations
- Provider uses good communication skills and avoids medical jargon and technical language
- Regularly scheduled visits

- Provider recommends culturally sensitive self-management strategies

Negative Influences

- Conflict by not being honest or limiting communication with a provider [†]
- Language barriers (not speaking or reading English) [‡]
- Inadequate time to discuss changes in plan of care [‡]

* Brand et al., 2010; JoWu, Chang, & McDowell, 2008; Lundberg & Thrakul, 2011; Ploughman et al., 2012; Vest et al., 2013; Wu et al., 2011.

[†] Lundberg & Thrakul, 2011; Newcomb et al., 2010.

[‡] De Brito-Ashurst et al., 2011; Griva et al., 2013.

coordinated care has risks for preventable health complications, conflicts among health care providers, increased stress for the individuals and their families, unnecessary hospitalizations, added expenses, and even death. Persons who experience even a single chronic illness can receive conflicting information, numerous diagnoses, or multiple medications by different health care providers. Nurses are in a position where they can facilitate care management, help individuals and family members sort out the conflicting information or directions, and develop a family-focused management plan. By helping the family to develop a management plan, the nurse empowers the family and the person with the chronic illness to participate in and control self-care, with the goal of improving health outcomes for all members of the family.

Family Adaptation

Living with chronic illness is described by Arestedt et al. (2013) as an ongoing process of adaptation, cocreating ways for the family members, both individually and as a family, to achieve a sense of well-being. By using this in-depth research methodology (i.e., phenomenological hermeneutic analysis), nurses can work with families to help them adjust to everyday living by developing a new rhythm of adaptation. (Hermeneutic phenomenology is a qualitative research methodology whose basic tenet is that our most fundamental and basic experiences of the world have meaning.

Phenomenology is a method for studying the individual and how the individual ascribes meaning to an experience.)

With many chronic illnesses, the family is continually shifting between illness being the primary focus of the family and wellness being the primary view of the family. For example, when there is an exacerbation of the illness that requires the family member to be hospitalized, the family is reminded that the illness is present and requires attention. At other times, the family is focused on the wellness of everyone by, for instance, having family dinner together once a week. Cocreation of ways the family adapts and flows with this movement allows for some overlapping of these two situations. Nurses working with families living with chronic illness who understand this process of evolving family adaptation empower families to move from a viewpoint of "victim" of circumstances to a viewpoint of "creator" of circumstances (Arestedt et al., 2013).

Nursing Interventions to Assist Families Living With Chronic Illness

One person's chronic condition has great potential to influence the lives of many others. Those living with a family member with a chronic disability can become fatigued by the constant vigilance required to perform normal everyday activities of daily living (ADLs) and the stress of uncertainty (Brown et al., 2020; Hummel, 2019b). This fatigue is influenced by the volume of help required, the emotional strain that accompanies the daily hassles, and the relationship strain of constantly giving to another. The following nursing interventions assist the family with adaptation to living with chronic illness.

- *Cocreating a context for living with illness:* When families are confronted with the reality of living with a family member having a chronic illness, they spend time learning how to develop different ways of accomplishing the tasks of the family and meet the needs of the family members. They accomplish this through discussion of the situation. After this initial adjustment and the establishment of how to maintain daily functioning, families report that the illness and situation are not always on their minds.
- *Communicating the illness within and outside the family:* Families learn to balance discussion about the illness, the situation, and the future with chronic illness with other life events for the individual family members and the family as a whole.
- *Cocreating alternative ways for everyday life:* Families learn to operate at a slower pace than before chronic illness. Families note that they are more focused on the present because there is an ever present awareness of an uncertain future.
- *Altering relationships:* The members of the family develop or adapt their relationships to include chronic illness because they have to get to know each other in a different way. In some situations, family members are interacting more often than before the onset of the chronic illness. In other situations, families report being stronger and pulling together more when the illness has exacerbations.
- *Changing roles and tasks:* All roles in the family require adjustment when living in the midst of chronic illness. The family struggles to reestablish a balance in getting the needs of the family accomplished.

One aspect of family nursing that is crucial to helping these families is assisting the family members to adjust to new roles, such as caregiver and care receiver. Nurses can help families explore who does what role in the family and how to use resources to help the family function well by using outside resources to fill some of the family roles. See Chapter 5 for more detail about role negotiation when working with families.

Social Support

Social support can be categorized into four types of supportive behaviors: emotional, instrumental, informational, and appraisal (House, 1981). The family's capacity to mobilize social support to manage crisis periods and chronic stressors related to a family member's health condition contributes to the well-being of all family members (Bellin & Kovacs, 2006). Table 10-5 provides examples of the four types of social support for families that have a member with a chronic illness condition.

Community contexts, such as the neighborhood, school, or church, support the family's development of positive values and foster strengths (Bellin & Kovacs, 2006). Social capital is a concept that can be useful in understanding the community context of health for those with chronic illness and their families. Similar to social support, social capital is about resources that come from relationships with other people and institutions. Social capital includes features of social life, such as norms, networks, and trust, that enable people to act together toward shared objectives (Putnam, 1996). Looman (2006) defines social capital in terms of investments in relationships that facilitate the exchange of resources. For families who have a chronically ill family member, social capital is especially relevant.

Unique community-building activities, such as *support blogging*, are now possible through the internet and through social media. Huh et al. (2014) analyzed 72 vlogs on YouTube that were posted by users diagnosed with HIV, diabetes, or cancer and found that this unique video medium allows for intense and enriched personal disclosures to viewers, which in turn leads to strong community-building activities. They found that vlogs allowed small groups to form, providing implications on how future technologies can provide support for chronic illness management.

When an individual has a chronic illness, the members of the family (particularly caregivers) are required to engage with numerous professionals and institutions in the process of managing the condition and exchanging resources. The family members benefit when a mutual investment exists in their relationships with nurses, physicians,

Table 10-5	**Helpful Support for Families With a Chronically Ill Member**		
TYPE OF SUPPORT	**DEFINITION**	**ACTIVITIES**	**EXAMPLE FROM CASE STUDIES**
Emotional support	Provision of love, caring, sympathy, and other positive feelings	Listening Offering commendations Being present	The nurse working with the Yates family commends them by saying, "I am impressed by the commitment that your family has made to making life as 'normal' as possible for Chloe and her siblings."
Instrumental support	Tangible and intangible items, such as financial assistance, goods, or services	Assisting with household chores (e.g., laundry) Providing respite care Providing transportation Assisting with physical care	Devon's parents offer to take Chloe's siblings for a weekend, providing respite for the family and giving the siblings an opportunity to share time with their grandparents.
Informational support	Helpful advice, information, and suggestions	Sharing resources (e.g., books, websites, provider names) Educating family members on the health needs of the ill family member Informational support groups	Sarah's brother David, who also has type 2 diabetes, recommends a website that provides healthy recipes for individuals with diabetes.
Appraisal support	Feedback given to individuals to assist them in self-evaluation or in appraising a situation	Reviewing daily logs Sharing written feedback from providers (e.g., laboratory results)	The nutritionist provides appraisal support to Sarah during her regular appointments, offering feedback on how Sarah is doing with her lifestyle and dietary changes.

teachers, other families, and neighbors. For example, a mother might invest in her relationship with her child's teachers by providing them with information about her child's health condition or by helping the teachers understand the child's unique learning style. The teachers, in return, might invest in a relationship with the child's family by scheduling additional parent-teacher conferences or by learning more about the child's specific health condition. The benefit of this investment in the family-school relationship, where the common goal is the success of the student, is an exchange of resources. The benefit of this investment may also reach other students and families if this pattern of communication becomes a norm in the school and if the general level of trust among parents and teachers increases. In this way, social capital facilitates the family's ability to acquire emotional, instrumental, informational, and appraisal support in many contexts.

CAREGIVING IN FAMILIES

A caregiver, sometimes referred to as an informal caregiver, is an unpaid individual such as a spouse, partner, family member, friend, or neighbor who is involved in assisting with ADLs and with the management of an illness. According to AARP and the National Alliance for Caregiving (2020), approximately 53 million caregivers in the United States have provided unpaid care to an adult or child in the last 12 months. This amounts to more than one in five Americans (AARP & National Alliance for Caregiving, 2020) and one in four Canadians (Statistics Canada, 2020) providing unpaid care to an adult or child who has either health needs and/or functional needs. This unpaid labor force is estimated to be at least $470 billion annually in the United States (Reinhard et al., 2019). Evidence shows that most caregivers take on this role without having affordable and/or adequate resources, services, and support (AARP & National Alliance for Caregiving, 2020). Caregivers are at risk of experiencing emotional, mental, and physical health problems for themselves as well as financial strain from the demands of caring for family members. Higher levels of stress, anxiety, and depression are common among family members who are caring for a member with chronic illnesses. Twenty-three percent report that caregiving has made it difficult to take care of their own health and has made their own health worse. A growing proportion of individuals from African American and Hispanic populations are providing care to an adult relative. Hispanic and African Americans also report lower household incomes than White or Asian Americans, meaning that many individuals from these groups are providing the same care with less financial resources. Studies of caregivers show that caregivers who are people of color provide more care to families than their White counterparts and report worse physical health than White caregivers (Cohen et al., 2019). Additional findings indicate that Asian American caregivers made less use of professional support services than other groups of caregivers (McCann et al., 2000) and report higher levels of emotional stress (AARP & National Alliance for Caregiving, 2020). Caregivers from Hispanic, African American, and Asian American ethnic/racial groups more often report having no source for help or information (26%, 17%, and 12%, respectively) (AARP & National Alliance for Caregiving, 2020). Despite more hours of providing care and more intense care situations, Hispanic and African American (61% and 59%) caregivers report more often that providing care gives them a sense of purpose (White: 46%, Asian Americans: 48%). Nurses have an important role in identifying the caregiver and providing support and effective education when working with families who are living with a chronic illness.

Family Caregiving

Family caregiving is a crucial role that provides support for those living with chronic illness. Several chapters in this book touch on family caregivers caring for family members with chronic illness. Glasdam et al. (2012) reviewed 32 studies of professional interventions with family caregivers. Few studies targeted the caregivers of family members with cancer, cardiovascular disease, or stroke. They concluded that health care providers lack knowledge about the effects of interventions on caregivers. There is a need for accurate descriptions of the intensified interventions used with caregivers and the outcomes achieved in order to identify the benefits of nursing actions for caregivers. It is clear, however, that soon after the diagnosis of a chronic illness of a family member, caregivers must become proficient in many areas, including managing the illness, coordinating resources, maintaining the family unit, and caring

for self. Nurses assisting families can incorporate the following educational and counseling needs into a treatment plan, making clear who is responsible for what in the family:

- Monitoring conditions and behaviors
- Interpreting normal and expected behaviors from different and serious ones
- Providing hands-on care
- Making decisions
- Developing care routines
- Problem solving
- Teaching self-care management
- Identifying resources to assist with respite care

Child Caregiving for an Adult

One population that is growing around the world is that of young children providing care for a chronically ill adult. In the United States, there are approximately 3.4 million child caregivers under the age of 18 (AARP & National Alliance of Caregiving, 2020). The following list provides an estimated number of children providing care for adult family members in countries or commonwealths of the United Kingdom (Becker, 2007; Clay et al., 2016):

- *England:* There are nearly 5 million caregivers; of these, 166,000 are children ages 5 to 17.
- *Scotland:* There are 657,000 caregivers in Scotland; of these, 16,701 are children.
- *Wales:* There are 340,745 people who are caregivers; of these, 11,000 are children.
- *Northern Ireland:* There are 185,066 people who are caregivers; of these, 2,300 are children.

In Australia, it is estimated that there are 2.65 million caregivers; of these, about 235,300, approximately one in 11 caregivers, were under the age of 25 (Australian Bureau of Statistics, 2019). A 2010 Canadian high school study of 483 ethnically diverse students in grades 8 through 12 found that 12% of youth between the ages of 12 and 17, with a mean age of 14 years, self-identify as "young carers" (Marshall & Stainton, 2010). In response to a rising number of young caregivers, Canada created an action task force to investigate the invisible population of the young caregiver population and its needs (Bednar et al., 2013). In a similar study in the United States, Bridgeland et al. (2006) found that a third of high school dropouts (32%) said that they had to get a job and make money, 26% said that they dropped out because they became a parent, and 22% said that they had to care for a family member. Many of these young people reported doing reasonably well in school and had a strong belief that they could have graduated if they had stayed in school. Childhood caregiver statistics in the United States are as follows:

- Three in ten child caregivers are ages 8 to 11 (31%), and 38% are ages 12 to 15. The remaining 31% are ages 16 to 18 (Hunt et al., 2005). In addition, 12% to 18% of adult caregivers are emerging young adults aged 18 to 25 years (Levine et al., 2005).
- Child caregivers are almost evenly balanced by gender (male 49%, female 51%) (Hunt et al., 2005).
- Caregivers tend to live in households with lower incomes than noncaregivers, and they are less likely than noncaregivers to have two-parent households (76% versus 85%) (Hunt et al., 2005).
- Child caregivers are more common in non-White populations/families, where about one in five families have children helping in Hispanic (21%), African American (20%), and Asian American (17%) populations compared to White families (9%) (AARP & National Alliance for Caregiving, 2020).

There are both negatives and positives to being a young family caregiver. The positive effects are that they report feeling appreciated for their help and that they like helping their family member (Hunt et al., 2005). Negative outcomes from assuming the family caregiver role at a young age are reported in the literature, however. Young caregivers between 8 and 11 years old are more likely than noncaregivers to feel at least some of the time that no one loves them (Hunt et al., 2005). Additional studies found significant effects on caregiving teens' and emerging young adults' mental health, specifically, significantly higher risk for anxiety and depression (Cohen, Greene, et al., 2012; Greene et al., 2017). Nurses should be aware that several young caregiver support groups are offered online, and camps are offered for these children where they can have some carefree time away from

family responsibility. As child caregivers can often be overlooked, it is important for family nurses to inquire about the involvement of children and teens in caring for family members with chronic illness.

The population of young caregivers remains an invisible population, and the exact numbers are unknown. Some reasons this caregiver population is growing include the following:

- Decreasing family size
- Geographical dispersion of families
- High divorce rates
- Increasing number of single parents
- Multiple marriages and reconstituted families

These students and young caregivers live a stressful life with many more responsibilities when compared with peers. In addition, the young caregivers are found to have significantly more anxiety and depression and less satisfaction when compared with noncaregiving age-related peers (Cohen, Greene, et al., 2012). Risks for this population include invisibility due to lack of public awareness, not meeting school expectations, school dropout, and negative influence on the emotional well-being of youth with dual student/caregiver roles (Cohen, Greene, et al., 2012). Families may choose not to disclose child caregiving due to fear that the child may be removed from the home, and families may also not be aware of the negative impact caregiving may have on the child (Faraone et al., 2017).

Countries in the United Kingdom have several major national laws that provide for a wide range of services and programs that include financial allocations to assess vulnerable children and to provide community- and home-based services for care recipients, families, and youth; they also have several support programs and resources for youth caregivers. The United States has no national policies or programs to support this vulnerable population. The American Association of Caregiving Youth (2020) was established by Connie Siskowski, a nurse. This is the only program in the United States that addresses any concerns about this vulnerable population. She designed an after-school program to help these young caregivers meet others living in similar situations, learn how to provide care for their family member safely, and learn how to seek help or resources (American Association of Caregiving Youth, 2020). This nurse also designed a week-long onsite summer camp for these young caregivers to attend so they could experience a normal childhood event and get away from the stress of everyday caregiving.

As this population of vulnerable caregivers continues to grow, one role of the family nurse is to be alert and recognize when a young child is providing care for an adult in the family. When a child is in this situation is present, the nurse should work to find supports for this caregiver and remember that the caregiver is also a child or adolescent who has normal developmental needs in addition to this caregiving family role.

Families Caring for Children Living With a Chronic Illness

The most recent statistics indicate that 14.1 million adults care for children with health or functional needs between the ages of 0 and 17 years (AARP & National Alliance for Caregiving, 2020). According to the *National Survey of Children With Special Health Care Needs 2009–2010* (Child and Adolescent Health Measure Initiative, 2012), 14.6 million children from 0 to 17 years of age have special health care needs (SHCN), which translates to one in five American households. Children with SHCN have a wide range of conditions and risk factors that underlie many shared health conditions. Based on survey results, the six conditions that require the most average hours of caregiving at home each week are: (1) cerebral palsy, (2) muscular dystrophy, (3) cystic fibrosis, (4) traumatic brain injury or concussion, (5) intellectual disability, and (6) epilepsy or seizure (Romley et al., 2017). CYSHCN who are most likely to receive the greatest amount of family care at home are children with severe chronic conditions, children who are 5 years of age or younger, children in Hispanic families, and children in families that live below the poverty level. Health care costs for children who are medically complex range from $50 billion to $110 billion yearly (approximately 15% to 33% of health care spending for all children) (Cohen, Berry, et al., 2012; Neff et al., 2004; Lassman et al., 2014).

CYSHCN are similar to typical children in many ways: They are actively growing and developing, enjoy playing and being with peers, and thrive in cohesive family environments. Children with chronic conditions have limitations, however, that affect daily lives and contribute to challenges uniquely different from peers without chronic conditions. More than half of CYSHCN report that they experience four or more functional disabilities that are related to everyday living, such as respiratory problems, eating problems, vision issues, difficulty using their hands, and communication issues.

Out-of-pocket health care costs that exceed $250 are often perceived by the family as burdensome, and even lower amounts affect families with lower socioeconomic status (Lindley & Mark, 2010). Twenty percent of families of CYSHCN report that they spend 2 to 7 hours a week providing health care for the child at home, and 14% spend more than 11 hours a week. Parents caring for a child with chronic conditions are less likely to work more than 20 hours per week, and they are more likely to have casual employment rather than regular employment (Kish et al., 2018). Caring for the child at home is associated with a significant increase in the odds of having a family member reducing or quitting employment outside the home because of the child's health care needs (Looman et al., 2009).

Families with CYSHCN have many needs, caregiving and otherwise. Studies have shown that mothers of chronically ill children often have greater levels of distress, anxiety, and depression than fathers, a concern thought to be related to the greater care demands placed on the mothers (Spilkin & Ballantyne, 2007; Cohn et al., 2020). Mothers of children with some types of chronic illnesses, such as those with congenital anomalies, also experience greater risk of mortality and poor physical health, such as cardiovascular disease (Cohn et al., 2020). It is also not unusual for parents to differ in their perceptions about the impact of the chronically ill child on the family as a whole and on the marital relationship. Although mothers may find that caregiving demands influence their role performance, fathers may perceive the impact most in their expression of feelings and emotions (Rodrigues & Patterson, 2007). A study of 173 parent dyads of children with chronic conditions found that mothers' marital satisfaction was influenced more than fathers' by perceptions about the effects of their child's condition on the family (Berge et al., 2006). Parents' perceptions of the negative effects of the child's chronic condition were measured in terms of family social strain, role strain, and emotional strain. If parents differed in perceptions about the effects of the illness on the family or marital relationship, an increase in stress and frustration resulted. Nurses can assist couples to identify differences in perception between parents and help facilitate discussions about the effects on roles and the benefits of sharing caregiving tasks (Berge et al., 2006; Spilkin & Ballantyne, 2007).

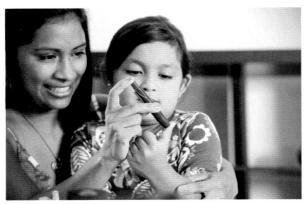

Source: © iStock.com/Fertnig

Family-focused care involves active participation between families, nurses, and other health care providers. Family-focused care supports partnering or collaborative relationships that value and recognize the importance of family traditions, beliefs, and management styles. For the general population of CYSHCN, approximately 35% of them received care that lacked one or more of the essential components of family-centered care (USDHHS, Health Resources and Services Administration, Maternal and Child Health Bureau, 2008).

In general, families raising children with chronic illnesses face the joys and challenges that most typical families face and are as unique and varied as families of typically developing children (Drummond et al., 2012). These families want their children to be happy, have a high quality of life, and grow and develop into caring adults who can live independently and contribute to society. These families face additional stressors, and many researchers acknowledge that the children and parents in these families who care for their children at home are at increased risk for stress-related health conditions and psychosocial problems (Barlow & Ellard, 2006; Berge et al., 2006; McClellan & Cohen, 2007; Meltzer & Mindell, 2006; Mussatto, 2006). Box 10-2 provides a list of stressors likely to

be experienced by families caring for a chronically ill child. Despite the risks for problems, however, most children with chronic conditions and their families, including siblings, demonstrate incredible resilience and capacity for finding positives amid the challenges.

One approach to working with these families is to help them understand the concept of normalization. Normalization is a lens through which families of children with chronic conditions focus on normal aspects of their lives and deemphasize those parts of life made more difficult by chronic conditions (Bowden & Greenberg, 2013; Protudjer et al., 2009; Rehm & Bradley, 2005). The following five attributes of normalization for families of children with chronic conditions offer foundational knowledge for nurses working with such families (Deatrick et al., 1999):

- Acknowledge the chronic condition and its potential to threaten the family's lifestyle.
- View all the management of the chronic illness as just normal daily activities in the family.
- Engage in parenting behaviors and routines that are consistent with a normalcy lens.

BOX 10-2

Potential Stressors When Raising a Child With Chronic Health Conditions

- Care regimen in meeting daily caregiving demands
- Grief about the loss of anticipated child events or activities
- Financial and employment strains
- Uncertainty about future
- Access to specialty services
- Reallocation of family assets (e.g., emotional, time, financial)
- Recurrent crises and crisis management
- Forgone leisure time and social interactions
- Social isolation because of stigmatizing policies and practices
- Challenges in transporting disabled children (e.g., when architectural and other barriers restrict their inclusion)
- Physiological stress of caregiving
- Fragmented health care systems
- Planning for additional space if health-related equipment is required (e.g., wheelchairs)
- Multiple medical, home health care appointments
- Respite care needs for caregivers

- Develop treatment regimens that are consistent with normalcy.
- Interact with others based on a view of the child and family as normal.

Although normalization is a useful conceptual and coping strategy for many families of children with chronic conditions, in families whose children have both complex physical and developmental disabilities, normalization as a goal may be neither possible nor helpful (Rehm & Bradley, 2005). When developmental delays compound the effects of a child's chronic physical conditions, a family's ability to organize and manage its daily life is affected significantly. In this case, parents often recognize normal and positive life aspects, acknowledge the profound challenges faced by their family, and accept a "new normal" (Rehm & Bradley, 2005). This capacity to normalize adversity and to define challenging experiences as manageable and surmountable fosters family resilience. Family relationships and support are another aspect to building resilience in parents, siblings, and the child with the chronic illness (Nabors et al., 2019). Positive relationships. particularly among the siblings, is supportive of resilience. In these cases, the siblings are often viewed as protectors and friends. Helping to support and foster these relationships is an important nursing intervention.

Families with members with chronic conditions, especially those whose conditions are complicated and require care from multiple specialists, often spend a great deal of time interacting with multiple specialists and systems. For example, a family who has a child with Down's syndrome may require regular visits for cardiac, ophthalmological, developmental, and immunological evaluations; physical and occupational therapy; and orthopedic assessments. In addition, parents typically spend a significant amount of time and energy advocating for their child within the school system, attending individualized educational program meetings, meeting with academic support professionals, and coping with worries about what is occurring when the child is out of sight (National Association for Down Syndrome, 2012).

In addition, children with chronic conditions still need well-child care similar to those without such an illness. These children are more susceptible to other infectious diseases or risks for injuries. It is important for children with chronic conditions to receive regular health maintenance visits with a primary health care provider for anticipatory guidance, routine illness, and injury prevention discussions. Parents of children with chronic conditions expect to discuss illness concerns during the well-child care visit. Many primary-care providers report that they are coordinating care in their practices. However, evidence indicates that coordination that involves distributing tasks across personnel is not an effective approach (Looman et al. 2013). Instead, research indicates that coordinating care with nurses who have content expertise, interpersonal skills, and knowledge of systems is essential to the success of care coordination as an important intervention for CYSHCN and their families (Looman et al., 2013). For parents of CYSHCN and other parents, as more illness topics were discussed, more prevention topics were also discussed.

Whether the chronically ill person is a child or an adult, family members require useful information that can be applied directly to real family needs. A trusting environment must exist, with easy information exchange, communication directed toward meeting individual and family needs, and respect.

Families want information that will help them provide adequate care for their member with chronic illness and that will help them to anticipate future needs. A decade ago, Ray (2003) noted that excellent informational resources are available but are not used by families because professionals assume that someone else has provided the information to the family. Parents' and others' need for information and support change over time as they move through phases of the illness and the family life cycle (Nuutila & Salantera, 2006). At the time of diagnosis, parents want clear and consistent information and possibly a more directive approach from the provider. For example, when a child with Down's syndrome is born, the parents may want to know the immediate implications for the child's health and how that will affect their ability to care for the child at home. As the child grows older and the family gains experience in the care of the child, parents may want a less directive approach from the provider and more of a mutual exchange of information in a collaborative partnership (Nuutila & Salantera, 2006). The nurse who encounters this family at a 3-year well-child examination, for example, should acknowledge the parents' intimate understanding of the child, her reactions to the environment, and her unique needs during the clinical encounter. At this point, the most helpful advice from the nurse is likely anticipatory guidance and planning for entry into the school system. Nurses must recognize that individual and family needs will greatly differ for this child as she becomes 16, 28, or 46 years of age.

Adolescents With Chronic Illness Transition to Adult Services

Transition-of-care issues have been discussed in the health care industry for decades, but little attention was given to this area prior to the 2011 report published by the American Academy of Pediatrics (AAP) (2011). Transitions occur in health care in a variety of ways: for example, when a patient moves from one health care provider to a different provider, a person is sent home from the hospital, a person who lives in a nursing home needs to be hospitalized, or a person must switch from private pay to being on Medicaid. Basically, a transition is any time there is a major change in health care management and, according to the 2016 National Survey of Children's Health, 83% of youth age 12 to 17 years with special health care needs are not receiving the recommended transition preparation needed to be successful (Lebrun-Harris et al., 2018).

Transition-of-care issues for adolescents, who are required to switch from pediatric health care providers to adult providers of care, is a global health care problem (Kralik et al., 2011; Lugasi et al., 2011; Sonneveld et al., 2013; Steinbeck et al., 2007, 2008; Wong et al., 2010). This process is a multidisciplinary approach that includes both pediatric and adult care clinicians such as physicians, nurses, social workers, and others (White et al., 2018). Family nurses are in a prime position to address transition issues because they work closely with families and children who have chronic illness (Jalkut & Allen, 2009). Survival rates have improved for many children who live with a chronic illness, and this aspect of family nursing requires even more focus. The transition is not just about the medical care from a pediatric physician to an adult specialist. The transition also needs to include psychosocial, educational, and vocational needs and cultural beliefs of the young adult. It also needs to consider the parents who, up until that point, have orchestrated management of the

illness, communicated with the health care team, made appointments, and interacted with school officials. The transition period causes anxiety for the whole family and involves leaving long-term health care provider relationships, developmental psychosocial stressors of adolescents, uncertainty about health insurance coverage and issues of the Health Insurance Portability and Accountability Act (HIPAA) relative to parental knowledge, and involvement in the care process and communication (Peter et al., 2009).

What compounds the difficulty of this transition period for the family and the individual members is the fact that the adult health providers who are assuming care of the young adults with chronic illness often lack understanding of normal adolescent growth and development (Bowen et al., 2010). This lack of understanding on the part of adult health care providers was recognized as a problem by AAP in 2011 and again in 2018 (AAP, 2011; White et al., 2018).

Osterkamp et al. (2013) developed an online educational program for nurses about the transition of care for adolescent patients with chronic illness. The modules in the program are HIPAA, family-centered care and its core concepts relative to transition of care of the adolescent patient, and healthy versus chronically ill adolescent development (including information about a decrease in adherence to medical regimens and feelings of isolation by being different than other teens). Box 10-3 lists the principles of successful transition to adult-oriented health services that were endorsed by the Society for Adolescent Health and Medicine (2021).

AAP, in collaboration with the American Academy of Family Physicians and the American College of Physicians, developed and updated the six core elements of a structured, customizable process for health care transition (White et al., 2018): discussion of transition policy, tracking progress, assessing skills, developing a transition plan, transferring to/integration in adult-centered care, and confirming completion of transfer and eliciting consumer feedback. These elements include age ranges and specific tasks spearheaded by a health care professional for both the adult and adolescent (Figure 10-5 and Table 10-6). Nurses have the potential to play a crucial role within many of these elements.

Nurses who work with families and their teenagers with chronic illness should establish a

BOX 10-3

Principles of Successful Transition to Adult-Oriented Health Services

1. Health care services for adolescents and young people need to be developmentally appropriate and inclusive of the young person's family where appropriate.
2. Young people with chronic illnesses and conditions share the same health issues as their healthier peers. Therefore, health services need to be holistic and address a range of concerns, for example, growth and development, mental health, sexuality, nutrition, exercise, and risky behaviors such as drug and alcohol use.
3. Health care services require flexibility to be able to deal with young people with a range of ages, conditions, and social circumstances. The actual process of transition needs to be tailored to each individual adolescent or young person.
4. Transition is generally optimized when there is a specific health care provider who takes responsibility for helping the adolescent or young person and his or her family through the process.
5. Active case management and follow-up help optimize a smooth transfer to adult health services and promote retention within adult services.
6. Engagement with a general practitioner can address holistic health care needs and help reduce the risk of failure of transfer to adult services.
7. Close communication between pediatric and adult services helps bridge the cultural and structural difference of the two health systems, resulting in a smoother transition of young people to adult services.
8. An ultimate goal of transition to adult health care services is to facilitate the development of successful self-management in young people with chronic conditions.

Sources: Adapted from: Nakano, K. T., Crawford, G. B., Zenzano, T., & Peralta, L. (2011). Transitioning adolescents into adult healthcare. *American College of Preventive Medicine.* http://www.medscape.com/viewarticle/755301_1; Rosen, D., Blum, R., Britto, M., Sawyer, S., & Siegel, D. (2003). Transition to adult health care for adolescents and young adults with chronic conditions. Position paper of the Society for Adolescent Medicine. *Journal of Adolescent Health, 33,* 309–311.

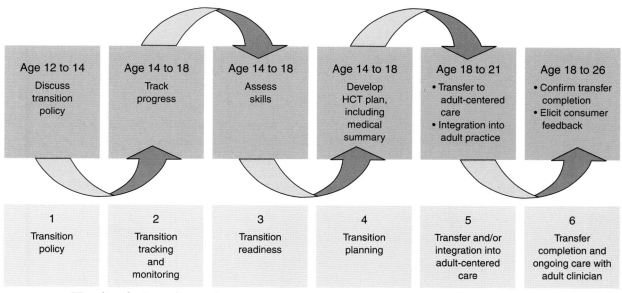

FIGURE 10-5 Timeline for Introducing the Six Core Elements into Pediatric Practices *Source: White, P. H., & Cooley, W. C., Transitions Clinical Report Authoring Group, American Academy of Pediatrics American Academy of Family Physicians, & American College of Physicians. (2018). Supporting the health care transition from adolescence to adulthood in the medical home.* Pediatrics, 142(5), e20182587.

process of getting ready for the transfer at least a year or so in advance—long before the situation occurs (van Staa et al., 2011)—and work with the family to design a well-thought-out, purposeful plan of transition. One difficult part of this care process is working with the family and the health care team to determine when is the best time for the transition to occur. To base this transition

Table 10-6 Summary of Six Core Elements Approach for Pediatric and Adult Practices						
PRACTICE OR PROVIDER	**NUMBER 1: TRANSITION AND/OR CARE POLICY**	**NUMBER 2: TRACKING AND MONITORING**	**NUMBER 3: TRANSITION READINESS AND/OR ORIENTATION TO ADULT PRACTICE**	**NUMBER 4: TRANSITION PLANNING AND/OR INTEGRATION INTO ADULT APPROACH TO CARE OR PRACTICE**	**NUMBER 5: TRANSFER OF CARE AND/OR INITIAL VISIT**	**NUMBER 6: TRANSITION COMPLETION OR ONGOING CARE**
Pediatric	Create and discuss with youth and/or family	Track progress of youth and/or family transition preparation and transfer	Conduct transition readiness assessments	Develop transition plan, including needed assessment skills and medical summary; prepare youth for adult approach to care; and communicate with new clinician	Transfer of care with information and communication, including residual pediatric clinician's responsibility	Obtain feedback on the transition process and confirm young adult has been seen by the new clinician
Adult	Create and discuss with young adult and guardian, if needed	Track progress of young adult's integration into adult care	Share and discuss welcome and questions from young adult and guardian, if needed	Communicate with previous clinician, ensure receipt of transfer package	Review transfer package, address young adult's needs and concerns at initial visit, update self-care assessment and medical summary	Confirm transfer completion with previous clinician, provide ongoing care with self-care skill building and link to needed specialists

Providers that care for youth and/or young adults throughout the life span can use both the pediatric and adult sets of core elements without the transfer process components.

Source: White, P. H., Cooley, W. C., Transitions Clinical Report Authoring Group, American Academy of Pediatrics, American Academy of Family Physicians, & American College of Physicians. (2018). Supporting the health care transition from adolescence to adulthood in the medical home. *Pediatrics, 142*(5), e20182587.

decision solely on chronological age is not sufficient (van Staa et al., 2011). The abilities of the young adult to demonstrate responsibility and to participate as much as possible in self-care management (self-efficacy) are better predictors than is age for readiness to transfer (AAP, 2011; van Staa et al., 2011), although the six core elements provide suggested age ranges for transition activities to take place (White et al., 2018). Other factors that nurses need to consider and address besides self-efficacy and age in this transition plan are the adolescent's attitude toward transition and the complexity of the illness and treatment plan. The transfer plan should also entail the following:

- Introduce the concept of transition early in the care relationship with the family. Stress that the transfer is a normative process that reflects achievement of an additional developmental task (Lugasi et al., 2011).

Assure the family that transition is not a form of abandonment.

- Hold family meetings to discuss expectations regarding the move to adult care. Explore what the family members think will be the same or different. Discuss the timing of the transfer. Use these meetings to uncover concerns and needs of the family and each family member about the transition process (Lugasi et al., 2011).

- Assess the adolescent's ability to provide self-care (Lugasi et al., 2011).

- Design educational programs to meet the needs of the adolescent/young adult as they relate to the illness, how to self-monitor, how to self-manage illness and situations, and how to ask for help when needed. This should include helping the young adult to learn how to develop communication skills.

- Hold discussions about the adult health care environment, insurance coverage, and health policy changes that will affect the care once the adolescent becomes 18 years of age and is considered a legal adult. This discussion should include differences between pediatric and adult health models of care.
- Hold discussions about how the parents may need to move from acting as the primary decision makers to a more supportive and collaborative model of decision making with the young adult.
- Provide the family with a list of adult health providers that they may want to consider in their selection process.
- Introduce independent visits with the pediatric health care provider without the parents present.
- Arrange for an introductory visit with the adult provider so that the first interaction is not about an exacerbation of the chronic illness but about health maintenance. If possible, plan for a joint visit of the family, the pediatric health care team, and the adult health care team.
- Identify a transition coordinator or someone in the adult health care team who can serve in this role for the family and young adult (Lugasi et al., 2011).

Siblings of Children With Chronic Illness

Younger siblings often strive to model the behaviors of older siblings, including illness behaviors. A study focusing on participants who identified themselves as growing up with an ill sibling found they reported acting out and alienation behaviors as well as social withdrawal. However, the majority of participants also reported that the experience affects their lives positively, with a greater appreciation of life and a greater awareness of family bonding and support (Fleary & Heffer, 2013). While some siblings of children with chronic illness show anxiety, jealousy, worry, fear, anger, and sadness, many siblings benefit from the closer family relationships required to care for family members with chronic illness (Havill et al. 2019; Nabors et al., 2019). They often report positive reflective emotions, including pride and protection

(Havill et al., 2019). When these relationships occur, families show positive coping and resilience (Nabors et al., 2019). Focus groups held with parents, siblings, and health care providers resulted in a comprehensive list of psychosocial concerns specific to the experience of school-age siblings of children with chronic illness (Strohm, 2001). These conversations identified seven significant feelings of siblings of children with chronic health care conditions (Strohm, 2001, p. 49):

- Feelings of guilt about having caused the illness or being spared the condition
- Pressure to be the "good" child and protect parents from further distress
- Feelings of resentment when their sibling with special needs receives more attention
- Feelings of loss and isolation
- Shame related to embarrassment about their sibling's appearance or behavior
- Guilt about their own abilities and success
- Frustration with increased responsibilities and caregiving demands

Other studies reveal more positive sibling outcomes, pointing out that siblings develop improved empathy, flexibility, pride in learning about and caring for a chronic illness, and understanding of differential treatment from parents based on ability and health. Siblings are noted to be more caring, mature, supportive, responsible, and independent than their peer counterparts who do not have siblings with chronic conditions (Barlow & Ellard, 2006). Siblings are reported to have high levels of empathy, compassion, patience, and sensitivity (Bellin & Kovacs, 2006). Siblings demonstrate learning about the disease and being supportive of their ill brother or sister and sometimes assume parental roles (Wennick & Hallstrom, 2007; Havill et al., 2019). Children who learn about their sibling's chronic illness and its mechanisms tend to feel more confident and competent in their ability to support their sibling and have a better understanding about why their lives have been disrupted (Havill et al., 2019; Lobato & Kao, 2005; Wennick & Hallstrom, 2007).

Families face the challenge of balancing the needs of the child with a chronic condition with those of the surrounding family, including siblings. It has long been demonstrated that parents of siblings of children with disabilities often lack the ability to give needed time and attention to siblings because of the demands of caring for the child with a disability; this sometimes results in siblings resenting the child with disabilities (Rabiee et al., 2005). Some parents rely on siblings to entertain or assist in the care of the child with disabilities, an action that puts additional stress on the other children and can have both negative as well as positive outcomes.

FAMILY NURSING INTERVENTION DURING CHRONIC ILLNESS

The role of the family nurse is to assist multiple family members to interact in ways that optimize abilities and strengths. Although chronic illness care requires consideration of individual outcomes, it must be addressed within the family environment, with consideration of long-term caregiver needs and family outcomes. Across the life span, families use management styles, functional processes, and family health routines to address actual problems, minimize risks, and maximize potentials. Nurses who assess for these styles, processes, and routines and who then tailor their interventions accordingly to empower and collaborate with families will be most effective in meeting chronic care needs.

Nurses assist families by discussing factors such as family strengths, couple time, balancing illness and family needs, developmental milestones, sibling needs, economic constraints, and caregiver well-being (Kieckhefer et al., 2013). Family-focused nursing care should also address prevention or reduction of additional health risks; maintenance of optimal wellness levels for all family members; development of therapeutic care management routines; goal setting that enhances individual and family well-being and integrity; assessments of ethnocultural influences, including macro- and microsocial factors; and accommodating unplanned changes. FHM (Denham, 2003) suggests that families have *core processes* (i.e., caregiving, cathexis, celebration, change, communication, connectedness, coordination) or ways families interact with one another. Nurses can use these ideas as guides to working effectively with families who have a member with a chronic illness (see Tables 10-2 and 10-3).

In chronic disease management, family-focused care needs that equip these individuals and their families with knowledge and tools to be effective self-managers have long been lacking (Wagner et al., 2001). Use of an empowerment model and integrative processes to respond to unique needs has been most successful (Phillips et al., 2015; Tang et al., 2006). An empowerment model involves the following types of care:

- Patient-centered care
- Problem-based care
- Strengths-based care
- Evidence-based care
- Culturally relevant care

Empowerment acknowledges that the person is central to chronic care self-management. As nurses seek to empower families for chronic illness management, they should encourage flexibility, coordinate the actions of multiple caregivers, use evidence-based guidelines, help families identify community resources, and provide education that builds confidence and skills in multiple family members. A need exists for more evidence about empowerment interventions (Henshaw, 2006; Hummel, 2019a).

Family nurses should keep in mind that families typically vary in four systematic ways in their abilities to incorporate medical regimens into their daily routines: remediation, redefinition, realignment, and reeducation (Fiese & Everhart, 2006). *Remediation* refers to a need to make slight alterations in daily routines to fit illness care into preexisting routines. *Redefinition* refers to a strategy whereby the emotional connections made during routine gatherings need to be redefined. *Realignment* occurs when individuals within the family disagree about the importance of different medical routines, and routines need to be realigned in the service of the child's health. *Reeducation* occurs when the family has little history or experience with routines and family life is substantially disorganized (Fiese & Everhart, 2006).

Research about family health suggests that structural behaviors or family health routines are visible activities that family members can readily recall and discuss from multiple perspectives (Denham, 1997, 1999a, 1999b, 1999c). Although family members may report similarities in routines, unique variations are common. The nested family context is a powerful, persuasive, and motivating determinant that influences ways health information is shared within a family and then incorporated into daily routines. Routines have unique characteristics; they vary in rigidity and timing, and family members have different expectations because of response to member beliefs, values, and perceived needs. Information that fits with perceived family needs is probably the most likely to be incorporated into daily actions. Thus, nursing assessment of chronic-care management extends beyond the disease and should also include ways family members interact and the life patterns already established.

Family health routines include several categorically different foci. Self-care routines involve habits linked with usual ADLs such as hygiene. Safety and prevention routines are primarily concerned with health protection, disease prevention, prevention of injury, and avoidance of unsafe situations. A nurse assessing this routine area might also be interested in discerning less healthy habits and considering the impact of high-risk behaviors, such as smoking, alcohol use, and use of other substances, on a chronic condition. Mental health routines are related to self-esteem, personal integrity, work and play, shared positive experiences, stress, self-efficacy, individuation, and family identity. Family-care routines are related to valued traditions, rituals, celebrations, vacations, and other events tied to making meaning and sharing enjoyable times. Illness-care routines are related to decisions about disease, illness, and chronic health care needs and often determine when, where, and how members seek health care services and incorporate medical directives and health information into self-care routines. Family caregiving routines pertain to reciprocal member interactions believed to assist with health and illness care needs and support during times of crisis, loss, and death.

Families use routines to arrange ordinary life and cope with health or illness events (Fiese & Wamboldt, 2000). These routines are embedded in the cultural and ecological context of families and highlight ways to focus on family processes and individual and family dynamics (Fiese et al., 2002). Nurses aiming to provide education and counseling to individuals with a chronic illness need to understand the unique family routines of multiple household members and the ways chronic care management will alter patterns that are revered, cherished, and comfortable. Nurses who collaborate with families during assessment, goal setting, and outcome evaluation increase the likelihood of providing effective nursing actions that get results that are sustainable over time.

CASE STUDIES: FAMILIES LIVING WITH CHRONIC ILLNESS

It is important to recognize that all chronic diseases are not the same. When diagnosis differs, individual and family needs can differ as well. Other factors are also in play. For example, race/ethnicity, primary language, cultural background, age, gender, educational level, socioeconomic factors, health resources, health and illness beliefs, health practices, and availability of family members can be critical factors in the ways that diseases are managed in family situations.

This section explores the ways that the Yates and the Current families address chronic illness management. (For a comparison of these two families and their differences using the ECGNM, see Table 10-7.) The Yates family represents a diverse family unit, with three generations living together. The father is White, the mother is Latina of Mexican origin, and the grandmother recently moved into the household. The family is focused on the young daughter, who has been diagnosed with type 1 diabetes, and the family has been living with this situation for a while. The second family, the Currents, provides an example of a rural working family with an older member living with Parkinson's disease. Although these two chronic diseases share some similar characteristics for the families living with chronic illness, some unique qualities also emerge. The values and beliefs about illness and ways for managing illness need to be explored. The timing of diagnosis can differ, and access to health care, treatment options, and financial and other resources can also be different. Living with the disease for several decades could mean that new treatments become available. Families living with these two conditions often face different challenges because of individual motivation and knowledge, demographics, family member characteristics, family developmental stage, and family community resources. Family-focused nurses recognize that multiple factors enter into understanding why some individuals manage their disease successfully whereas others may not, and reasons why they are at risk for complications.

Table 10-7 Select Features of ECGNM: Comparing the Yates and Current Families

ECGNM ELEMENTS	CASE STUDY 1: CHLOE YATES FAMILY (SELECTED PRIMARY DIMENSIONS FOR THIS FAMILY)	CASE STUDY 2: BEN CURRENT FAMILY
Macrosocial (Outside) Influences		
Political/world climate	Uncertainty with new political administration, new type 1 research.	Uncertainty with new political administration, new Parkinson's disease research.
Economic climate	Two working parents. Three children in private schools.	Ben is retired and his health insurance and family's financial status need to be explored.
	Explore implications of adding a maternal grandmother to the household.	Financial struggles prevent family from hiring a full-time caregiver.
Public policy	Safety requirements at school. Policies at school with syringes. Providing EMS services with hypoglycemic events.	Ben agrees to stop driving and surrender his license.
Climate: stereotypes, attitudes, ascriptions	Child/adolescent with type 2 diabetes.	What are Ben's beliefs regarding assisted living? How does Grace, his sister, feel about providing personal hygiene?
Perception of discrimination, illness, self-care	Assess Chloe's perception of her illness among her peers.	Stigma of Parkinson's disease in the community?
Cultural/historical traditions	Multicultural household. Role of grandparents. Mix of American and traditional Mexican diet.	Explore Ben's belief and values systems as his elder role is compromised. Close-knit family. Patriarch structure now shifting, with grandsons taking a caregiving role.
Gendered experience	Bonita raised in traditional Mexican household, adjusting to her mother and caregiving role, adjusting to having a parent living in the home.	Ben as a patriarch and provider of family.
Cohort influence (generational, etc.)	Maternal grandmother primarily Spanish speaking. Children may or may not speak Spanish.	Multigenerational home: grandsons and sister living on ranch
Microsocial (Personal) Influences		
Sociodemographics; income comfort, caregiving structure	Need to assess multicultural personal influences for the father, mother, and grandmother. How will caregiving be affected by adding a grandmother to the household?	Need to assess shift in roles with Ben needing assistance from grandsons. Daughters, sister, and grandsons take on role of caregiver. Who takes leadership?

Health dimensions; comorbid conditions	Hyperlipidemia is common with diabetes. Annual checkups to assess for retinopathy, nephropathy, and neuropathy.	Scheduling and coordinating continued evaluations for nonmotor Parkinson's disease symptoms: depression, constipation, sleep changes.
Biological variations	Latinx at higher risk for delayed diagnosis of diabetes and complications. Will need to assess nutritional practices further.	Parkinson's disease is a genetically heterogeneous condition and most likely accounts for about 30% of familial Parkinson's disease. Complex disorder.
Personal/Family Experiences		
Communication	Language: grandmother speaks Spanish; what is the language of children at home? What resources are used for communication? Who communicates with the providers? Can Chloe communicate with the providers?	What resources are used for communication? Who communicates with providers? Can Ben communicate with providers?
Resources: Additional Considerations for the Yates and Current Families		
Sociocultural, including economics	Who provides education regarding hypoglycemia to Chloe's peers? Who provides language-appropriate educational material for the grandmother?	Who manages Ben's bank account? Who has executive function?
Others: chronic illness focus	Explore cross-cultural beliefs and practices, grandmother's perspective. Explore younger children's beliefs and knowledge about diabetes and family risk.	Explore the family's perspective and practices with progressive chronic illnesses. Discuss concerns with possible familial/genetic component to Parkinson's disease.
Health insurance (private, state aid, etc.)	Two working parents: need to explore options.	Need further exploration of insurance coverage, referral services.
Employment		
Family structure	Multigenerational household, roles and responsibilities need to be assessed.	Multigenerational household, roles and responsibilities need to be assessed.
Caregiving support	Explore if grandmother drives and if she is a participant in the child's care and medical appointments.	Explore if all members have transportation and who takes responsibility for getting Ben to his appointments.
Transportation needs	Parents and grandmother may need to be included in nutritional guidance appointments.	
Housing/space	Housing: Is additional space needed for extended family members? Explore parental, mother, and grandmother roles. Determine space needed to accommodate adolescents.	Home needs to be assessed for potential fall risk for Ben, with resources to keep him safe, such as rails in the bathroom.
Equipment needed for health care	Assess knowledge of glucometers and potential insulin pump use.	Assess knowledge and use of CPAP machine, battery, and maintenance.

Case Study: Yates Family

Chloe Yates, age 13, was recently admitted to the pediatric intensive care unit with ketoacidosis, a complication of type 1 diabetes. She passed out at school after vomiting and complaining of fatigue and was transported to the hospital via ambulance. On her hospital admission, her serum glucose level was 350 mg/dL. Her glycosylated hemoglobin (Hba1c) was 11%, indicating poor metabolic control during the past 3 months. Chloe has been in the hospital for 2 days and is getting ready to be discharged home today.

   Chloe's parents, Devon and Bonita Yates, were surprised when they found out how poorly Chloe's metabolic control had been before her admission. (See Figure 10-6 for a detailed Yates family genogram.) They believed that their family had open communication and that they knew what was happening with their children. Chloe told her parents that her glucose levels were "fine." Chloe is an honor roll student at school, active in basketball and soccer, and well liked by her peers. Devon, a white male, is college educated and works for a thriving law firm. Bonita, a college-educated female, is a first-generation Mexican American and is employed as a business manager in a large firm.

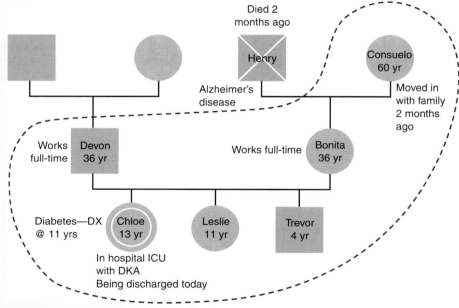

FIGURE 10-6 Yates Family Genogram

   The Yates family recently experienced several stressors besides this new hospitalization. Bonita's father, Henry, passed away 2 months ago after a long bout with Alzheimer's disease. Bonita's mother, Consuelo, is now living with them. The family recently moved into a new and larger home in a racially diverse urban neighborhood. The children are enrolled in a private school, so the move did not affect their school relationships. Chloe and her younger siblings, Leslie and Trevor, appear to have adjusted to the new living location and seem content with their new neighborhood friends. Chloe has continued to receive primary-care services in the clinic where the long-term pediatric nurse practitioner has come to know the family quite well.

   Chloe was diagnosed with diabetes 2 years ago and was 11 years old at the time. When diagnosed, she spent several days in the hospital. Bonita accompanied her to a series of diabetes education classes, and they shared what they learned with the rest of the family. Chloe easily assumed responsibility for monitoring her glucose levels and administering her insulin when she was diagnosed. At first, the family struggled to make needed changes to their family health routines based on Chloe's medical needs.

   The family recently started "highlight/lowlight" time at dinner, during which each family member shares one high point and one low point about his or her day. Chloe's highlights have focused on her new friend at school, Brian. Her lowlights have focused on the "hassle" of checking her glucose and having to eat differently than her friends, something she is finding embarrassing. Having Consuelo move in with the family added some stress to the family, but the children are enjoying having their grandmother present when they come home after school.

Case Study: Yates Family—cont'd

Leslie and Trevor are staying at home with Consuelo while Bonita and Devon prepare to take Chloe home from the hospital today. Leslie and Trevor have been asking about Chloe for several days because they are worried about her "sugar." Leslie, age 11, has been especially concerned about Chloe. She and Chloe have been arguing lately, and Leslie feels it might be her fault that Chloe became ill. Trevor, age 4, has been asking if he can use Chloe's "finger pokers" and saying, "I have diabetes too!" Devon and Bonita share with the nurse their beliefs that he wants some of the special attention that his sister is getting at the hospital. These parents are worried about being "spread too thin" as they try to fulfill their employment responsibilities, attend to each child's unique needs, understand Consuelo's emotional needs after the loss of her husband, and also provide Chloe with the medical care she needs to manage the diabetes. Bonita is also concerned that her mother may not be ready to assist with Chloe's medical management so soon after caring for her husband for several years before he died from Alzheimer's disease.

Chloe's parents are meeting with the nurse today as they prepare for Chloe's discharge home. When the nurse asks whether they thought Chloe fully understood how to manage her diabetes, Devon said, "She not only understands, she could teach it! We just can't figure out why she had such a setback recently." This family is experiencing a transitional stress that is typical of adolescent behavior and also typical of adolescents living with a chronic illness.

Family Nurse's Reflection on the Yates Family Using Evidence-Based Practice
Adaptation to type 1 diabetes is more effective when there is ongoing communication between parents and children regarding treatment management. Continued involvement of parents in treatment management is associated with better health and psychosocial outcomes in children and adolescents (Jaser, 2011). See Figure 10-7 for an ecomap of the Yates family.

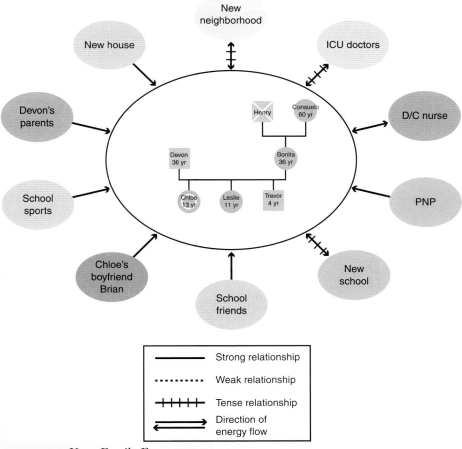

FIGURE 10-7 Yates Family Ecomap

(continued)

Case Study: Yates Family—cont'd

Questions for reflection on the nursing care of the Yates family:

1. What priority nursing assessments will the nurse obtain before Chloe's discharge from the hospital to inform discharge planning and prevent recurrent hospitalizations?
2. What types of adaptation strategies would be important for the nurse to recommend to the family given the recent stressors?
3. As an 11-year-old newly diagnosed with type 1 diabetes, what challenges and adaptations would the nurse anticipate Chloe and the family may experience, and what type of support and/or resources would be anticipated by the nurse?
4. As Chloe and her family prepare for her discharge home, the nurse anticipates a multidisciplinary approach. What resources would the nurse discuss with the family? What are some cultural aspects that should be considered when assessing and developing a plan of care for the family?
5. What are some family strengths?
6. What socioeconomic and multicultural factors influence self-management and family adaptation to a family member living with a chronic illness?
7. Using ECGNM, identify the macro- and micro social aspects that may be influencing the family and adaptation to Chloe's ongoing health care needs.
8. What aspects of the FMSF would be useful for the nurse to assess?

Case Study: Current Family

Ben Current, a 68-year-old White widower, was diagnosed with Parkinson's disease at the age of 58. He owns and farms his 500-acre family ranch in eastern Oregon, where he raises cattle and hay. Several years ago, Ben managed a small group of cattle, which provided the family income. Since his wife Sarah's death 2 years ago, the number of cattle decreased, as well as the household income. This case study is presented through the lens of Rolland's (1987) Chronic Illness and the Life Cycle Conceptual Framework.

Illness Onset

Parkinson's disease is a slow, progressive neurodegenerative brain disorder with motor symptoms of slowness, rigidity, and tremor. There are also a host of nonmotor symptoms that include autonomic, neuropsychiatric (e.g., dementia and depression), and sleep complaints. The cause of Parkinson's disease is not known, and treatment is aimed at minimizing disability and maintaining optimal quality of life. At his most recent visit to the Movement Disorder Clinic, Ben presents with several motor and nonmotor concerns. In addition, he has low adherence to treatment recommendations, and his family is expressing strain from the growing burden of care.

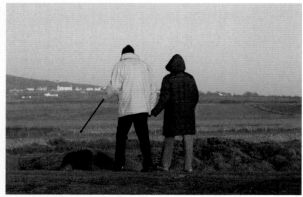

Source: © iStock.com/tirc83

Case Study: Current Family—cont'd

Course of Illness

When individual family members have a progressive chronic illness, such as Ben with Parkinson's disease, the increasing disability requires families to make continual changes in their roles as they adapt to the losses and needs of the family member. Ben's family is at the Movement Disorder Clinic today to seek help with Ben's increasing symptoms. Several family members express feelings of stress and are exhausted with the routine and ongoing demands of his progressive symptoms.

One assessment scale used to evaluate the needs of a Parkinson's patient is the Unified Parkinson's Disease Rating Scale. This scale is a detailed instrument that assists family nurses to assess the daily needs of the ill family member and the family caregiver in six areas of function: functional status, level of ADLs, motor function, mood, cognition, and treatment-related manifestations.

Outcome—Trajectory of Illness and Incapacitation

Typically, people with Parkinson's disease can live 20 years or more from the time of diagnosis. Death is usually secondary to complications of immobility. It is the 14th leading cause of death in the United States. There is currently no cure for Parkinson's disease, and it is progressive in nature. The focus of this visit is to minimize Ben's disability through symptom management and to help the family find resources in the local community to support Ben and minimize caregiver strain. If these interventions improve his adherence to medication, the family may maintain Ben's current level of functioning.

Time Phase: Brief Review of Ben's Initial Diagnosis

At initial diagnosis, Ben, 58 years old, was, in his words, "just not doing well." He was worried about a tremor in his left hand, but at that point it did not interfere much with his daily work or activities. Sarah, his wife, had taken over writing the paychecks for their three ranch hands and all the bills because Ben's handwriting had started to deteriorate. He noticed that he was slowing down, but attributed his increasing stiffness of legs and arms to "getting old" and his demanding physical lifestyle. What brought him in to see his health care provider was dizziness and falls. Sarah was worried that he would get dizzy while operating the farm machines. When he came home with a cut lip, swollen ankle, and scraped-up shoulder, Sarah demanded he see the family nurse practitioner (FNP), who was located 50 miles from his ranch. The FNP suspected Ben had Parkinson's disease but sent him to the Movement Disorder Clinic and specialists in Portland, Oregon, which was 330 miles from where Ben lived.

Mid–Time Phase and Family Functioning

Ben and his extended family have been living and adapting to his progressive Parkinson's disease for 10 years. The adaptation was relatively smooth initially because Ben responded well to medication intervention, and his wife Sarah was the major support person. The family experienced a major change in the family involvement and management of Ben's illness when Sarah died 2 years ago from a heart attack at age 66. Since that time, 27-year-old Logan, Ben's grandson, has been living at the ranch and helping to provide support and care for Ben.

Julie, the nurse practitioner (NP) in the Movement Disorder Clinic, consulted the detailed family genogram in the chart and updated it at this time. Figure 10-8 shows the current family genogram. At this visit, the family members who were present include Ben; his daughter Kathleen; his daughter Carole; and his grandson Logan, who is the primary caregiver. Logan expresses feeling overwhelmed with his caregiver role and work-time conflict. He feels that Ben needs more assistance. Because both Kathleen and Carole are worried about Ben's safety while Logan is working on the ranch during the day, they report alternating days when they come to spend time with Ben.

The family decided to have Aunt Grace (Ben's sister) come for a trial run to help with Ben's care. The family determined that they would also explore having a home health aide come to the ranch a couple of days a week to help with Ben's hygiene.

After a visit to the physical therapist during their time at the Movement Disorder Clinic in Portland, Logan was excited about the possibility of all the grandsons working together to build a flat walking trail not far from the ranch house for Ben that would incorporate many of the physical therapy exercise strategies that may help strengthen his muscles, improve agility, and help decrease the freezing episodes. They would put several logs at varying heights for him to practice high stepping. They could increase his stride by placing stepping stones across the creek. They would make the trail so that it had several direction changes and have Ben walk between two trees that were shoulder width. Logan agreed that he would spearhead this venture with all the grandsons.

Julie worked with Logan and Ben on medication reconciliation. Together they designed a medication administration chart to help the family caregiver and Ben improve medication adherence. For a complete Parkinson's assessment using the Unified Parkinson's Disease Rating Scale, family concerns, and interventions, see Table 10-8.

(continued)

Case Study: Current Family—cont'd

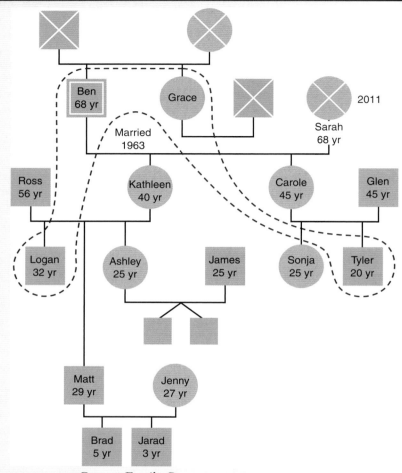

FIGURE 10-8 Current Family Genogram

Interventions implemented by Julie include the following:

- Making a referral to speech therapy to assist Ben with his soft voice (hypophonia). Kathleen agreed to accompany Ben to this part of the visit in an attempt to relieve Logan of some caregiving responsibilities.
- Making recommendations to the FNP (Ben's primary-care provider) to make a referral to the sleep clinic to evaluate the need for a continuous positive airway pressure (CPAP) mask to address Ben's sleep problems

Ben agreed to stop driving and surrender his license only if he could still drive on the ranch. See the Current family ecomap in Figure 10-9.

An ethnocultural approach begins by first desiring the knowledge and actively engaging in cultural encounters with patients from diverse backgrounds. The Current family is a ranching family living in rural Oregon. Their daily lifestyle choices and problem-solving approaches to chronic illness concerns may differ from those of a family living in an urban setting. Nurses must self-reflect and acknowledge biases and discriminatory practices that prevent meaningful communication and interaction with unfamiliar community members.

The nurse working with Ben and his family must assess his family's long-standing culture-bound traditional beliefs and practices. The various political, economic, and public policies that have an impact on this family's chronic illness management also need to be examined. Changes to the Affordable Care Act may influence the medical benefits that affect Ben's ability to continue seeing Julie, the NP specialist in the Movement Disorder Clinic in Portland, and possibly having access to management strategies beyond the scope of practice of his primary-care provider. See Table 10-7 for a comprehensive ECGNM evaluation sample.

Case Study: Current Family—cont'd

Table 10-8 **Presentation of Ben's Mid-Phase Parkinson's Disease Symptoms Using Unified Parkinson's Disease Rating Scale**

	BEN'S PRESENTATION AND SCORE	FAMILY CONCERNS/ PROBLEMS	SUGGESTED ACTIONS
Mentation, Behavior, and Mood			
IQ impairment	Score of 2: moderate memory loss with disorientation and moderate difficulty handling complex problems: needs prompting for some ADLs.	Ben wants to continue to drive during the day to do some errands, especially as Logan works during the day on the ranch. Ben is not driving safely, especially with skills such as pulling out on the highway or turning left when traffic is present. In addition, Ben got lost on the ranch last week while trying to check on an area of fencing.	Discuss Ben surrendering his license. Allow him to continue to drive during daylight on the ranch as long as someone is with him.
Thought disorder	Score of 0: no problems.		
Depression	Score of 2: sustained depression (1 week or more). When asked, Ben reports feeling sad and depressed. He has made several statements of low self-esteem and how he is useless on the ranch anymore.	Family asks if Ben should be started back on an antidepressant medication. He was taking one right after Sarah, his wife, died 2 years ago, but he stopped quite a while ago.	Start on a selective serotonin reuptake inhibitor (SSRI) medication. The prescription has been faxed to the local pharmacy in Joseph, Oregon, and will be there for the family to pick up when they get home. Need to build this into daily medication schedule.
Motivation, initiative	Score of 1: less assertive than usual; more passive. See the previous entry. Ben does report feelings of anxiety at times.	Logan reports that Ben repeatedly asks about the same aspect of work on the ranch, such as completing the corral repair.	Consider adding an anxiety medication but will hold off for now. Discuss next visit or during phone call with local FNP.
Activities of Daily Living			
Speech	Score of 2: when "on" and "off" or at end of dosing period as Ben has hypophonia because of his Parkinson's disease.	Family reports that Ben is hard to hear and they feel as though they are always asking him to repeat what he says.	Referral to speech therapist during this visit to review with family some simple vocal exercises that will help Ben speak louder.
Salivation	Score of 1: slight but definite excess of saliva in mouth; has nighttime drooling.	Ben says this is annoying but not a problem.	Suggest Ben chew gum or suck on hard candy if this bothers him because either option stimulates swallowing.
Handwriting	Score of 3: severely affected; not all words are legible.	Kathleen has assumed bookwork for the ranch.	No further interventions at this time.
Cutting food and handling utensils	Score of 2: can cut most food, although clumsy and slow; some help needed; this is becoming more of an issue and before, Ben didn't need any assistance from Logan.	Logan and Ben eat breakfast and dinner together. Logan helps Ben when this is an issue. Logan has been doing all the cooking.	Kathleen and Carole agree to bring homecooked meals for Logan to heat up. Kathleen and Carole take turns food shopping.

(continued)

Case Study: Current Family—cont'd

Table 10-8	Presentation of Ben's Mid-Phase Parkinson's Disease Symptoms Using Unified Parkinson's Disease Rating Scale—cont'd		
	BEN'S PRESENTATION AND SCORE	**FAMILY CONCERNS/ PROBLEMS**	**SUGGESTED ACTIONS**
Dressing	Score of 2: occasional assistance with buttoning, getting arms in sleeves.	Logan helps Ben in the morning and at night with changing clothes. Ben struggles some at home in getting pants zipped and buttoned after toileting.	Suggest overalls that don't require buttons or pants with Velcro closures. Use slip-on shoes. Because of balance concerns, suggest Ben sit down when dressing.
Hygiene	Score of 2: needs help to shower or is very slow in hygienic care.	This is a new development. Logan is embarrassed by having to help his grandfather shower. In addition, this adds increased caretaking time to Logan's day.	Discuss safety adaptations in the shower (i.e., chair, grab bars). Discuss not bathing every day. Refer to occupational therapy to see if there are assistive devices for brushing teeth.
Turning in bed and adjusting bed clothes	Score of 2: can turn alone or adjust sheets, but with great difficulty.	Logan was concerned as he didn't even think about this aspect of help that his grandfather might need.	He will use silk pajama bottoms to decrease the friction of turning. Explore if a bed rail can be placed on the bed. Discuss the weight of the covers or blankets used at night.
Falling	Score is between a 2 and 3: Ben falls often but not daily. Sometimes he has fallen more than once in a day. Ben reports being dizzy when he stands (orthostatic hypotension).	All family members are very concerned about Ben falling and the difficulty he has getting up from the fall. Ben walks on a regular basis. He has not kept up with his physical therapy in the last year. Ben seems to be stiffer and has more abnormal movements even on his medications.	Family will increase fluids and get some support stockings to keep blood from pooling in his extremities. Have Kathleen and Carole complete a fall safety check in the home environment to identify hazards. Check that Ben has his cell phone on him or a cordless phone is within reach so he can call if he falls when alone.
Freezing when walking	Score of 3: Ben frequently freezes and occasionally falls from freezing.	See the previous entry. Explore more to see when Ben is freezing, such as during a turn, going through doorways, at the start of walking, or when he is doing something that requires him to take a step back.	Review strategies with Ben to help him get going when he freezes while walking.

Case Study: Current Family—cont'd

Table 10-8   **Presentation of Ben's Mid-Phase Parkinson's Disease Symptoms Using Unified Parkinson's Disease Rating Scale—cont'd**

	BEN'S PRESENTATION AND SCORE	FAMILY CONCERNS/ PROBLEMS	SUGGESTED ACTIONS
Walking	Score of 2: moderate difficulty. Ben refused to use a cane, but his grandson Tyler made Ben a walking stick, which he now uses. Ben has bradykinesia with a weak push-off, reduced leg lift, small stride length, lack of right arm swing, and a narrow stance.	See the previous entry. After much discussion, Ben admitted that he had trouble following his medication regimen during the day, when Logan was at work. He also noted that he had been taking more Sinemet when he wanted to go out.	See the previous entry. Refer to physical therapy (PT) for mobility evaluation and assistance in walking.
Pain	Score of 2: Ben complains of numbness, tingling, and frequent cramps and constant ache in his calves and lower back.		Starting Ben on SSRI for depression may help decrease pain sensations. Stretching and heat may relieve pain in calves.
Other Complications			
Sleep	Ben reports that he has insomnia. He has difficulty staying asleep. Before being diagnosed with Parkinson's disease, Ben was assessed for sleep apnea in a sleep clinic. He reports that he dislikes the CPAP machine and the mask on his face, so he does not use it. He thinks he sleeps about 4 hours a night. He has daytime sleepiness.	Logan hears Ben up at all hours of the night, which interferes with Logan's sleep. Ben has fallen at night too, which adds to Logan's vigilance of getting up to check on Ben.	Will discuss with FNP about having Ben reassessed for sleep at the sleep clinic in Pendleton, Oregon. Have Ben keep a simple sleep log if possible. Check on medications that Ben is taking and make sure that the timing of medication intake is not affecting sleep.
Excessive sweating	Ben reports that he has had periods of excessive sweating, similar to being caught in a rainstorm.		Check the timing of medications because these periods of excessive sweating may be happening as the dosing is ending or during the off periods.
Constipation	Ben has a long history of constipation, even before diagnosis.		Because Ben is sweating excessively at times, consider that he may be dehydrated. Set up a plan so that he drinks about 1,500 mL of fluids a day. Continue daily dose of Miralax.
Urinary problems	Ben reports nocturia, which might contribute to his insomnia.	Note that Ben was given a diuretic for hypertension. Explore the time of day when he is taking this medication.	Be sure there is a night-light and rugs in the bathroom.

(continued)

Case Study: Current Family—cont'd

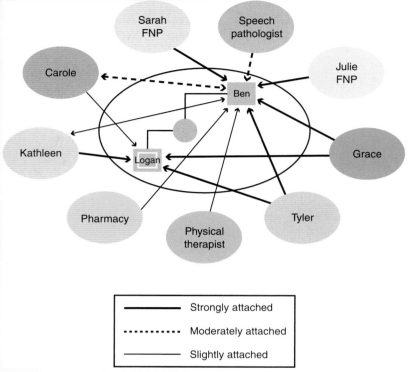

Strongly attached
Moderately attached
Slightly attached

FIGURE 10-9 Current Family Ecomap

Questions for reflection on the nursing care of the Current family:

1. Because Parkinson's disease has a progressive course, what challenges will the nurse anticipate the family will experience as the disease course progresses?
2. During the initial diagnosis time phase, what were some challenges and barriers Ben and the family might have experienced that the nurse should address?
3. How can the nurse facilitate assessment of family stressors as well as Ben's current medical condition?
4. What interventions can the nurse implement to help the family find balance and alleviate stress?
5. What alternative care options can the nurse discuss with the family to decrease care burden?
6. What home adaptations and/or assistive devices could be considered to provide care successfully in the home?
7. Ben has decided to surrender his driver's license. What implications might this have for Ben and his family that the nurse needs to consider?
8. What ethical issues might arise for Ben, the family, and the nurse throughout the trajectory of Ben's illness?

SUMMARY

A family focus on care should not be considered optional when it comes to chronic illness. The long-term effects of chronic health conditions affect individuals and families differently than acute health events.

- Although the needs that families experience may be similar initially, the duration of the illness alters the ways that care is managed and perceived during a long life course.
- The severity, complexity, and longevity of care needs associated with chronic conditions can alter a desired or expected

future into one that dramatically revolutionizes the lives of entire households.

- Financial costs and family resources are often highly taxed by years of debt and stress that would not have been expected if a chronic condition had not occurred. Some conditions may worsen over time or require endless amounts of attention that can become especially burdensome as the chronically ill person ages and economic or family resources are exhausted.
- Some CYSHCN and adults may require extraordinary adaptations by parents, siblings, and others that strain relationships.
- Although the chronic illnesses of children may be primarily genetic or environmental in nature, many adult chronic conditions are linked with lifestyle behaviors.
- Healthier lifestyles can reduce risks for some chronic conditions and can prevent or delay many complications from these diseases.
- Family-focused care aimed at meeting family needs when a member or members have a chronic illness requires nurses equipped with knowledge about families and their interactions.
- Optimal nursing care for those with chronic illness involves nurses who are knowledgeable about developmental alterations, willing to hear and listen to the voiced needs without judgment, and able to become collaborators that empower multiple household members to reorganize routines and manage existing resources.

chapter 11

Families in Palliative and End-of-Life Care

Kimberley A. Widger, PhD, RN, CHPCN(C)

Melissa Robinson, PhD, RN

Ridwaanah Ali, MSN, RN

Critical Concepts

- Palliative care is both a philosophy and a type of care.

- Palliative care is whole-person care that involves a focus on quality of life, or living well, for all family members when they are dealing with a life-limiting illness. It can start long before the end-of-life period, as early as the time of diagnosis of a life-limiting illness, and extend beyond death to bereavement.

- The principles of palliative care are applicable in a sudden, acute event—such as an accident, suicide, or myocardial infarction—although the context is different because there is a shorter time span in which to work with a family. A palliative approach complements the disease orientation that is often the focus of acute care.

- The majority of palliative care is provided by family caregivers.

- Skilled nursing interventions and relationships between nurses and families are crucial in creating positive outcomes in palliative and end-of-life care.

- Interprofessional teamwork is essential in palliative and end-of-life care, and the team includes family members.

- People who have advanced, life-limiting illnesses worry about being a burden on their families and about the consequences of their death on their families. Family members worry about burdening their ill member. Everyone involved is often afraid. This fear can lead to communication problems, isolation, and lack of support within the family.

- Barriers to nurses providing quality end-of-life care may be ameliorated when the nurse understands palliative care principles.

- Nurses need strong patient and family communication, assessment, and intervention skills to provide optimal palliative and end-of-life care.

- End-of-life decision making is a process that involves all relevant family members identified by the individual and evolves over time. Advance care planning is an important part of this process.

- A "good" death is one that happens in alignment with patient and family preferences.

Nurses encounter families who are facing end-of-life issues in almost all settings of practice. From newborns to older adults, people die, and their families are affected by the experience. Nurses are in an ideal position to influence a family's experience and to facilitate a positive experience for families, one that will bring them comfort in the future as they recall the situation when their loved one died. Depending on the circumstances and the support that is available to families when a loved one is at the end of life, the experience may also come with challenges. This is particularly true if the family experiences complex challenges during the course of illness, such as significant symptoms due to disease or challenges due to family caregiving in the home. Being a witness to the suffering and losses experienced by individuals and families can be stressful. Yet palliative and end-of-life nursing can be extremely rewarding and professionally fulfilling. It offers an opportunity for personal growth in patients, families, and health care providers; interactions among all can be especially meaningful (Davies et al., 2017). In a study that highlighted the experiences and coping strategies of palliative home-care nurses, Kaup et al. (2016) found that nurses felt great admiration for individuals and their families during such a vulnerable time, and they felt rewarded when their work was recognized and appreciated by family members.

The delivery of palliative care and the ongoing improvement of the quality of palliative care should be goals for all nurses, regardless of educational level. As more people live longer with chronic, life-limiting conditions, nurses increasingly require knowledge and skills in palliative care, particularly because nurses spend the most time with patients and families compared with any other health care providers. At all levels of nursing education, including undergraduate, nursing students require education about palliative care so they can deliver quality care (Ferrell et al., 2016; Negrete & Tariman, 2019).

This chapter details the key components of providing palliative and end-of-life nursing care, as well as families' most important concerns and needs when a family member experiences a life-threatening illness or is dying. The chapter also presents concrete strategies to assist nurses in providing optimal palliative and end-of-life care to all family members. More specifically, the chapter begins with a brief definition of palliative and end-of-life care, including its focus on improving quality of life for patients and their families. This is followed by a discussion of the principles of palliative care and ways to apply these principles across all settings, regardless of whether death results from chronic illness or a sudden or traumatic event. As the chapter closes, the concepts of family-centered palliative and end-of-life nursing care are applied in three case studies.

PALLIATIVE AND END-OF-LIFE CARE DEFINED

Palliative care and *end-of-life care* are not synonymous terms. Palliative care encompasses end-of-life care and aims to improve quality of life and reduce suffering in people living with a serious, life-limiting illness (Government of Canada, 2019). Palliative care may be provided from the time of diagnosis over many months, even years (especially in children), and can coexist with treatments aimed at curing an illness (World Health Organization [WHO], 2021). Palliative care includes bereavement support for the family (Government of Canada, 2018). The purpose of palliative care is to provide the individual and family with support for controlling symptoms and comfort throughout their illness while supporting them so that they experience optimal quality of life. End-of-life care is a component of palliative care that focuses on the care of persons who are nearing the end of life (Krau, 2016). Although it is difficult to predict and very unique to each person and their specific set of circumstances and conditions, end-of-life care is typically provided in the last days, weeks, or months of life. End-of-life care is focused on maintaining quality of life and allowing people to die with comfort and dignity (U.S. Department of Health and Human Services [USDHHS], 2017). A related term is hospice care which has slightly different meanings in Canada and the United States. In Canada, hospice typically refers to a community-based facility where residential respite, symptom management, and end-of-life care may be provided in a home-like setting. Hospices may also provide out patient services, respite in the home, bereavement support, or other services along the continuum of palliative care (Government of Canada, 2019). Children, in particular, may receive respite care in a hospice for years before their death. In the United States, a person may receive hospice care once attempts at curative treatments have been discontinued, and the person is expected to die within 6 months. Hospice may be provided in the home, hospital, or nursing home (USDHHS, 2017).

The difference in meaning may be confusing to health care providers, patients, and families if they share the common misconception that palliative care is equivalent to end-of-life care, a misconception that underpins the significant problem of late referral and acceptance of palliative care (Fox et al., 2016; Mulville, 2019). Another misconception, identified previously, is that health care providers cannot actively treat disease while concurrently engaging in palliative care. Palliative care focuses on improving the quality of life of patients and their families facing problems associated with life-limiting illness. Palliative care helps families in these situations live well by preventing and relieving suffering through early identification and excellent assessment and treatment of pain and other physical, psychosocial, or spiritual problems (WHO, 2021). If employed with a team approach, palliative care offers a support system to help patients live as actively as possible and to help families cope during the patient's illness and their own bereavement. Life is affirmed and dying is regarded as a normal process (Radbruch et al., 2020).

Family-centered care is a key principle in palliative care. Nowhere is this more evident than when a child is the patient. Support targets both individual family members and the family as a whole. The age range of patients receiving pediatric palliative care, typically 0 to 19 years of age, requires that children's developmental, social, educational, recreational, and relational needs be considered. The developmental stage of the family must also be considered, regardless of the patient's age.

Palliative care in adults developed primarily around care for patients with cancer. The current trend in palliative care, however, is an expanded focus on life-threatening illnesses beyond cancer. Life-threatening illnesses are conditions with the possibility for cure or remission, including physical traumas, infectious diseases, and cancer diagnoses (Witt et al., 2017). *Life-threatening illness*, *life-limiting illness*, and *serious illness* are terms often used interchangeably. *Life-limiting illness* refers more specifically to conditions that can be expected to cause death in the foreseeable future,

whereas *serious illness* is defined as a condition with a high risk of mortality and impairment of daily function and quality of life (Canadian Hospice Palliative Care Association, 2021; Lee et al., 2019). *Life-threatening illness* is often used to encompass both definitions of life-limiting and serious illness. Patients and their families have similar needs for information, care, and support in a wide variety of illnesses, for example, cardiovascular disease, cancer, chronic respiratory diseases, AIDS, diabetes, multiple sclerosis, Parkinson's disease, and neurological diseases. Palliative care may also be appropriate when patients are simply of an advanced age or failing to thrive (WHO, 2021).

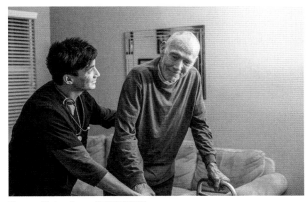

Source: © istock.com/LPETTET

Palliative care is about nurturing and maintaining quality of life from diagnosis of life-limiting illness through bereavement. Palliative care principles, listed in Box 11-1, can be applied to nursing care in any setting with any family, regardless of how long a person has to live or how sudden the death is. An awareness of illness trajectories and decline as people approach the end of life can also help nurses recognize when palliative care could be introduced. Trajectories of dying have been used to map the course of illness and the experience of dying, and a few are more relevant to palliative interventions than hospice care (Ballentine, 2018).

The sudden death and catastrophic event trajectories may be followed by periods of acute illness or result from an accident, injury, or violence, and they leave little to no time for individuals and families to prepare or benefit from support or advance care planning (Ballentine, 2018). Families experience shock, devastation, and grief, and they can benefit from support in the acute phases of loss.

Palliative Care Principles

- Palliative care can begin as soon as there is a diagnosis of life-limiting illness.
- Palliative care can occur concurrently with care that is curative in intent.
- The focus of palliative care is on supporting and enhancing quality of life.
- Patient- and family-centered care is the priority approach to care.
- Attention is paid to the needs of the patient and family, including their physical, developmental, psychological, social, and spiritual needs.
- Education and support of patient and family are crucial.
- An interprofessional approach is required.
- Care extends across inpatient and community-based settings.
- Bereavement support is an essential component of quality palliative care.

The terminal illness trajectory follows the diagnosis of a life-limiting illness such as cancer or heart disease and includes stages of disease progression, the need for close management of symptoms, and the support of family and loved ones (Ballentine, 2018). If early palliative intervention is available, individuals and families benefit from advance care planning and physical, emotional, and spiritual support.

At some point in the illness trajectory, the primary goal of care shifts from curative to palliative. This point often occurs when there are no available curative treatments, or treatments are no longer effective or are associated with a burden that is no longer tolerable to the patient. It is well recognized that communication about the transition of care from curative in nature to comfort or palliative is difficult but crucial. It requires discussion about shifting the focus to quality of life rather than quantity of life. When a sudden or traumatic event occurs, there is little time to hold such discussions. But when someone has a protracted illness, this discussion can be introduced gradually and can be repeated over time.

In many clinical settings, unfortunately, the option for palliative care is raised only in the last few days or weeks of life, even when death has been anticipated (Widger et al., 2016; Odgers et al., 2018). The late introduction of palliative care results in limitations for delivering the full potential of palliative care for both patients and family members (Hawley, 2017). For example, British Columbia's Fraser Health palliative care program cares for a population that experiences approximately 10,000 deaths per year; the average length of stay of patients on the program has dropped from 108 days in 2007 to 68.5 days in 2016, with a median length of stay of just 22.5 days (as reported by Director N. Hilliard), which unfortunately demonstrates delayed palliative care referrals (Hawley, 2017, p. 2). Some of the reasons for delayed referrals, which are well documented, include lack of access to palliative care, not knowing what resources exist, and misunderstandings about the differences between palliative care and end-of-life or hospice care (De Lima & Pastrana, 2016).

The introduction of palliative care is particularly challenging for health care providers when patients suffer from illnesses that are difficult to prognosticate, such as advanced lung, heart, and liver disease. One way of determining if a patient and family need palliative care is to use the so-called surprise question: "Would I be surprised if this patient died in the next 12 months?" (Weijers at al., 2018). Research has shown that this simple question may help identifying patients who are at higher risk of dying (Downar et al., 2017). When the answer is no, these patients and families should be a high priority for initiating conversations about palliative care and offering palliative interventions. It is important to ensure that patients, family members, and health care providers are aligned in their goals for care, such as to prolong life or to focus on comfort care (Hanson et al., 2017), and have a common understanding of what *quality of life* means for the patient and family. Goals of care and the meaning of *quality of life* will be unique in each situation, and care should be tailored to the needs of each particular family (Hanson et al., 2017).

Death occurs in many settings, from various causes, and across the life span. Some differences can be expected in families' experiences depending on the context, for example:

- Where the death takes place (e.g., home versus intensive care unit [ICU])
- The cause of death (e.g., natural progression of a chronic illness versus an unexpected, acute event)

- The dying trajectory (e.g., over a period of years versus sudden)
- The age of the family member who is dying (e.g., a 3-year-old child versus an 85-year-old adult)
- The cultural and spiritual backgrounds of families

No matter the context, the principles of palliative care should be consistent, with implementation tailored to address the particular family and the context of the family's experience. Consistent use of these principles contributes to high-quality palliative and end-of-life care.

Identifying Relevant Literature

The amount of research about the provision of palliative and end-of-life care to adults is growing. Research in pediatric palliative care is much more limited, but many of the reported issues for families are similar across the life span. The literature review updated for this chapter includes exploration of palliative and end-of-life nursing care for individuals and families experiencing life-limiting diseases and conditions, different causes of death (sudden deaths, deaths after illness), different care settings (long-term care, acute hospital care, critical care, home, and hospice), and who are at different stages of the life span (pediatric to older adult patients). Significant variation exists related to the beliefs, preferences, and needs across cultural groups as well as within individual families (Weerasinghe & Maddelena, 2016). Therefore, one cannot determine from the literature what the exact needs of specific individuals in certain settings will be, yet research does highlight key considerations for providing individualized palliative and end-of-life care, including important areas for nursing assessment and interventions. The literature found through these searches, plus seminal articles, forms the evidence base for this chapter.

KEY CONSIDERATIONS IN PALLIATIVE AND END-OF-LIFE CARE

In order to provide optimal palliative and end-of-life care, key areas must be considered, such as the following: nurses' own personal assumptions and biases about death and dying, nurses' personal assumptions about people and their backgrounds, the involvement of the family in all aspects of care, the involvement of the interprofessional team, the inclusion of bereavement care as part of palliative care, and potential barriers to optimal palliative and end-of-life nursing care.

Personal Assumptions and Biases About Dying and Death

To provide optimal palliative and end-of-life care, nurses need to be aware of their own assumptions and biases about dying and death. As a nurse, it is important to explore personal beliefs and attitudes and personal and professional experiences to understand how they may influence attitudes toward death, dying, and bereavement. For example, if a nurse believes that a family member should be physically present with someone who is dying, she or he may find it difficult to work with family members who choose not to be present.

Nurses may feel inexperienced when they encounter dying and death, no matter their level of expertise. They may be afraid, nervous, or anxious when faced with a dying patient and grieving family. Some nurses experience great satisfaction when working with dying patients. In fact, some have reported that their perspectives on life were enhanced through communication with patients about death, and some have grown in their own awareness of their mortality and personal beliefs (Rodenbach et al., 2016). Nurses who have developed their palliative care knowledge and skills, not simply through caring for many dying patients but through reflecting on their experiences with those patients and in their personal lives, may experience growth related to the meaning of life and death and on how both affect their own behavior (Hendricks-Ferguson et al., 2015). They are able therefore to provide competent physical care and be a supportive and therapeutic presence to those who are dying and to their family members. All nurses, from novice to expert, should develop basic competencies in the area of dying and death, from how to provide effective symptom management, using both pharmacological and nonpharmacological approaches, to being comfortable enough with dying and death that they can be present for family members. See Box 11-2 for some key areas of focus when seeking education about palliative and end-of-life care.

BOX 11-2

Key Areas of Focus for Education in Palliative and End-of-Life Care

In the *International Affairs Best Practice Guidelines*, the Registered Nurses' Association of Ontario (2020) recommends that entry to practice nursing programs and postregistration education should incorporate specialized end-of-life care content that includes the following areas:

- Dying as a normal process, including the social and cultural context of death and dying, dying trajectories, and signs of impending death.
- Care of the family (including the caregiver).
- Grief, bereavement, and mourning.
- Principles and models of palliative care.
- Assessment and management of pain and other symptoms (including pharmacological and nonpharmacological approaches).
- Emotional, spiritual, and existential issues and care.
- Decision making and advance care planning.
- Ethical issues.
- Effective and compassionate communication.
- Culturally safe care and ongoing assessments of expectations and preferences about illness and death.
- Advocacy and therapeutic relationship building.
- Interprofessional practice, model of care, and competencies.
- Self-care for nurses, including coping strategies, mitigation of compassion fatigue, and self-exploration of death and dying.
- End-of-life issues in mental health, homelessness, and the incarcerated.
- The roles of grief and bereavement educators, clergy, spiritual leaders, and funeral directors.
- Knowledge of relevant legislation and health services.

Source: Registered Nurses' Association of Ontario. (2020). Best practice guidelines: End-of-life care during the last days and hours. Toronto, ON: Author. http://rnao.ca/sites/rnao-ca/files/End-of-Life_Care_During_the_Last_Days_and_Hours_0.pdf

Nurses can develop these competencies by building on personal strengths and learning ways to become more comfortable with dying and death. It is often helpful to begin with reflection on personal experiences surrounding loss, death, and dying. Reflecting on personal beliefs about life and death helps clarify understanding of and appreciation for the human condition—the only thing certain in life is that everyone will die. Reflection can lead to deeper knowledge, personal growth, and strength, particularly through the discomfort of palliative and end-of-life care experiences (Carvalho, 2020). Professional development activities related to dying and death and to providing care at life's end, such as attending workshops or conferences and studying best-practice guidelines, or by reading books and even watching popular movies, can support nurses' development as palliative care clinicians. Gaining knowledge through formal education such as professional certification or academic study can also help improve knowledge and comfort with providing skilled care to patients and families facing a life-limiting illness. See Table 11-1 for a list of professional development opportunities for nurses.

Nurses often remember their first experience of patient death, and that memory can have a lasting impact, both personally and professionally. Preparing for this experience in advance through education, seeking out a supportive mentor and peer support at the time of a death, taking time to participate in debriefings that may be offered following the death, and reflecting on the experience can all facilitate a more positive experience that offers the opportunity for personal and professional growth, reduced anxiety, and development of positive attitudes to care of the dying (Hendricks-Ferguson et al., 2015; Nunes & Harder, 2019).

Personal Assumptions and Biases About People

An underlying principle in palliative care is respect for persons. It is helpful for nurses to be aware of the assumptions and stereotypes about the people cared for because assumptions and stereotypes get in the way of person- and family-centered care. Part of quality palliative and end-of-life care is recognizing that every person is valuable in his or her own right; however, this is sometimes negatively influenced by judgments about a particular person's or family's worth, background, or circumstances. Valuing appreciates the possibility that every human being has the potential for actualization or optimal development (Widger et al., 2009).

Assumptions and biases about people sometimes relate to their cultural or spiritual background. Similar to exploring personal assumptions and biases about dying and death, it is important to recognize one's personal cultural or spiritual background or previous experiences with other cultures and how they might influence practice, as well as one's expectations of others (Weerasinghe &

Table 11-1	**Professional Development Opportunities for Nurses**
ACTIVITIES	**ORGANIZATIONS, RESOURCES THAT SUPPORT PALLIATIVE CARE**
Advocacy, Best practice, Guidelines, Certification for nurses, Health policies, Membership for nurses, Research opportunities	Canadian Palliative Care Nursing Association (CPCNA)
	Hospice and Palliative Care Nurses Association (HPNA)
	International Association for Hospice and Palliative Care (IAHPC)
	Registered Nurses' Association of Ontario
	National Hospice and Palliative Care Organization (NHPCO)
Conferences and workshops	Canadian Hospice Palliative Care Learning Institute
	Canadian Hospice Palliative Care Annual Conference
	End-of-Life Nursing Education Consortium (ELNEC)
	National Hospice and Palliative Care Organization (NHPCO)

Maddelena, 2016). For example, if the importance of an Aboriginal smudging ceremony to a family is not understood, the nurse may be unwilling to create an environment that allows for such a ceremony within a hospital setting. The cultural and spiritual implications discussed elsewhere in this text also are relevant to quality palliative care. Effectively implementing the palliative care philosophy means that nurses must be sensitive to the needs of patients and their families who may be from a different culture or spiritual background than their own in order to integrate their beliefs, preferences, and practices into the patients' treatment plan (Cain et al., 2018). While some family members may find strength and renewed connection to their cultural or spiritual background, others may question previously held beliefs. Cultural beliefs, as well as spirituality, spiritual beliefs, or faith, inform people's worldview, including their response to advanced illness (Cain et al., 2018; Swinton et al., 2017). For example, advance care planning (see the section called Advance Care Planning later in this chapter) is an intervention developed primarily in Western cultures and it may not be appropriate or viewed as necessary in other cultures (Menon et al., 2018). It is very important that nurses avoid imposing their own beliefs on the patient and family or making assumptions about what a family might want or not want based on a particular background; instead, nurses should determine what is most important to the family (Bloomer et al., 2019).

It is also important to remember that there may be a great deal of diversity *within* cultures or faiths. There will never be a single approach that is appropriate for all people from a particular culture or faith group, so one of the best strategies is to ask families about the significance of dying and death within their spiritual or cultural traditions, their own beliefs, and their preferred ways of doing things (Dennis & Washington, 2018; Swinton et al., 2017). Personalized care, ethical practice, compassion, and empathy can guide palliative care, particularly when navigating differences (Ortega-Galán et al., 2019). From this place of understanding, nurses can negotiate care so that it aligns as closely as possible with the family's values and beliefs and demonstrates a fundamental respect for people.

Assumptions and biases may also relate to a person's sexual orientation or gender identity. LGBTQ+ persons often fear mistreatment and discrimination when accessing palliative care services (Hunt et al., 2019; Pang et al., 2019). Misconceptions on the part of health care providers and community members contribute to feelings of fear and prejudice, as well as inadequate access to services at the end of life (Hunt et al., 2019; Seelman et al., 2018; Stein et al., 2020).

A key principle of palliative care is patient- and family-centered care and the awareness that every person has the right to define their family and who can be involved in their care planning. This aligns with the concept of chosen family, or family of choice, wherein LGBTQ+ individuals construct familial and relational ties with chosen family members in addition to biological family members (Cloyes et al., 2018). Chosen families may include partners, spouses, friends, and biological and adopted children, and they are no less strongly bonded or significant than traditional forms of family. Chosen families are family and consist of whomever the individual identifies as family, including during palliative and end-of-life care interactions, where individual autonomy, respect for decisions, and compassion are prioritized.

It is important for nurses to be sensitive to the needs of members of underrepresented communities and to acknowledge how personal judgments can influence interactions when providing care. Strategies to promote inclusivity include creating a safe environment for open communication, demonstrating respect for differences, recognizing strengths, using appropriate and inclusive language on intake forms, using preferred pronouns, and incorporating sexual orientation and gender identity in care discussions when appropriate (Cloyes et al., 2018; Lowers, 2017; Stein et al., 2020).

Involvement of the Family and Family Caregiving

Life-limiting illness affects all family members, not just the patient. The effects of life-limiting illness on family caregivers, in particular, varies and is highly individualized depending on the situation (Committee on Family Caregiving for Older Adults, 2016). If the individual is in emotional or physical pain, has a low quality of life, or has difficulty coping with the illness, the caregiver's suffering dramatically increases as well, both during the illness and during bereavement (Hashemi et al., 2018). Siblings too may suffer if parents are too focused on the ill child to meet sibling needs (Eilertsen et al., 2018; Lövgren et al., 2017). Therefore, interventions directed at one family member can also be supportive of other family members, whether the individual is a child or an adult. Family members feel supported when they believe that professionals have the best interests of their loved one at heart. Therefore, nurses need to ensure that the patient is well cared for but also keep in mind that interventions directed at the family unit, as well as individual family members, can be effective. It is also important that nurses consider family caregivers as essential members of the health care team. Family caregivers are performing increasingly complex tasks and managing complex health conditions, and nurses can lead the way in supporting them (Reinhard & Brassard, 2020).

Among the top concerns of dying patients is the well-being of their family members in terms of caregiving burden and their ability to cope after the death (Gudat et al., 2019). Even children experiencing life-limiting illness may make decisions based on what they believe is best for their family rather than on what they particularly want (Weaver et al., 2016). Patients do not want to become a burden to their families (Gudat et al., 2019). If patients know that their families are well supported, it may reduce their own suffering.

Family members provide the majority of care for persons with life-limiting illness, and a home death relies on their strong involvement (Morris et al., 2015; Robinson et al., 2017). Family members carry a variety of burdens when a family member is dying (Totman et al., 2015), including compromises in their own health (e.g., depression, back pain, shingles, difficulty sleeping, and preexisting chronic illnesses), conflicting family responsibilities (e.g., caring for the ill parent or spouse plus caring for their own children), little time to meet their own needs, cumulative losses, fear, anxiety, insecurity, financial concerns, loss of physical closeness with a spouse, and lack of support from other family members and health professionals (Boersma et al., 2017; Washington et al., 2018).

The work of caregiving can be both physically and mentally exhausting (Boersma et al., 2017). There also may be an ambivalent sense of waiting for the person to die but not wanting the person to die. Family members may experience these issues whether their relative is mostly at home (Totman et al., 2015) or in an institutional setting (Martz, 2015). They often have increased responsibilities and may view the situation as burdensome (Hudson et al., 2019). Yet family caregivers are often more concerned about the care of the dying person than about their own health (Hashemi et al., 2018) and do not want to burden the patient or take focus off the patient. Supporting the family members to grow in their ability to be competent caregivers can help them significantly. It may also be helpful to facilitate communication among the family caregivers and the patient because they may each be over- or underestimating the level of burden or distress that each is experiencing. Sharing perspectives and their respective experiences may help improve understanding and support of themselves and each other (Leroy et al., 2016).

Although patients may want to remain at home, family members often have to assume extra responsibilities, such as administering medications, which can lead to a great deal of anxiety (Boersma et al., 2017; Robinson et al., 2017; Washington et al., 2018). When patients choose to receive care or die at home—perhaps to increase their quality of life through greater normalcy; increased contact with family, friends, and pets; and the familiar, comfortable surroundings (Benson et al., 2018; Robinson et al., 2017)—this location may not be the caregiver's first choice. For some families, a home death brings additional burdens, worry, and responsibility, and the home may feel like an institution or even a prison (Natsume et al., 2018). The caregiver may for go breaks in caregiving in order to honor the patient's desire to stay at home. Decisions related to care location must be made with family members because the course chosen has a profound impact on the well-being of both the patient and the family (Ates et al., 2018; Benson et al., 2018). Recognize too, however, that family caregivers often do not express their preferences if they differ from those of the individual and may need assistance from a nurse to navigate the competing demands and priorities (Petursdottir & Svavarsdottir, 2018).

Family members may not be available or able to give care at home. Patients and family members may believe that hospitals and hospices can provide a higher quality of end-of-life care than can be given at home or that the patient may pefer nonfamily providers of care. Some family members may experience profound guilt if they are not able to provide end-of-life care at home. Health care providers can alleviate some of this guilt if they alert patients and families early that plans for location of care may have to change over time to ensure provision of the best possible care that meets the needs of all family members, not just the dying person (Martz, 2015).

Burnout from caregiving is a common risk if family members are not able to cope with the caregiving requirements (Benson et al., 2018). The risk may be increased by the physical and emotional demands of the patient; reduced opportunities for the caregiver to participate in usual activities; and feelings of fear, insecurity, and loneliness (Ates et al., 2018; Totman et al., 2015). Caregiver strain may increase when patients need more assistance with activities of daily living or have greater levels of psychological and existential distress. Differences may exist in needs based on age and sex, with younger caregivers having more concerns about finances and maintaining work schedules, social activities, and relationships compared with older caregivers, who may be experiencing health-related concerns (Vick et al., 2019). While the challenges of caregiving vary widely, particularly among family caregivers, some include physical strain, disruption in sleep, financial strain, social isolation, stress, and coping challenges.

On the other hand, many people report positive aspects of caregiving, such as feelings of satisfaction, greater appreciation for life, greater purpose and meaning to life, increased closeness and intimacy, newfound personal strength and ability, and the opportunity to share special time together and show their love for their dying family member (Benson et al., 2018; Collins et al., 2016). Even bereaved siblings report positive outcomes from the experience, such as strengthened family bonds, increased maturity, and personal growth (Eilertsen et al., 2018). Some family members may view care provision as an opportunity and a privilege (Benson et al., 2018). It is important, therefore, to help families uncover the positive aspects and recognize the value in what they are doing because it may contribute to their overall well-being and may enhance their experience. Similarly, bereaved parents have consistently identified health care professionals and the care institution as having an impact on their grief journeys. Parents have emphasized the importance of developing strong relationships, providing high-quality communication throughout the care experience, and preventing negative experiences during their child's illness (Snaman et al., 2016). Nurses are in an excellent position to identify and foster a family's strengths and to identify, prevent, and alleviate many of the negative aspects of caregiving. Through provision of optimal palliative and end-of-life care, nurses can have a significant, lifelong effect on the well-being of family members.

Involvement of the Interprofessional Team

Although the focus of this chapter is on the role of the nurse, provision of care through an interprofessional team approach is one of the principles of palliative care (Kelley & Morrison, 2015). The composition of the team may look quite different depending on the care setting. For example, in a rural setting, the team may be comprised of a family physician and a nurse, whereas in a large urban setting, there may be a team of palliative care specialists, including palliative physicians, advanced practice nurses, psychologists, spiritual care advisers, pharmacists, social workers, and volunteers. In all settings, nurses are core team members. The *interprofessional team approach* focuses on health care providers collaboratively working with each other and with a patient and family members as members of the team to develop a plan of care to achieve common goals (Kelley & Morrison, 2015). Despite sharing common goals, each team member will bring different ideas and skills to the team, which is both the strength and the challenge of the interprofessional team approach. Multiple perspectives contribute to holistic care and the ability to meet the multiple complexities of the patient and family needs that arise in palliative care. The challenge is how to make best use of each health care provider's and family member's contributions while negotiating differences in perspective and respectfully managing tensions around professional and personal boundaries and expertise. Palliative care is known for blurring of team member roles in order to meet the current needs of the patient and family members.

For nurses, being an effective member of an interprofessional team often means that they share information and consult with others on the team; mediate on behalf of patients and families when necessary; and act as a liaison between various members, institutions, and programs. Novice nurses can contribute effectively to the interprofessional team by eliciting and understanding the patient's and family members' hopes, preferences, beliefs, fears, and goals and sharing this understanding with the team. Knowledge about group dynamics is invaluable in learning how to become a successful team member. Everyone needs to know and accept that each member of the team is unique and valuable, and good communication skills are crucial so that supportive rather than defensive communication can be fostered. A lack of communication among health care providers is common and frustrating for families because they then receive conflicting information or need to repeat information and relay decisions that have been made already (Caswell et al., 2015; Widger & Picot, 2008).

Bereavement Care

One of the principles of palliative care is that care continues after the death of the patient and into the bereavement period. The need for follow-up with the family after the death of their loved one by involved health care providers is considered by many families to be a crucial component of end-of-life care, but unfortunately one that is often missing (McAdam & Puntillo, 2018; Widger & Picot, 2008). Families sometimes feel abandoned after the death, which adds to the grief they experience (Widger & Picot, 2008). Bereavement care is important because family members that lack sufficient support have a higher risk of developing physical health problems, post-traumatic stress disorder, anxiety, depression, and prolonged grief (McAdam & Puntillo, 2018). Family caregivers may have additional risks related to physical exhaustion, difficulty sleeping, and the aftermath of the demands of caregiving. It is not unusual for family members to express some feelings of relief that the patient's suffering has ended or to worry that everything possible was done to keep them comfortable. Having a supportive presence to acknowledge their feelings can make a significant difference. After the death, some caregivers may be at risk for impaired quality of life and physical or mental health challenges. Support for families after the death may help prevent or alleviate prolonged suffering. Specific interventions for bereavement care are highlighted later in the chapter and in the case studies.

Barriers to Optimal Palliative and End-of-Life Nursing Care

A major barrier to optimal palliative and end-of-life care for patients and their families arises from the limited formal education and clinical training that nursing students and medical residents receive (Hawley, 2017). Although some improvements have been made, historically little attention has been given to palliative and end-of-life care in nursing and other health care providers' curricula. Health care providers report being unprepared to treat pain and symptoms effectively, emotionally support the dying person and his or her family, or deal with the ethical issues that may be present at end of life (Hussin et al., 2018). Health care providers may be uncomfortable or too afraid to initiate conversations about palliative care because they feel unprepared and are concerned about diminishing the patient's or family's hope (Fox et al., 2016). However, research has shown that even difficult conversations about preferences for care at the end of life do not disrupt hope (Delgado-Guay et al., 2016; Konietzny & Anderson, 2018).

Another barrier to optimal palliative care is the availability and use of palliative services. Specialist palliative care services may not be available in all care settings, particularly at home or in rural and remote areas, to provide support to practicing health care providers in addressing the learning needs of or providing care to patients and families (Hawley, 2017). Even when appropriate hospice and palliative care services are available, a lack of understanding of palliative care on the part of health care providers can lead to delayed services or even a lack of referral to these services.

Involvement of the patient and family members in the interprofessional team is a critical component of palliative care, yet barriers may exist that limit this involvement. In many cases, the program setup and lines of communication do not allow for families to be included to the extent they could and should be, nor do they allow for provision of bereavement care by the health care professionals who provided care before the death. Although work has to be done to remove the identified barriers, it is possible for nurses to practice high standards within constraining contexts. It is important to seek opportunities to improve your knowledge and skills in palliative and end-of-life care and to be an advocate for the needs and views of patients and families regardless of the barriers that may be present.

A different type of barrier that can be even more challenging to manage is the moral distress that can arise for nurses when they provide end-of-life care to patients and their families. This can occur when nurses do not feel prepared to provide palliative or end-of-life care to patients, when the care is perceived as inadequate, or when access to care is limited (Wolf et al., 2019). Moral distress occurs when a person is powerless to carry out an action that he or she believes to be ethically appropriate. Some situations common to the provision of palliative care that may cause moral distress include the following:

- Patients receive medical treatments that are believed to be inappropriate and/or contribute unnecessarily to patients' suffering (e.g., a ventilator, providing artificial nutrition and hydration) (Cheon et al., 2015).
- Inadequate management of pain or other symptoms (Gagnon & Duggleby, 2014).
- Lack of communication with family members about prognosis (Kerr et al., 2019; Odgers et al., 2018).
- Provision of false hope to family members.
- Difficulty providing palliative care in acute-care settings because of organizational constraints (e.g., task-oriented curative culture of care that devalues the emotional dimension of care, lack of time, and poor communication within the interprofessional team) (Gagnon & Duggleby, 2014)

Work-related moral distress can lead to compromised health status for nurses, reduced productivity, and a risk to patient safety. Ultimately, it can affect nurses' job satisfaction and their physical and psychological well-being, and lead to burnout and leaving the work environment (Christodoulou-Fella et al., 2017).

FAMILY NURSING PRACTICE ASSESSMENT AND INTERVENTION

Nurses must possess strong patient and family assessment skills if they are going to provide optimal care (e.g., excellent pain and symptom management, psychosocial support) because the most appropriate interventions can be designed and implemented only once a family's needs and goals have been assessed accurately. A nurse's assessment helps determine what a specific family or family member needs, and the care can then be tailored with an individual approach in consultation with the family. Assessment and intervention are therefore intertwined and are discussed together in the following sections.

Assessment should be ongoing and sequential, building on what is known about the family and shaping interventions to meet the family's changing needs and preferences throughout the palliative care and end-of-life process. This section is organized around interventions that may be helpful to families. The interventions discussed are informed by existing research evidence and have been used successfully in the authors' clinical practices. The most important thing to remember is that each family is unique. Although practice should be informed by evidence, it is important to apply theory and research critically and in alignment with individual family needs. What works for one family or family member may not be right for another (Hill et al., 2017). The need to assess and critically analyze each situation on its own merits and actively involve the family in the process is especially important in palliative care. Because a nurse cannot know in advance if an intervention will be useful to a particular family, interventions should always be offered tentatively and then evaluated regularly from the patient's and family's perspective. An intervention is only helpful if a patient or family member experiences it as helpful.

It is not possible to cover every potential scenario in palliative and end-of-life care; therefore, the focus is on discussing the main assessment and intervention concepts needed for palliative and end-of-life care. Most deaths encountered when providing end-of-life care occur as the result of chronic disease rather than an acute event. Therefore, these situations are the focus of the remaining discussion and the case studies.

Connections Between Families and Nurses

The relationships that families develop with health care providers have a significant effect on how families manage palliative care and end-of-life events, as well as how they cope after the death (Davies et al., 2017; Sopcheck, 2019). In nursing education, characteristics of a helping or therapeutic relationship are often discussed, but in practice, nurses often speak of their "connections" with families rather than their "relationships" with families. Making a connection with family members helps uncover what is meaningful to them and builds a bridge between the nurse and the family member as human beings (Davies et al., 2017).

Understanding the family's situation apart from the illness is important. Asking about the family's previous experiences with death, any recent or concurrent life changes (e.g., new job, new house, new baby), or work and school responsibilities (e.g., self-employed, supportive work environment, nearing final examinations) may allow a more in-depth understanding and appreciation of the complex influences on the family's experience.

Connecting allows a nurse to apply general palliative knowledge in ways that are more likely to be successful for individual patients and their families. Connecting is a two-way process where both the nurse and the patient and family members get to know one another as individuals and begin to establish reciprocal trust (Robinson, 2016). With trust comes a greater sense of comfort and ease for the family and an increased ability for nurses to offer effective interventions and to act as advocates (Davies et al., 2017).

Communication and interpersonal skills can facilitate or hinder connecting with patients and families (Davies et al., 2017; Kerr et al., 2019; Odgers et al., 2018). Therefore, nurses need to be aware of how their personal styles of interaction and communication can make, sustain, and break connections. These connections have to be attended to and nourished over time. Families typically are not used to talking about dying and death. The presence of a mutual, trusting relationship is foundational to palliative assessment and intervention (Davies et al., 2017; Robinson, 2016; Widger et al., 2009) and is crucial to providing a safe environment for difficult and emotional conversations to occur.

Nursing interventions that promote connections and trusting relationships include careful listening to the family's experience with illness and suffering, valuing their expertise as caregiver, asking effective questions that encourage family members' understanding of the differences in their perspectives, demonstrating compassion by showing that the nurse is touched by the family's suffering, remaining nonjudgmental, offering a new perspective or information through open and honest communication, working *with* the family, acknowledging family strengths, and being reliable and accessible (Davies et al., 2017; Kerr et al., 2019; Robinson et al., 2019; Sopcheck, 2019). It is important for nurses to show families through attitude and behavior that they not only have the knowledge to assist them but are also willing and able to do so. The sense of security and trust a family experiences in relationships with health care providers can add to and strengthen the family's resources. Simple acts, such as addressing family members by name; smiling; making eye contact; showing emotion; and appropriate physical contact, such as a hand on the shoulder, can foster connections between family members and the nurse (Butler et al., 2015; Davies et al., 2017). Family caregiving in palliative care is emotionally and physically challenging for family members, so responsive empathetic communication is essential when providing support.

Nurses are responsible for taking the lead in developing a trusting relationship with families and providing an environment of openness where all family members feel comfortable asking questions (Robinson, 2016). Completion of a brief family genogram is one effective way of learning family members' names; their relationships; and their level of involvement in care, including decision making. Social support, including shared caregiving, is a key aspect of managing well, yet primary family caregivers may be reluctant to ask for help (Wittenberg-Lyles et al., 2014). When working with families, nurses may find creating a genogram and ecomap can help identify gaps in support.

Getting to know each family member demonstrates respect for the patient's and family members' individuality, dignity, needs, concerns, and fears (Gordon et al., 2009; Sopcheck, 2019). It also enables recognition of differences within the family. Box 11-3 provides some questions to help open up communication and learn about family members' perspectives to build connections with the family.

Making a connection does not necessarily happen instantly, nor does it have to take a lot of time; however, it does require attention and cannot be taken for granted (Davies et al., 2017). Sometimes a connection between a nurse and a family is easy to make; other times, the nurse may need to make an extra effort to get to know the family and to establish a relationship. The nurse may need to "prove" their trustworthiness to the family (Robinson, 2016) or set aside their own negative reaction to a particular family or family member. Developing a reflective practice and consulting with experienced professionals may be helpful when making connections proves difficult (Hendricks-Ferguson et al., 2015).

All too often, unfortunately, families report lack of support, not being valued and respected, and a poor sense of connection with a nurse, which in turn can contribute to negative experiences and dissatisfaction with care. Even single incidents related to poor communication and interpersonal skills on the part of health care providers can contribute to intense emotional distress in family members, including anxiety, depression, and guilt, often long after the event occurred (Odgers et al., 2018; Widger & Picot, 2008). Understanding this pattern leads some nurses to worry about saying the wrong thing. Listening carefully may assist in knowing where to start. Sometimes there are no "right" words to say, but simply being present and staying with the family can be helpful.

Humor may be another way to facilitate a connection with families, but it is important first to assess their openness to humor. Obviously, this is much easier when families demonstrate humor in their interactions, which can indicate that they will be receptive when humor is initiated by nurses or other health care professionals. The use of humor can provide respite from thinking about the illness, relieve tension, and demonstrate respect for the patient and family members as people if it fits with their way of being. Palliative care nurses have reported that humor often has a meaningful impact on families and can be a way to facilitate meetings with patients and their family members (Kaup et al., 2016). In a study that examined the experiences of palliative home care nurses, a participant shared the following:

> When you work in palliative care, the rules are already given: You know the patient will die—the worst is already known—and we are asked to make the best of the situation, and we can often do that. (Kaup et al., 2016, p. 566)

Some strategies that nurses can use to make a connection between themselves and patients and families are provided in Box 11-4.

Relieving the Patient's Suffering

What do dying people want? They want adequate ways to control their pain and symptoms, prepare for death and avoid inappropriate prolongation of dying, achieve a sense of control, live a meaningful life, relieve burdens for their loved ones, and strengthen relationships with loved ones (Kastbom et al., 2017). Concern about becoming a burden to their family may keep dying people from talking to family members about their fears. At the same time, family members are worried about burdening the dying person. These types of worries can create silence that contributes to a sense of isolation and aloneness for dying people and their loved ones. One of the ways nurses can be helpful is to assess who is talking to whom, who knows what, and what is holding people back from having conversations that nurture and strengthen the relationships that are often deeply desired within

BOX 11-3

Key Questions to Ask Families to Open Up Communication and Obtain Family Members' Perspectives

Questions to open up communication and obtain family members' perspectives ideally should be asked with all involved family members present, including the patient. Keep in mind, however, that family members may not want to burden their ill member with their emotions and concerns, so you may find that some of these questions need to be asked of family members when they are alone. You will need to finesse questioning depending on where the ill family member is in the palliative care experience.

Start by saying, "I'd like to understand what it has been like for your family to live with [illness]." Then, use the following key questions to invite communication and obtain family members' perspectives. It is often helpful to indicate that you expect different family members to have different views about different topics, so you may need to ask a question multiple times in order to have all family members' views.

- What is your understanding of what is happening with [ill family member]?
- What experience do you have as a family in dealing with serious health problems? With death and dying?
- If you were to think ahead a bit, how do you see things going in [the next few days, the next few weeks, the next few months: use the time frame that is most appropriate]?
- How are you hoping this will go?
- What is most important for me to know about your family?
- What are you most concerned or worried about?
- When you think about your loved one getting really sick, what fears or worries do you have?
- I've found that many families caring for someone with this condition think about the possibility of their loved one dying. They have questions about this. Do you have questions?
- Who is suffering most?
- How do they show their suffering?
- How are you managing?

- I understand that different family members have different talents or strengths: How do you most want to be involved?
- How can I be most helpful to you at this time?
- How does your family like to talk about challenging issues?
- How have you been talking about the situation you find yourselves in? Who has been involved?
- Is there anyone involved who is important and who I haven't met?
- How are important decisions made in your family? How would you like important decision making to go now?
- Families often find it helpful to talk about the care they want at the end of life. Have you been able to have a conversation about this? I wonder if I might be able to help you start this conversation.
- Do you have any cultural beliefs, rituals, or traditions around illness and end of life that I should be aware of?
- What have you found most helpful or useful to you as a family at this time?
- What do you most need to manage well?
- What has not been helpful?
- What sustains you in challenging times?
- What is going well?
- What do you most want to be doing at this time? What brings you joy [or what helps you get out of bed in the morning]?
- If your loved one were to die tonight, is there anything you have not said or done that you would regret? If so, how can I help you do or say what you need to do? [Ask this of the patient as well, that is: If you were to die suddenly, is there anything you would regret not doing or saying?]
- In families, many things are often happening apart from the illness that we do not know about. Is there anything going on that is adding to what you are already coping with?

the family. Suffering can be alleviated by inviting and assisting families to come closer together and to engage in meaningful conversations (Konietzny & Anderson, 2018).

Meaningful conversations are not possible, however, unless the dying person is physically comfortable. Controlling pain and symptoms is a high priority for individuals who are approaching

the end of life. This is also a priority for family members, who often step in to provide skilled palliative care for their loved ones. Witnessing the suffering of their dying family member when there is uncontrolled pain and symptoms is traumatic for family members. Therefore, the control of pain and symptoms is truly the foundation of quality family palliative and end-of-life care. Nurses need

BOX 11-4

Establishing and Sustaining Connections With Families

To establish and sustain connections with families, do the following:

- Patients and families need to know who you are; when you meet a patient and family for the first time, make them feel welcome, introduce yourself by name, then find out who they are and learn about them as people as well. Ask them how they would like to be called (e.g., by full name or first name). Ask them about their relationship to one another (e.g., to find out whether they are partners, sisters, friends). This is a good time to begin a genogram, which can be supplemented over time.
- Begin any interaction by clarifying your role and telling the patient and family about your "professional" self so you can establish your credentials. For example, "Hello, Mr. Li. My name is Rose Steele. I'm a third-year student nurse. Sandyha Singh, the registered nurse supervising me, and I are taking care of your wife today. I'm working until 3:30 p.m. today and will also be here tomorrow, so I'll be her nurse then too. I have worked on this unit for the past 3 weeks, so I am pretty familiar with all the routines, but I'm really interested in finding out how we can fit in with what you and Mrs. Li want."
- The best approach is not "This is how we do it here," but rather "How do you like to do this?" and "How can we find a way to do that in this context?" Sometimes we cannot do it exactly the way the patient and/or family would like, so then we need to ask about what the most important pieces are so that we can come as close as possible to the desired result.
- Ensure a comfortable physical environment; let patients and families know the routines and how they can get help as needed to provide a sense of familiarity and help you begin to make the connection.
- Privacy is often an issue, and it is critical to some of the sensitive discussions that occur in palliative and end-of-life care. Try to find a private location before broaching sensitive issues.
- Describe who the other team members are and what their roles are so families understand the context. Family members often do not know who to ask for what.
- Attend to the patient's and family's immediate state of well-being; it is impossible to connect with someone when you have not attended to their basic needs first. If a patient is lying in a wet bed or is in pain, family members will not be open to a "connecting" conversation with the nurse. When you demonstrate good assessment and intervention skills that result in enhanced comfort, your practice invites trust.

- Be sensitive to an individual's particular characteristics, such as cultural or gender differences; making eye contact is a useful strategy for connecting in many cases, but a First Nations person, for instance, may be uncomfortable with direct eye contact. Touch is often welcome but is not universally experienced as supportive. You may need to ask about what provides comfort to the patient and family members.
- Be aware of your own assumptions and biases, and guard against "operationalizing" your biases—for example, do not assume that an older adult is hard of hearing.
- Be sensitive to a person's way of being. Some people are outgoing and talkative; others are more withdrawn. It is a good idea to check your observations rather than simply assuming that your interpretation of what you are seeing is correct. For example, some people become very quiet and stoic when in pain. This approach may be their way of managing pain and not their usual way of "being." Humor may be appropriate for some people or situations but not for others. Responding to people in ways that match their style enhances their comfort level. Another useful habit is to use the family's language. If you need to use medical terms, be sure to explain them. Sometimes family members use incorrect words (e.g., *prostrate* instead of *prostate*). Generally, the best way to handle it is to use the correct word in a matter-of-fact way and say something similar to, "Oh yes, I understand that the problem is prostate cancer."
- Not all people will want the same level of connection; you need to respect where the person is coming from and not try to force a deeper relationship. Families dealing with prolonged, life-threatening illness often have negative health care encounters that lead them to be wary of new health care providers and make them careful in how much, and in whom, they trust. Sometimes it takes time and the repeated demonstration of trustworthy behaviors before they are willing to begin to trust a new health care provider.
- Patients and families differ in their expectations of what health care providers should provide; some only want information, some expect only physical care, and still others expect more of a supportive relationship. The key here is in asking for expectations. This does not mean that you can meet the expectations, and you may want to preface the request with a statement such as, "To be most helpful to you, I need to know what you would like. I may not be able to do things exactly as you prefer, but we can work together to get as close as possible."

(continued)

BOX 11-4

Establishing and Sustaining Connections With Families—cont'd

- You may find that when you simply meet the patient's and family's expectations without imposing your own, further opportunities for connecting may evolve.
- Once the connection has been made, it is important to pay attention to nurturing it so that it is sustained over time.
- Sustaining the connection allows you to learn even more about the patient and family so you can continually adapt your care according to their needs; it is also a way of demonstrating your trustworthiness by inviting the patient and family to get to know and trust you. When you are well connected, you are more likely to offer useful interventions that the family will accept.
- Ways of sustaining the connection include spending time with the patient and family, asking effective questions, noticing what they are doing that is positive or helpful, and being available. Sometimes the only thing we can do is to stay with patients and families as a witness to their suffering.
- Making and sustaining the connection is a two-way process that has to do with sharing parts of yourself with patients and families as you seek a common bond. This process may mean revealing some personal details about your life. There are a few circumstances when it is appropriate, for example, when the patient or family ask you a direct question about yourself or when you have had an experience that helps you understand what the family may be experiencing. Revealing personal details can be helpful in inviting trust, but they should be brief and should not take the focus away from the patient and family.
- Continuity of care, such as having the same nurse be in contact with the same patient during some period of time, is important. It is critical that team members communicate effectively with one another to support continuity of care.
- It is not just the quantity but also the quality of time we spend with a family that makes the difference.

For example, if you clear your mind before coming into the room, come to the bedside, and are calmly attentive to the patient rather than doing multiple tasks while also talking, the encounter will seem longer and be more satisfying to the patient.
- The "best" nurses are those who give the impression of "having all the time in the world," even when they are really busy. One way of doing this is to come into the room and sit or stand by the bedside, even if only briefly.
- Taking the time to be there for patients and families instead of being in a rush maintains the connection. This requires you to be mindful and to let go momentarily of all the demands that compete for your attention.
- Even when you are not actually with patients and families, it is important that they feel as if you will be available when they need you; simple things such as saying hello and goodbye at the beginning and end of shifts and also at breaktimes help them know your availability. Let the patient and family know how long you are available and when you will be back; for example, "I'm just popping in to see how your pain is and won't be able to stay long, but I'll be back in about half an hour and will be able to spend more time with you then."
- Informing patients and families so they know what to expect and keeping your word, such as being there when you say you will be, also sustain the connection.
- Instead of having your routine set for the day, adapt your routine to what the patient and family need at the time.
- Be flexible because you are always working under constraints; share these constraints with patients and families, and tell them if you need to change the plan you have made with them.
- Changing plans often requires the support of colleagues who can take over for you or help out as needed.

to understand the variety of symptoms common to patients at the end of life so that they can anticipate, prevent when possible, recognize, assess, and effectively manage pain and symptoms with both traditional and complementary therapies. Key to this is regular, systematic assessment using standardized assessment tools, such as the revised Edmonton Symptom Assessment System, which is used worldwide in both clinical practice and research for skilled symptom management (Hui & Bruera, 2017). Involving the dying person as much as possible in planning and treatment decisions supports the need for achieving a sense of control as more and more of their life feels out of control.

Relieving suffering results in improved quality of life, but no single definition exists for the most important factors that contribute to a good quality of life. Only the individual and family members know what constitutes quality of life for them. Individual needs must be assessed. Higher patient quality-of-life ratings have been associated with a variety of activities, such as playing music that was meaningful to the patient, attending a place of worship, having a familiar health care team available (for patients at home), and having individual preferences respected (Norris et al., 2007). Other components predictably contributing to better quality of life include valuing everyday activities; maintaining a positive attitude; relieving symptoms; feeling in control; and feeling connected to and needed by family, friends, and health care providers (Lewis et al., 2018; Park et al., 2018).

Empowering Families

Family palliative and end-of-life care is a strengths-based approach. It is about building and nurturing family strengths to ensure that quality of life, as defined by the family, can be achieved as closely as possible. Rather than solely focusing on deficits or areas that the nurse perceives as problematic, palliative care emphasizes empowering families to manage this challenging time in their own unique way by noticing and building on strengths while at the same time effectively addressing problems. All the empowering strategies require good communication skills. The focus should be on maximizing the patient's and family's capacity to use their own resources to meet their needs and respecting their ability to do so. Nurses empower patients and families by creating an environment in which their strengths and abilities are recognized, encouraging them to consider various options, assisting them in fulfilling their needs and desires through the provision of information and resources, and supporting their choices. Several specific interventions that empower families are commending families, educating families about clinical options and constraints, and helping families to help themselves. The Carer Support Needs Assessment Tool (Aoun et al., 2015) is both an assessment and an intervention resource that has been shown to engage family caregivers effectively in conversations about their needs, priorities, and solutions.

Family members appreciate being recognized for being close to their loved one and for their caregiving ability. Nurses can facilitate this appreciation by commending the work of the caregiver.

Commending patients, families, and individual family members is a powerful intervention (Wright & Leahey, 2012), especially in the presence of the individual being cared for. Caregivers may be better able to cope with caregiving when the nurse recognizes and appreciates their role. Effective commendations involve making specific observations of patterns of family strengths that occur across time (Wright & Leahey, 2012). Similarly, parents appreciate recognition of their parenting role and skills. Complimenting the work of parents can strengthen parents' confidence and even their relationship with their child. Empowering patients and families with knowledge of the resources available to them, as well as some of the constraints of clinical care, can prepare them to make choices that are most appropriate for them (Robinson et al., 2017).

Engaging both the patient and involved family members in discussion about preferences for care, preferences for place of death, and available resources may assist negotiations regarding decisions that can be simply taken for granted when family members automatically step forward to take on the role of caregiver. Families feel empowered when they are involved in care decisions and attention is paid to their personal choices and preferences.

Strain on families, also referred to as caregiver burden, may be reduced when families feel more

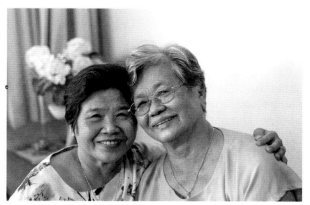

Source: © istock.com/Pornpak Khunatorn

capable in their ability to provide and manage the patient's end-of-life care and better able to attend to their own self-care needs, which in turn may also have an impact on their grief and difficult emotions or interactions (Dempsey et al., 2020). Nurses need to assess families for their knowledge, skills, and concerns and then offer appropriate interventions, such as providing required information, teaching family members how to provide adequate care to their loved one, and providing the needed instrumental support (e.g., referring to appropriate resources such as a social worker who can arrange for respite care) (Dempsey, 2020). Encouraging family members to share their emotions and then validating these feelings can also help to reduce strain on the family (Hudson et al., 2019).

Empowering patients and families may include helping them to do what they themselves want and need to do rather than health care providers taking over and doing it for them (Davies et al., 2017). For example, although it may appear quicker and easier for the nurse to assist a patient out of bed, it may be important that the patient moves by herself or that a family member is taught to assist. Sometimes the nurse needs to be creative in finding ways to empower patients and families. Consulting and collaborating with other team members can help identify creative ways to empower family members across diverse environments and situations.

It is important to assess the capacity of patients and families to do for themselves and then find ways of supporting them when hopes and expectations exceed capability. Careful assessment of the situation is central to knowing when to act on behalf of patients and families and when to encourage them to manage themselves because if the nurse "does for" patients and families when they can care for themselves, their sense of competency may be diminished, which can be disempowering. Family members and caregivers can feel insecure and anxious about their abilities and what to expect during uncertain times (Ortega-Galán et al., 2019), so the nurse's assessment is critical to understanding the needs of the family.

Providing Information

Effective communication is essential to providing quality end-of-life care, enabling patients and families to understand what is happening and to adjust to the situation as it changes (Caswell et al., 2015). Families need information, but they may not know what questions to ask. A lack of knowledge and feeling uninformed can leave people feeling isolated, frustrated, and distressed. There is also significant variation among individuals and families regarding what type of information they want

from clinicians. In a study conducted to understand possible barriers to preparedness among caregivers of elders with dementia, researchers identified dramatic differences. Participants identified indirect communication and a lack of communication as major barriers in their ability to prepare for prognosis, death, and what to expect, sharing that the clinicians would "beat around the bush" (Hoveland & Kramer, 2019, p. 61). Others admitted, "I didn't want to hear that," when clinicians tried to inform them, and they were not willing or able to receive the information due to a lack of acceptance (Hoveland & Kramer, 2019, p. 62). Some families want a great deal of detailed information, whereas others feel overwhelmed with too much information and find that it interferes with their ability to live as normal a life as possible. Therefore, ongoing assessment of how much and what types of information families want is important (Chi et al., 2018). This assessment should also include how much information should be offered directly to the patient, especially a child, and if there are cultural beliefs and norms for communication that affect the preferences of the family (Cain et al., 2018). By communicating with the family about their responsibilities for communication, nurses can initiate an open dialogue about the importance of communication. One way of approaching this is to ask the patient and family whether they want information about the patient's condition and, if they do not, who in the family should be given information.

As a family nurse, it is important for you to know what information can be offered that is likely to make a positive difference for family caregivers. Nurses are in one of the best positions to understand and appreciate the challenges for family members to take on the job of caregiving. Family members who do not have a background in health care may not know what to expect when they take on the role of caregiver. They may not know how to provide basic care effectively, such as assisting the individual in activities of daily living, for example, toileting and bathing; assisting the individual to move without causing more pain; managing symptoms such as nausea and breathlessness; or even safely working with equipment such as an oxygen tank. It is important for caregivers to be prepared with the knowledge and skills in anticipation of the changing needs of their family members. Noticing what the individual experiencing illness needs, anticipating future needs, and listening to both the individual and the family caregiver can assist the nurse to identify priorities for the family. The nurse can help them negotiate how care will be done at home, work directly with the family caregiver to provide knowledge and model essential skills, and determine available resources, which are some examples of interventions that may prove supportive.

Timing is important—information and teaching have to be provided proactively, before a crisis occurs, and at a time that is meaningful to the family. Listening carefully to both the individual and the family can help the nurse support them in meeting mutual goals. At the same time, it is important to recognize and assist with strategies to maintain "normal" roles within a family, such as parent or spouse (Hardy et al., 2014). Family caregivers have reported that interventions aimed at separating them from their dying family member, such as exhortations to leave the bedside and get some sleep, are often not helpful and can be experienced as disrespectful (Robinson et al., 2017). Family caregivers may see these interventions as evidence that nurses really do not understand their commitment to the dying person and to providing care, regardless of the personal consequences.

When patients and family members are empowered with the amount and kind of information they want and at the time they need it, the result is more effective partnerships with health care providers. Nurses are in a key position to act as a liaison between the health care team members and the family. Patients and families should be encouraged to ask questions, and these questions should be answered with full explanations and support. Nurses can create an environment that allows family members to speak openly without fear or anxiety.

Nurses may sometimes be reluctant to invite questions from families because they are concerned that they may not have an answer. Simply knowing the questions that the family would like answered is valuable information, and many times the questions do not have clear answers. For example, the question, "When will my family member die?" cannot be easily answered. Nurses may not know the answer, and it is acceptable to let families know that some things are not known. When possible, however, nurses can show their trustworthiness by seeking the information and providing it in a timely fashion.

Overall, families need to have honest and understandable information about a variety of areas, including the following:

- The patient's condition
- The illness trajectory
- Prognosis (keeping in mind that prognosis is inherently uncertain because we cannot predict when death will occur)
- Symptoms to expect and treatment options
- How to provide physical care
- What to expect (including signs of impending death, which allow family members the opportunity to say final goodbyes)
- Ways of coping (including helping families become aware of possible strategies, such as respite and mental pauses)
- The dying process
- How to access additional support
- What aids (e.g., wheelchairs, beds, lifts) may be helpful and where to get them
- The care system in which this all occurs

Provision of this type of information is linked to reduced caregiver burden, improved coping, greater self-efficacy, increased hope, reduced anxiety, and enhanced quality of life (Shin & Choi, 2020). The way in which information is shared is as important as the content of the information. Critical components of the process of sharing information include timing; pacing; and both verbal and nonverbal conveyance of respect, empathy, and compassion (Davies et al., 2017). The timing and pacing in particular are important because they allow families to absorb the reality of the situation and to make informed decisions (Davies et al., 2017). Not rushing families to make decisions is important; however, giving information as early as possible to allow for ongoing discussions and decision making is most effective. The use of simple, jargon-free language is also helpful. In emotionally intense situations, little information is absorbed, and it must be repeated over time, so nurses should be willing to clarify repeatedly for family members without becoming impatient. Asking clarifying questions of all family members to ensure that information is being understood is also important (Davies et al., 2017). Nonverbal communication is also important to consider when working with families. For instance, watching the person's face to determine if she looks confused, upset, or comprehending can help ensure that information is being understood and welcomed. The nurse's body language can also aid communication. For example, standing close to a family member when talking about care rather than standing in the doorway of a patient's room gives the impression of having the time to talk and listen rather than being in a hurry to move on. Moderation of the tone of voice can change a statement from sounding annoyed or without compassion to respectful and empathetic (Davies et al., 2017).

Through learning about other families' experiences, patients and family members can better understand their own experience. Nurses can share insights gained from other families both from practice and research. For example, a nurse may share the following: "Other families have told me that talking about what their child's death might be like was one of the hardest things they ever had to do, but once they knew there was a plan in place for how to handle the possible symptoms or issues that may happen, they were able to stop worrying about all the 'what-ifs' and just focus on having the best time possible with their child." Having information about other families going through similar experiences enables patients and family members to connect better with health care providers, which in turn enhances decision making and planning for the future.

Balancing Hope and Preparation

A fair amount of ambiguity always exists when working with families at the end of life, regardless of whether the situation is acute or chronic. Nurses need to become comfortable with the inherent uncertainty and help families live well within an uncertain context. One common ambiguity surrounds prognostic uncertainty. Given that we cannot predict when death will occur, families need to be encouraged to attend to what they view as important and to take advantage of the moment. When a patient or family member asks, "How long?" the nurse might reply by asking, "What would you be doing differently now if you knew that the time was very short?" Suggesting that they do whatever "it" is and that getting to do "it" again next week or next month or even next year would be a bonus may help family members achieve what matters most in the difficult circumstance of advanced illness.

As a patient's condition changes and deteriorates, the hopes and expectations of the patient and family may change as well. Hope often shifts from a more global perspective—such as hope for a cure—to a more focused or specific perspective, such as a hope to live long enough to see a grandchild who is due in a few months. Nurses can help facilitate this change in hope by asking powerful questions, such as, "If your loved one were to die tonight, is there anything you have not said or done that you would regret?" or "If you were to die suddenly, is there anything you would regret not doing or saying?" Such questions encourage patients and families to consider what is most meaningful to them and allow them to shift their hope to areas that may be more attainable. Nurses who participate in these discussions can help maintain hope for some things while not providing false hope. They can also offer to help patients and families do or say what they need to do.

For some families and in some cultures, they need to keep fighting for every chance at life, hoping for a miracle, until the last possible moment, even when they may know this is considered medically unrealistic (Robinson, 2012). A nurse must find the balance between supporting families in their hopes and still being comfortable talking about death and preparing the patient and family for what is to come, including advance care planning (Robinson, 2012; Sussman et al., 2017). Therefore, when preparing the family for what is to come, the nurse must provide the information in a sensitive and compassionate manner that also inspires hope. One way of doing this is to use a hypothetical question (Wright & Leahey, 2012), such as, "If things don't go as we hope, what is most important for you to have happen?"

Parents of dying children identify a need to balance hope and despair and appreciate when health care providers support hope without offering false hope (Verberne et al., 2017). Lack of discussions about the possibility of death are closely linked to parents' belief that health care providers sometimes give false hope that the child will survive the illness (Gordon et al., 2009). False hope may be detrimental to parents' ability to prepare for the child's death, so nurses need to be mindful of what they say and how they say it. Honest acknowledgment of the severity of the situation is important.

Facilitating Choices

A major role for nurses is to be an advocate for patients and families and to facilitate their choices.

But to do so, nurses need to know what the patient and family want. One specific intervention is to encourage advance care planning so that everyone is clear about the patient's preferences regarding end-of-life care (Hopeck & Harrison, 2017). A related area for discussion with patients and families is goals of care and, in some cases, discussion of physician-assisted suicide or medical assistance in dying (MAID) is appropriate. Other interventions include assessing the extent of both the patient's and family members' desire for involvement in decision making and then respecting that desire, assessing their awareness about the possibility of death and opening lines of communication, and identifying and then building on the patient's and family's strengths in order to optimize choices (Gallagher et al., 2015; Odgers et al., 2018).

Advance Care Planning

At the end of life, patients may be unable to participate in making decisions about their care, leaving family members to make decisions based on their understanding of what the patient would want if he were able to participate. One way in which families can prevent misunderstanding and promote facilitation of choices is by discussing wishes and desires in advance. Advance care planning is a process that involves reflection and communication. It is a way of letting others know personal future health and care preferences so that, if the individual becomes incapable of consenting to or refusing treatment, others—especially a designated substitute decision maker or the person who will speak for a person when that person cannot—will make decisions for that person that reflect his values and wishes, regardless of their own desires. Advance care planning often involves not only discussions with family and friends but also writing down end-of-life wishes; it may even involve talking with health care providers and financial and legal professionals. The Canadian Hospice Palliative Care Association (2021), in collaboration with the National Advance Care Planning Task Group, provides several valuable online resources about advance care planning, including a workbook to guide writing the plan.

An *advance directive* specifies the medical treatments an individual does or does not want at the end of life, for example, resuscitation if her heart stops. It is usually a legally binding document, but nurses must be aware of the legal requirements within their own workplace jurisdiction (e.g., state or province). If someone has written an advance directive, their substitute decision maker should have a copy. It is important that health care providers are made aware of a patient's advance directives and, preferably, have a copy in the patient's chart. Nurses need to make themselves familiar with such advance directives so that they can advocate for the patient as needed when decisions are being made.

Advance care planning is a process that is best initiated early in the illness experience and revisited as the illness progresses, because preferences can change over time. Parents of children with life-limiting conditions have indicated a need to keep options open and to revisit plans as the child's condition changes because it can be hard to envision how they will feel in the future about a particular situation (Beecham et al., 2017). Some of the topics that may be discussed as part of advance care planning include location of care, location of death, and the types of treatments that may or may not be wanted (Beecham et al., 2017). These types of conversations are difficult to have among family members, and families may appreciate assistance to initiate and facilitate the conversation. Nurses can facilitate the process and empower both patients and families by encouraging them to talk about end-of-life issues and preferences long before they are faced with the situation. By initiating discussions about substitute decision making, the choice of a substitute decision maker, and the legalities of representing the patient's wishes, decisions can be well thought out rather than crisis-oriented. The process of substitute decision making can be a very demanding one for families, particularly if they have not had discussions about the patient's preferences (Ohs et al., 2017; Yamamoto et al., 2017). Having a written advance care plan and/or an advance directive assists family members by helping them understand the patient's wishes, which can then inform decision making (Hopeck & Harrison, 2017; Ohs et al., 2017). Documentation of wishes and preferences is also helpful when there are differences among family members about what they think is best for the individual. Family members often appreciate acknowledgment of the difficulty of their role in making decisions, and the nurse's attentive, respectful support throughout the process can be very helpful.

Goals of Care

Goals of care are related to but not synonymous with advance care planning. In long-term care settings, discussions about barriers to goals of care may include the substitute decision maker's difficulty in recognizing the person's poor prognosis, lack of understanding of the potentially negative impact of some life-sustaining therapies, lack of prior advance care planning or documentation of previous discussions, and lack of time for discussion (Siu et al., 2020).

Physician-Assisted Suicide and MAID

One aspect of advance planning may include a patient determining when and how she will die, within specific legal contexts. Several countries legally allow people who are suffering to arrange for their own death as a medical intervention. In the United States, the state of Oregon enacted the Death with Dignity Act in 1997, which allows individuals with a terminal illness to end their lives through the voluntary self-administration of lethal medications that are expressly prescribed by a physician for that purpose. Currently, eight states and Washington, DC, have enacted death and dignity laws. The state of Montana does not currently have a statute safeguarding physician-assisted death; however, in 2009 Montana's Supreme Court ruled that nothing in the state law prohibited a physician from honoring the wishes of a terminally ill patient, and a mentally competent patient could request prescription medication to hasten death (Death with Dignity National Center, 2021). To qualify legally for a prescription under Physician Assisted Suicide/Death (PAS/D) legislation, individuals must be a resident of the applicable state, be at least 18 years of age, be mentally competent to make and communicate their own health care decisions, and be diagnosed with a terminal illness that, if allowed to take its natural course, would lead to death within 6 months (Oregon Health Authority, 2020). In addition, individuals must be able to self-administer and ingest the prescribed medication.

The American Nurses Association (ANA, 2019) prohibits nurses' participation in assisted suicide, or euthanasia. ANA refers nurses to their statutory body (e.g., the Oregon Nurses Association) for guidance on how to proceed. The delivery of high-quality, compassionate, holistic, and patient-centered care is central to nursing practice (ANA, 2019). End-of-life care that includes respect for patient self-determination, nonjudgmental support for patients' end-of-life preferences and values, and prevention and alleviation of suffering are priorities for nursing practice (ANA, 2019).

On June 17, 2016, the federal government of Canada received formal approval for amendments to the criminal code so that MAID, under certain circumstances, would no longer be considered a criminal offense. Nurses in Canada must now be familiar with the wording of Bill C-14 (an act to amend the criminal code and to make related amendments to other acts [medical assistance in dying]) and must work within both this legislation and their relevant regulatory standards. An important limitation to the nursing role expressly requires that only a physician or nurse practitioner administer the substance that will bring about death. Therefore, most nurses may assist (e.g., by preparing medication), but they must not actually administer the medication. Similarly, if a patient is given a prescription to self-administer the medication, then nurses should not assist with the administration of the medication. Nurses must ensure that their practice is consistent with not only the law and the guidelines from their regulatory bodies but also their employer's position on whether or not MAID is permitted within the setting and, if so, the policies and procedures that outline how and by whom MAID may be undertaken. It is also important to note that the amendments to the criminal code do not impose an obligation for nurses to participate in MAID. However, nurses continue to have a legal duty of care to patients and must not abandon them. Therefore, it may be necessary to refer to or involve other health care providers in certain circumstances. Regardless of where a nurse is practicing, it is critical that nurses understand and practice within all appropriate laws, rules, and standards. If something is not clear, then nurses should seek advice, including legal advice as necessary, to ensure that they understand the consequences of the actions they are contemplating—whether choosing or refusing to participate in MAID or PAS/D.

In Canada, debate continues over whether MAID is part of or separate from palliative care. Proponents of MAID suggest that it offers an alternative that facilitates a "good death," while others note that part of the definition of palliative care is neither to postpone nor to hasten death, and thus MAID should be a separate option. Access to

MAID is a right that is available to all Canadians over the age of 18 years who meet the criteria. Individual nurses have varying personal beliefs about MAID; however, recent research suggested that, regardless of their beliefs, nurses must focus on providing nonjudgmental care and on the patient's right to choose his or her care (Beuthin et al., 2018). Nurses who chose to be part of the delivery of MAID noted that they employed the same competencies described throughout this chapter to support the patient and family, such as communication, information sharing, and care after the death (Beuthin et al., 2018).

Involvement in Decision Making

Families may be facing their first experience with death and dying, and they often depend on nurses to help them in their process. Families may not know what they need or what might be possible, or they may expect health care providers to bring up issues at the appropriate time. Therefore, it is important for nurses to open the conversation by assessing and respecting the patient's and family's desired level of involvement in discussions about the end of life and in decision making. In some families, based on their experiences or culture, discussion of the end of life may be equated with giving up, or family members may be the preferred decision makers rather than the patient (Menon et al., 2018). Rather than making assumptions about preferences or beliefs, nurses should ask questions such as, "How are important decisions made in your family?" and "How would you like important decision making to go now?" so that they understand the family's approach and can facilitate appropriate interactions that respect family choice.

Some patients and families may want full responsibility for decisions; some may want to be involved but not make final decisions; some may want the physician to take the initiative and make all decisions (Selman et al., 2007); some patients want their family members to make decisions (Ohs et al., 2017). Some parents feel that making decisions for the child is inherently a parental role, but not all parents want to have complete responsibility for final decisions (Hardy et al., 2014). Again, assessment of preferences about decision making is important. Nurses can use questions such as, "I understand that different family members will have different talents or strengths; how do you most want to be involved?" to uncover family members'

preferences so that they can work with the family in ways that facilitate choice.

Regardless of their actual role in the decision-making process, parents want to be recognized as the experts on their child and as the central, consistent figures in their child's life (Hardy et al., 2014; Sullivan et al., 2014). As such, they want health care providers to seek out and respect their knowledge, opinions, observations, and concerns about their child (Butler et al., 2018; Davies et al., 2017; Verberne et al., 2017). Therefore, nurses should verbally acknowledge that the parent's input is critical; seek to work collaboratively with parents as members of the health care team; and aim to support parents' choices, regardless of their own beliefs (Butler et al., 2018).

The involvement of family members in discussions about end-of-life care and decision making can have a lifelong effect on the well-being of family members (Ohs et al., 2017), such as through decreasing rates of depression or less complicated grief in bereaved family members (Yamaguchi et al., 2017). These types of discussions may be associated with higher-quality end-of-life care and a good death (Yamaguchi et al., 2017). Therefore, nurses must foster good communication to ensure that the patient's and family's needs and wishes are understood and supported within a caring relationship that is based on collaboration within the relationship between health care professionals and families. Occasionally, health care professionals block families from participating because they feel that they know what is best or because they are trying to protect families. But effective end-of-life care is not possible unless open and mutual communication occurs between families and professionals and unless families participate in shared decision making to the extent they desire (Robinson, 2012). Questions and statements such as, "If you were to think ahead a bit, how do you see things going in the next few weeks?" and "Families often find it helpful to talk about the care they want at end of life. Have you been able to have a conversation about this? I wonder if I might be able to help you start this conversation" can be used to learn what a patient and family want. See Box 11-3 for other questions that may help nurses learn a family's choices.

Awareness of the Possibility of Death

Lack of early information about the possibility of death makes it difficult for family members to come to terms with decisions such as the withdrawal of life-sustaining therapy or the use of cardiopulmonary resuscitation (CPR). Families faced with these types of decisions usually place great value on open, honest, and timely information, but they also need the opportunity to share their knowledge of the patient and their wishes. It is crucial to prepare the family for what to expect when life-sustaining therapy is withdrawn. For example, families need to be aware that death may occur very quickly or may take hours or days. When decisions are made, such as about withdrawal of life-sustaining therapy, any delays or changes in the plan of care may increase the family's anxiety or grief. Therefore, it is important for nurses to keep the family informed about the reasons for any changes to the plan and to be available to talk with family members when needed.

Building on Strengths

Nurses need to recognize the dying person's and family members' rights and abilities to make their own decisions and then try to find out what is important to them. It is crucial to focus on what patients and families *can* do rather than on what they cannot do. Nurses can reinforce those aspects of the self that remain intact and assist patients and families to recognize their own strengths and abilities. Individual and family strengths can be built on, which in turn can smooth the way for patients and families to meet their own needs. Nurses can work with patients and families by making suggestions, providing options, and planning strategies that allow them to achieve their goals. Professional knowledge may be invaluable in guiding families to consider options and possible routes of action that they might not have considered. Nurses may have a clearer sense of the consequences of certain choices, which again is extremely valuable information. At the very least, nurses can seek out answers to families' questions and be a resource for families.

Facilitating choices also means identifying and accepting a patient's and family's limitations and finding ways to work with them so they can achieve an outcome that is both positive and satisfactory for them. One example is suggesting new activities that are appropriate for the patient's current capabilities. It is important that relationships remain mutual and reciprocal, and patients in particular need to experience their positive contribution to their family members. Thus, as a patient's

condition declines, her or his contribution will look different and may focus on such things as words of wisdom rather than concrete actions.

Offering Resources

One nurse cannot be all things to every patient and family. It is important to be aware of and utilize the support of other palliative care team members, including spiritual or pastoral advisers, social workers, hospice caregivers, and others who may be available to provide support to the family. The nurse should be knowledgeable about hospital and community-based resources such as hospice or privately paid caregiving agencies that may be able to support families. Nurses can offer these other resources and services to families, but each family will decide what will actually be helpful for them. For some families, using inpatient respite services during the last year of life may help relieve their burden, if only for a short time; other caregivers may experience feelings of guilt and increased stress caused by worrying about the quality of care provided during respite (Robinson et al., 2017). Caregivers may be supported in their role simply by knowing there are other resources and support readily available, even if they do not make use of them.

Encouraging Patients and Families

Patients and family members often seek approval and encouragement from professionals as they make decisions about how to meet their needs. Offering encouragement is an important strategy in empowering patients and families to do for themselves. This means verbally and nonverbally supporting patients and families in their choices, providing reinforcement for each individual's ideas, and demonstrating support by finding ways to facilitate their choices. Encouraging does not necessarily mean that the nurse *agrees* with the choice, merely that the nurse supports the patient or family member in finding ways to enact the choice. At the same time, encouraging does not mean that the nurse abandons her or his expertise, which is complementary to the expertise of the family. Sharing professional knowledge and perspective contributes to fully informed decision making.

Nurses can sometimes think that they know what is best for patients and their families. As caring professionals, nurses have families' best interests at heart and want to protect them as much as possible. Even as nurses value each person as a worthwhile individual who has the right and ability to make his or her own choices and decisions, they may find that the patient's and family's choices conflict with what they believe is "best" based on their experience. This can cause moral distress as nurses struggle with feeling there could be ways that the situation might be improved, which they base on previous experiences and knowledge, such as when families choose to continue medically futile interventions over comfort care (Wolf et al., 2019). The ethical challenges that arise can be difficult, and sometimes nurses feel conflicted with a patient's or family's wishes. Some nurses describe their bottom line as "ensuring patient safety," and unless the patient's physical safety is compromised, they support the patient's choice, even when they disagree with it. Another example of conflicting decisions can be when a patient and family decide to continue care in the home setting when the nurse believes admission to hospice or a hospital is the best option. It is important for nurses to support families to find solutions to do what is most important for them in the best way possible.

Managing Negative Feelings

End-of-life care is not all encouragement and positive feelings. Many patients and family members also have negative feelings that influence their experiences. Talking with patients and family members (often individually) about their negative feelings gives them permission to have, experience, and deal with them. For many people, negative feelings, such as guilt or anger, are suppressed or internalized. Others openly express their anger but displace it onto someone else, often the nurse or other family members. The ability to diffuse a situation effectively requires nurses to learn how to accept someone else's negative feelings in an open and nondefensive manner. It means not taking their words as a personal attack but realizing that patients and family members simply need a safe outlet for their frustrations and negative feelings. The nurse's role is to listen in an accepting way, and allow them to express themselves. It can be hard to face an angry tirade, but most people will calm down once they have said what they need to say and they realize that the listener values their feelings even if they are negative ones. Questions that are often useful include "How can I help?" or "What needs to be different?"

Sometimes people will remain angry or guilty, however, despite best efforts; diffusing will not always be successful. Some people are so angry about what is happening to their loved one and their family that they cannot move to any other emotional state. During these instances, it is best to accept that this is their reality and find ways to work with them. This is often a time when nurses need the support of colleagues, and a team approach may help to lessen the effects of working with patients and families that may be in crisis or suffering (Hendricks-Ferguson et al., 2015). An important role for nurses includes coordinating support from the palliative care team (e.g., social work, pastoral care) and making referrals to community resources as needed (e.g., mental health or counseling providers, support groups).

Facilitating Healing Between Family Members

Negative feelings and misunderstandings can cause or expand rifts in families. If nurses can facilitate healing between family members that unifies the family or involve palliative care team members in the process of supporting the family, the family members may be able to achieve a higher level of function during the dying process. The nurse can help mend relationships or reduce conflicts by interpreting family members' behaviors to one another and helping them to see each other's point of view (Hudson et al., 2019). Sometimes an outsider can bring clarity to a situation that is impossible for those who are enmeshed in it. An assessment question that may be useful is: "Is there anything that is unsaid or undone in the family that needs your attention?" Be careful that questions are not aimed at "fixing broken families." It is important to avoid interactions that may give families the impression that they are dysfunctional or not normal or that they need to change. Every family is quite unique and diverse in their own ways, including how they function as a family. They will not accept attempts to "fix them" and, indeed, may find concerns about the family intrusive. Relationships develop over many years and yet interventions occur in a relatively short period. Large changes in family dynamics cannot often be expected during the short time that a family works with the nurse. Rather, seeds are often planted, and when the family is motivated to make changes, improvements in family function will occur. Sometimes all that can be done is to acknowledge that certain things cannot be altered, and often genuine and empathetic presence is the best intervention that can be offered. Level of family functioning will have to be attended to carefully, and the expectation that a family will pull together to cope with the process of dying may be unrealistic. Noticing the family members' love for the individual experiencing illness and acknowledging their mutual desire for the best outcome (even though there may be quite different ideas about what is best) is sometimes helpful.

Family Meetings

Family meetings typically involve the patient, those family members desired by the patient, and the relevant health care providers. Family meetings are important when there is a change in condition, if the patient is experiencing a transition in living situation or transferring care, or if there are complicated factors involved in the care situation (Kallianis et al., 2017). Family meetings should routinely offered be on admission to palliative or hospice care and can be requested by family members and coordinated by members of the interdisciplinary team. If there are challenges with family members being able to attend family meetings onsite, it is important to arrange for virtual or phone access to the meeting (Siu et al., 2020). Rather than being reserved for crisis situations, family meetings may be part of an initial meet-and-greet for family and staff to get to know each other and share understanding of the situation and the expected course for the illness (Forbat et al., 2018), as well as to clarify patient and family preferences and identify goals for care. Family meetings enable patients, family members, and health care providers to discuss issues involved in the plan of care and to improve the experience.

As coordinators of care, nurses are ideal partners to lead end-of-life family conferences. In all settings, the nurse can assist families in preparing for the meetings by helping them to write down questions that they want to raise at the meeting and informing the family about what to expect during the conference. Family satisfaction can be enhanced when clinicians allow family members to speak about what they have been experiencing, facilitate

shared decision making, and express support for the family's decisions (Sullivan et al., 2015). It is helpful to begin by eliciting the family's understanding of the situation, as well as pressing concerns, before moving to the health care providers' perspectives. Different family members and providers will have different ideas, so it is useful to request different perspectives. Afterward, discussing with the family how the conference went, the changes in the patient's plan of care and what they mean, and how the family feels about the conference as well as the changed plan of care helps to solidify decisions made during the family meeting (Sullivan et al., 2015). Summarizing decisions that were made and then supporting the family in these decisions can help strengthen the family's trust in the care plan.

More than one family meeting may be necessary as the patient's condition changes or if the family needs time to think or discuss issues in more depth before decisions are made (Hudson et al., 2008). Allowing family members to talk and share their experiences during family meetings can increase family satisfaction and decrease conflict between families and health professionals. It is important to ensure that families do the majority of talking during family meetings. Nonverbal communication is an important cue for nurses when working with families and is particularly powerful when the topics are emotional. For example, arms wrapped tightly around the body may indicate anxiety, whereas interrupting may be a sign of impatience. By listening and engaging with a kind and compassionate presence, the nurse can learn more about what the patient and family need and want.

Finding Meaning

For some, caring for the spiritual needs, or caring for the human spirit, of patients and families can be the most challenging (Starck, 2017). When recovery is impossible, nurses must consider their role in helping patients and families find meaning in the experience as they care for and assist families. Patients and families may struggle to understand why the patient is dying. They try to make sense of the experience, and they search for ways to make the patient's life and inevitable death meaningful. Their search for meaning may involve examining intrafamily relationships, their religious or spiritual beliefs, or even certain events or experiences during their life. Some people are more successful at finding meaning than others, and sometimes the process may not occur until long after the death (Widger et al., 2009). The process of reflecting on the meaning and purpose of one's life can bring closure and comfort to those involved and can even lead to peace and fulfillment for some (Starck, 2017).

Nurses may assist in this process of finding meaning by truly listening and hearing what family members have to say. Engaging in a relationship and dialogue is empowering and can help families create meaning even in a difficult situation (Davies et al., 2017). There are many different ways of finding meaning, and not all individuals will overtly search for meaning. However, nurses have the opportunity to accompany people as they try to make sense of their situation. No one can find meaning for someone else; each individual seeks her or his own meaning in her or his unique way. Some may be very articulate about their beliefs; others may talk about these issues in more concrete terms, perhaps rarely having articulated their thoughts and feelings. Still others may talk through their actions or the experiences in their lives. Finding meaning gives strength to people; therefore, nurses may find the experience empowering for families. Nurses who examine the concepts of the meaning of illness and dying with patients may gain a deepened understanding of the patients' experiences, which can help them improve their approach to providing care. Open-ended, compassionate questions can help nurses understand the patient's experience, examples include: "Can you tell me what it is like to be at this point in your life?" or "What has this experience been like for you?"

Care at the Time of Actively Dying

Patients who are dying are often most concerned about how they will die. This is sometimes even more of a concern than the fact that they are experiencing a terminal phase of their illness. Excellent pain and symptom management is critical because uncontrolled pain or symptoms, such as nausea and breathlessness, create suffering for *all* family members. A "good death" may contribute to family members feeling more at peace with the death (Martz, 2015), as well as having a sense of satisfaction and accomplishment (Witkamp et al., 2015). Thus, facilitating a good death is an imperative for nurses (Gagnon & Duggleby, 2014). What constitutes a good death, however, is not always well understood.

For nurses, a good death (or "dying well") includes the involvement of patients and families in decision making, the family's presence with the patient, dignity and respect for the patient's wishes, physical comfort, being at peace, being in an appropriate environment, and acceptance of death (Becker et al., 2017; Gagnon & Duggleby, 2014).

When a cure is not possible, families often react to the news with a blanket statement: "We want everything done." But that may not be what they mean literally. Sometimes families may believe their loved one will be abandoned if they agree to palliative care; they may think that treatment and comfort will be withheld simply because the patient is terminal and death is expected. Delaying palliative care compromises the ability to achieve a good death and a level of comfort for both patients and families. Clear discussions are needed about the continued provision of active care with a shift in emphasis to quality of life instead of prolongation of life. Such discussions reassure families that, indeed, everything is being done and they are not being abandoned.

No matter the setting, family members are often afraid of the actual death event and require education and support on what the process of dying is like. There are four dimensions to preparation: (1) medical, which relates to receiving clear prognostic information as well as information about the physical and psychological changes that signal death is approaching; (2) psychosocial, which entails saying goodbye, sharing intimate time, and resolving conflicts; (3) spiritual, which may involve a religious aspect as well as time to reflect on the meaning of life and death; and (4) practical, which focuses on completing unfinished business (Sopcheck, 2019; Swinton et al., 2017). Nurses can help alleviate families' fears by finding out what they know and what they need (Becker et al., 2017). They can then prepare families for the death and act as a coach during the dying process (Martz, 2015) to help them recognize the signs of imminent death so that they are aware of what will likely happen when the signs appear (see Box 11-5). This preparation may be even more crucial for families in the home, who may be alone as death approaches. It also is important in the ICU and emergency department to tailor information to the situation (Peden-McAlpine et al., 2015). For example, a patient's breathing will not change if they are on a ventilator. Creating a sacred space to facilitate saying goodbye may be a very helpful intervention (Peden-McAlpine et al., 2015).

BOX 11-5

Signs of Imminent Death

Signs of imminent death include the following:

- Decline in physical capabilities
- Decreased alertness and social interaction
- Decreased intake of food and fluids
- Difficulty swallowing medications, food, and fluids
- Visual or auditory hallucinations; near-death awareness experiences
- Confusion, restlessness, agitation, or delirium

Physical changes as death nears include the following:

- Circulation gradually shuts down; hands and feet feel cool, and a patchy, purplish color called *mottling* appears on the skin; heart rate speeds up but also weakens so that the pulse is rapid and may be difficult to palpate.
- Bowel movements and urine production decrease as less food and fluid are taken in; there may be no urine output in last day or two of life; constipation is not usually an issue to be managed in the last week of life; loss of bladder or bowel control can be managed with frequent skin care and the use of adult incontinence products, or a urinary catheter if needed.

Changes in breathing often provide clues about how close someone is to death. As the automatic centers in the brain take over the regulation of breathing, changes generally occur in the following ways:

- The rate of breathing tends to be more rapid.
- The pattern or regularity in breathing becomes irregular, almost mechanical.
- The depth of breaths (may be shallow, deep, or normal) tends to become shallower. There may be periods of apnea where breathing pauses for a while. When the pauses in breathing appear, a

noticeable pattern often develops: clusters of fairly rapid breathing that start with shallow breaths that become deeper and deeper, and then fade off, becoming shallower and shallower; there may be 5 to 10 breaths in each cluster, and each cluster is separated by a pause that may last a few seconds or perhaps up to 30 seconds. This is called the Cheyne-Stokes pattern of breathing and is occasionally seen in healthy older adults as well, especially during sleep.

- The kinds of muscles used in breathing may change; the person may start to use the neck muscles and the shoulders; although it may look as if the person is struggling, unless he or she is agitated, it is simply "automatic pilot."
- The amount of mucus or secretions that build up because the person is unable to cough can be noisy (rattling or gurgling) and sometimes upsets people at the bedside, even though it is unlikely to be distressing to the dying person, who is usually unconscious. Some people call it the death rattle, and it can be treated by medication to dry up the secretions. Because the term *death rattle* may cause strong emotional reactions, the term *respiratory congestion* is now recommended.
- The pattern of breathing in the final minutes or perhaps hours of life takes on an irregular pattern in which there is a breath, then a pause, then another breath or two, then another pause, and so forth. There may be periods of 15 to 30 seconds or so between final breaths.
- After the last breath, very slight motions of breathing may happen irregularly for a few minutes. These are reflex actions and are not signs of distress.

Generally, an illness begins to weaken the body when a person is nearing death. Some health conditions affect vital body systems, such as the brain and nervous system; lungs; heart and blood vessels; or the digestive system, including the liver and bowels. As illness progresses, the body becomes unable to use the nutrients in food, resulting in weight loss and a decline in appetite, energy, and strength. More time is spent resting, and in the final few days before death people usually sleep most of the time. If families are aware of this natural progression, they may be less distressed, for example, when their loved one stops eating. One common end-of-life phenomenon, delirium, poses unique relational challenges and can be distressing

for family members. Sedation at the end of life may be necessary to control severe symptoms, such as terminal restlessness that accompanies delirium.

Communication and relationships continue to be important as death approaches (Generous & Keeley, 2017; Odgers et al., 2018). Many family members want to be present when their loved one dies; however, it may be more important to have the opportunity for meaningful conversations and to say goodbye than to actually be there at the moment of death (Otani et al., 2017). Thus, it may be important for nurses to facilitate conversations where families can say goodbye to their loved one and potentially resolve unfinished business (e.g., sharing honest feelings, saying thank-you or apologizing, discussing funeral arrangements) (Yamashita et al., 2017). Given the difficulty of predicting when death may occur, nurses can encourage family members not to wait to have these conversations. Even if the patient is nonresponsive, however, nurses can encourage family members to continue talking to their loved one because they may still be able to hear. Nurses can model compassion through continuing to communicate to the patient, even though she or he is not responsive, and by treating the patient with dignity throughout the dying process. During this time, the nurse can also demonstrate respect for family members and their intimate knowledge of the patient by seeking their advice on things that were soothing or calming to the patient in the past, such as particular music, foot rubs and back rubs, or a particular way of arranging the pillows, and then following these suggestions and encouraging the family to do so as well (Sopcheck, 2019).

Nurses should be aware ahead of time about a family's wishes to be present at the time of death and ensure that members are called if there is a change in the patient's condition. However, it is impossible to predict exactly when a patient may die and despite best efforts, death sometimes happens when family members are not present. Sometimes the patient dies when the family member has nodded off to sleep or stepped out of the room for a cup of tea. When family members wish to be present, it is important to talk about the possibility that this may not happen. It may be helpful to suggest that if death occurs when family members are not there, it may be the patient's way of protecting the family from that sad moment. Family members express a variety of emotions and challenges during those final days and final hours of life. It can be helpful to engage them in discussion about their wishes but also to encourage them to care for themselves. In a recent news article, Dr. B.J. Miller (2019), hospice and palliative medicine physician at the University of California San Francisco (UCSF) Helen Diller Family Comprehensive Cancer Center, encouraged caregivers and loved ones to consider leaving the room:

> As any hospice worker can tell you, this is also a well-known phenomenon. It's almost as if the presence of others—especially deeply loved ones—gets in the way of the dying person's final step. That big moment may need to happen alone. What dying people seem to need at the very end is to know that the people they love are going to be OK; that life will go on and that you—the person they care for—will be able to take care of yourself. So, the kindest thing you can do is to demonstrate that care by leaving the room when you need to. Just be sure to give a kiss and know that it may have to be the last. (para 11)

For parents of an ill child, the days, hours, and minutes leading up to the death may be seen as the last opportunity to be a good parent to the child. Their ability to be physically present, emotionally supportive, and an effective advocate for their child is often key to viewing themselves as good parents in the years after their child's death (Rini & Loriz, 2007). "Normal" parent activities such as bathing, feeding, or holding the child, even in the midst of technology that is being used to support the child's life, allow parents to develop or continue their bond with their child and sometimes to be able to say goodbye (Butler et al., 2018; Rini & Loriz, 2007). Nurses can facilitate parents' wishes at this time and provide an environment that allows for parents to fulfill their parental role.

Bereavement Care

Once the patient dies, the nurse continues to work with the family. Several family members may be present for the death, all of whom may need support, advice, information, and time to begin the grieving and healing process. Family members may wish to stay by the bedside and say whatever words seem appropriate. Both before and after the death, there may be important cultural or religious rituals that the family may wish to conduct. It is important for the nurse to determine in advance what these rituals are and how they can be facilitated in the particular setting where death occurs. Facilitation of these rituals may require advocating at the organizational level to remove any potential barriers (Bloomer et al 2019; Jones et al., 2018). Some families may want active involvement in caring for the patient's body or at least to know the body will be cared for in a respectful manner (Widger & Picot, 2008). There is no harm in touching the person's body, and there should be no rush to move the person until any rituals can be completed and everyone has had a chance to say their final goodbyes.

Family members who were not present for the death may need to be contacted and may wish to see the patient before he or she is taken to the morgue or a funeral home. Family members can be encouraged to be together if they wish and to take as much time as needed after the death. The nurse's presence as family members express their emotions may help them to create meaningful final memories and begin to process their experience (Rini & Loriz, 2007). Additional team members, such as pastoral care and social workers, may need to be contacted to assist in supporting the family. Some families appreciate assistance with or information on arranging funerals.

Particularly when the patient who has died is a child, families may appreciate receiving a collection of mementos such as pictures, locks of hair, and handprints or footprints (Rini & Loriz, 2007; Tan et al., 2012; Widger & Picot, 2008). Some families later regret not taking mementos, but others may be distressed if mementos are taken, especially pictures, against their wishes (Blood & Cacciatore, 2014). Therefore, determining what each family wants and needs requires sensitivity and a careful approach.

In some cases, autopsy and organ or tissue donation may be possible. Nurses and other health care providers sometimes view such discussions as an intrusion and, thus, because of their own discomfort, they do not approach families about these topics. Parents in particular may have lingering regrets, however, if they miss an opportunity to help another child or to receive answers to some questions about their own child's death (Widger & Picot, 2008). Therefore, these conversations can be very beneficial should they be indicated. It is also important to make sure that when autopsies are done, families are given the results in a timely and compassionate manner (Rini & Loriz, 2007). Families may want to meet with health care providers to discuss autopsy results, clarify the events leading to and the circumstances of the death, and be reassured that everything possible was done and the right decisions were made (Milberg et al., 2008).

It was previously thought that healing meant a person got over the loss and severed ties with the deceased. It is now known that people never fully get over the loss of a loved one; rather, they will always have memories and bonds with the person they lost. Nurses can facilitate a healthy start to family members' grieving journey and help them find meaning in death; in fact, nurses' actions at the actual death event are critical. Family members vividly remember the moment of their loved one's death. They often remember who was present, what

was said, what was done that was helpful, and what was not so helpful. Many remember that it was the nurse who was with them at the moment of death or that the nurse was the first to respond to the family's call about a change in their loved one's condition. More often than not, families clearly recall the nurse's words and actions. What is done for and with family members at the time of their loved one's death can have a profound and long-lasting impact on them. It is important to remember that, although the death may be one of many for the nurse, it may be the first for the family; therefore, a person's death should never be treated as "just a job" on the part of the nurse. Clichés such as "This was meant to be" or "He [or she] is in a better place," or referring to the deceased person as an angel may make families feel that the death is minimized, as is the impact of the death on the family. Simple expressions, such as "I am sorry for your loss" (Bloomer et al., 2019, p. 26), are more often appreciated.

Nurses should understand loss, know how to support families in grief, and be able to provide quality bereavement care. Beginning nurses often worry about showing emotion, such as crying, in the presence of family members. Family members are often deeply touched when they see a nurse's genuine emotional response (Butler et al., 2015), but it is critical that the family not be put in the position of caring for the nurse.

Provision of bereavement care by the nurse offers the opportunity for continued contact with the family and signifies the importance of the family to the nurse (Collins-Tracey et al., 2009; Davies et al., 2017). Follow-up activities that many families appreciate include calls, cards, attendance at the funeral, and offers to make referrals to additional sources of support as needed (Boyle, 2019; Butler et al., 2015). Families may appreciate written information on practical issues, such as what to do next, and about grief or other sources of support (Boyle, 2019), as well as information to share with extended family and friends on how to offer effective support. Depending on the setting, bereavement care may continue for a period of time in the community and helps family caregivers adjust to the new normal in their lives. Sometimes health care providers call or send a card to families on the first anniversary of the patient's death, especially if it was a child who died. This simple contact acknowledges that the grieving process takes time and can make families feel really cared for, once again highlighting the importance of the patient and family to the health care provider (Collins-Tracey et al., 2009).

Special Situations

Some situations can be challenging for nurses to consider and deserve additional attention. More specific assessment and intervention tools may be required in order to offer optimal care in these special situations.

Children's Developmental Levels and Facilitating Grieving

Children tend to express some common behaviors and emotions, depending on their developmental level. However, it is still important to recognize that everyone grieves differently. Generally, children aged 2 to 4 years do not yet completely understand that death happens to everyone and that it is permanent. They may use play to work out their thoughts and may ask questions such as, "Daddy died? When will he come home?" Regression in behavior, crying, general anxiety, and temper tantrums are all common responses. Children of this age need consistent routines and short, honest answers to help them feel safe and to ensure that they do not develop incorrect ideas about death. It is important not to use euphemisms because, for example, a child who is told that she has lost her father may start searching for the lost person and not learn that death is permanent (Dougy Center, 2017).

Children aged 5 to 8 years are concrete thinkers who may use magical thinking. They often still see death as reversible, and they can feel responsible that their thoughts or wishes caused the person's death. They typically ask repetitive questions and worry about abandonment and safety. These children may also regress and may show somatic signs of grieving (e.g., headaches, stomachaches). Honest explanations and avoidance of euphemisms are needed with this age group, and the children need to be allowed to talk about their experiences and ask questions (Dougy Center, 2017).

As children mature, they begin to understand abstract ideas such as death and grief, and they realize that death is permanent. Children aged 8 to 12 years may still have some concrete thinking, but they also start to think about how the loss will affect them. Some children may feel regret and guilt,

believing that their thoughts or actions led to the person's death. These children need to have safety and predictability reestablished in their lives, and they should be offered various ways to express themselves (Dougy Center, 2017).

Teenagers, 13 to 18 years old, understand that death is permanent, but they sometimes struggle with more existential questions about the meaning of life and death. Withdrawing from family is common because children in this age group tend to rely more on peers. Safety and security continue to be issues for some, yet teenagers may also increase their own risk taking (e.g., drug and alcohol use), and thoughts of suicide or self-harm may appear. Some teenagers may feel responsible for caring for younger siblings or other adults, whereas others may push themselves to be perfect. Patience, reassurance, and nonjudgmental listening are all important (Dougy Center, 2017).

Facilitating Connections for Children When a Family Member Is Critically Ill

When a family member is critically ill, families and health care providers may have a concern about the importance and impact of bringing children to visit, whether at home, in the ICU, or in any other setting. Yet these visits may reduce feelings of separation, guilt, abandonment, fear, loneliness, and worry for the child (MacEachnie et al, 2018). Children can generally decide for themselves if they wish to visit and, where possible, families and health care providers should respect their decision. Younger children visiting a relative may be most interested in the equipment, whereas older children may spend more time focused on the person they are visiting (Knutsson et al, 2017). The visit can also benefit the patient by acting as a diversion, offering hope, and bringing a sense of normalcy. Thus, nurses should offer families the option of bringing children in to visit loved ones.

Talking with the patient and family about previous experiences with children visiting can be helpful. Some examples for starting conversations included the following: "Sometimes family members are afraid that a child will be very upset to see grandpa looking so sick. Are you worried about that possibility?" and "In my experience, children are very curious as well as resilient. They often suspect that something bad is happening, and they imagine terrible scenarios. Being truthful and also letting them see for themselves what is happening can be very beneficial." It is important to support families by preparing children ahead of time about what to expect. Being present during the visit to support family members in answering questions can make the child feel welcome and an important part of the family. It is important that everyone realizes a child's reactions are somewhat unpredictable; one child may seem unaffected, whereas another may be upset and crying. Nurses should acknowledge that every reaction is normal and work with the child in a way that meets his or her needs at the time. Although it may be difficult for a critically ill patient when a child chooses not to visit, you can help the patient understand by sharing your knowledge about how children need to make their own decisions, and you can offer ways to assist in maintaining connections between the child and the ill family member through cards, calls, and frequent updates about how the patient is doing.

When Death Is Sudden or Traumatic

Unlike with chronic illness, a sudden or traumatic death leaves little time for families to come to terms with the situation. The frequently chaotic environment of a traumatic or sudden death may contribute to a lack of communication between health care providers and families. It is important that the information given to families includes the big picture; otherwise, families often receive different pieces of information from each health care provider and may have trouble putting it all together to understand that it actually means the patient is dying. This may be more of an issue in situations when there is a sudden illness or injury because the family did not know what to expect and may be unprepared for what is happening (Odgers et al., 2018). (Refer to Chapter 16 for more detailed discussion about supporting families when the death of their loved one is sudden or traumatic and occurs in an acute care setting.) However, many of the principles of palliative care still apply, and it is possible to facilitate aspects of a good death by respecting families' wishes, providing excellent pain and symptom management, facilitating family presence or being present with the patient if the family is not able to be there, and preserving dignity (Stokes et al., 2019).

Dying at Home

Families need professional support, particularly in the area of symptom control, to facilitate a home death (Lewis et al., 2018; Spelton et al., 2019). Caring for a dying family member at home can be extremely demanding work—physically, emotionally, psychologically, and spiritually. Caregivers report feeling isolated and left on their own to navigate their way through the health system to access appropriate supports, work with health professionals who came to the home to ensure that quality care was provided, seek information about what to expect at the time of death, and manage all of the administrative details after the death occurred (e.g., arranging for the death certificate, transporting the body, arranging the funeral) (Mohammed et al., 2018). The primary caregivers require support and resources to reduce isolation and help them be successful. First and foremost, the family and the nurse need to discuss the dying process, existing resources, and present and future needs. Then together they can develop a plan that anticipates changes. For example, symptom crises, such as escalating pain, must be anticipated and addressed in advance. When the family is committed to supporting death at home, it can be devastating when a symptom crisis results in death in the middle of a busy emergency department. Box 11-6 provides some practical suggestions about what you need to consider and perhaps facilitate when someone is dying at home.

PALLIATIVE AND END-OF-LIFE CARE FAMILY CASE STUDIES

Three family case studies are presented in this section to demonstrate the art and science of family nursing in palliative and end-of-life care. The Jones family was introduced in Chapter 2 and is reintroduced here to demonstrate family care when the person who is dying is the mother. Please return to Chapter 2 and reacquaint yourself with the family and familiarize yourself with the Jones family genogram in Figure 11-1. The Garcia family case study illustrates how a student nurse working with a preceptor assists a young family during and following the death of an infant. The Wall family case study illustrates the importance of involving extended family and family traditions in the care of a Native American family when they experience the death of an elder.

BOX 11-6

Practical Considerations When Someone Is Dying at Home

The following are considerations for in-home care of the dying person:

- Involvement of expert resources, such as hospice, and an interprofessional team, including volunteers.
- Symptom management plan, including anticipating changes such as the inability to swallow and the need for parenteral medications, as well as management of breathlessness and agitation.
- Advance care planning, including the presence of a DNR or Physician Orders for Life Sustaining Treatment (POLST) order if necessary.
- Home medical equipment such as a hospital bed, bedside commode, personal-care items.
- Identification of willing informal support persons (friends, church members, extended family members).
- Development of a list of things that volunteers and friends can do, for example, a calendar for preparation

of meals, house cleaning, and/or someone to visit so the caregiver can take a walk.

- Respite service options that could be arranged to allow the caregiver time away during the day or overnight.
- Financial implications and available support, for example, compassionate benefits program.
- Resource list for services and support, including contact numbers.
- Discussion of unfinished business to enable a peaceful death.
- Discussion of alternative options for care in case dying and death or caregiving becomes too difficult or impossible in the home.
- Discussion and provision of written, detailed instructions for what to do and who to contact when the person dies.

Case Study: Jones Family

Linda, the mother in the Jones family, has been living with multiple sclerosis (MS) for 13 years. (See Figure 11-1 for the family genogram.) Early in the illness, Linda experienced relapses where her symptoms worsened, but these were followed by periods of

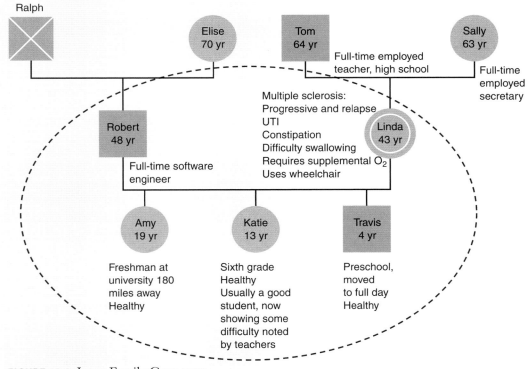

FIGURE 11-1 Jones Family Genogram

(continued)

Case Study: Jones Family—cont'd

remission where she recovered back to "normal." Since Travis's birth, her relapses have become more frequent, and although her symptoms sometimes improved a little, her condition steadily worsened.

Before Linda's discharge from the hospital, where she was treated with antibiotics for pneumonia after aspiration, the primary nurse, Catherine, initiated a family meeting with Linda, Robert, and Linda's physician Dr. Brooks. Catherine had noticed Robert's fatigue and his repeated questions about whether Linda was really ready to come home. Catherine had also noticed Linda's reluctance to take medications (particularly for pain), her determination to walk with her cane despite serious unsteadiness, and the deepening silence between the husband and wife.

Catherine began the conversation by asking Linda and Robert about their understanding of the MS at this point. Linda quickly responded, saying that the pneumonia was really an unusual one-time problem, and although it had set her back, it would not be long before she was back on her feet. Robert worried out loud that it seemed things were getting progressively worse. He was concerned about how Linda would manage at home alone in the mornings and with Travis in the afternoon when he returned from preschool. Noticing the difference in perspective, Catherine acknowledged that she could see how there might be differences because MS is, indeed, a tricky illness that is difficult to predict. She asked Linda and Robert to think back to how things were a year ago and to what had happened during the last year. Both noticed that the hospitalizations had become more frequent, the recoveries were more difficult, and Linda was not doing as well overall. Dr. Brooks, who had been listening quietly, remarked that, although MS was often an unpredictable disease, it seemed that Linda's MS had changed into a different kind of illness than it had been at first. He agreed that now the MS was progressing more steadily and that it seemed things were getting worse more quickly. Linda said that she could see this but kept hoping that the situation would turn around.

Catherine then asked what the family's goals for care were. Linda was quick to answer, "Remission—I want full remission." Robert was slower to reply. He said, "I am so tired, and it hurts me so much to see you suffer. I want you to be comfortable, to be free of pain, to enjoy the kids rather than snapping at them . . ." Linda said, "I'm just trying so hard to get back to normal. I always thought that a wheelchair would be the end for me. And I'm just so tired." Catherine acknowledged that MS often creates profound fatigue in many family members and wondered which of the children might be most affected. Both Linda and Robert agreed that, of the children, Katie was suffering the most from tiredness. She picked up a lot of the pieces of Linda's work in the home, beginning supper preparations and looking after Travis. Often, she would be up late at night working on homework, but her grades had been slipping and she had been crying more. Linda worried that Amy was also tired because she spent a great deal of time driving home on weekends to care for the family.

Dr. Brooks interjected at this point to say that their primary goal for care during this hospitalization had been to cure the pneumonia. He noted that, although they were successful, they had not been able to assist Linda toward a remission of her MS. He remarked that, with the change in the MS, it seemed that the hope for remission might not be possible. He then asked, "If things continue the way they are going, where do you think you will be in 6 months?" Linda began to cry and said that she was thinking she might not be alive. The pneumonia scared her, and she was frightened about aspirating again, so she had been decreasing what she ate and drank. Robert was worried about how he could continue to work full-time supporting the family and also care for Linda at home, especially as it seemed there was so little he did that was right for Linda.

Catherine replied that the "new" MS was clearly creating challenges for the family and wondered if the time had come to shift the focus of care more toward comfort and quality of life for all family members while at the same time working to prevent problems such as aspiration. She explained that as illness gets more demanding, additional supports are needed. She also explained that as illness becomes intrusive, attention must be given to what is most important to living well for all family members. Linda was getting tired at this point and having a lot of difficulty holding her head up, so Catherine asked if they could schedule another meeting. Robert and Linda readily agreed, saying that they knew they needed to talk about these things but just did not know how. Catherine asked each of them to do some homework: to identify their biggest concern as well as what was most important to living well at this time. They were asked to find this out from the children too, and a meeting was scheduled for the next day. Dr. Brooks let them know that he wanted to speak with them about Linda's preferences for care should she have another experience with pneumonia.

The next day, Linda, Robert, Catherine, and Dr. Brooks all met again. Linda began the conversation, saying that she had done a great deal of soul searching and was most worried about suffering from unmanageable pain and being a burden to her family. She was wondering if perhaps she should not go home but should be admitted into a care facility. Robert was most

Case Study: Jones Family—cont'd

worried about burning out and not being able to support Linda and the children as he wanted. They had had a three-way conversation with each of the children last evening. Amy was most worried that her mother was going to die, and she let her parents know that she was planning on leaving university to move back home. Katie was most troubled by her lack of friends because they were no longer including her in their activities. Travis missed his mother and wanted her to be able to read stories to him and play with him more.

The things that were most important to Linda's quality of life were reducing her pain, having Amy continue at university, being more involved in Katie's and Travis's everyday lives, being able to attend a service at her church on a weekly basis, and reconnecting with Robert. She said her greatest hope was to be at home as long as possible. Robert wanted to be able to sleep, to go to work without constantly worrying about Linda, and to reconnect with Linda. He too wanted her at home as long as possible. Both Linda and Robert agreed that for them to live well, they needed more help in their home. Options were discussed, including the possibility of Elise (Robert's mother) moving in to assist and preplanned, short stays in hospice for respite. Linda did not want Elise doing her personal care, so again, they discussed their options. Dr. Brooks and the family developed a systematic plan for pain management. During the assessment process, he learned that Linda was refusing her medications because she was concerned that they were contributing to her irritability with Robert and the children. He was able to reassure her that this was not the case; in fact, her unmanaged pain was more likely a major negative influence. They devised a plan for long-acting pain medication so that Robert would be able to sleep through the night. They consulted a dietitian regarding ways to manage swallowing problems and scheduled a home assessment by the team physiotherapist to maximize Linda's mobility with safety in mind.

Both Catherine and Dr. Brooks commended Linda and Robert on the deep love they saw between them and how effective they were at problem solving, systematically working through their issues until they achieved a mutually satisfying outcome. Finally, Dr. Brooks raised the topic of what Linda's preferences for care would be if she should experience development of pneumonia again. He explained that this was a real possibility because Linda's respiratory muscles were weakening. Dr. Brooks understood that both Linda and Robert wanted her home as long as possible, so he was curious about whether she would want to come to the hospital to be treated with intravenous antibiotics, as she had during this hospitalization. Linda stated this would be her preference, especially if she was likely to be able to go home again after the treatment. Dr. Brooks explained that as her muscles become weaker, she might need the assistance of a breathing machine (ventilator) to give the antibiotics time to work against the infection and asked whether she would want that. Linda was not sure what her preference would be in this situation, but she was very clear that she did not want to be "kept alive on a machine." She and Robert wanted more time to discuss this question, and they wanted to consult with their pastor, so they agreed to continue the conversation at the next doctor's appointment. Robert and Linda agreed to visit the local hospice to explore respite opportunities, as well as end-of-life care, should staying at home prove too difficult.

Three weeks later, at the scheduled appointment with Dr. Brooks, Linda let him know that many things were going better with Elise in the house and home visits from Catherine, as well as a personal care aide. Amy agreed to stay in college with the promise from her parents that she would be told immediately if Linda's health changed. All family members were feeling less tired. Linda stated that she was not ready to leave Robert and the children but was in a dilemma about the use of a ventilator if she developed pneumonia. She continued to worry that she might be kept alive on the machine, which to her would not be considered living. Dr. Brooks explained that, if necessary, one possibility was a time-limited trial of a ventilator to determine whether the antibiotics would work. Both Linda and Robert agreed. This was a difficult discussion, and Linda expressed distress about her loss of independence and her deep sorrow about the possibility of leaving her children. She admitted to swinging between despair and anger, and that both made it hard for her to enjoy her days. This was new information to Robert, who had noticed her struggling but thought things would work out over time. Through assessment, it became apparent that Linda was experiencing depression. She agreed to try an antidepressant medication and to join a local MS support group.

Eight Months Later

Linda experienced fever, congestion, and shortness of breath after aspiration. The health team initiated antibiotics and managed symptoms to relieve pain, breathlessness, fever, and constipation. Linda occasionally had periods of acute shortness of breath during which she worried that she might not be able to take her next breath. The fear served to make the breathlessness worse, so the visiting nurse showed both Linda and the family how to slow and deepen breathing by consciously breathing together. Dr. Brooks made a home visit and asked Linda about admission to the hospital. When he could not assure her that she would get off the ventilator, Linda declined, saying she wanted to stay with her family. Robert agreed. A family meeting with Catherine and

(continued)

Case Study: Jones Family—cont'd

Dr. Brooks was held at Linda's bedside to discuss what the family would experience if the pneumonia progressed. They developed a family ecomap (Figure 11-2), and they increased support services with more frequent visits from the nurse, care aide, and friends (particularly from Linda's support group). They discussed a move to hospice, but all agreed that home was the best place for Linda and that death at home was their preference.

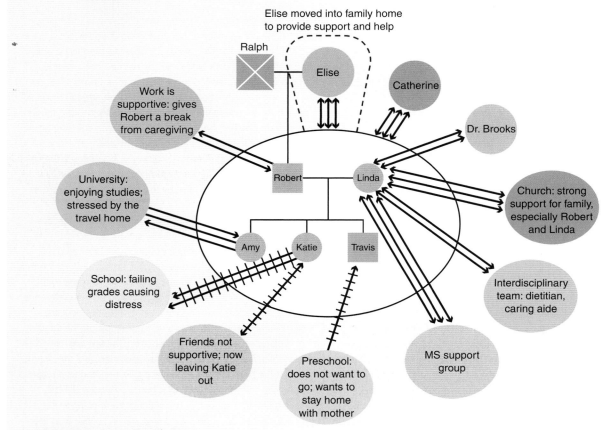

FIGURE 11-2 Jones Family Ecomap

Linda engaged in one-on-one time with each of her children. They talked about their best memories together, what they most loved about each other, and their hopes and dreams for the future as the children grow up. Robert participated by videotaping the conversations. Each child was given a journal, and together with Linda, they drew pictures, wrote notes, and gathered mementos to capture these conversations. She organized gifts for their birthdays and for Christmas in the upcoming year. It was not that she knew that she was dying, but she had been encouraged to plan for the worst and hope for the best, and to do the things that needed doing. The family received the same encouragement, so they were all able to have special time with Linda during the last few months. Linda died surrounded by her family.

Six Weeks Later

Catherine visited the family 6 weeks after Linda's death and found them managing well. Pictures of Linda were everywhere. Elise continued to live with the family, and they thought this was the best plan for the time being. Robert had taken some time off work to be with the children after Linda's death, but shortly afterward all went back to work and school. Amy still came home on some weekends. Robert, Amy, and Katie talked of their sense of having done the very best they could to honor Linda's preferences. They took comfort in the fact that she died at home. They marked the 1-month anniversary of Linda's death with a visit to her

Case Study: Jones Family—cont'd

grave site, taking flowers and a picture Travis had drawn of his mother. Family members drew support from different sources: each other, friends, their pastor, and some of the people from the MS support group who continued to visit. The children continued to read and reread the letters Linda had written; for Travis, this was part of his bedtime ritual. They were sad, and some days were better than others, but they had a sense that the weight of their grief was lifting.

Questions for reflection on the nursing care of the Jones family:

1. What actions demonstrated collaboration with members of the team to support the patient and family? What are the priorities for nursing assessment in this case?
2. Are there special considerations for working with children who are experiencing the life-limiting illness of a family member?
3. How can family meetings be used to support palliative and end-of-life care?

Case Study: Garcia Family

You are a nursing student in your final clinical placement. Your preceptor is a clinical nurse specialist (CNS) on the palliative care team in a children's hospital. You asked for this placement as a final-year nursing student because you have come across several situations during your student experiences when you wished you knew how to talk and be with a patient and her family when the patient was dying. You realize that all nurses, from novice to expert and in all areas of nursing practice, need to develop skills in the area of death and dying. Please acquaint yourself with the Garcia family genogram in Figure 11-3. Consider what it would be like if you were the student working with this family.

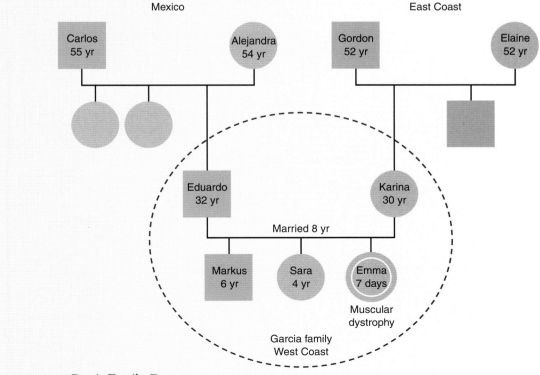

FIGURE 11-3 Garcia Family Genogram

Case Study: Garcia Family—cont'd

We have received a new consultation to meet with Emma and her parents, Eduardo and Karina Garcia. We learn that Emma is 7 days old and is a beautiful little baby with a perfect little face, big dark eyes, and lots of dark hair. Emma is on a ventilator because she has severe congenital muscular dystrophy and is unable to breathe on her own. Babies with severe disease, such as Emma, have a very limited life expectancy, typically only a few weeks. Her severe muscle weakness means she is not able to breathe on her own for any length of time. We have been asked to meet with Emma and her family because the parents have decided, in consultation with their health care team, to withdraw ventilator support. As part of the palliative care team, we have been invited to assist Eduardo and Karina to decide how, when, and where the withdrawal might occur.

Before meeting with this family for the first time, we realize how important it is to prepare ourselves. We know that we need to pause for a moment and consider how we might begin this conversation with Eduardo and Karina. We also want to ensure that we have in place whatever we might need to facilitate this first meeting.

We decide to meet with Eduardo and Karina in a quiet, private room where we will not be interrupted. Pagers are turned off, and other staff members are covering for us so that we will have time to sit with the parents and really listen to what they have to say. Given that there will be several challenging topics to discuss, we invite the neonatal intensive care unit (NICU) social worker, who already has a relationship with the family, to join us for this meeting.

Before meeting the family, we spend some time talking about different ways to begin the conversation with the parents. This is the beginning of what we hope will be a therapeutic relationship during one of the most difficult times a family can experience. Eduardo and Karina need to know who we are. It is often hard for parents to keep track of health care providers—who we are, what we do, and how we can be helpful. This is especially true in highly emotionally charged situations. So we typically start with brief introductions. Rather than starting the conversation by saying why we are here, it is sometimes helpful to gain an understanding of why the parents think we are meeting and then continue from there.

We start the meeting by each introducing ourselves. Then one of us says, "Tell us your understanding of why we are meeting today." To facilitate our connection with this family, we also ask Eduardo and Karina to tell us about Emma—*not* her medical condition but what they, as parents, have noticed about her or experienced in their relationship with Emma. One of the things Karina tells us is that she thinks Emma has Eduardo's eyes. Eduardo has noticed that she follows Karina with her eyes and he says, "She really knows her mom."

We learn that after talking with both sets of grandparents (mostly by telephone because Eduardo's family is in Mexico where he and Karina met, and Karina's parents live across the country), the health care team, and their priest, Karina and Eduardo have indeed come to the decision that the most loving thing they can do as parents is to withdraw Emma's ventilator and allow natural death. We encourage them to discuss their concerns, fears, and hopes for the time they have now with Emma. There is much silence and tears as the parents try to put into words all the thoughts swirling in their heads. They tell us that their focus is on having Emma experience as much of normal newborn life as she can, and they want to touch her and care for her. They want her to spend time with her 4-year-old sister, Sara, and 6-year-old brother, Markus; to be in her car seat; to be bathed, cuddled, and have her diaper changed by both her mom and dad; to be baptized; and most of all to see the sun. We learn that it was the middle of the night when Emma was born, after which she was immediately transferred from her small community to our tertiary urban hospital 3 hours away, so she had seen the moon but not the sun. Eduardo is a forestry worker, and the family loves to be outdoors. They cannot believe that one of their children will never spend any time outdoors. Neither Karina nor Eduardo had been able to hold Emma before she was whisked away. Karina has held her in the NICU, but Eduardo has been reluctant because of all the tubes. He is feeling sad that her pervasive muscle weakness means she cannot grab onto his finger the way Sara and Markus did as babies and he is searching to find another way to connect with Emma. Both parents express worry about how to help Sara and Markus understand what is happening in a way that does not frighten them. Although both Karina and Eduardo are committed to their decision, they are afraid that Emma may suffer when the ventilator is withdrawn. They are worried about watching her struggle for breath. The parents ask us for a week to have these experiences with Emma; they also want time for additional family members to visit and to plan for withdrawal of the ventilator.

Following our meeting with Eduardo and Karina, we meet with the involved NICU staff members, who are quite concerned with the proposal that we wait a week to discontinue the ventilator. This is not the way it usually happens, and they worry the family will only become more attached to Emma, finding it harder and harder to let her go, or that something will change in Emma's health status that may lead to an earlier death than what the parents expect. We provide further explanation and facilitate

Case Study: Garcia Family—cont'd

a meeting between the parents, Eduardo and Karina, and the NICU staff. At the meeting, NICU staff members can express their concerns and the family can respond, as well as talk about their wishes. Hearing each other's fears and hopes is helpful, and there is now agreement and support for the parents' request. Eduardo and Karina understand that it is possible something could happen unexpectedly with Emma and, although everything possible will be done to ensure that she is comfortable, the staff will not provide CPR if her heart stops.

Emma and her parents move into one of the private family rooms in the NICU. Karina's parents, Elaine and Gordon, who came to care for Sara and Markus in the family home, bring them to stay in a nearby hotel. This proximity enables them to visit often and to get to know the newest member of their family. Before their first visit, we spend time talking with Eduardo and Karina about how to prepare the siblings for seeing Emma and explaining similarities and differences in how Sara and Markus may understand what is happening. Another member of the team, a child life therapist, spends time with Sara and Markus individually and together to assess and support their understanding and coping with Emma's illness. Eduardo and Karina join some of the discussions and have some of their own time with the child life therapist. They learn how young children come to understand serious illness and death and that Sara and Markus will likely have questions about Emma for many years. They are happy about the picture books and other resources on how to support their children over time.

During the week, even in the midst of the technology that is still needed to keep Emma breathing, Eduardo, Karina, Grandma Elaine, Grandpa Gordon, Sara, and Markus do all the things that families with newborns usually do. The family is given the opportunity to say hello and goodbye to their new family member all at the same time. Eduardo holds Emma for the first time, and they take many, many pictures and videos. They give Emma her first haircut, and each saves a tiny lock of hair tied with a ribbon. Sara and Markus each create a memory box with drawings, the locks of hair, Emma's hand- and footprints, and copies of the photos. They also help the child life therapist make molds of Emma's hands and feet, as well as their own. Eduardo's parents arrive from Mexico, and several close family members and friends come to meet Emma and witness her baptism in the hospital chapel. The list of hopes and dreams for this time gets ticked off. Eduardo and Karina also use this time to contact a funeral home in their home community and plan for Emma's wake and funeral with their priest.

One day we take Emma, her parents, her siblings, and her grandparents outside to the hospital's play garden where it is beautifully clear and sunny with a gentle breeze blowing. Hospital security has closed the garden to other families and staff members so it is intimate and peaceful. Emma is able to feel the sun on her face for the first time. The child life therapist is there to support Sara and Markus. They both seem to enjoy this family outing; they run over to see Emma, give her a kiss, and then head off to explore the sandbox and the swings before coming back again for a hug from their parents. Eduardo and Karina ask if we think that Sara and Markus really don't understand the situation and that is why they keep running off to play. The child life therapist reassures them that this is a typical way for children to cope and essentially, they are just taking in what they can handle at their own pace. The child life therapist continues to follow the children's lead in supporting whatever they want to do and wherever they want to be in the garden. A nurse from the NICU stays close to Emma to assist her to breathe while she is being held by her parents and grandparents. Everyone relaxes and shares stories about Karina's pregnancy, the labor and delivery, and the things they have learned about Emma during the last few days. We take more family pictures and video to send to the rest of the extended family that night. To our surprise, the parents feel so comfortable in the garden that they ask if the ventilator can be discontinued in the garden. We set about making this request happen.

Eduardo, Karina, and Elaine meet with us, the neonatologist, the NICU CNS, and the NICU social worker; we explain how we will keep Emma comfortable when the ventilator is withdrawn. The family is reassured to learn that there are medications that will ensure that Emma does not struggle for breath and that we will not allow her to suffer. Eduardo asks what it will be like when the ventilator is taken away. We are able to help them understand that we do not know how long Emma will be able to breathe without assistance, but it could be minutes to hours; her breathing will slow, become irregular, and then stop. Her color will change and she will feel cool. Eduardo and Karina decide that they would like to be by themselves with Emma when she dies. Sara and Markus will stay at the hotel with their grandparents and then may come back to see Emma before she is taken to the funeral home.

Both parents seem to be coping fairly well with the situation, with Eduardo taking on the role of the "strong one" and Karina appearing more fragile. On the day of Emma's death, however, we are surprised at the reversal of roles: Eduardo looks disheveled and distressed, whereas Karina has done her hair and makeup. She is wearing a special outfit and seems "in control." You

(continued)

Case Study: Garcia Family—cont'd

comment to her parents that Emma has seen the moon and the sun and now she is experiencing a true West Coast day—foggy and gloomy! Emma is given some medications so she won't experience any pain or distress and is settled with her parents in a secluded corner of the garden. The priest performs last rites. The nurse removes all the tape and then the endotracheal tube while Emma remains peaceful in her parent's arms. We give the family private space to be together but we and other members of the team (the priest, the NICU social worker, and the NICU nurse) are available in the play garden, with additional medications ready in case Emma experiences any distress.

The play garden is on a busy street, and we are concerned that the level of traffic noise might be disturbing to the family. Our concerns are heightened when the siren starts at the nearby fire hall and the fire truck roars past; Emma's dad simply walks over to the fence and lifts her up to see her first fire truck. Emma and her parents walk the paths of the garden. Although there is still bustle and noise around them, it is clear that Emma and her family are in their own little world. Although they had opportunities to do "normal" family things during the last week, this is the first time Emma and her parents experience each other without interference from machines, tubes, wires, or other people.

Emma lives for another 2 hours. After she dies, her parents continue to hold her for another hour. Both sets of grandparents return with Sara and Markus to say goodbye to Emma. Although the children were both told how Emma would look and feel after she died, Markus in particular has many questions about whether or not she is hungry, why she is cold, and if she is just sleeping. Karina responds gently to all their questions to help them understand what has happened. When the family is ready, Sara and Markus spend some time with the child life therapist while a senior nurse, Patrick, partners with you to help Karina and Eduardo prepare Emma's body. Patrick asks the parents if they have any special rituals they would like to do and he also explains about what has to be done to meet the hospital rules. Everyone works together and, though it is sad, there is also a peacefulness as Karina and Eduardo talk about how happy they are to have done things the way they wanted to. They thank you and Patrick and say how grateful they are that the staff made it possible for Emma to die in peace in such a beautiful setting; Karina and Eduardo say that they will never forget what the staff did. With one last kiss on Emma's forehead, they leave for home with the rest of their family.

Patrick assists you to complete all the charting and necessary paperwork related to Emma's death. Because Eduardo and Karina decided against having an autopsy, Emma does not need to go to the hospital morgue. Patrick calls the funeral home and accompanies you as you carry Emma's body in a special softly colored and patterned bag to meet the funeral home director at the staff entrance to the hospital. You return to the unit and spend some time talking with Patrick and me. We make sure that you have a way home and a friend available to spend the evening with you. I also contact your clinical coordinator to let her know about the day's events to make sure that you have some ongoing support from the faculty. A few days later, I invite you to attend a special debriefing session to be held with NICU staff members.

The funeral is held 3 hours away, so you are unable to attend. I suggest that you may want to send a note to the family and offer to review it if needed (Box 11-7).

BOX 11-7
Example Follow-Up Note to Family From Student Nurse

Dear Eduardo, Karina, Markus, and Sara,

It was my privilege to get to know all of you and to meet Emma. She had the most beautiful expressive eyes and so clearly looked at each of you when you spoke to her. It was amazing to watch all of you together and to see Emma experience so much life in such a short time. Your love for her and for each other was evident in everything that you did.

I learned so many things about how families can be together and live life to the fullest even in the midst of such difficult circumstances. I know my experience with your family will make me a better nurse with other families in the future. Emma and all of you will forever remain in my thoughts.

All my best,

[Name of Student Nurse]

Case Study: Garcia Family—cont'd

One Month Later

Emma's death was not the end of our relationship with the Garcia family. We make a home visit a month after Emma's death where we learn about the funeral. Karina and Eduardo remark that they were very happy when two of their favorite NICU nurses came to Emma's funeral. They tell us about how moved they were when they received notes from you and some of the other nurses, as well as a card from the NICU staff. They tell us that it helps them to know that Emma touched the hearts of those who looked after her. We discuss how Karina and Eduardo are managing as a couple and as parents. Eduardo is back at work; Sara and Markus are back at preschool and school. Both sets of grandparents have gone home. At this point we draw an ecomap of the family's community connections (see Figure 11-4), discuss their experiences of grief, and work together to find local avenues of support. We let Karina and Eduardo know that they will receive a letter with an appointment to see a geneticist in about 6 months. Because there was a genetic component to Emma's diagnosis, they may want to explore genetic testing and understand any possible risks for future pregnancies. A follow-up visit with the NICU neonatologist, CNS, and social worker will be coordinated to occur on the same day to respond to any questions the parents may have about Emma's illness and death, as well as to see how they are all coping. They are invited to bring Sara and Markus at that time to meet with the child life therapist.

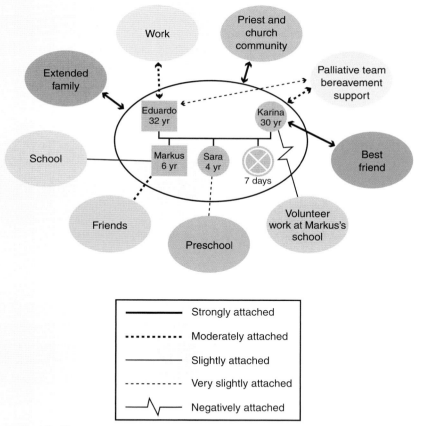

FIGURE 11-4 Garcia Family Ecomap

We also let them know that the NICU has a formal program where, with the parents' permission, staff nurses are supported to contact families at regular intervals in the first year after the death and then send a plant on the 1-year anniversary. Karina and Eduardo express their appreciation for such a program and say that they can only imagine how hard it will be on the anniversary of Emma's death; to know that the NICU staff who looked after her will be thinking of them gives them great comfort.

(continued)

Case Study: Garcia Family—cont'd

Questions for reflection on the nursing care of the Garcia family:

1. Reflect on the challenges of end-of-life communication. What strategies did the team utilize to support the Garcia family during difficult communication?
2. What rituals and activities did the team suggest during Emma's transition? What are the short- and long-term benefits of those activities?
3. What elements of patient- and family-centered care were included in the plan of care that can be applied to the care of others?
4. How can nurses utilize bereavement support to enhance the quality of care for individuals in palliative and end-of-life care?

Case Study: Wall Family

Robert Wall was a 78-year-old divorced man. He lived in rural Montana and was a member of the Confederated Salish and Kootenai Tribes. He lived alone in his home in the small town where he was born and raised. He was recently taken to the hospital after he suffered a fall in his home. In the local emergency room, bone fractures and other musculoskeletal injuries were ruled out. During his examination, he was diagnosed with severe weakness, difficulty breathing, recent weight loss, and severe dehydration. For many years he had been using various inhalers for his breathing and has reported more difficulty with his breathing lately. An initial reading of the chest x-ray showed a mass in his right lung. He refused hospital admission for further workup of his symptoms but agreed to follow up at the tribal health clinic the next day.

Tribal Health Clinic Visit

Robert presented to the tribal health clinic a couple of days after the tribal health nurse called to ask if he needed a ride to the clinic. She had reviewed his records from the emergency room visit, including the chest x-ray report and his refusal for hospital admission. On the phone, he mentioned that he had not yet come to the clinic because he was not feeling well enough to leave the house. His brother gave him a ride and provided him with assistance to walk into the clinic, where he was treated by the tribal health nurse and physician.

Medical and Social History

Upon assessment, Robert was vague about his medical and social history. His tribal health record confirmed chronic asthma and emphysema, hypertension, and alcoholism. His lung condition was exacerbated by decades of smoking one pack or more of cigarettes per day. He reported that he drank several beers each day "when I feel good enough" and he denied illicit drug use. Approximately 30 years ago, he was involved in a near-fatal car crash and had "hardware" in both hips that caused significant pain in his legs and lower back. He had multiple surgeries following his accident. He reported taking pain pills from time to time and an occasional sleeping pill to manage his symptoms, although he had no current prescriptions. He was not currently taking any medications or supplements regularly except a Tylenol "every so often."

Robert was one of three remaining (five total) male siblings in his family. He had been married and divorced "too many times" and had two daughters who lived locally, a son and a daughter who lived in another state, several grandchildren, multiple nieces and nephews, and several extended family members and friends in the community. (See Figure 11-5 for the Wall family genogram.) He spent several decades living in California but returned to his home community approximately 15 years ago. He was an avid antique gun collector and enjoyed traveling to gun shows across the state.

Condition, Health Beliefs, and Trajectory of Illness

Robert admitted to the tribal health physician that he had not been feeling well for several weeks. He reported that it had been months since he had been able to attend a gun show or go out for his daily lunch with friends at the local Veterans of Foreign Wars bar. He was hoping to get some medicine that might make him feel better so he could go home. Again, he declined admission to the hospital, stating that it was not something he would ever want. After some discussion, he was willing to accept home health visits from the tribal health nurse. He was prescribed hydrocodone/acetaminophen for pain and lorazepam for anxiety and/or sleep. The nurse provided him with a written plan for the medications and for possible symptoms of alcohol

Case Study: Wall Family—cont'd

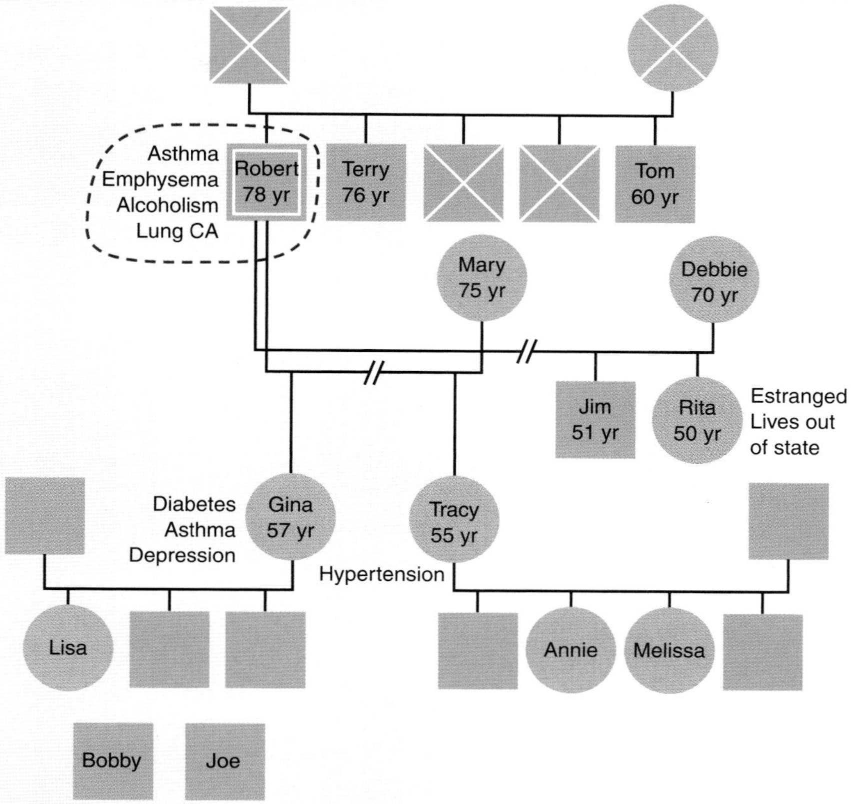

FIGURE 11-5 Wall Family Genogram

withdrawal. He agreed to have the nurse visit on Monday following the weekend. He agreed that his brother would check on him throughout the weekend.

On the morning of the home visit, Robert had declined significantly. When the nurse arrived, she observed that he was much weaker, less communicative, and more dyspneic. He was now confined to the couch in his living room and had been incontinent of urine. He was no longer able to perform activities of daily living or get himself to the bathroom. His oral intake was poor, and it was not clear that he understood how to take his medications. After confirming his wishes not to go to the hospital, the nurse called the tribal health physician to report his condition and discuss a referral to hospice. Robert was agreeable to this approach and asked the nurse to call his brother and his daughters.

Admission to Hospice

By the afternoon, the family had gathered at Robert's home to meet with the hospice nurse. The tribal health nurse also attended the admission visit in order to continue to provide support for the patient and family in a collaborative manner with the hospice team. It was also important to continue support from the tribal health team because of the trust the team had developed with Robert. A primary goal for the visit was to engage in communication with the patient and family about the patient's terminal condition and his choices for care. Because the conversations between palliative care clinicians, patients, and families that focus on transitions to hospice and palliative care often signal the beginning of the dying process, it was important to have in the home those family members identified by the patient as important for decision making (Kirby et al., 2014). A family-centered approach to the hospice admission that addressed the following priorities was utilized:

1. *Decision making:* It was important to discuss with the family what was currently known about Robert's condition in order to clarify his choices for care. He was considered appropriate for admission to hospice because of the physician's certification of

(continued)

Case Study: Wall Family—cont'd

terminal illness and his preference for comfort care rather than curative treatment. It was important to consider his personal cultural beliefs when discussing his illness with the family. The hospice team secured the patient's signature for a do not resuscitate (DNR) order (called a Comfort One order in Montana) that documented his wishes. Family discussion centered on ensuring that his wishes were carried out and making sure other family members were given accurate information.

2. *Comfort care/pain and symptom management:* A complete pain and symptom assessment was completed to understand the patient's current condition and potential sources of suffering. Medication reconciliation helped the nurse identify the patient's needs for medication refills and additional recommendations for the primary provider.

3. *Family support:* Robert lived alone and would need to rely on family support to provide personal and comfort care in his home (Figure 11-6). As his disease progressed, he would require bathing, medication administration, and other personal-care needs. His daughters, brothers, and granddaughters were willing to provide care so that he would not be alone.

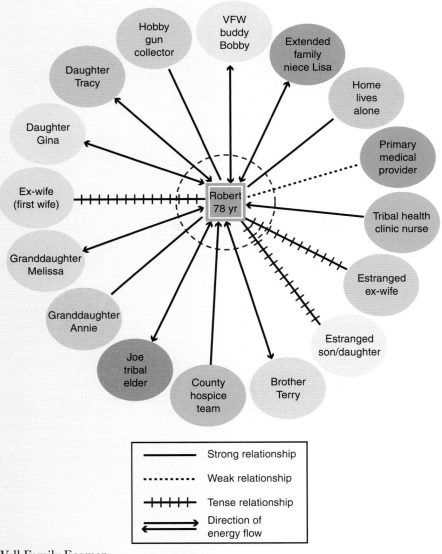

FIGURE 11-6 Wall Family Ecomap

Case Study: Wall Family—cont'd

4. *Home safety:* A safety assessment included making an agreement with the patient and family that Robert's guns would be locked away during the period of home visiting to ensure safety of the patient, family, and staff. Assessment of fire hazards in the home and education on oxygen precautions were completed. Durable medical equipment was ordered to support safe care for the patient (e.g., hospital bed, wheelchair, bedside commode).

5. *Culture and traditional practices:* An assessment of the patient's and family's traditional practices was an important priority. The patient declined chaplain support but did request that his extended family and friends be allowed to visit the home and support his family. His daughters requested a Catholic priest to pray with them.

Outcomes and Family Functioning

Once Robert was admitted to the hospice program, his condition progressed rapidly. His decline was difficult for his family, particularly his daughters, who had spent the majority of their lives estranged from their father. During this time, they provided loving care and shared close communication with their father. The hospice team and the tribal health team worked collaboratively with the family to care for Robert in his home until his peaceful death. At the time of his death, he was surrounded by his family. Each family member felt that he or she had been able to share special moments with him and to say goodbye.

Questions for reflection on the nursing care of the Wall family:

1. Reflect on the importance of patient autonomy in this case. What is the value of patient autonomy in palliative and end-of-life care? What is the role of the nurse when it comes to patient and family choices?

2. What is the nurse's role in preparing individuals and families for what to expect? How was this done in Robert's case?

3. In this case, how were Robert's cultural beliefs and preferences for care honored? Are there additional ways that nurses can address the diverse and unique preferences of individuals approaching the end of life?

SUMMARY

Nurses are in a unique position to help families manage their lives when a loved one has a life-limiting illness or faces an acute or sudden death. Providing palliative and end-of-life nursing care as you accompany a family during this intense period is a privilege that should not be taken lightly. The importance of the nurse-family relationship in affecting and effecting positive outcomes cannot be overstated; this relationship can make the difference between a family who has good memories about their loved one's death and a family who experiences prolonged suffering because of a negative experience. Open and trusting communication; physical, psychological, and spiritual support; respect for the families' right to make their own decisions; and support to facilitate these decisions are essential components of quality palliative and end-of-life care. The following points highlight the concepts addressed in this chapter:

- Palliative care and end-of-life care are inherently patient and family-centered.
- The principles of palliative care can be enacted effectively in any setting, regardless of whether death results from a chronic illness or a sudden or traumatic event.
- Interprofessional team collaboration is essential in palliative and end-of-life care; the team includes the patient and family.
- Nurses in all settings should develop competencies in the area of death and dying.
- Effective patient and family-centered communication, assessment, and intervention skills can help nurses provide quality palliative and end-of-life care.
- Therapeutic nurse-patient and nurse-family relationships are central to quality palliative and end-of-life care.
- Nurses who incorporate the principles of palliative care are more effective in tailoring their nursing practice and family interventions.

chapter 12

Trauma and Family Nursing

Deborah Padgett Coehlo, PhD, C-PNP, PMHS, CFLE

Melissa Robinson, PhD, RN

Critical Concepts

- Trauma is a key experience affecting individuals and the family system.

- Trauma-informed care (TIC) is an important part of nursing care for all clients, including families, to improve outcomes, avoid biased and inaccurate assessments and interventions, and prevent unethical decision-making processes.

- Bronfenbrenner's Ecological Systems Model (Bronfenbrenner, 2005; Guy-Evans, 2020) can guide nurses in applying TIC.

- Post-traumatic stress disorder (PTSD), a medical diagnosis, is based on a cluster of symptoms in response to trauma that can be an acute stress reaction or a chronic condition and can occur months, or even years, after a disaster or traumatic event.

- Adaptive responses to trauma are more likely to become problematic when resilience traits are underdeveloped.

- When one or more family members are traumatized, all family members and family relationships can be affected.

- Perpetrators of trauma can experience trauma themselves. Nurses who focus on TIC can address the dilemmas of caring for perpetrators through mandatory reporting and family-focused care.

- Secondary or vicarious trauma can occur whenever a family member or caring provider is exposed to victims of trauma and is affected by the victims' response to the traumatic event(s).

- The family's response to the trauma of one or more of its members cannot be understood or treated by focusing on individual family members alone.

- Family members can provide key contextual information about past traumatic events and experiences that help explain current responses, offer support, and address their own reactions to trauma.

- Community systems can prevent, treat, and measure negative outcomes of traumatic events. If community agencies are not well trained and prepared, communities suffer.

- Larger political and social systems can influence and be influenced positively and/or negatively by individual, family, and community trauma.

- Nursing focuses on the individual, family, community, and societal reactions to trauma in order to optimize positive outcomes and prevent or treat problematic stress responses.

- Nurses have an essential role in supporting health and resilience rather than focusing on the pathology of a trauma response.

Trauma has been an increasing area of attention across the field of mental health for the past three decades. With the advanced understanding of brain function, general physiology, and the mind and body response to severe and/or prolonged stress, and the increase in traumatic stress experienced by families through war, natural disasters, and personal and family violence, the need to understand, prevent, treat, and monitor the effects of trauma on individuals and families has never been more vital. In addition, the effects of trauma transcend individuals and families and affect communities and the broader society. Trauma affects future generations as the effects influence individual family genetics, community, and societal cultures. The negative effects of trauma are most profound during early childhood development, touching every domain of growth, with the potential of negative outcomes in adulthood, such as higher rates of mental illness, unemployment, poor health, substance abuse, and failed relationships.

The care by nurses of families experiencing traumatic stress revolves around preventing trauma when possible; supporting the development of resilience; and, when not preventable, working toward positive outcomes. This chapter focuses on the current knowledge about trauma and nurses' key role in the field of trauma-informed care (TIC). TIC emphasizes the importance of prevention, early intervention, and encouraging resilience and the ability to make meaning out of negative events. This chapter also stresses an understanding of secondary trauma, or the negative effects of witnessing the trauma of others, whether that other person is a stranger, family, or fellow professional. This discussion is particularly salient for nurses because they are among the most likely health care providers to encounter traumatized victims in their everyday practice. Nurses are also among the professional groups most likely to experience vicarious or secondary trauma as a consequence of their exposure to traumatized clients.

POST-TRAUMATIC STRESS DISORDER (PTSD)

The diagnosis of PTSD has grown significantly during the past two decades, as has the understanding of differences in symptoms across developmental ages and stages and the types of trauma.

The key symptoms of reexperiencing the trauma through painful memories and nightmares, hypervigilance, and emotional instability are common to adults, but children are more likely to react with withdrawal and mood dysregulation. Different types of trauma have different rates of severity and incidences of PTSD symptoms, with sexual assault causing more severe, chronic, and frequent symptoms than other forms of trauma, especially in cases of repeated sexual assault (Hamrick & Owens, 2019). The symptoms cross ethnic groups, ages, and time. The number of individuals with PTSD in turn affects communities. Larger cultures and societies shift as the number of trauma victims grows, adding other negative consequences that include poor health, higher rates of other mental health disorders, and an increase in family violence (Hamrick & Owens, 2019).

The American Psychological Association (APA) first recognized PTSD as a diagnosis and began to categorize symptoms of this disorder in 1980. Since that time, researchers and clinicians have identified the complexity of this disorder and the lifelong, intergenerational impact of repeated and prolonged trauma experienced by individuals, families, communities, and societies. Over time, researchers have attempted to clarify and expand the diagnosis to cover different categories of trauma, such as combat, horrific accidents, and child abuse; different contexts such as domestic violence, natural disasters, and war; and differences across cultures, such as victims of genocide and of natural disasters across cultures and historical contexts across time (Friedman, 2021).

The *Diagnostic and Statistical Manual of Mental Disorders (DDSM-5)* (APA, 2013) has taken PTSD out of the category of anxiety and developed a separate category titled Trauma and Stressor Related Disorders (Pai et al., 2017). The scope has been expanded to include both experiencing a traumatic event and witnessing or repeatedly hearing about or watching a traumatic event. The *DSM-5* has also included four categories of symptoms:

1. Intrusion of thoughts about the trauma
2. Avoidance of discussion or other stimulus reminding the person of the trauma
3. Increased arousal or sensory sensitivity
4. Negative cognitions and moods (APA, 2013)

Today, it is estimated that up to 10% of the general population around the world meets the criteria for a diagnosis of PTSD, with areas experiencing war or severe natural disasters experiencing the highest rates of community trauma. When further divided between geographical areas, ages, and genders, the prevalence rates vary, with risks higher for women and adolescents and lower risks in Asian countries (U.S. Department of Veterans Affairs, 2020a). When considering children and adolescents, it is important to note that most PTSD is caused by (1) abuse and neglect across time, (2) witnessing violence within the home and/or neighborhood, and (3) experiencing single-incident traumatic events such as motor vehicle accidents and natural disasters (Hamblen & Barnett, 2021).

The number of studies on individual trauma and outcomes has increased in the past two decades, as has awareness that PTSD is not limited to individuals but rather affects individuals, families, communities, and societies. The understanding of the political and societal influences on the diagnosis, treatment, and continued research in this area explains in part the continued need to explore trauma and its relationship to family health. The extent of damage to physical and mental health caused by trauma has now been realized.

This chapter uses the Ecological Systems Model (Bronfenbrenner, 2005) to explore current understanding of risk and protective factors of PTSD, and uses that knowledge to further understanding of the multidisciplinary approach to TIC that goes beyond the medical model of diagnosis and treatment. Family nurses are in a key position to understand, recognize, prevent, and treat trauma at multiple levels. Case studies throughout this chapter illustrate the complexities of trauma and its effect on all family members, and the strong influence nursing care can have on short- and long-term outcomes.

THEORIES APPLIED TO TRAUMA-INFORMED CARE (TIC)

Understanding of TIC has progressed significantly during the past two decades, with a plethora of studies published to clarify evidence-based practice across cultural groups, ages and genders, geographic areas, and types of trauma experiences. Health care providers historically considered trauma to be a form of hysteria, meriting ineffective treatments as severe as hysterectomies. Current treatment approaches recognize the modern understanding of trauma as a complex stress disorder with several applicable underlying theories. For the purposes of this book, we delve into trauma understanding and care using the Substance Abuse and Mental Health Services Administration's (SAMHSA) Guide for TIC in Behavioral Health Services (2015), the Ecological Systems Model (Bronfenbrenner, 2005; Bronfenbrenner & Lerner, 2004), and Family Systems Theory (Bowen, 1978) as the underlying models to guide practice.

TIC

TIC has emerged as a leading guideline for those health care providers, including nurses, who care for and are affected by trauma in their clients. SAMHSA (2014) has been on the forefront identifying six key principles guiding TIC, including:

1. Safety
2. Trustworthiness and transparency
3. Peer support
4. Collaboration and mutuality
5. Empowerment and choice
6. Cultural, historical, and gender issues

Following a review of literature investigating interventions that worked with trauma survivors across traumatic experiences, Watkins et al. (2018) found across studies that outcomes were better when trauma-focused strategies were used over non-trauma-focused interventions. Investigators reviewed studies on the use of Prolonged Exposure Therapy (PET), Cognitive Behavioral Therapy (CBT), and Trauma-Focused CBT with comparisons to non-trauma-focused strategies including relaxation strategies, psychopharmacology, and non-trauma-focused support. Studies indicated success immediately following treatment and up to 10 years, using the following strategies:

1. Providing a safe strategy for reviewing the trauma, such as imaginal exposure, writing a narrative story, and/or reading the traumatic memory out loud.
2. Emotional reprocessing of the trauma that explores how the individual experiencing the trauma makes sense of what happened to him- or herself, to others involved, and to the individual's worldview.
   - The individual often assimilates the experience by trying to fit the traumatic

event into previous beliefs (i.e., "I should have been stronger and braver to prevent this from happening") or accommodates the experience into previous beliefs (i.e., "while I am usually a strong person, there is no way I could have overcome the attackers"), or overaccommodates the experience (i.e., "I can never trust going out alone again").

- The individual experiencing the trauma often makes errors in memory due to missing context (i.e., place, age, time), associative memory and strong perceptual priming, or reacting to perceptions from the trauma that occur in the present but trigger the past memory. This can be helped by using then-and-now exercises and helping the individual identify traumatic memories versus misinterpreted associations (i.e., if the trauma occurred in January, rhe individual might feel that January is a dangerous month).

3. Identifying dysfunctional thoughts and thinking errors and replacing them with alternative thoughts, especially reappraisal of self, the trauma, and the impact on current emotions (Watkins et al., 2018).

The TIC approach is consistent with the foundational principles of the nurse-client relationship, including patient safety, respect and compassion, and collaboration. By using these guiding principles, it is believed that victims of trauma who suffer from mental health issues, such as substance abuse, depression, anxiety, eating disorders, and social isolation, will be better served because there will be understanding of how the trauma has affected the trajectory of a person's life. By working with individuals, families, and communities that have experienced trauma, health care providers can build a more collaborative approach to care. Several evidence-based approaches to working with victims of trauma include strategies for individual therapy (e.g., Eye Movement Desensitization and Reprocessing [EMDR]) and group therapy (e.g., Trauma, Addiction, Mental Health, and Recovery [TAMAR]). Other approaches include changes to the treatment environment to prevent retraumatization, such as eliminating the use of restraints and isolation as punishments for individuals struggling with emotional dysregulation (Substance

Abuse and Mental Health Services Administration [SAMHSA], 2014). TIC is a shift away from pathology of trauma to recognition of the physical, relational, and emotional changes that occur in response to trauma. The questions for clients shift from "What is wrong with you?" to "What happened to you and how is it affecting your life?" (Evans & Coccoma, 2014; SAMHSA, 2014, 2015). TIC is also one of the few models that embraces working with survivors of trauma and their families (SAMHSA, 2014).

Bronfenbrenner's Ecological Systems Model

Bronfenbrenner (1996) identified four systems that interact together in the Ecological Systems Model: the *microsystem*, *mesosystem*, *macrosystem*, and *exosystem*. He later added the system of time, or the *chronosystem*, to describe the impact of history and time on individuals, families, communities, and societies. Time is integrated as a concept within each of the four other ecological systems. Understanding the impact of trauma on the micro- to exosystem levels helps health care providers and policy makers understand the interconnections of trauma and abuse with individuals, families, communities, and societies, and the impact of that trauma across time, generations, and geographical and cultural systems. Trauma tends to be repeated if nothing intervenes to stop the pattern. Interventions intended to stop and/or alter these patterns are much more effective when chosen and implemented with the complexity and interconnections between systems in mind. See Figure 12-1 for a visual portrayal of Bronfenbrenner's Ecological Systems Model.

Microsystem

The microsystem involves the individual and the systems within that individual, including physiological (i.e., respiratory, cardiovascular), developmental, and psychological (i.e., sensory perceptions, memory). The role of trauma in violating and damaging physical and mental well-being and negatively affecting development of children and adults is no longer questioned. The negative impact of trauma, particularly violence against children or witnessed by children, on children and adolescents ranges from interference with healthy development of attachment to physical and mental

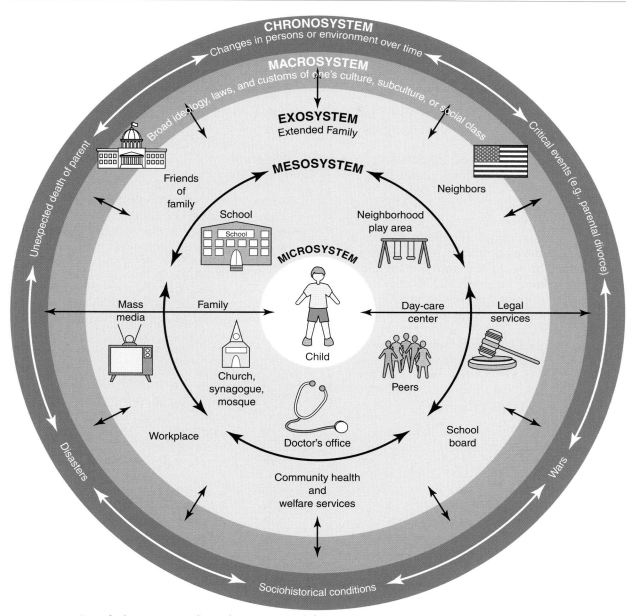

FIGURE 12-1 Bronfenbrenner's Ecological Systems Model

illness across the life span (Malti, 2020). Although understanding the impact of trauma on individuals is important to understanding family trauma, care of these individuals in isolation is less effective than providing care within the context of the family. The microsystem provides a beginning knowledge to family trauma, but the mesosystem adds a deeper understanding.

Mesosystem

The effect of trauma on any one individual within the family has a significant impact on family development and family functioning. The stress response from trauma is felt from experiencing, witnessing, or being informed about an act of violence against others. Younger children and those with intellectual disabilities who do not have the ability to process or understand the traumatic events are more vulnerable to developing problematic stress responses. This is also the case when the trauma is repeated and unpredictable (Maeng & Milad, 2017). This traumatic stress response is experienced by family members directly or witnessed by other family members, expanding the experience beyond the micro level to the meso level of reaction. For example, children's reactions to trauma and their resilience skills are shaped in part by family experiences and reactions as well as cultural experiences. The act of witnessing trauma includes direct observation as well as hearing about traumatic events repeatedly from family members. How family members react to a traumatic event has a direct impact on how other family members respond. For example, if parents cannot regulate their own reactions and cannot support the child because of their own physical, mental, or emotional difficulties, then their child is at higher risk for developing mood dysregulation and an inability to develop healthy attachments. If parents lack support and positive coping strategies, they are less likely to be able to provide support to their child.

Macrosystem

Trauma at the macro level includes all trauma within a community. This level of trauma not only influences individuals (micro) and families (meso) but also has an impact on how a community reacts and recovers from trauma. During the past two decades, the growing disparity between mental health and access to mental health services within a community has been well documented (Friedman, 2021). Traumatic events within schools, for example, have increased the awareness of the need for more in-depth and comprehensive mental health services to prevent these events and to be available to treat the victims and perpetrators (i.e., bullying) following these events. Schools have been identified as key community systems that can provide both prevention and treatment services. More than 60% of schools already attempt to address trauma at a community, or macrosystem, level through prevention services; community preparedness, such as town meetings and educational programs; provision of temporary food and shelter following a disaster; counseling services; and/or behavioral programs (Nealey-Oparah & Scruggs-Hussien, 2018). Using TIC when working with schools

experiencing trauma (e.g., school bullying, school shootings, or school suicides) improves outcomes, especially for traumatized youth (Nealey-Oparah & Scruggs-Hussien, 2018).

Exosystem

The exosystem includes the larger culture and government or laws and justice within a culture. The exosystem is touched by and touches on individuals, families, and communities. For example, the cultural reactions and legal responses to a natural disaster have grave implications for individuals, families, and communities. Consider the stress in many communities brought about by the wildfires on the West Coast of the United States during 2020, with over 8 million acres burned, including over 4 million acres in California. Many families who lost their homes relied on donations and federal aid programs to obtain emergency housing and financial support. While this aid was helpful, most families had to wait up to five months for their application for support to be approved. Additional complications arose due to the fires occurring in the midst of the COVID-19 pandemic, making congregate housing options too much of a risk. The need for rehousing, income recovery, and support for vulnerable populations lagged behind. In addition, many of the fires occurred in agricultural centers, leaving undocumented citizens without support (Center for Disaster Philanthropy, 2020). Researchers have explored the dysregulation and hyperarousal of individuals during crisis periods within American culture. For example, the accumulated stress experienced by many during the Great Recession of 2007–2009 resulted in a nation experiencing trauma. Judith Warner (2010), in a 2010 *New York Times* article, observed that the large-scale dysfunction of federal regulatory systems, including the banking meltdown, collapse of the housing market, and high unemployment rates, resulted in the United States—as a country—struggling with symptoms of PTSD for several years after the big financial bailout. The current COVID-19 pandemic has had a global impact, with loss of life, high rates of unemployment and business closures, and reactive demonstrations and divides across political and cultural lines as nations struggle with the trauma of a pandemic. Traumatic events, such as the pandemic, are situations that are different than our everyday experiences and they are out of our control, causing us to feel that our lives may be in danger (Brown, 2021).

The incidence of diagnosed PTSD for veterans has increased significantly during this time, from 0.7% of all military personnel diagnosed with PTSD in 2004 to 8% of all military personnel diagnosed with PTSD in 2012 (Institute of Medicine [IOM], 2014), and 11% to 20% of veterans serving in Iraq or Afghanistan currently suffering from PTSD (U. S. Department of Veterans Affairs, 2020a). Currently, it is estimated that 60% of men and 50% of women will experience at least one traumatic event in their lifetime, with men more likely to experience trauma through accidents, physical violence through combat or altercations, or witnessing violence or death, whereas women are more likely to experience trauma through sexual assault or child abuse. Of these individuals exposed to trauma, 10% of women and 4% of men will develop symptoms consistent with a diagnosis of PTSD (U.S. Department of Veterans Affairs, 2020a).

While abuse, assault, injury, and violence are commonly known triggers for PTSD, a growing body of literature is identifying medical illness as a risk factor for PTSD. For example, a meta-analysis of 38 articles investigating the incidence of PTSD in people living with HIV found that 28% of individuals met the criteria for PTSD (Tang et al., 2020). The risk of PTSD is being investigated for those surviving COVID-19 as well. Kaseda and Levine (2020) reviewed the risk of PTSD in those recovering from COVID-19, comparing their symptoms and incidence of PTSD with other, similar illnesses such as severe acute respiratory syndrome (SARS) and Middle East respiratory syndrome (MERS). Because of severe negative impacts of COVID-19, including near-death experiences from hypoxia, intubation, prolonged stays in the ICU with related risks of ICU psychosis, numerous and prolonged painful medical procedures, and the increased risk of PTSD with brain injuries, those surviving severe COVID-19 infection are at a higher risk for PTSD than the general public. The estimate is that up to 30% to 80% of individuals suffering from acute respiratory distress syndrome (ARDS) will have neurological and PTSD symptoms up to a year after recovery from COVID-19 (Kaseda & Levine, 2020).

Family Systems Theory

Family Systems Theory focuses on the interaction between family members and the impact of an individual's health and behavioral responses on other family members, as well as other family members' reactions and health impact on individuals. The metaphor of a wind chime is commonly used to describe Family Systems Theory, with one chime, or individual family member, being struck by other chimes, or other family members, to make music or cacophony. The wind flowing through the wind chimes represents the stressors that flow through every family. The wind can be a gentle breeze, or low stress level, or a high-speed wind, similar to high stress and less controlled stress levels. Family Systems Theory, when considered through an ecological lens, can help explain the impact of trauma within and surrounding families.

The remainder of this chapter examines the types of trauma that individuals, families, communities, and societies at large currently face, along with implications for nurses.

EARLY TRAUMA

Early trauma shapes early attachment, developmental progress, and early brain development, which can be understood through the lens of the Ecological Systems Model. By considering the individual's and family's experiences, nurses can better understand the progression of trauma and its impact on childhood development.

Attachment

Because early trauma has been shown to interfere with healthy development of attachment, attachment theories are used as a basis for research and understanding. Failure to develop healthy attachments during childhood is commonly linked to later issues with developmental growth and physical and mental well-being. Bowlby (1973), an early researcher and theorist in the area of attachment, identified the importance of early attachment for healthy development. During healthy attachment, infants learn to trust their caregiver and develop the ability to compartmentalize isolated threats or fears. When severe abuse or neglect occurs, infants learn to mistrust their caregivers and view the environment as unsafe and threatening. This process destroys the infants' ability to compartmentalize threats, leading to the inability to self-regulate emotions, behaviors, and physiological processes (i.e., sleep and elimination) (Breiner et al., 2016; Evans & Coccoma, 2014).

Developmental Trauma Theory

Heller and LaPierre (2015), in describing their Developmental Trauma Theory, categorized this early traumatic interference with attachment by describing five core areas of concern: (1) interference with connection to others, (2) lack of attunement or ability to recognize physical and emotional needs, (3) lack of trust in caregivers and the environment, (4) difficulty with boundaries between self and others, and (5) difficulty developing a sense of love and healthy sexuality. Table 12-1 describes the Neuroaffective Relational Model Five Core Needs developed by Heller and LaPierre (2015). More specific symptoms of failure to develop healthy attachments related to experiencing trauma include the following:

- *Absence of self-regulation:* inconsistent and unpredictable patterns of eating and sleeping, and mood regulation.
- *Lack of response to caregivers:* poor eye contact, lack of response to consoling measures, withdrawal, and isolation.
- *Lack of response to the environment:* inability to pretend-play, interact with toys, and/or experience shared pleasure with others (Heller & LaPierre, 2015).

If untreated, children experiencing trauma struggle in cognitive, emotional, and social development. The Developmental Trauma Theory proposed by Heller and LaPierre (2015) also describes the survival strategies that individuals (micro level) learn to cope with traumatic experiences, thereby expanding the understanding of the negative impact of trauma on attachment. These coping strategies interfere with healthy development. For example, whenever an individual experiences a severe threat, the sympathetic-adrenal-medullary (SAM) axis is triggered. This reaction is followed by a release of catecholamines, norepinephrine, and epinephrine, which in turn trigger the hypothalamic-pituitary-adrenal (HPA) axis. The hypothalamus in the brain works during this process to regulate heart rate, respiratory rate, and blood flow, and stimulates the amygdala to store the memory and the response for quick reaction to future threats. The adrenal gland then releases cortisol, the stress hormone, that eventually allows activation of the fear extinction process, or eventual recovery from the stress (Evans & Coccoma, 2014). When repeated trauma occurs, a state of constant fear develops, causing distinct physiological and psychological changes.

Research during the past 50 years has explored why prolonged or repeated trauma results in a different response in individuals compared with a typical stress response from isolated threats. Three areas of the brain have been identified as key factors in altering a healthy stress response to a trauma-related response that in turn causes chronic physical and mental disorders (Evans & Coccoma, 2014):

- *Amygdala:* With prolonged trauma, the amygdala becomes hyperactive, which interferes with the ability to process trauma memories appropriately and decreases the function of the prefrontal cortex, causing a decreased ability to think about the response to present traumas and problem-solve appropriate reactions.

Table 12-1	Neuroaffective Relational Model Five Core Needs
CORE NEED	**DESCRIPTION**
Connection	Lack of ability to form healthy connection with caregivers or significant support people
Attunement	Lack of ability to recognize physical and emotional needs
Trust	Lack of ability to trust others
Boundaries	Difficulty setting healthy boundaries
Deep sense of love and sexuality	Inability to form deep loving relationships and, as adults, to connect deep love with healthy sexuality

Source: Heller and LaPierre (2015).

- *Hippocampus:* The hippocampus is responsible for changing explicit memories, or new memories, into implicit memories, or patterns (i.e., driving a car, riding a bike, or skiing change from an awkward new skill to an automatic skill that takes little conscious thought). Severe or prolonged trauma interferes with this process, resulting in feelings of inadequacy and doubt. The hippocampus is also responsible for differentiating past experiences from present experiences. With severe and prolonged trauma, this ability to differentiate is damaged, causing an individual to respond to a memory, or a similar sensory trigger (e.g., vision or sound), as if the trauma were repeating itself in the present. Finally, the hippocampus is responsible for repeated memories retrieved for a variety of cognitive, physical, and emotional functions. In the context of severe and repeated trauma, however, this process results in intrusive memories interfering with function.
- *Prefrontal cortex:* This part of the brain is responsible for cognitive processing of traumatic memories. Without prefrontal cortex functioning, *fear extinction*, or the resolution of the SAM axis response, cannot occur. With hyperactivity in the amygdala, the prefrontal cortex cannot be fully functional, resulting in unresolved traumatic memories.

These three areas, when affected by severe and repeated trauma, have an impact on an individual's ability to process, store, and appropriately retrieve memories. In turn, the neurological system alerts the brain to stay in survival mode. Because this system is activated continuously when repeated trauma occurs, the individual's ability to feel safe is threatened, resulting in a state of constant hyperarousal. This constant state of arousal causes an individual to become overwhelmed, leading to an abrupt shift to the parasympathetic system, and the individual shuts down, withdraws, becomes numb, disassociates, or falls into sleep. Sleep, eating, and digestive patterns are affected, and excitable behavior builds again with the next remembered or experienced trauma. Emotions range from the hyperstimulated, such as demonstrating hysteria or excessive, inconsolable crying, to numbness or demonstrating no reaction at all to the environment. Without resolution, the individual develops a state of fear and gradually loses the ability to regulate emotional and autonomic reactions. If these processes are uninterrupted, the young child develops secondary complications, including anxiety, shame, isolation, mood dysregulation, and uncontrolled anger or explosive outbursts (Evans & Coccoma, 2014).

As children develop into adulthood, they may try to adapt to those feelings by abusing substances or avoiding emotions (Evans & Coccoma, 2014; Heller & LaPierre, 2015). The underlying fear remains; the threat to self and to the ability to survive is not over. Symptoms emerge over time, including the following (Heller & LaPierre, 2015):

- Lack of affect
- Feelings of shame
- Separation from others
- Avoidance of emotionally disturbing situations or people
- Overintellectualizing and avoiding emotions
- Lack of attunement or awareness of bodily and related needs
- Fear of being alone while at the same time feeling overwhelmed by others
- Fear of death and illness
- Fear of their own anger
- Fear of intimacy
- Strong need to control
- Desire for altered states and disassociation
- Cognitive impairments, including difficulty with auditory processing, memory, and attention
- Feelings of helplessness
- Hypo- or hypervigilance

Physical symptoms of prolonged and repeated trauma in childhood may include the following:

- Disrupted sleep
- Eating disorders
- Panic disorders
- Obsessive-compulsive disorders
- Rage
- Depression
- Addiction
- Cardiovascular disorders
- Autoimmune disorders

A pattern emerges across time. Figure 12-2 illustrates the developmental pattern of maladaptation to early trauma.

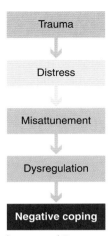

FIGURE 12-2 Developmental Pattern of Maladaptation to Early Trauma

Environmental Trauma

Studies on the impact of war, terror, and unexpected natural disasters on children have resulted in the identification of the term *disaster syndrome.* Adams et al. (2009) and Smith (2013) described this syndrome as a combination of symptoms of PTSD, including anxiety, dissociation, and depression. The loss of personal connections, support, routines, and assumptions regarding safety and regularity, as well as parental response, all affect the severity of a child's response. Parental response is influenced by parents' prior diagnosis of mental illness, prior coping strategies, and number of past traumatic experiences. Children respond to their family members' emotional and physical changes related to trauma. When an individual (micro level) experiences trauma over time, her or his interaction with others (meso level) and her or his ability to interact in a functional manner with the surrounding community (macro level) are altered. One distinct difference between children and adults experiencing trauma through environmental events is that adults tend to have less PTSD because of the support of the community and decreased feelings of isolation; children feel more isolated during these events because of profound fear of losing their supportive loved ones (Evans & Coccoma, 2014).

The human desire for regulation of the autonomic nervous system, with a return to balance, is strong. Individuals are highly motivated to find this balance and will pursue strategies to achieve this goal through either positive measures

(e.g., healthy patterns of sleep, eating, exercise, meditation, yoga, and spiritual connection) or negative measures (e.g., drug-seeking behavior, obsessive thinking patterns, or avoidance patterns) (Evans & Coccoma, 2014). These negative patterns interfere with every stage of development, primarily altering cognitive, emotional, communication, and social domains. Although young infants cannot consciously think about their reactions to trauma, their emotions and related autonomic reactions are affected in a measurable way (Evans & Coccoma, 2014; Heller & LaPierre, 2015). Infants have bottom-up responses, or responses starting with brainstem or autonomic reactions to external threat, moving up toward emotional responses. Adults, in contrast, experience trauma initially from thought, or the cortex of the brain, and move down to emotional response and finally to autonomic or brainstem reaction, what is considered a top-down reaction. Another important difference between infants and adults is that infants tend to have a broad interpretation of experiences, whereas adults are able to separate experiences and feelings between experiences. The difference in reaction is caused by the difference in development of pathways from the frontal cortex to the brainstem as the brain develops across time. The pathways are reinforced by experiences and interactions in the environment (Heller & LaPierre, 2015). Figure 12-3 illustrates bottom-up and top-down responses to trauma.

This variance in response to trauma is important to understand. Adults who experience trauma can make a distinction between different experiences in their lives and therefore *feel* badly about a specific experience. Infants and young children cannot differentiate between experiences; therefore, when they experience trauma, they tend to think *they* are bad (Heller & LaPierre, 2015). Young children and adults, however, if left untreated following a trauma, can regress back to thinking and feeling they are bad as a global response to trauma.

Early Trauma and Brain Development

The understanding of the impact of early trauma on brain development has led to detailed study of the impact on brain development and plasticity, or the ability of the brain to recover from injury. When considering trauma or major stress, the body is governed by two main systems: the

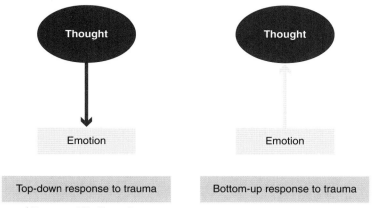

FIGURE 12-3 Top-Down and Bottom-Up Reaction

neurological system and the endocrine system. These two systems ensure survival of the individual through stimulation of the sympathetic nervous system when the individual is threatened, and the parasympathetic nervous system when the individual is safe and relaxed. Hans Selye (1976), a renowned theorist on stress, identified the connection between the hypothalamus, the pituitary gland, and the adrenal glands, now commonly referred to as the HPA axis. To summarize this process, the hypothalamus links the nervous system to the pituitary system, which secretes hormones that regulate homeostasis. If homeostasis is not reached, the adrenal glands secrete the stress hormones epinephrine and norepinephrine. These hormones stimulate the sympathetic nervous system, and the result is increased heart rate, dilation of pupils, relaxation of bronchial tubes, increased blood flow to large muscles that can cause blood pressure to rise, and initial stimulation of the prefrontal cortex through a surge of dopamine, followed by bypassing the prefrontal cortex to the amygdala.

This bypass process encourages rapid action based on the previous experience of threats and on the assumption that the same threat has occurred and the same action for survival is needed. When this process is stimulated repeatedly and without resolution, the connection between the limbic system (where automatic actions based on emotions and repeated actions rather than thought occur) and the cortex (or the thinking part of the brain that includes judgment, creativity, and prediction of action on future consequences) is pruned (i.e., cut). When the connection is pruned, sensory perception becomes scattered and disorganized.

By bypassing the prefrontal cortex, the individual exchanges accuracy, judgment, and the ability to learn for speed. The bypassed prefrontal cortex provides the individual with the executive functions of detailed assessment, regulation of emotion or thought, inhibition of inappropriate responses, expressive speech, and problem-solving skills. Over time, an individual constantly facing threat through trauma develops a fearful identity, avoids relationships because of previous threats, has uncontrolled emotional outbursts or withdrawal, disassociates from the present, and/or experiences depression.

The hippocampus, which is key in neuroplasticity or the ability to generate new neurons and new neuron pathways (known as neurogenesis), is impaired. This process explains why many who experience prolonged and repeated trauma struggle with cognitive impairments, such as poor short-term memory; difficulty concentrating; difficulty learning new skills; and poor sensory integration, especially auditory processing (Maeng & Milad, 2017). This process has been found to be more severe in both children and adults experiencing relational trauma, or trauma inflicted by people in a position of trust (meso level), than in those experiencing trauma from inanimate objects (e.g., motor vehicle accidents) or environmental trauma (i.e., natural disasters) (Evans & Coccoma, 2014). This process is most damaging when the trauma experienced occurs early in life and continues throughout childhood, causing initial and prolonged damage to normal brain development (Evans & Coccoma, 2014). For family nurses, it is important to assess the start and duration of any family trauma occurring to a child or young adult.

Early Childhood Trauma

The impact of early trauma and the negative long-term outcomes has led to further study of the effect of childhood trauma on health and well-being later in life. The Centers for Disease Control and Prevention (CDC)–Kaiser Adverse Childhood Experiences (ACE) Study, conducted from 1995 to 1997, was one of the largest studies on childhood adversity and later life health. The study was conducted by surveying over 17,000 health maintenance organization (HMO) members from Southern California about their childhood experiences, and adult physical and mental health variables (CDC, 2020a). The results revealed a relationship between the number of adverse childhood experiences, such as childhood abuse and household dysfunction, and the number of comorbid outcomes, including adulthood depression and mental health disorders, substance abuse, high-risk behaviors, and domestic violence (CDC, 2020a). The findings of the CDC–Kaiser study led to a more in-depth understanding of the cumulative effect of repeated traumas experienced during childhood and the effect on brain development. More recent studies have identified that long-term effects are associated with the occurrence of one or more chronic illnesses in adults. Figure 12-4 illustrates the relationship between the occurrence of adverse childhood experiences and the diagnosis of comorbid conditions such as coronary artery disease, stroke, asthma, chronic obstructive pulmonary disease (COPD), cancer, kidney disease, diabetes, and depression.

During the 2015–2017 collection of the Behavioral Risk Factor Surveillance System (BRFSS) survey conducted annually, data from participants from 25 states were analyzed that answered additional questions to assess exposure to eight types of adverse childhood experiences: abuse (physical, emotional, and sexual) and household challenges (substance misuse, incarceration, mental illness, parental divorce, or witnessing intimate partner violence) before the age of 18 years old (Merrick et al., 2019). Respondents were classified into categories based on the number of adverse childhood experiences reported: zero, one, two, three, and four or more. Of 144,017 participants, nearly 16% of adults reported four or more types of adverse childhood experiences that were significantly associated with poorer health outcomes, health risk behaviors, and socioeconomic challenges (Merrick et al., 2019). Females and members of racially diverse and underrepresented groups were at greater risk for experiencing four or more adverse childhood experiences (CDC, 2020a). Preventing adverse childhood experiences could reduce health conditions significantly, including up to 21 million cases of depression, up to 1.9 million cases of heart disease, and up to 2.5 million cases of overweight and obesity (Merrick et al., 2019). Ultimately, raising awareness of about the causes of childhood adversity and promoting strategies that prevent them can lead to better health and social outcomes:

1. Shift the focus from individual responsibility to community solutions.
2. Reduce the stigma of needing help for parenting skills, substance misuse, depression, and suicidal ideation.
3. Promote safe, stable, nurturing relationships and environments where children live, learn, and play.
4. Adopt evidence-based strategies to strengthen economic support for families.
5. Provide support for quality care and education in early childhood.
6. Enhance connections to caring adults, and support emotion and conflict management among parents and youth.

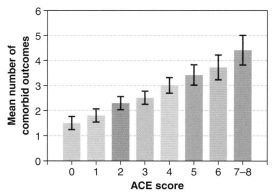

FIGURE 12-4 Relationship Between Adverse Childhood Experiences and Comorbid Conditions. Adverse childhood experiences include verbal, physical, or sexual abuse, as well as family dysfunction (e.g., an incarcerated, mentally ill, or substance-abusing family member; domestic violence; or absence of a parent because of divorce or separation) *Source: Anda et al., 2006.*

7. Develop partnerships in the community that support programs and policies that provide safe and healthy conditions for all children and families.
8. Intervene with support to reduce harm, mitigate risks, and prevent child maltreatment. (CDC, 2020a; Sulaski Wyckoff, 2019)

Clearly, understanding the effects of early childhood adversity and trauma helps health care providers address the long-term health effects on adults. Studies have found that resilience is one factor that determines which adults continue to suffer from childhood trauma versus those who overcome traumatic experiences. One factor affecting the complexity of childhood trauma includes continued reexposure in adults, such as in the experience of intimate partner violence and adult sexual assault, which is more common in women. A case study describing the harrowing events of domestic violence and rape from one woman's point of view brings this pattern to life (Barnes, 2018). A woman named Sophia was repeatedly beaten, raped, and strangled by her boyfriend before she fled for her life. Her recovery was slow because she was easily reminded of her trauma every autumn, with a reminder of what cold air felt like on her bruises, certain sounds, and certain smells that were present during the abuse. Through a combined therapy approach that was trauma-focused and supportive, she was slowly able to reclaim her life.

Resilience

Through the improved understanding of childhood trauma and related reactions, the concept of resilience, or why some who experience the same or similar events adapt without any measure of physical or emotional damage or even report growth, is more fully understood. APA (2014, para. 4) defines resilience as "the process of adapting well in the face of adversity, trauma, tragedy, threats, or even significant sources of stress." A more thorough consideration of biological, psychological, social, and cultural factors is also important to understanding how resilience is determined or revealed in an individual (Southwick et al., 2014). As resilience continues to be studied, multiple definitions make sense. Dr. George Bonanno asserted that resilience is "a stable trajectory of healthy function" (Southwick et al., 2014, p. 6). Others have identified it as a more multidimensional construct called

holistic wellness (Strout et al., 2016). Resilience is associated with a variety of health and social outcomes, including:

- Healthy coping mechanisms
- Optimism and a positive attitude
- Positive self-esteem and a strong sense of self
- Supportive family and peer relationships
- Social connectedness and engagement
- Success with hobbies, school, work
- Competent, positive parenting
- Moderate, well-balanced temperament
- Compassion, gratitude
- Trusting others to help
- Recognizing meaning and purpose in life
- Strong self-efficacy and determination (Gartland, 2019)

The Holistic Wellness Model integrates characteristics from biological, psychological, and social aspects of development across the life span. Qualities added to the above list, using the Holistic Wellness Model, include being realistic and being adaptable to change, in addition to physiological attributes such as being free of chronic conditions, genetic longevity, functional health, and independent skills.

Research on resilience continues as an important shift from focusing on the negative outcomes of adversity to instead focusing on those individuals who do not show any negative outcomes after facing adversity. The many examples of adverse events studied range from parental mental illness and abuse; low socioeconomic status; chronic and life-threatening illnesses; natural and human-made disasters; loss and grief; discrimination; and chronic, repeated, and/or prolonged stress. Past studies have defined resilience as a dynamic process that changes across developmental stages, personalities, and qualities of the adverse event(s) (Karaırmak & Figley, 2017). Karaırmak and Figley studied 300 undergraduate students enrolled in social work courses to investigate whether personality proved more influential in identifying those with stronger resilience traits compared to other characteristics, including gender, ethnicity, and the number or severity of past adverse events. Their findings indicated that there were no differences in resilience based on gender or the number of negative life events. African American students were more positive than White American students. The authors stated that although this study should be replicated across other groups, positive traits (e.g., optimism and adaptability) in an individual's personality seemed to be a very important factor in predicting resilience. Looking at resilience from a different angle, Deblinger et al. (2014) studied 250 youth in an inpatient treatment program for children who had experienced sexual and physical abuse. They confirmed that those individuals with the highest vulnerability scores and the lowest resilience scores had the highest scores for depression. Resilience traits, therefore, should be assessed by family nurses to determine the traits that were present before the trauma and reinforced versus those that are lacking and should be taught and supported. Resilience can buffer the negative impacts of trauma on the individual's brain development.

Recent studies have shifted from individual traits of resilience to family traits of resilience, recognizing that close family support has a significant influence on both the genetic influence on resilience as well as the environmental influence on learning and using resilience traits (Walsh, 2016). This emphasizes the strength of using Bronfenbrenner's Ecological Systems Model when assessing and treating not only trauma but also family resilience.

Resilience has moved beyond just preventing negative outcomes following a traumatic event to understanding why some individuals and families report growth or positive meaning after a traumatic event or events. This phenomenon was first described by Antonovsky (1987) following his research on Holocaust survivors. He identified three characteristics of those who were healthy following prolonged trauma:

1. Finding solutions to problems (engaging cognitive functioning in the prefrontal cortex)
2. Identifying supportive resources
3. Identifying capacity (engaging motivation)

Later research by Antonovsky (1993) included the development of the Sense of Coherence Scale, which has been translated into several languages and is now commonly used to assess survivors of trauma. This scale measures well-being or health following trauma rather than pathology. Shakespeare-Finch and Armstrong (2010) used this research to guide research on post-traumatic growth (PTG). They studied survivors of motor vehicle accidents, bereavement, and sexual assault and found that those sexually assaulted had the lowest scores for PTG compared with the other two groups. They proposed that personal trauma, such as sexual assault, is experienced in isolation and surrounded by shame, whereas other types of trauma are often accompanied by societal support and are without social stigma. Others have confirmed this idea, with sexual assault across the life span having higher levels of PTSD when compared with natural disasters, accidents, or other types of physical abuse (Evans & Coccoma, 2014).

Resilience in war victims offers further understanding into who will develop PTSD versus who will not. Studies have shown that women and children, and those vulnerable within a population, often suffer more in a war than soldiers. Evans and Coccoma (2014), after their review of the literature, felt that part of this pattern is the increased isolation and lack of support for women and children; also part of this pattern is the praise and acknowledgment of soldiers, with honorary rituals for their service, while women and children remain silent and anonymous victims. Children respond differently than women, and up to 90% of children experience some type of trauma in their lives (Horner, 2015). The degree to which children survive trauma without negative consequences depends on the nature of the threat, their stage of development and degree of cognitive awareness of the event, previous trauma experience, cultural beliefs, the quality of support, the proximity to the event, healthy self-esteem, increased cognitive ability, and developing locus of control (Evans & Coccoma, 2014; Horner, 2015).

These studies help nurses realize the importance of making sure that trauma survivors are not left alone and isolated but rather supported and respected and that care is developmentally appropriate. Following a review of four decades of research on resilience, Horner (2015) concluded that nurses can intervene to build resilience by encouraging supportive relationships between parent and child; anticipatory guidance for parents to prevent trauma, including positive parenting skills; referral to evidence-based therapies, including trauma-focused psychotherapy or EMDR; and team efforts to prevent future traumatization, such as referral and support of violence prevention programs.

FAMILY TRAUMA

Families experience trauma as a family, and family members experience it individually. This section discusses both (1) family trauma through disasters and war and (2) individual experiences of trauma and their effect on family members. Each member of the family experiences trauma differently, with different symptoms, reactions, and needs for recovery. For example, both parents and children experience similar symptoms of PTSD, but adults are more likely to reexperience the event through nightmares and flashbacks, whereas children are more likely to avoid similar experiences (e.g., avoiding riding in a car after a car accident) or avoid talking about the event. Both children and adults experience hyperarousal, or the HPA axis response to stress (Evans & Coccoma, 2014; Heller & LaPierre, 2015). When this occurs, parenting often becomes overwhelming because children overreact to environmental stimuli and parents overreact to the stressors of parenting. Each family member in turn can easily be misdiagnosed as depressed, anxious, or having attention deficit-hyperactivity disorder (ADHD), and the opportunity for effective and comprehensive treatment is therefore lost. The National Center for PTSD (2016) has identified 10 key areas that affect family functioning when one or more members are diagnosed with PTSD:

1. Increased sympathy by family members, which may provide support for the family member with PTSD or prolong feelings of victimization.
2. Increased negative feelings about the person with PTSD. These feelings are often triggered by changes in the person with PTSD, including changes in mood regulation, depression, and explosive outbursts. The person is no longer the same as the person they knew before.
3. Avoidance is a common reaction by individuals with PTSD and by family members. Family members often circumvent talking about anything related to the trauma and may dodge other topics hoping to avoid angry outbursts. Individuals with PTSD tend to avoid social situations because of fear of not fitting in or being questioned about the trauma. This in turn leads to social isolation of all family members as they try to support the individual with PTSD.
4. Depression is common among individuals with PTSD and their family members. The longer the symptoms of PTSD last, the more likely family members may lose hope that their family member will ever get back to normal.
5. Anger is common among family members as they struggle to cope with changes in the person with PTSD and with expectations not being met.
6. Guilt and shame are common for family members because they feel helpless to change negative family functioning and find themselves feeling angry about the individual's illness.
7. Health problems increase in individuals with PTSD and their family members, including substance abuse; reduction in healthy immune response; and negative effects of poor eating habits, poor sleep, smoking, and lack of healthy exercise.
8. Fear and worry develop as the worldview of the person suffering from PTSD changes given the intimate knowledge that terrible things can happen. Family members may also worry about symptoms of anger and unpredictable behavior that is manifested by the person experiencing PTSD.
9. Drug and alcohol abuse occur as a way to escape negative feelings.
10. Sleep problems develop, especially for the trauma survivor.

These outcomes can leave parents feeling inadequate and spouses feeling angry, guilty, and disillusioned. Nurses are often at the forefront of trauma care because they encounter family members during traumatic events such as war, natural disasters, family violence and abuse, severe illness, and unanticipated accidents. The nurses' role with families facing PTSD in a loved one include education of the outcomes of PTSD, support for all family members, advocacy for families, and referral for appropriate counseling and support resources for both the individual experiencing PTSD and the family members.

Families Affected by War

Since the turn of the century, the nature of war has changed dramatically. Warfare in the 21st century rarely involves confrontations between professional armies. Instead, wars typically are fought as grinding struggles between military personnel and civilians, or groups of armed civilians in a city environment rather than in distant battlefields. Thus, civilian fatalities from battles fought in towns and cities have increased in the 21st century. The effects on children are devastating. Worldwide, approximately 31 million children had been forcibly displaced by the end of 2018, including 13 million child refugees, 1 million asylum-seeking children, and an estimated 17 million children displaced within their own countries due to violence and conflict (UNICEF, 2021). In 2018, the government of Uganda published results from the 2016–2017 National Labour Force Survey, which estimated that 2,057,000 children were in child labor that included gold mining, fishing, agriculture, and more. The government indicated that this was a low estimate because those involved in the worst forms of child labor, such as child sex trafficking and those required to serve as soldiers, are not included (Bureau of International Labor Affairs, 2018). In the United States, the impact of war on families, other than for refugees, is limited to wartime separation and reunion.

In 2017, the suicide rate for veterans was 1.5 times the rate for nonveteran adults, and a total of 919 suicides occurred among never federally activated former National Guard and Reserve members (U.S. Department of Veteran Affairs, 2019). Firearms were the method of suicide in 70.7% of male veteran suicide deaths and 43.2% of female veteran suicide deaths in 2017 (U.S. Department of Veteran Affairs, 2019). The risk for female veteran suicide is 2.5 times higher when compared to U.S nonveteran women (Office of Public and Intergovernmental Affairs, 2017).

During Operation Iraqi Freedom, thousands of family members were deployed. This war brought to light the effects of the trauma of war on families. This war resulted in 6,364 fatalities and 48,296 wounded U.S. troops. Two million children were affected by separation from parents, changes in health status of parents, and/or loss of parents because of this war. Forty-four percent of these children were under 6 years of age, and thus they were particularly prone to the effects of trauma from coexperiencing family trauma (Smith, 2013). As evidence of the difficulty these families face, the telephone calls to the 24-hour helpline Military OneSource, which provides counseling to veterans

and their families, numbered more than 100,000 in the first 10 months of 2005; the calls increased by 20% in 2006. More than 200,000 antidepressant prescriptions were written for military families and service members during a 14-month period in 2005 to 2006. In addition, unidentified and untreated PTSD presented special risks for family reintegration and put the veterans and their families at higher danger for maladaptive responses to stress, such as alcoholism, depression, and family violence (U.S. Department of Veteran Affairs, 2018). Most soldiers have transient symptoms of stress following a traumatic event. These symptoms resolve for most when stability and routine are restored. This is the same pattern for children. But the risk for trauma-related symptoms in children from their parents' traumatic experiences increases with prolonged separation from parent(s) and decreased time between recovery from one traumatic event to onset of another (i.e., repeated deployment, or repeated terror associated with war) (Foran et al., 2017). Because of the increased understanding of the risk of trauma to family members, the military has funded numerous studies to identify effective strategies to prevent PTSD in soldiers and their family members. One program, entitled Building Resilience And Valuing Empowered Families (BRAVE Families), employs strategies used for families experiencing effects from urban violence, Hurricane Katrina, and the 9/11 terrorist attacks. These strategies include individual and family education and support about PTSD, art and play therapy for children, parenting guidance, and group therapy and support (Smith, 2013). The goal of programs designed to reach PTSD at the meso level is to reach more families experiencing trauma early rather than waiting for families to experience pathology first.

Family Violence and Trauma

Family violence is generally divided into three categories: physical violence, emotional violence, and sexual abuse. The cause of family violence is well studied and is considered multifaceted, with influences ranging from multigenerational trauma, social and cultural learning, and parental mental disorders (Lunnemann et al., 2019). Lunnemann and colleagues studied 101 fathers, 360 mothers, and 426 children (mean age of 7 years) to determine if a history of child abuse and neglect and current symptoms of PTSD are mediated by intimate partner violence in mothers and if children's PTSD symptoms are mediated by mother's or father's trauma symptoms. Their findings indicated that fathers and mothers who experienced child abuse or neglect during their childhood were related to adult trauma symptoms and increased the risk of PTSD in their children. This was mediated by mothers' intimate partner violence, indicating that mothers who had a history of child abuse and/or neglect and were victims of intimate partner violence were more likely to have trauma symptoms than those without intimate partner violence.

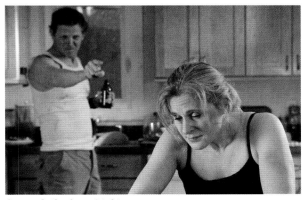

Source: © iStock.com/ejwhite

Domestic violence not only increases the risk for PTSD, it is also a cause of PTSD for both the victims and witnesses of the violence. The incidence of witnessing domestic violence by children and related trauma continues to be a major public health problem. Approximately 45 million children will be exposed to violence, at least one violent event, during their childhood, which is approximately 10% of all children annually (Huecker et al., 2021). These children have a higher risk for repeating violence toward their partners as adults, and they are at higher risk for becoming a victim to intimate partner violence. For example, if a young boy sees his mother abused by her partner, he is ten times more likely to abuse his partner as an adult (Office of Women's Health, 2019).

The experience of trauma, especially repeated traumas, increases the risk of long-term negative outcomes for children and adults. Each family member exposed to abuse; neglect; and major transitions and loss, such as divorce, is at risk for PTSD, as well as continuing the cycle of violence within

families, with repeated events increasing that risk (McLaughlin et al., 2017). As noted earlier, family resilience traits can alter these outcomes significantly, with the result that, for most individuals who experience negative and traumatic events and have strong personal and family resilience traits, these individuals and families do not develop negative health outcomes or repeat the family pattern of PTSD (Walsh, 2016). These findings clearly support the need for trauma-focused family care and interventions by nurses and other health care providers to prevent family-centered trauma.

Families Affected by Disasters

Disasters are events that cause widespread destruction of property, dislocation of people, and immediate suffering through death or injury. Disasters interrupt basic daily needs, such as obtaining food and shelter, for an extended period, making recovery difficult.

Natural disasters kill an average of 60,000 people per year around the world. The deadliest natural disasters over the past century have been earthquakes. Yet the death rate from earthquakes has dropped from a high of 276,974 deaths in 1976 to 4,321 in 2018. Disaster deaths disproportionately affect the poor, with low- to middle-income countries faring the worst. This is largely due to poor infrastructure that does not protect populations from natural disasters, in contrast with earthquake-proof buildings, which do protect. Protection from floods, with better water control mechanisms, has greatly reduced the number of deaths from floods, from a high of 3.7 million in 1931 to 2,869 in 2018 (Ritchie & Roser, 2019).

Disasters are classified as either natural or humanmade. Natural disasters include weather and seismic events such as floods, hurricanes, and earthquakes. Humanmade disasters include events such as fires, building collapse, explosions, acts of terrorism, and war.

Natural disasters are the most frequently occurring type of disaster. In the last 10 years, the International Red Cross reported that 1.1 million people around the world were killed by natural disasters (e.g., hurricanes, tornadoes, earthquakes, storms, tsunamis, and volcanic eruptions) (International Federation of Red Cross and Red Crescent Societies, 2016). An additional 100,000 people were killed worldwide from technological disasters, ranging from industrial accidents to transportation accidents (International Federation of Red Cross and Red Crescent Societies, 2016).

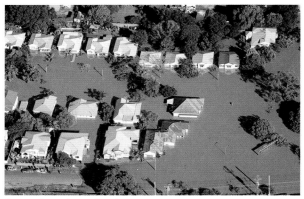

Source: © istock.com/On-Air

Regardless of the type of event, families are affected in multiple ways when disasters strike. Some of the many stressors that occur include loss of significant others, injuries to self or family members, separation from family, or extensive loss of property. These losses result in heightened feelings of stress, with many families experiencing symptoms of PTSD. The most vulnerable suffer the most. For example, children often display sleep disturbances, depression, and anxiety, with symptoms increasing the closer the child is to the disaster and the greater the perceived threat to self and loved ones (Evans & Coccoma, 2014).

Family Functioning and PTSD

Trauma-related reactions have a negative impact on family functioning. Studies conducted among combat veterans, including those who served in the Vietnam War, showed that PTSD symptoms are associated with poor family and couple functioning, problems with marital adjustment, and emotional strain on relationship partners (Campbell & Renshaw, 2018; Yambo & Johnson, 2014). Relationship strain was identified in the spousal relationships of first responders of the 9/11 terrorist attacks. In a sample of 49 first responders working after the attacks, 34.4% disclosed a PTSD diagnosis, and another 22.7% mentioned experiencing at least one trauma symptom (Hammock et al., 2019). As partners of responders found themselves actively managing the trauma-related symptoms (e.g., anger, guilt, feelings of isolation)

on their own, the strain became too much to handle and they began to seek help, even years after the symptoms started (Hammock et al., 2019). In a review of literature related to family relationships and PTSD, Blow et al. (2015) reported a similar pattern for veterans returning from Iraq and Afghanistan, with the added negative effects of traumatic brain injuries and multiple deployments. The PTSD symptoms of avoidance and emotional numbing have deleterious effects on parent-child relationships (National Institute on Mental Health, 2020). Among Iraq and Afghanistan veterans, trauma symptoms such as sleep problems, dissociation, and severe sexual problems predicted lower marital satisfaction for both the veteran and his or her partner (Blow et al., 2015). When looking at other causes of trauma in parents, the relationship between parental PTSD and child outcomes continues to be explored. Samuelson et al. (2017) studied 52 low-income mothers living in an urban setting who had experienced repeated traumas, including community violence, intimate partner violence, and childhood sexual abuse. The severity and number of traumas, parenting stress, childhood trauma, and observation of parenting skills were evaluated by looking at the direct and indirect influence of parental PTSD and stress on children's outcomes. The results indicated that these mothers perceived their parenting skills as negative, but they were more engaged and responsive than perceived. The biggest threat to children's emotional and behavioral regulation was the combination of parental PTSD mediated by high levels of parental stress. These findings indicate the importance of supporting mothers who have experienced trauma to decrease future exposure and decrease ongoing stress in order to improve children's health outcomes.

Gewirtz and colleagues (2019) found that deployment to war continues to disrupt children due to their parents' dysregulated emotions and the impact of this on parenting skills. They studied 181 fathers who had returned from deployment from Iraq or Afghanistan and had a child between the ages of 3 and 14 years. After enrolling fathers in a parenting program designed to help with emotional regulation and comparing them to a control group of fathers, they found that emotional regulation improved with the intervention over 24 months (Gewirtz et al., 2019). Their study and review of the literature amplifies the importance of continued attention to supporting parents after deployment in order to decrease the negative impact of emotional dysregulation on parenting.

Secondary Traumatization

The impact of trauma is not limited to the traumatized persons themselves. Spouses of the injured persons seem particularly susceptible to a phenomenon called *secondary traumatization* (Bachem et al., 2018). Secondary traumatization as a clinical finding has received only limited research and is not yet a separate diagnostic category in the *DSM-5* (APA, 2013). Rather, secondary PTSD is included under both PTSD and acute stress disorder and is described as learning that a traumatic event occurred to a close family member or experiencing extreme details of a traumatic event (e.g., professionals hearing of child abuse). The Cognitive-Behavioral Interpersonal Theory of PTSD (Monson et al., 2010) has helped describe the relationship between PTSD and relationship difficulties with family members, including cognitive and behavioral changes that occur as family members avoid communication about traumatic events and the resultant change in communication and behavior, which in turn leads to decreased ability to support the traumatized parent, problem-solve challenges, and model resilience characteristics. Using this model, Bachem et al. (2018) studied 123 veterans and their spouses and offspring from the 1973 Yom Kippur War. The results of this study indicated that veterans who experienced the most severe trauma tended to talk less about their trauma and had poorer relationship quality with their spouses. The spouses also developed symptoms of PTSD, and the spouse's stress response had a negative effect on the children's stress level. Another study using this same data from the longitudinal study on the psychological implications of war among veterans from the 1973 Yom Kipper War and their spouses was completed by Lahav and Solomon (2018). This study found that the more severe the PTSD symptoms in the veteran, the higher the risk of PTSD symptoms in their spouses and the higher the incidence of intimate partner violence. This pattern showed a dual risk for partners of veterans with PTSD, including both secondary trauma and exposure to firsthand trauma through intimate partner violence. Both of these studies further support the importance of using the Family Systems Model when caring for individuals experiencing trauma.

This pattern is not limited to family members caring for veterans with PTSD. Other studies have looked at nonfamily members, including health care professionals. Researchers have attempted to define this phenomenon, using terms such as *compassion fatigue, professional burnout, secondary traumatic stress,* and *vicarious trauma* (Meadors et al., 2009; Newell & MacNeil, 2010; Taylor et al., 2016). Each definition describes the psychological and physical response to the experience of caring for victims but not directly experiencing trauma or being exposed to traumatic events from others. More recently, the term *secondary traumatic stress* (STS) has been used to define trauma experienced by health care workers who are repeatedly exposed to their patients' trauma (Roden-Foreman et al., 2017). In their review of literature on STS, Roden-Foreman and colleagues identified risk factors for those helping professionals who develop STS response, including working against natural circadian rhythms (i.e., working the night shift), having high patient-provider ratios, and having limited resources while making critical decisions. Of note is that up to 33% of emergency room nurses showed symptoms consistent with a diagnosis of STS. Based on this review, Roden-Foreman and colleagues studied 118 emergency room providers working in several trauma centers and found that 12.7% had symptoms consistent with a diagnosis of STS (APA, 2013). Participants with high resilience scores were less likely to have symptoms of STS. The results did not vary by gender, time spent with traumatized patients, or neurotic personality traits. While their percentage was lower than previous studies, the authors offered an explanation that those working in trauma centers may represent professionals who have developed more resilience skills compared to those choosing other career paths.

The recent COVID-19 pandemic has placed added pressure on all health care workers, including nurses. The stress of caring for patients with COVID-19 is made harder than usual because of the following factors: the lack of personal protective equipment, uncertain outcomes and mixed messages from the government, patient isolation from families and separation from staff due to isolation procedures and protective equipment, staffing shortages, high levels of dying patients, demands from professional duties often conflicting with self-care abilities, and the fear of disease exposure for self and family members. Several strategies decrease the risk of stress-related disorders such as vicarious trauma for nurses, including strategic staffing to utilize those whose job duties have decreased (e.g., elective surgeries); collaboration with interdisciplinary experts; planning and implementing self-care activities on the job, such as social support and emotional/psychological support following repeated loss of patients; and continually planning for the future (Akgün et al., 2020).

COMMUNITY AND TRAUMA

The community response to trauma can have a major impact on the degree of traumatic stress experienced by individuals, families, and the community. The community has a key role in the prevention and treatment of trauma. Child welfare services often respond to threats of trauma from abuse and neglect, and police services often respond to threats of domestic or community violence. Nurses as a professional group are mandatory reporters. Every state in the United States and every province in Canada has enacted legislation governing the reporting of child abuse and elder abuse. Reporting requirements can differ from one country to the next, and each health care provider is responsible for knowing which conditions require reporting to appropriate authorities.

It is incumbent on all agencies that work with victims of trauma to become well versed in TIC. Agencies that work with trauma victims have a responsibility to be trained for their role in trauma care. For example, if child welfare workers are not properly trained in the area of trauma, they may not support foster parents in appropriate reactions to children with trauma-related behaviors. This lack of support may lead to placement failure and result in children being retraumatized by multiple interruptions in attachment, initiating a dangerous cycle (Richardson et al., 2012).

Consider the following scenario. A 13-year-old child who has been sexually abused by her father is placed into foster care. During counseling, she is encouraged to retreat to a quiet place when chaos from the crowded foster care becomes too much. Because of lack of training and poor communication with the counselor, her foster mother scolds her for "being too isolated." When she goes to school, she becomes overwhelmed by fear and retreats to the library to regain her homeostasis. Because her teachers are untrained and unaware of her needs, she is again punished. She begins to distrust her counselor, foster parent, and teachers and relapses into fear, disconnection, and dysregulation. She retreats into rigid boundaries. This short vignette illustrates the importance of educating community-based service providers about TIC and to integrate and collaborate services to promote positive rather than dangerous and negative outcomes.

SYSTEMIC TRAUMA

The symptoms of PTSD cross individual, family, and community boundaries. Many argue that the United States is suffering from PTSD from repeated traumatic events such as wars, natural disasters, economic recessions, the COVID-19 pandemic, the killing of citizens by police, and demonstrations surrounding the Black Lives Matter (BLM) movement. Some of these events have lasted a long time without resolution. This has resulted in a nation with trauma symptoms, including depression; intrusion of unwanted and negative thinking patterns; hyperarousal, especially to perceived threats from others, intense focus on news and other sources of feared information; and related health decline in individuals and families. One clear symptom of this premise is the decline in the general health of U.S. citizens, not unlike the health of individuals suffering from PTSD. Americans have the shortest life span of any industrialized nation, with almost half of American adults struggling with hypertension, high cholesterol, diabetes, or all three. In addition, 42.4% of adults and 19% of children ages 2 to 18 years are obese (CDC, 2018). An increasing number suffer from stress-related illnesses stemming from or causing mental illness, substance abuse, and domestic violence, as well as several different physical illnesses. Infant mortality is dismally high, with the United States ranking lower than 55 industrialized countries of the world and with a recent rate of 5.8 deaths per 1,000 births, compared to Japan at 2.4 deaths per 1,000 births (World Fact Book, n.d.). Child abuse rates in the

United States are also high when compared with other nations (Pritchard et al., 2019).

Approximately one-quarter of children in the United States take prescription medications. Mental health disorders among children are described as changes in the way that children learn, behave, or handle their emotions that result in challenges in multiple areas of their lives (CDC, 2020b). The more common mental disorders among children include ADHD, anxiety, and behavior disorders. This is compounded by the fact that more than two-thirds of children reported experiencing at least one traumatic event by the age of 16 (National Child Traumatic Stress Initiative, 2020). The statistics demonstrate symptoms of a country experiencing dysregulation from systemic trauma.

The high obesity rate in the United States is a clear example of a nation experiencing dysregulation and fear. The lack of healthy foods, safe neighborhoods that support outdoor activity, high levels of stress, and the presence of early and repeated trauma are key factors in causing obesity and related chronic health conditions (Masodkar et al., 2016). Yet the response to obesity is not centered on trauma-focused interventions but instead on unsuccessful dieting and major surgeries.

Another indicator that the United States as a nation is struggling with high levels of trauma and related stress symptoms is the increasing rate of substance abuse. Although nicotine addiction is at an all-time low, addiction to other substances, such as alcohol and opiates, is continues to be high (National Institute on Drug Abuse, 2020). Researchers have found that those struggling with food cravings leading to obesity and those struggling with drug addiction both exhibit decreased dopamine levels. Overeating and drug use temporarily raise dopamine levels. A lack of dopamine, particularly in the prefrontal cortex, is caused by early trauma more often than genetics (Karr-Morse & Wiley, 2012; De Bellis & Zisk, 2014). A country experiencing repeated trauma without resolution quickly fills with individuals, families, and communities that are highly stressed and traumatized, with a resulting increase in stress-related illnesses.

Chronic stress is toxic stress. *Toxic stress*, as defined by the Center on the Developing Child at Harvard University, is when an individual experiences strong, frequent, and prolonged stress such as chronic child abuse or neglect without adequate support (Center on the Developing Child, 2021).

Toxic stress interferes with the ability to learn, be creative, stay healthy, and experience joy. Countries that experience toxic stress through natural disasters, war, or dysregulation of major systems also experience a drop in the ability to learn, be creative, have healthy citizens, and experience joyous outcomes. Robin Karr-Morse and Meredith Wiley, the authors of *Scared Sick: The Roles of Childhood Trauma in Adult Disease* (2012), compared our body's response to stress with the U.S. Department of Homeland Security. Both systems are aimed at a complex and integrated system that maintains safety. When part of that system is overtaxed or disconnected, safety is threatened. Threats to the larger system, whether real or imagined, can further overwhelm the system and lead to disease. Reviewing the outcomes to date on the challenges faced by the United States because of the COVID-19 pandemic compared to other industrialized nations is further evidence that United States is a system under stress.

The greater culture and societal laws and policies can influence the incidence and the treatment of trauma. Countries riddled with war, poverty, and disease have higher incidents of stress-related symptoms, whereas countries that support policies that decrease violent solutions to problems, provide broad access to preventive and primary health care, and decrease poverty levels have lower incidences of stress-related symptoms. For example, the incidence of PTSD in New Zealand is estimated to be 6.1% of the population (U.S. Department of Veterans Affairs, 2020a), whereas the incidence of PTSD in the Gaza Strip was found to be 53.5% of 11- to 17-year-olds exposed to the ongoing Israeli-Palestinian conflict (El-Khodary et al., 2020). The extent to which countries can prevent and/or treat the causes of post-traumatic stress early clearly influences the health of the citizens in every country.

Many argue that the traumatic events experienced over the course of the last two decades in the United States were too rapid to resolve and caused a chronic state of fear in the country. For example, in 2020 and 2021 the United States experienced a COVID-19 pandemic with over 600,000 deaths (death rate continues to climb), record numbers of hurricanes, economic recession, a record number of raging wildfires in California and Colorado, and numerous police-related deaths. U.S. citizens watched these disasters unfold with little support or education on how to process these events to avoid post-traumatic stress symptoms.

Today, many individuals talk about feeling numb to the disasters that they see on television and online, and have increased fear related to travel, economics, and routine activities such as attending school. The management of trauma symptoms has to expand beyond individuals, families, and communities to include national and international traumas and the impact on a nation as a whole. See Box 12-1 for risks associated with trauma.

BOX 12-1
Risks Associated with Trauma

Severe risks and risk factors are associated with both adults and children exposed to traumatic events. Nurses should be aware of them, including the following:

- *Suicide risk:* because of feelings of numbness, disconnection from support people, chronic fear and anxiety, and feelings of hopelessness and helplessness.
- *Danger to others:* ask about firearms or weapons, aggressive intentions, feelings of persecution.
- *Ongoing stressors:* stressors include changes that have occurred at home, marital discord, problems at work.
- *Risky behaviors:* risky behaviors include risky sexual adventures, nonadherence to medical treatment, substance use and misuse.
- *Personal characteristics:* past trauma history, coping skills, relationship attachment.
- *Limited social support:* the individual's lack of willingness to accept help and inclination to isolate.
- *Comorbidity:* coexisting psychiatric or medical problems such as depression and chronic widespread pain (CWP).

Child risks associated with PTSD include the following:

- *Dysregulation:* unpredictable or irregular sleep and eating patterns, and difficulty regulating moods and emotional responses.
- *Poor connection:* difficulty forming or maintaining relationships, with a tendency to be alone, have poor eye contact, and resist connection with others.
- *Poor cognitive development:* difficulty with attention, short-term memory, problem solving, creativity, and play. High incidence of learning disabilities, particularly auditory processing disability.
- *Poor attunement skills:* difficulty recognizing and asking for needs.
- *Inability to trust:* difficulty forming relationships, oppositional behavior, sleep problems.
- *Hyperarousal:* increased response to environmental stressors or memories, with rage, anger, or severe anxiety.

NURSES AND TRAUMA

Nurses are key to helping with the diagnosis and treatment of trauma-related illnesses in individuals and families. Their presence at the forefront of emergency and intensive care of victims of trauma and their help throughout the healing process render nurses important members of the interdisciplinary team that prevents, treats, and evaluates care for individuals and families affected by trauma-related illnesses. This section outlines the nurse's role in the prevention, identification, and treatment of these conditions as part of an interdisciplinary team.

Trauma-Informed Nursing Assessment and Intervention

Trauma-related illnesses, including PTSD, can develop after a traumatic event or events at any age. To be diagnosed with PTSD, a person has to have been exposed to a traumatic event; experience intense feelings of fear, helplessness, or horror (for preverbal children, the feelings of helplessness are commonly seen as withdrawal, and feelings of fear are commonly seen as intense emotional arousal); reexperience the event through flashbacks, dreams, or disturbing memories; avoid any stimuli associated with the event; avoid any reminders, thoughts, or feelings about the event; be hypervigilant; have difficulty falling or staying asleep; possess an exaggerated startle response; and have symptoms that last longer than one month and that cause significant distress or impairment in functioning (U.S. Department of Veterans Affairs, 2019).

The role of nurses is to assess for symptoms of PTSD. There are simple methods to screen patients who may have undetected PTSD. One easy-to-use tool is the Primary Care PTSD Screen (Prins et al., 2016), which consists of five questions preceded by an introductory question:

Sometimes things happen to people that are unusually or especially frightening, horrible, or traumatic, for example:

- A serious accident or fire
- A physical or sexual assault or abuse
- An earthquake or flood
- A war
- Seeing someone be killed or seriously injured
- Having a loved one die through homicide or suicide

Have you ever experienced this kind of event?
Yes/No

If no, screen total = 0. Please stop here.

If yes, please answer the following questions.

In the past month, have you:

1. Had nightmares about the event(s) or thought about the event(s) when you did not want to?
   Yes/No

2. Tried hard not to think about the event(s) or went out of your way to avoid situations that reminded you of the event(s)?
   Yes/No

3. Been constantly on guard, watchful, or easily startled?
   Yes/No

4. Felt numb or detached from people, activities, or your surroundings?
   Yes/No

5. Felt guilty or unable to stop blaming yourself or others for the event(s) or any problems the event(s) may have caused?
   Yes/No

(Source: Prins et al. (2016). *The Primary Care PTSD Screen for* DSM-5 *(PC-PTSD-5)*.

The screen is positive if the patient answers yes to any three items.

It is also important for nurses to assess risk factors and provide families with protector factors or positive coping strategies and enhancement of resilience characteristics (Garland et al., 2019; Warner, 2010). See Box 12-2 on vicarious trauma.

The best evidence-based nursing treatments for individuals with PTSD include both psychotherapeutic interventions—such as CBT and family therapy—and education and monitoring of medications, primarily serotonin reuptake inhibitors (SSRIs) (U.S. Department of Veterans Affairs, 2019). CBT is one type of counseling. Research shows it is the most effective type of counseling for PTSD. The U.S. Department of Veterans Affairs (VA) is providing two forms of CBT to veterans with PTSD: Cognitive Processing Therapy (CPT) and PET.

BOX 12-2

Vicarious Trauma

Trauma clearly transcends individuals, families, communities, and greater societies across time and across cultures. Nurses are often the front-line health care providers to identify and intervene when acute and chronic trauma occurs. There is evidence to suggest that health professionals, including nurses, are skilled at emotional regulation and reflection that may protect them against vicarious trauma; however, there is still significant risk for clinicians exposed to trauma (Taylor et al., 2016).

A real risk for nurses is the development of the attunement survival style described by Heller and LaPierre (2015). This style of coping is characterized by attuning to others' needs and neglecting one's own needs, which is an apt description of the lived experiences of many nurses. If nurses identify themselves as givers yet neglect their own needs, they are at high risk for vicarious trauma, or the development of PTSD symptoms from caring for or witnessing trauma in others. This condition is also referred to as *compassion fatigue* and *secondary trauma* in the literature (Afifi et al., 2009).

This term has evolved as health care providers were identified as being at high risk for negative psychological reactions to their job, with early descriptions of burnout. Symptoms of burnout include feeling overwhelmed, hopeless, helpless, unmotivated, and unappreciated. The result of burnout and secondary trauma for health care professionals can be damaging. If unrecognized or untreated, members of the workforce are at risk for real suffering, including depression, emotional trauma, and suicide (Kelly, 2020). Although burnout can be caused by repetitious and emotionally exhausting work, it can also be caused by vicarious trauma. Prevention of vicarious trauma is possible through education, avoiding professional burnout, reaching out for peer support, and engaging professional support when needed during and after caring for traumatized patients (Taylor et al., 2016; Kelly, 2020).

Prevention is the goal, with primary treatment of potential post-traumatic stress response; several programs start interventions at the time of the traumatic event rather than waiting for symptoms to develop. Sufficient evidence for psychological first aid is widely supported by available objective observations and expert opinion and best fits the category of "evidence informed" but without proof of effectiveness. An intervention provided by volunteers without professional mental health training for people who have experienced a traumatic event offers an acceptable option.

Once symptoms develop, outcomes improve with a combination of individual and family therapy, and with appropriate medication management of symptoms when needed. For example, in a study of seven children following a bus accident, the combination of individual and family therapy with SSRIs resulted in a remission of PTSD symptoms, whereas the control group that received only medication without family therapy still had symptoms 3 months later (Stankovi et al., 2013). In the cases where medication and family therapy were used, researchers used Systematic Family Therapy (SFT), a structured family therapy protocol, to facilitate family involvement and family-directed interventions. It proved effective in preventing chronic PTSD in victims.

Secondary Family Traumatization Assessment and Intervention

To help the traumatized family, nurses should first realize that traumatized families rarely seek family-focused intervention. Instead, they often present with problems that are not immediately related to the traumatic events they have experienced (Figley & Barnes, 2005). Nurses should learn the parallel processes of individual and systemic stress reactions that follow a traumatic event. Figley and Barnes (2005) offer suggestions to help clinicians recognize family responses to traumatic events and offer some interventions to help patients and families affected by these events. For example, families are affected by an individual family member's symptoms of PTSD. They know the story of the trauma, witness the symptoms, and want to help in some way. Therefore, the family spends more and more time caring for the traumatized member. While the traumatic event is being persistently reexperienced by the exposed family member, the other family members are responding to this individual's expressed need for support. As the primary affected family member tries to avoid stimuli and reminders of the trauma, the other family members must devote increased time, energy, and problem solving to avoid conversations, people, places, and things that might stimulate memories. They must cope with withdrawal and numbing that goes along with the primary affected family member's diminished interest in usual activities, refusals to see friends, and

inability to express love and caring. The family becomes increasingly more isolated. Family members must manage problems with sleep, outbursts of anger and rage, exaggerated startle responses, and hypervigilance about safety. These factors increase the risk of secondary traumatization or symptoms of trauma reaction in family members from witnessing the traumatic stories and the negative impacts on the primary family member.

Nurses applying TIC by using the Ecological Systems Theory Approach to Trauma Treatment begin the treatment by correcting interrupted trust and attachment (Heller & LaPierre, 2015). Infants and young children who experience rejection and abuse early in life often expect that same experience from present and future caregivers. A trusting and therapeutic relationship must form. This process is slow because the child or adult who has learned to avoid feelings and relationships will first resist and then struggle with moderating those feelings and relationships, and then, if successful, learn to trust. The initial steps of treatment are as follows:

1. Move slowly. Building connections can be terrifying to a traumatized individual.
2. Build trust. Building a therapeutic relationship depends on being predictable and trustworthy.
3. Be empathetic. You may be the first kind person in your patients' lives.
4. Help children and adults listen to and explore their new skills at identifying emotions, organizing thoughts and emotions, and learning different reactions and responses to their emotions.
5. Help build self-esteem through teaching top-down thinking. For example, if an adult has always felt he was bad because of traumatic events in his life, help him rethink that the events are bad instead.
6. Gradually support and encourage connection with patients' own feelings, then their body responses and reactions, and finally connection to other people. The connection to other people should also be gradual, starting with close caregivers or family members and advancing, as tolerated, to outside peers and associates.
7. Be available to help the child or adult explore feelings of rejection, anger, abandonment, and fear. Many individuals

who have experienced trauma have survived by becoming numb. As this numbness fades, survival feels threatened. During this transition from numbness to feeling, many may withdraw for varying periods of time. Therapeutic nurses can recognize this pattern and avoid judging the traumatized individual during these phases.

8. Help children and adults connect with others because support has been found to be a key factor in successful treatment of trauma (Evans & Coccoma, 2014).

The nurse working with a traumatized family needs to explore each family member's perception of what happened both before and after the event. The family may block the telling of trauma if the family was the cause of that trauma. Listening to individuals and observing for signs of secondary trauma can be critical to getting help for all family members. Nurses need to recognize that the family's worldview was altered by the traumatizing events and that its attitudes and beliefs may have shifted from safety to suspicious, distrustful attribution regarding the motivations of others, including helping health care providers. Hypervigilance and controlling behaviors may interfere with the family getting the help it needs. In addition, if the stressors impinging on the family go unattended, a pattern of poor communication and blaming may become the central family dynamic. Also, the roles in the family may shift, with some members becoming more enmeshed with the traumatized member and others withdrawing from the family system. Children may have to take on the role of emotional caretaker for the parents and thus be compelled to hide their own feelings and fears, while other siblings act out to express anger, leading to more parenting stress. Most emerging trauma treatment has as its main shortcoming the focus on the individual rather than the family system. Careful implementation of interviewing techniques and the exploration of the family life experience through ecomaps assist nurses in accessing the complex relationships and characteristics of families living with trauma or post-traumatic complications. Nurses are also key in finding resources for families that use a family approach to trauma care.

The nursing role also includes looking at community actions and societal responses to trauma at personal, family, community, and societal levels and how that trauma affects health. Becoming involved with prevention strategies, such as community preparedness for disaster, can lead to improved community health. Working with national organizations to provide organized community-based interventions for traumas can be an important step to preventing negative long-term consequences. Participating in research and implementing research findings that demonstrate the impact of trauma at all ecological levels can help improve treatment plans and outcomes. Finally, shaping policies at the national level that support families in need, by decreasing poverty, improving access to health care, supporting parents with improved child-care options and improved parenting education and support, and reducing environmental stress, can be important steps to reducing the impact of trauma in children, adults, families, communities, and nations.

Case Study: Knoll Family

This case study offers an example of a family that experienced trauma and demonstrates the impact of individual trauma and family trauma on all family members. The events that occurred within this family illustrate the complexities of prolonged and repeated trauma, as well as resilience characteristics touching the individual, family, community, and nation.

Family Members

- Mother: Laura (age 45)
- Father: Victor (age 46)
- Oldest daughter: Natalie (age 24 years)
- Middle daughter: Kimberly (age 23 years)
- Youngest daughter: Taylor (age 22 years)

(continued)

Case Study: Knoll Family—cont'd

Figure 12-5 shows the Knoll family genogram.

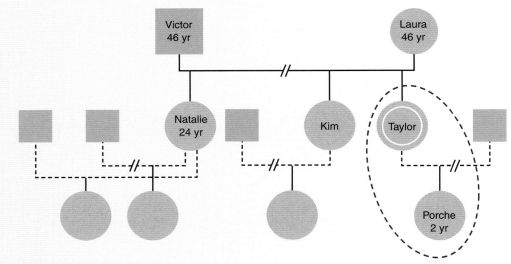

FIGURE 12-5 Knoll Family Genogram

The Knoll family initially sought care at a multidisciplinary clinic because of increasing concerns about their youngest daughter, Taylor. They started this care when Taylor was 15 years of age and complained that Taylor was refusing to attend school, using marijuana and alcohol on a daily basis, and was currently dating a man who was 20 years older. When they threatened to call the police, Taylor stated that she would "run away and never return."

Family Development

The mother, Laura, has a history of intimate partner violence from her husband, causing her to escape across the country when her daughters were ages 3, 4, and 6, respectively. She remarried when her daughters were ages 8, 9, and 11, respectively. All three girls did well until adolescence, with participation in sports, family activities, and school. Her youngest daughter abruptly stopped all participation in school and sports at age 13 years and began befriending peers who were involved in drugs. Her mother sought treatment through her primary-care physician, who recommended residential care. In spite of 3 months' residential treatment, the same problems continued. When Laura's oldest daughter disclosed memories of sexual abuse from her biological father when she was in preschool, Laura became overwhelmed. She had just asked her ex-husband to take care of her younger daughter because she did not know how to help her. With her ex-husband being an active alcoholic and having a history of physical violence and now under suspicion of sexual abuse of her oldest daughter, this decision brought more guilt and shame to Laura. However, Taylor insisted on going to live with Laura's ex-husband and did not believe he sexually abused her sister. Taylor came back after 6 months. Laura tried other resources and agonized as she watched her youngest daughter struggle through years of methamphetamine and heroin addiction. Her ex-husband moved to town when her daughters were 18, 19, and 21, respectively. This added to her stress because he demanded participation in family activities and celebrations and demanded rides from all family members because he did not have a driver's license. This caused strain in Laura's current marriage. Today, Laura works full-time and cares for her four grandchildren on a regular basis. She has recently started counseling because of feelings of depression and being overwhelmed with family responsibilities.

The father, Victor, lived across the country from his family from the point of divorce until 5 years ago. Divorce occurred against his will when his three daughters were ages 3, 4, and 6, respectively. Although he has had other partners, he continued to try to get back together with his ex-wife, trying to convince her that the domestic violence was only caused by his heavy drinking. He denied any sexual abuse of his daughter. He continued drinking alcohol in spite of being diagnosed with hepatitis C and cirrhosis

Case Study: Knoll Family—cont'd

of the liver. He was agreeable to having his youngest daughter come live with him when she was 14 years of age, which lasted 6 months. Taylor left her father's home because of his "constant drinking." Two years later Victor moved to the same town as his children and ex-wife. He currently joins the family for all family events and celebrations. He maintains employment off and on and relies on his daughters for transportation to his job because he does not have a driver's license; he has received repeated citations for driving under the influence (DUI).

Natalie grew up with her mother and two sisters from the time of her parents' divorce to her mother's remarriage when she was 10 years old. She then lived with her mother, stepfather, and two sisters. She did well in school and participated in activities throughout her school years. When she was 17 years old, she disclosed memories of sexual abuse. She was distraught to learn that her siblings did not believe her, and her mother told her to "forgive your father; that was a long time ago." She sought counseling on her own but now notes that she continues to pick abusive men as partners. She has two children from different fathers, and both fathers are incarcerated for drug sales. She is completing her college degree in counseling.

Kimberly, the middle daughter, grew up with her mother and sisters until her mother remarried when she was 8 years of age. She then lived with her mother, stepfather, and two sisters. She did well until high school, when she developed incapacitating panic disorder. This caused her to avoid school. She received antianxiety medications for approximately 1 year and reported feeling better. She received her GED when she was 20 years of age and now works as a housecleaner. She has had the same partner for the past 4 years, and they have one daughter together. Her partner is concerned about her alcohol abuse and has threatened to leave if she does not seek treatment.

Taylor is the identified patient. She stated that she did well in school and with peers until she was 13 years of age. She states that she became very depressed at that time and lost interest in all that she previously cared about. She remembers being in residential care and being diagnosed with bipolar disorder. She was given medications, but she refused to take any of the medications once she left the treatment facility. Upon return home, she returned to using drugs as a strategy to "feel something" and "have the energy to do anything." Taylor spent 6 months with her father at age 14 years but returned stating that he "drank too much." Taylor then went back to residential care for 6 months, followed by 3 years of methamphetamine and heroin addiction. She earned her GED and has been fully employed in computer technical help for the past 5 years. She gave birth to her daughter, Porche, 2 years ago. Porche's father was trying to get custody because of Taylor's drug use, so Taylor reentered drug treatment. During this treatment time, she experienced a flood of memories of her father sexually abusing her during her preschool years. She stated that she remembered her father getting drunk and sexually abusing her in a closet in their old home. She stated that she felt shame and extreme guilt that she did not believe her sister when her sister disclosed the same abuse, that she did not know how to set boundaries with her father to this day, and that she requested help keeping her father out of her life. Currently, her father calls her almost daily and demands help with transportation three to five times per week.

Function

Communication within the family started out as avoidant, with each family member feeling unable to share thoughts and feelings with other family members. Boundaries were blurred and unclear (i.e., mother being unable to say no to having her daughter live with a suspected sexual abuser, and Taylor being unable to say no to seeing her father in spite of memories of sexual abuse). Through intensive counseling and parent coaching within the clinic and through home visits, the family now participates in healthier communication patterns, nonviolent problem solving, and shared positive experiences. Each family member, however, continues to show signs of chronic PTSD caused by repeated and severe traumas within the family. When asked about traumatic events, the family summarized the following:

- Intimate partner violence
- Alcohol addiction of father
- Sexual abuse of two daughters by father (father denies this)
- Drug addiction by Taylor

Laura was asked about resilience skills for both herself and her daughters. She felt she had positive support through her parents, a strong religious affiliation including daily prayer, the absence of any substance abuse, and the ability to adapt to the

(continued)

Case Study: Knoll Family—cont'd

many changes and traumatic events occurring across time. She noted that her daughters were her support as well as her burden. She stated that they were very adaptable at times to big changes. Areas where this family lacked resilience included optimism, self-efficacy, and ability to set healthy boundaries.

Nursing Interventions

Microsystem: The individuals within this family needed a thorough and comprehensive assessment of symptoms of trauma-related health concerns given the history of repeated and prolonged trauma. The mechanism of prolonged stress for Taylor started in early childhood, given her symptoms of mood dysregulation, attention deficit disorder, depression, and drug addiction. Her older sister, Natalie, also experienced early childhood trauma, but her symptoms and outcome were different. She struggled more with relationships, choosing men who would abuse her and desert her, similar to her biological father. Taylor's middle sister, Kimberly, denied any memories of sexual abuse. She did show signs of trauma, however, through her panic disorder and alcohol dependency. Given that two out of three daughters remembered being abused, it is likely Kimberly experienced abuse, too. Laura struggled with her own abuse. She suffered from intimate partner violence, which is often accompanied by sexual assault (Evans & Coccoma, 2014). She also witnessed all of her daughters struggle through adolescence and young adulthood because of their past abuse and her difficulty setting boundaries.

   The understanding of each of these individuals' experiences and related traumas helps the nurse identify the need for individual care for each family member. The daughters and mother started family care with individual counseling. They soon built a trusting relationship with the therapist and learned across time to become more attuned to each of their own needs, learned to ask for help with their needs appropriately, and discovered how to regulate their responses to emotions.

Mesosystem: Family-centered care was instituted after 3 months of individual counseling to improve family development and functioning. Family self-care strategies were initially implemented to stabilize and organize the family, followed by family meetings to address communication and problem-solving skills, as well as ways to build positive connections between and among family members. During the family meetings, family members also discussed the effects of trauma on the family, especially the difficulty all members had in setting healthy boundaries with Victor. The family is now currently preparing to meet with Victor and enforce clear boundaries to prevent further trauma.

Macrosystem: This family struggled with finding supportive community resources. See Figure 12-6, the Knoll family ecomap, which depicts the subsystems. This family experienced trauma care at a time when addiction services were separated from TIC. Therefore, Taylor did not address her own trauma until early adulthood. Her siblings and mother did not receive TIC until almost two decades after the trauma occurred.

Exosystem: This family was affected by societal rules, culture, and policies. The availability of health care through the state allowed services to this family but limited those services to weekly contacts with specified providers rather than the family being able to pursue professionals skilled in TIC.

Outcome Following Treatment

Following 1 year of TIC, this family is no longer demonstrating symptoms of PTSD. Each family member is experiencing positive connections within and outside the family. During this treatment period, the family worked with the same nurse, with interventions focused on ongoing family assessments, care coordination to facilitate better relationships across the family care–provider ecology, improving family communication and closeness through the use of rituals and routines, and individually targeted development of resilience characteristics. All family members, except the biological father, are sober, and all members report more energy, ability to express emotions, and decreased hyperarousal toward Victor, the biological father and ex-husband.

   Questions for reflection on the nursing care of the Knoll family:

1. What characteristics are identified in individuals who are resilient?
2. Following treatment, what signs of resilience were demonstrated by the Knoll family?
3. How can nurses and other health care professionals help individuals develop resilience even when faced with adversity?

Case Study: Knoll Family—cont'd

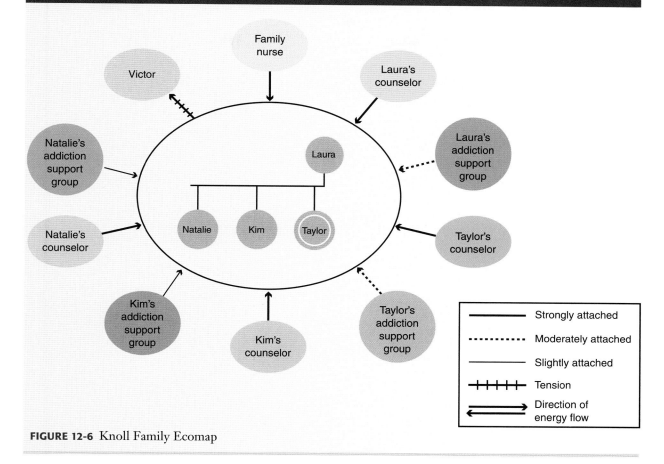

FIGURE 12-6 Knoll Family Ecomap

Case Study: Caldwell Family

Mr. Caldwell, a 47-year-old National Guard soldier who is in the hospital for a hernia repair, had returned home from a 12-month deployment to Iraq, where he had his first exposure to combat in his 18 years of National Guard duty. Before deployment, he worked successfully as a firefighter/paramedic and was a happily married father with two children. He and his wife were socially outgoing, with a large circle of friends from the same rural area in which they both grew up. They have been married since high school. See a genogram and ecomap for the Caldwell family in Figures 12-7 and 12-8, respectively.

While in Iraq, and as the noncommissioned officer in charge of the battlefield medical aid station, Mr. Caldwell had extensive exposure to other soldiers' combat injuries. His unit treated the severe, crippling injuries of soldiers en route to the trauma hospital. The aid station was often overrun with multiple casualties. He treated soldiers from patrols and convoys in which improvised explosive devices (IEDs) destroyed vehicles and wounded or killed people. Although he did not have to kill enemy combatants, he agonized that he may also have been responsible for the deaths of some soldiers because he simply did not have enough personnel or resources to treat all the casualties adequately. When asked about the worst moment during his deployment, he readily stated it was when he was unable to intercede while a Humvee with a bleeding soldier draped over the hood and several wounded soldiers in the back drove by the aid station because the driver's view was blocked by blood gushing on the windshield and the driver could not see him waving the Humvee to safety.

(continued)

Case Study: Caldwell Family—cont'd

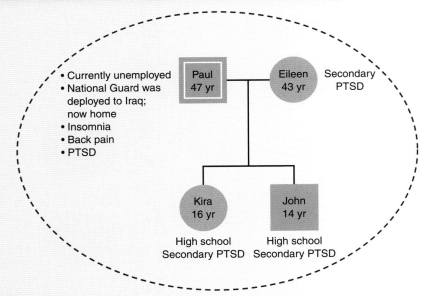

FIGURE 12-7 Caldwell Family Genogram

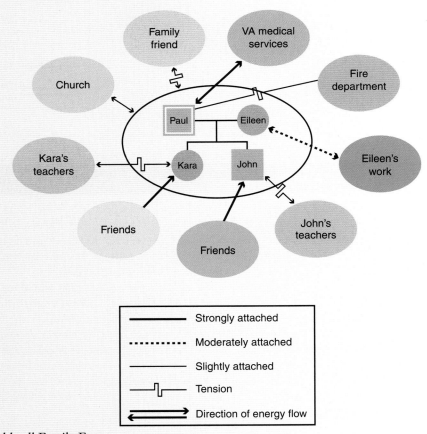

FIGURE 12-8 Caldwell Family Ecomap

Case Study: Caldwell Family—cont'd

When he first returned home, things seemed to be okay. But more than 2 years after coming home, he has had more and more difficulty relating to his wife. He reports feeling angry all the time and that no one will listen to him. Sleep has become difficult. He has to sleep on the recliner in the living room because his back hurts so badly that he cannot lie flat. When he does sleep, he has a recurring, vivid nightmare about turning a corner outside a building in Baghdad where he encounters an insurgent with a rifle who shoots him. His daughter complains that he has become so overprotective that he will not let her go out with any friends, much less any boys. His wife reported that he has been emotionally distant since his return. His employer, who initially supported him, has reported that his work at the fire department has suffered dramatically. During a recent burning motor vehicle extraction drill, one of the car's tires exploded. The unexpected explosion rattled him so much that he became unable to go to work anymore.

Mr. Caldwell says that since his deployment, he no longer has an identity—he cannot work, and he no longer feels like he can fulfill his obligations as a husband and father. He reports that he sometimes experiences strong surges of anger, panic, guilt, and despair and that at other times he has felt emotionally dead, unable to return the love and warmth of family and friends. He does not want to get a divorce but fears this will happen. Although he has not been actively suicidal, he reported that he sometimes thinks everyone would be better off if he had not survived his tour in Iraq. He is currently on several medications for back pain from his on-the-job injury at the fire department. He is complaining of a lot of postoperative pain.

This composite case illustrates several kinds of war-zone stressors. Mr. Caldwell felt helpless to prevent several deaths. In addition to that feeling of helplessness, he had to witness the horror of many people dying and had to respond to emergencies on a very unpredictable basis. Nurses who are taking care of patients who have had a difficult return to civilian life need to be aware of the complicated nature of readjustment. This case also illustrates the prevalence of PTSD and that it may increase considerably during the 2 to 6 years after veterans have returned from combat duty (Hermes et al., 2015).

The Caldwell family is dealing with the chronic problems that occur when a veteran returns home with significant PTSD. The care for this family, when delivered from the perspective of Family Systems Theory, will have to address Mr. Caldwell's PTSD as well as the family's ever-increasing secondary traumatization from his stress responses.

Theoretical Perspective

Using a family systems theoretical approach, the plan of care for Mr. Caldwell includes referral for his PTSD and providing the family members with education and resources about what they can do to address their own secondary trauma as well as support his recovery. As part of the plan, the nurse can help the Caldwell family by drawing a family ecomap that shows resources currently being used.

Mr. Caldwell has been traumatized by his experience with war and ultimately all his family members and family relationships are affected. Mr. Caldwell's war experience was his alone, but his wife is being affected by the symptoms he is experiencing, symptoms that will get worse as she takes on even more of a caregiving role following his surgery. The children are baffled by the changes in their father and do not know quite what to do. Because Mrs. Caldwell is so involved with caring for him, the children do not feel like they can go to her with their problems. In addition to their parents not being available to them emotionally, both children have had to take on family roles that their parents used to manage. For example, the daughter, Kira, now must do more of the family meal preparation and house cleaning. The son, John, has to do all the yard work, which has made it harder to spend time with his friends. Both teenagers are starting not to do as well in school because of the constant tension in the home and their fears that their parents may divorce. Because Mr. Caldwell's trauma is so severe, it is highly likely that the other members of the family suffer from secondary traumatization.

This family's response to the war trauma of Mr. Caldwell cannot be understood or treated by focusing on just his care (microsystem). His family members (mesosystem) can provide key contextual information about past traumatic events and experiences that can explain current responses. In fact, they are a central reason why Mr. Caldwell wants to get better and resume more of his leadership roles within the family. As he has spiraled downward, the rest of the family has followed, and all now report deteriorating mental health.

The boundaries for this family may be protective, but they may also act as a barrier to seeking help. It may be that Mrs. Caldwell feels it is disloyal to talk about her husband's problems with an outsider. Mr. Caldwell has many fears about admitting his difficulties and feels ashamed about how his problems have affected his wife. Mrs. Caldwell is afraid to ask for help because she does not want her husband to feel any more embarrassment than he does already. They are both suffering in silence, reluctant

(continued)

Case Study: Caldwell Family—cont'd

to talk to each other or to anyone else. The nurse will have to create a trusting relationship to overcome this natural reluctance to share family secrets. One of the things that may help is to explain how providing this information may enhance the medical team's ability to provide quality care.

In this case, the spousal relationship has suffered because of Mr. Caldwell's trauma. Wartime separation and reunion, and then later problems with PTSD from combat, have created some marital dysfunction that was not present before Mr. Caldwell's deployment. In this situation, the marital relationship as a subset within this family is the most problematic area. By helping this family improve this one area of its family functioning through appropriate referral, the nurse could have a great impact on the rest of the family subsystems. Because PTSD therapy is a new experience for Mr. and Mrs. Caldwell, they are not quite sure how to deal with it, plus they are reluctant to seek outside help at this time.

Assessment and Intervention Considerations

The assessment and intervention for the Caldwell family focuses on PTSD and secondary trauma. Although Mr. Caldwell's traumatic exposure occurred some time ago, undiagnosed or inadequately treated PTSD could complicate his surgical recovery, as shown clearly from this case study. PTSD is associated with more physical health problems and somatic symptom severity (Hoge et al., 2007). Although chronic widespread pain (CWP)—defined as pain in various parts of the body and fatigue that lasts for 3 months or longer—has thus far been documented only in veterans from the first Gulf War, the potential for this phenomenon to emerge in current combat veterans is high. CWP is associated with greater health care utilization and a lower quality of life (Forman-Hoffman et al., 2007).

In this instance, Mr. Caldwell may be having more problems postoperatively with pain perception, pain tolerance, and other kinds of untreated chronic pain. In addition, PTSD symptoms may make it difficult for the nurse to communicate with the patient, may reduce the patient's active collaboration in evaluation and treatment, and reduce patient adherence to medical regimens.

Assessment

Because trauma is underrecognized, patients with PTSD are not properly identified and are not offered education, counseling, and/or referrals for mental health evaluation. Simple methods are available to screen patients who may have undetected PTSD. As noted, one easy-to-use tool is the Primary Care PTSD Screen (Prins et al., 2016).

Next, assess the family for possible symptoms of secondary trauma. How are Mr. Caldwell's wife and children responding to his symptoms? What symptoms are they experiencing in relation to his difficulties? Identify how roles may have shifted for this family given Mr. Caldwell's current circumstances. Is the family still functioning as a strong cohesive unit? How have things changed? How open is this family to working with the nurse? What might help facilitate their cooperation with the nurse?

Nursing Interventions

Provide education about PTSD and secondary trauma. Because the family's participation is essential in identifying symptoms of PTSD and planning treatment, the nurse must create an environment that is supportive and inclusive of family members in order to work in partnership with the family. Several online sites can help the nurse develop educational fact sheets that can be shared with patients and families. The Veterans Affairs National Center for PTSD and the Defense Department's Walter Reed Army Medical Center collaborated to develop the Iraq War Clinician Guide. The next step that the nurse should take in intervening with the Caldwell family is referring all family members for further care. Set up a plan for referring to a PTSD specialist for those patients who show signs of potential PTSD and who are amenable to receiving additional evaluation or counseling. In this instance, the nurse could provide the family with a list of possible options. Many local areas have lists of returning veterans' counseling services that include counseling for couples and families. Involve the family in the plan of follow-up care.

Questions for reflection on the nursing care of the Caldwell family:

1. Reflect on the concept of secondary or vicarious trauma. In your own words, describe what this is and who may be affected.
2. As you provide education to the Caldwell family about PTSD and secondary trauma, what strategies can you encourage the family to use to minimize the impact of the trauma?
3. How can nurses and other health care professionals minimize the impact of secondary stress or vicarious trauma on themselves when working with individuals and families who have experienced traumatic events?

SUMMARY

In this chapter, we discussed trauma and how TIC may be employed with patients by family nurses. Key points include the following:

- Trauma affects the entire family system.
- Trauma-related illnesses are more likely to develop when resilience traits are lacking either before or after the trauma.
- Trauma-related illnesses can occur months or even years after a disaster or traumatic event such as war. Trauma-related illnesses, particularly PTSD, affect both children and adults, with adults more likely to have flashbacks of the incident and children more likely to develop hypersensitivity and avoidance of similar situations (e.g., avoiding cars after a motor vehicle accident).
- The Ecological Systems Theory can guide nursing assessment and interventions to help families cope effectively with trauma.
- When one or more family members are traumatized by an experience, all family members and family relationships are affected.

- The more severe the trauma that an individual family member suffers, the more likely the other members of the family are at risk for secondary trauma.
- The family response to trauma of one or more of its members cannot be understood or treated by focusing on individual family members alone. Family members can provide key contextual information about past traumatic events and experiences that help explain current responses.
- Community systems can prevent, treat, and measure negative outcomes to traumatic events. If community agencies are not well trained and prepared, the risks for undetected and untreated trauma-related illnesses increase.
- Larger political and social systems can influence and be influenced by individual, family, and community trauma. If a nation experiences severe trauma, it as a whole shows signs of trauma response.
- Nursing focuses on the individual, family, community, and societal reactions to trauma in order to optimize positive outcomes and prevent or treat negative implications.

chapter 13

Relational Nursing and Family Nursing in Canada

Colleen Varcoe, PhD, RN

Helen Brown, PhD, RN

Liz Cave, RN, MA

Critical Concepts

■ Relational inquiry rests in a socioenvironmental understanding of health and health promotion (World Health Organization, 2020). A socioenvironmental understanding of health incorporates sociological and environmental aspects, as well as medical and lifestyle choices. Thus, a person's or a family's capacity to define, analyze, and act on concerns in one's life and living conditions joins treatment, prevention, and health promotion as essential goals of nursing practice with families.

■ Families, health, and nursing are understood to be shaped by the unique historical, geographical, economic, political, and social features of the particular person's or family's context. By purposefully working with this diversity when providing care, nurses are prepared to consider the contextual nature of people's and families' health and illness experiences, and how their lives are shaped by their intrapersonal, interpersonal, and contextual circumstances to provide more effective and responsive care.

■ Context is not a circumstance outside or separate from people; rather, contextual elements (e.g., socioeconomic conditions, family and cultural histories) are literally embodied in people and within their actions and responses to particular situations.

■ Canada is prosperous, but the country has a significant and growing gap between high- and low-income segments of its population, along with a biomedical- and corporate-oriented health care system. These influences shape Canadians' health, experiences of family, and experiences of health care and nursing care. By understanding how these economic and political influences shape family experiences and nursing situations, nurses can promote health more effectively.

■ Dominant expectations and discourses about families in Canada are similar to those of other Western countries. These expectations and discourses shape Canadians' health, their experiences of family, and their experiences of health care and nursing care. By examining how families and nurses themselves draw on these expectations and discourses, nurses can improve their responsiveness to families.

■ Multiculturalism is part of Canada's national identity and is enshrined in Canadian state policy. Multiculturalism is understood in Canada to promote equality and tolerance for diversity, especially as it relates to linguistic, ethnic, and religious diversity. Tensions exist between this understanding and the lived experiences of families,

(continued)

Critical Concepts—cont'd

however, particularly those who are racialized, do not speak French or English as their first language, and are from nondominant religions. *Racialization* refers to the social process by which people are labeled according to particular physical characteristics or arbitrary ethnic or racial categories and then dealt with according to beliefs related to those labels (Henry et al., 2009; Little, 2014). In Canada, there is extensive evidence of systemic racism alongside claims to value diversity and fairness (Henry et al., 2009). Nurses who understand these realities and tensions and how they shape families and experiences are better prepared to provide responsive nursing care.

■ As a colonial country, Canada has an evolving history of oppressive and genocidal practices against Indigenous peoples and an evolving history of varied immigration practices. Understanding how migration and colonization affect both Indigenous and newcomer families and the health and lives of people within those families is fundamental to providing culturally safe and effective family nursing care.

■ Competent, safe, and ethical nursing care for families involves accounting for the intrapersonal, interpersonal, and contextual aspects of families' lives. Nurses also need to consider how their own contexts shape their understandings and responses to particular families and situations. Together, these actions enable nurses to reflect critically upon their nursing care, tailor it to the specific circumstances of families' lives, and thus mitigate making erroneous assumptions about the families they serve.

■ Without a careful consideration of context and its influence on families' health and illness experiences, nurses typically draw uncritically on stereotypes in ways that limit the health-promoting care for the families they serve. By inquiring into families' and nurses' own contexts, nurses are better able to provide responsive, ethical, and appropriate care.

For much of her life, Sarah has been acutely aware of her place within or distance from family. Shortly after she was born, she was removed from her mother's care; sometime later her mother died of drug poisoning. Since then, she has been parented by many people, including some who openly disparaged her mother's "choices." In Sarah's midteens, she dabbled in substance use; however, for the last three years she has diligently pursued abstinence from "hard drugs," echoing her caregivers' encouragement that "I am not my mom." Sarah is currently receiving the enthusiastic support of a health care team, living in a cozy "sober" housing placement, held up as a role model in her recovery community, and on track to receive a youth agreement that will provide a range of government supports for her to live independently. Sarah feels loved and cared for but at the same time conflicted.

Now, at age 18 (the same age her mother was when she was born), Sarah decided that she wanted to better understand her mother; she has been secretly going to the neighborhood that her mother called home and has started using substances while there. She feels more accepted by the community of people there than she has felt elsewhere, and she feels a renewed kinship with her mother. Part of her wants to be honest with her health care team because she relates to them like family, she is interested in pursuing harm reduction, and they will inevitably find out because of the level of police surveillance of the neighborhood where she is spending so much time. Nevertheless, she is ashamed and afraid because she knows that active substance use is incompatible with the relationships and resources of her abstinence-oriented life.

Sarah's relationship to family is and always has been intertwined with her engagement in health care. As a youngster, she noticed that it was never straightforward for her to get health care, and she is used to nurses stumbling over their realization that the caregivers accompanying her are not her guardians. Now that she is older, providers do not undergo these same contortions.

When nurses pause to locate Sarah in relation to her family, they are better able to see the risks of making assumptions, whether as a nurse who provides care to Sarah in the emergency department, sees her in an unexpected location while on outreach, or manages her care on a high-risk youth team. Indeed, given her needs for connection, income, shelter, and good health, it is apparent that Sarah has a lot to both lose and gain by connecting with her health care at this point.

While you may not know or work with anyone like Sarah, her story illustrates how a person's experience of family—as transient or permanent, as contingent or unconditional, as present or absent—influences her decisions and actions (Doane & Varcoe, 2005, 2006).

Enter relational inquiry, an orientation to nursing practice founded on complexity theory and an understanding that people and their environments are interrelated and continuously influencing one another (Doane & Varcoe, 2021). Relational inquiry rests on a socioenvironmental understanding of health and health promotion (World Health Organization [WHO], 2020). This understanding of health incorporates sociological and environmental aspects as well as medical and lifestyle (behavioral) ones. From this perspective, health is considered to be "a resource for living . . . a positive concept . . . the extent to which an individual or group is able to realize aspirations, to satisfy needs, and to change or cope with the environment" (WHO, 2020, p. 1). Promoting health and the capacity of people and families to understand, prioritize, and act on their concerns is the central goal of nursing care for families. Relational inquiry both focuses on relationships between and among individuals and places simultaneous attention on individuals' relationships with themselves and their environments, including their social, economic, historical, and language environments or contexts. *Inquiry*, then, from a relational orientation, refers to more than asking people questions; it involves asking questions of one's self continuously while also seeking to understand each person's and family's situation and how best to proceed toward optimizing health.

This chapter describes a relational inquiry approach to providing nursing care to families, with specific emphasis on the significance of context; that is, the interface of sociopolitical, historical, geographical, and economic elements in shaping the health and illness experiences of families in Canada and the implications for nursing and health care practice. This chapter begins with an explanation of family and nursing care of families and then turns to the integral role of context in providing care to families. The chapter then covers some of the key characteristics of Canadian society and how those characteristics shape health, families, health care, and nursing. Finally, a relational inquiry approach for responsive and effective nursing care for families is described.

EXPLANATION OF FAMILY AND NURSING CARE FOR FAMILIES

A relational inquiry approach for nursing care of families relies on critical analysis of what has been taken for granted in the very concept of family within the Canadian context. This requires reflecting on and questioning dominant ideas and ways of thinking about what family "is" and how family members may relate to one another in their specific contexts. For example, the concept of family is frequently sentimentalized through portrayals that imply positive experiences and that privilege blood relations for defining family relationships. These kinds of assumptions can limit a nurse's capacity for understanding and responding to diverse experiences. Sarah's experiences of family are diverse and dynamic, comprised of past, present, and future influences as she reconnects with her mother's life and navigates the present safety and connection she has experienced in her cozy "sober" shelter and moves into her future. When families are understood as diverse and dynamic and as places where both love and harm are possible, nurses are in a better position to provide care to families in a range of contexts, situations, and services. There is no one place where "family nursing" can be located, no "family nursing unit" like other specialized care areas. Whether literal family members are present or not, "family" is relevant to nurses practicing anywhere—in cancer care, long-term care, pediatrics, and the emergency department; however, family presence and care needs may be amplified in specific contexts. Relational inquiry requires questioning if any one specific practice context is more "family nursing" than others and helps nurses examine the consequences of always seeing family as relevant for providing care. All nurses, in varying ways and to different degrees and depending on specific situations, provide care to families; thus, *all nursing is family nursing*.

Relational inquiry enhances nurses' ability to encourage the capacity and power of people and families to live meaningful lives from their perspectives. Although this may involve treating and preventing disease or modifying lifestyle factors, the primary focus is on enhancing peoples' well-being, capacity, and resources for meaningful life experiences. Thus, relational inquiry focuses very specifically on how *health is a sociorelational experience* that is strongly shaped by contextual factors. Understanding and working directly with context provides a key resource and strategy for responsive, health-promoting care for people and families. Appreciating the range of diverse experiences; the different compositions of families; and the dynamics of geography, history, politics, and economics allows nurses to provide more effective care to particular families, better understand the stresses and challenges families face, and better support families to draw on their own capacities or access resources within their immediate environments. The starting point for appreciating the uniqueness and diversity *within* families requires that nurses inquire how their own lives and experiences influence their approach to nursing care for people and families.

CONTEXT IS INTEGRAL TO FAMILY NURSING

Context is often conceptualized as a sort of container of people, something that surrounds but is distinct and separate from people. This chapter, however, encourages readers to think of context as something that is integral to the lives of people, as something that not only creates people's circumstances and opportunities but also shapes their physiology at the cellular level. In other words, context is embodied. For example, if a person is born into a middle-class, English-speaking, Euro-Canadian family, the very way that person speaks—accent, intonation, vocabulary—is shaped by that context. The way that person's body grows is influenced by the nutritional value of the food and quality of water available, the level of stress, the quality of housing, and the family's opportunities for rest and physical activity. Each person's sense of self and expectations for his or her life is shaped by the circumstances into which that person is born. The individual's success in education depends not only on available educational opportunities but also on how the person comes to that education—for example, how well fed or hungry, how well rested or tired, or how confident and content they are—and the economic resources available that shape the school the person attends. It is also affected by how education is valued within the person's family and community. Thus, a person's or a family's multiple contexts cannot be left outside or cannot be understood as being outside or separate from one's self or as being under one's control. Rather, people and families embody their circumstances, and their circumstances embody them. Although people have some influence over their circumstances, such influence is generally more limited than we would like to imagine. In addition, the contextual elements and the experiences to which those elements give rise live on in people. That is, past contexts go forward within people, shaping how they experience present and future situations. For example, those descended from people who have experienced generations of persecution will experience life events differently from those who have not.

People are both influenced *by* and live *within* contexts. Throughout nursing careers, nurses provide care in specific contexts, and families live in their own diverse contexts. Consciously considering the interface of these differing contexts and how they shape families' health and illness experiences is vital to providing responsive, health-promoting care. Also foundational to this process is the need to inquire into how context shapes your own life and practice as a nurse. This enables you to choose more intentionally how to draw on those influences to enhance your responsiveness to families. For example, many nurses practice in health care settings, surrounded by well-educated and financially stable professionals. This context contrasts with many of their clients, who may lack education and live in low-income and unstable housing because of financial instability. When a nurse recognizes this difference, care includes sensitivity to the disparity between these two contexts.

CANADA IN CONTEXT

Canada is diverse in multiple ways. This section considers five key areas of diversity that are significant to families and family nursing: geographical, economic, ethnocultural, linguistic, and religious diversity. These contextual elements overlap and intersect, shaping health, experiences of family, and experiences of health care and nursing.

Geographical Diversity

Canada's varied geography, with its differing terrains and climates and ranging from dense urban settings to sparsely populated remote rural areas, shapes Canadian life. Across the prairies, the various coastal regions, the remote areas of the north, and the different mountain ranges are varied resources and climatic conditions that shape the lives of Canadians in differing ways. In 2011, Statistics Canada (2018) reported that fewer than 20% of Canadians (about 6.5 million people) were living in rural areas (areas located outside urban centers and that have a population of 10,000 or more people). According to the World Bank, historical data, development indicators, and census projections confirmed that estimate to be relatively unchanged in 2019, at 18.52% (Trading Economics, 2020). A continuing trend exists toward urbanization as more people move from rural settings to more urban communities, particularly in the southern part of Canada. As of 2018, approximately 26.5 million people were living in metropolitan areas, including in the three largest cities of Toronto, Montréal, and Vancouver (Whelan, 2020). Experts anticipate that the population in urban Canadian communities will continue to grow due to immigration patterns, better transportation, and the economy (Whelan, 2020).

Although the Canadian government committed to providing public, accessible, universal, comprehensive, and portable health care through the Canada Health Act of 1985, statistics show that people who reside in northern regions of the country have greater unmet heath needs than other Canadians (Government of Canada, 2020). People living in northern and remote regions of Canada were significantly more likely to die from cancer, injuries, and cardiovascular conditions than were people who resided in places where health care was more accessible (Young et al., 2016, 2019). This may be due to the increased time and distance people must travel to meet their needs, increasing their risk of accidents, or their inability to engage with health care or other strategies to mitigate acute and chronic conditions (Subedi et al., 2019). People's food security and access to culturally safe care is substantially reduced in the northern regions of Canada compared to urban centers and communities in southern Canada, and scholars have suggested that the government fund the provision of adequate and affordable food and housing for people (Young et al., 2016). Qualitative research also points to the importance of resisting the urge to import southern-style health care to remote communities (Burnett et al., 2020), or export people to the south of Canada for care (Kerber et al., 2019). They describe the inefficiency and burden on communities and individuals of transporting people and services, how this reintroduces colonial and imperialist logic, and how care could be better delivered to Indigenous people living in rural settings if it were more attuned to person, place, and community.

Urban settings also pose particular challenges to health. Urban contexts are typically divided into neighborhoods by levels of affluence that are in constant flux through processes of urban decay and gentrification. These divisions and processes both mirror and deepen health and health care inequities. For example, more affluent neighborhoods often support certain health resources and amenities (e.g., access to high-quality education) and block others (e.g., social housing) (Turner et al., 2018). Thus, it is not simply that urban contexts are more health promoting than rural contexts. For example, for Indigenous Canadians who do not live on reservations, living in an urban location was associated with negatively rating one's health; in contrast, those who resided in rural settings rated their health significantly higher (Bethune et al., 2019), demonstrating the complexity of social determinants of health. Perhaps Indigenous people have greater access to cultural and spiritual resources in rural settings and therefore experience a better quality of life (Bethune et al., 2019).

Geographical diversity shapes health through multiple pathways, including varied access to food, housing, and other health resources; the kinds of employment available; environmental conditions and hazards; and social patterns. The disparities in health care availability across geographical areas continue to be a challenge to the quality of nursing care. Health care services for people grappling with poverty and other forms of marginalization are often provided by the nonprofit sector, which cannot provide the level of services or wages and benefits of the public sector (Lavoie et al., 2018). Public health nursing care for families can be challenged by the distance between clients, the difficulty clients have in reaching health care centers (whether urban or rural), and a lack of resources needed to provide quality care. Nurses are often faced with having to provide care in an inadequate amount of time with limited resources in both community and hospital settings. Rural areas of

Canada in particular lack sufficient numbers of nurses to meet the complex needs of rural clients and clients with low incomes (MacLeod et al., 2017). If nurses recognize these challenges, however, they can work on a micro level to incorporate relational inquiry into even the briefest contact, asking family members how they support healthy living patterns, and they can work at a macro level by being advocates for improved health care across contexts.

Economic Diversity

Although Canada is a wealthy, developed nation, a large and steadily widening income gap exists between the rich and those with low income (Beach, 2016; Statistics Canada, 2020). Beach (2016) described how this trend can be seen through decades-long changes in characteristics of the labor market, including the progressive elimination of middle-income jobs; trends of "deskilling" and "upskilling," which make it harder for low-income people to qualify for high-income jobs; and the rise of gig, contract, and other precarious positions. As the job market has become increasingly polarized, Statistics Canada (2020) observed that many Canadians increasingly live in poverty. Indeed, as of 2018, 11% of the Canadian population lived below the poverty line, with 5.4% of Canadians reporting "deep poverty," or having incomes 75% below the poverty line. In the 2016 census, the occupants of 12.7% of Canadian residences were found to have inadequate or unaffordable housing. When families found themselves below the poverty line in 2018, the incomes they reported were on average 33.4% below this line: a greater poverty gap than was reported in 2017. The Canadian Community Health Survey revealed that between 2007 and 2018 a growing number of Canadians reported food insecurity (Statistics Canada, 2020). Other work puts Canada in global context. Since publishing its tenth report card on child poverty in the world's richest countries in 2012, UNICEF's Office of Research ranked the child poverty rate as 24th of 34 industrialized countries, or at the "top of the bottom third," compared to other affluent countries. More recently, in report card 15 on hunger among children in the world, Canada ranked 37th of 41 wealthy countries, because one in six children and four in six Inuit children do not have enough nutritious food, and one in three has an unhealthy weight (UNICEF, 2018). Thus, economic inequality is a feature of Canadian life.

The economic prosperity of Canada is disproportionately distributed, and the inequities between those who are wealthy and those who are low-income, and between those who are healthy and those who are not, continue to grow (Bezruchka, 2019; Nickel et al., 2018). People who are racialized in Canada are more likely to be economically disenfranchised. For instance, the 2011 National Household Survey found that 38% of Indigenous children resided in single-parent homes compared to only 17% of non-Indigenous children. More Indigenous people were also underhoused compared to non-Indigenous people; this was especially pronounced for Indigenous people living on reservations and Inuit people living in Nunavut (Statistics Canada, 2015a). The median after-tax income of people who identified as First Nations was $17,621 compared to $27,622 for non-Indigenous people (Statistics Canada, 2015a). Similarly, compared to people in Canada who do not identify as Black, people who are Black are paid lower wages, they are overqualified for the jobs they do, and their children are more likely to live in a low-income home. Significantly, compared to Black women and other groups, the median income of Black men declined from 2000 to 2015, which could be secondary to systemic racism (Houle, 2020). People who are newcomers to Canada and are members of underrepresented groups also have significantly lower incomes than those not so designated (Houle, 2020; Statistics Canada, 2017a).

Understanding the pervasiveness and distribution of income inequity is critical to nurses because income is a key determinant of health. People who are racialized, are new immigrants, live in rural settings, and have disabilities are more likely to be low-income and are therefore more affected by the health consequences of poverty. For example, the *2019 Report Card on Child and Family Poverty in Canada* (First Call, 2020) reported that, despite an overall national "child poverty" rate of about 18.6%, particular groups are at greater risk for poor health outcomes, including children of recent immigrants (35%), Indigenous children living on reservations (53%), and children who are racialized (22%). As with work that compared Canada with other Commonwealth countries (Nickel et al., 2018), First Call (2020) noted the history of colonialism and dispossession continues to disadvantage Indigenous people from accessing the social determinants of health. For example, young children living in poverty have diminished access to health, education, and long-term employment achievement (First Call, 2020). Substantial research shows that early adversity, including children living in poverty or suffering from abuse and neglect, is associated with diminished health and social opportunities across the life span (Metzler et al., 2017).

Ethnocultural Diversity

Canada is one of the most ethnically diverse countries in the world, and this diversity is increasing (Statistics Canada, 2017a). In 2016, there were approximately 2.1 million Indigenous people in Canada, comprising 6.2% of the Canadian population. Of the three Indigenous groups, First Nations people were the largest (1.5 million), followed by Métis (600,000), and Inuit people (79,125) (Statistics Canada, 2017a). More than 250 different ethnic origins were reported in the 2016 Canadian census (Statistics Canada, 2017a). In 2016, an estimated 20% of the Canadian population was born outside Canada (Evra & Kazemipur, 2019). Between 2011 and 2016, 1.2 million people immigrated to Canada, representing 16.1% of Canada's immigrant population (Statistics Canada, 2017b). Of the more than 13.4 million immigrants who came to Canada during the 20th century, the largest number arrived during the 1990s (Statistics Canada, 2016). The origins of immigrants to Canada have changed in recent decades, with increasing numbers coming from non-European countries. In the 2016 census, the majority of immigrants reported being born in Asia (70%), whereas only 15% of immigrants came from European countries (Statistics Canada, 2017b).

Although Canada has official state policy that advocates equality and promotes tolerance through multiculturalism, many argue that the rhetoric of multiculturalism authorizes inequities and discrimination based on ethnicity and racism by implying that inequality might be explained by apolitical cultural difference (Thobani, 2018). As discussed above, people who are Indigenous to Canada, who are newcomers, or who are visible minorities experience economic disadvantage. Nevertheless, visible minorities who are newcomers have been shown to report less experience with discrimination than their second-generation counterparts (Vang & Cheng, 2019). This may be because newcomers are not as aware of their subordinate position in society as their children, who can observe the disjuncture between the ideals taught in the Canadian school system and the opportunities available to them (Vang & Cheng, 2019). Indeed, studies have shown that many newcomer children and youth feel mistreated and isolated by both peers and teachers (Oxman-Martinez & Ri Cho, 2014; Oxman-Martinez et al., 2012). Henry and colleagues (2009) argue that in Canada a form of racism is practiced wherein policies and rhetoric promote equity and justice and simultaneously tolerate widespread discrimination.

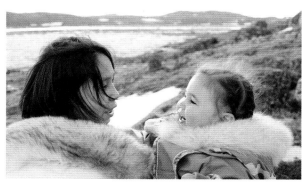

Source: © iStock.com/RyersonClark

Racism has significant health effects. Discrimination based on race has been linked with health outcomes such as hypertension and other chronic diseases (Siddiqi et al., 2017), mental health problems (Colizzi et al., 2020), low birthweight (Alhusen, 2016), and complications among childbearing people (Brennenstuhl, 2018). For example, Veenstra's (2009) analysis of the Canadian Community Health Survey found significant relative risk for poor health for people identifying as Indigenous, Indigenous/White, Black, Chinese, or South Asian that were not explained by socioeconomic status, gender, age, immigrant status, or location, suggesting that institutional and everyday racism and discrimination play an important role. This was confirmed by researchers who analyzed 28 studies (literature review and meta-analysis conducted between 2013 and 2019) that identified racial discrimination as an emerging risk factor for disease and as a contributor to racial disparities in health (Williams et al., 2019).

Changing immigration patterns and increasing ethnic diversity coupled with discriminatory policies and attitudes influence families' experiences and health. Migration processes are stressful, and this stress is intensified when combined with language barriers and downward economic mobility (Papademetriou et al., 2009) and racism. Nevertheless, the resilience of newcomer and Indigenous communities in Canada should not be underestimated. Indeed, forming friendships or having family in Canada prior to one's arrival is associated with higher employment income (Evra & Kazemipur, 2019), and connection to rural communities was also correlated with better health outcomes among Indigenous people (Bethune et al., 2019). These factors combined with structural barriers to care (cost, accessibility, transportation), health care providers' lack of understanding of people's circumstances, and clients' lack of familiarity with health care processes add to risks for poor health care. Nurses can minimize these risks by striving to understand families' circumstances, supporting families' navigation of health care contexts, and advocating for optimal care.

Linguistic Diversity

Consistent with its history as a colonial nation and destination for immigrants from around the globe, Canada is linguistically diverse. The 2016 census recorded more than 70 Indigenous languages, grouped into 12 distinct language families, and more than 260,550 people reported speaking an Indigenous language. While colonial efforts eradicated many Indigenous languages, the overall number of Indigenous language speakers grew by 3.1% in 10 years (Statistics Canada, 2017c). Most Canadians speak one or both of the official languages: French and English. Yet in 2016, about one of every five people reported having a mother tongue other than English or French (LePage, 2020). Of these, one-third reported that the only language they spoke at home was a language other than English or French, that is, a nonofficial language. During the past few decades, language groups from Asia and the Middle East increased in number, and Chinese is now the third largest language group after English and French (Statistics Canada, 2017c).

Language affects health in many ways. First, because language is connected to identity, reclaiming and revitalizing language is critical for cultural identity due to the ongoing impacts of colonialism for both Indigenous peoples and immigrants to Canada (McIvor, 2018). When individuals and families have their cultural identity erased through assimilation policies, they face increased risk of isolation and depression that can make accessing health care unsafe and initiate a cascade of related risks for secondary poor mental health outcomes. Second, language barriers profoundly affect access to employment and social resources and those related to health literacy. Finally, language barriers can be direct barriers when receiving health care and communicating with health care providers (de Moissac & Bowen, 2019; Wang et al., 2019; Government of Canada, 2016).

Some people who speak the dominant languages of Canada presume that everyone should learn French or English without considering the resources required and the barriers (such as poverty, transportation, discrimination, ability, accessibility) to doing so. Very limited supports are available for language acquisition, and in the case of immigrant families, the priority for who accesses language classes is often the person who is most likely to obtain employment. This pattern increases health risks for those who are unemployed and those without the ability to speak the dominant languages, including single parents, disabled adults, and children. Nurses can advocate by assisting families with the use of interpreters, connecting families to community resources that teach languages, and using visual pictures and icons to explain health care procedures rather than just verbal instructions.

Religious Diversity

Canada is also a country of considerable religious diversity. Historically, Canada has been predominately Christian, yet this pattern is changing. In a recent survey conducted by the Pew Research Center (2018), 55% of Canadian adults reported that they are Christian, including 29% who are Catholic and 18% who are Protestant. Approximately 8% reported being atheist, being agnostic (5%), or having no religious affiliation (16%). In addition, a rising number (8%) of Canadian adults identified with other faiths, including Islam, Hinduism, Sikhism, Judaism, and Buddhism, due in large part to immigration (Pew Research Center, 2018). Despite this changing profile, Christianity continues to dominate many Canadian public institutions, including health care (Smith, 2018).

Religious affiliation affects health in multiple ways, including fostering social inclusion and community support, and, depending on the religion, serving as a basis for discrimination and negative effects on health practices, access to care, and acceptance of care. While immigration to Canada by people from diverse religious backgrounds increases and anti-Semitism and anti-Muslim escalates globally, Canada has professed its tolerance for diversity. Religiously diverse individuals and families are at risk for violence, hate speech, harassment, discrimination, and vandalism (U.S. Department of State, 2019). However, between 2017 and 2018, religiously motivated hate crimes in Canada dropped by 24%, including a decrease of 50% in crimes against Muslims and a decrease of 4% in crimes against Jews (U.S. Department of State, 2019).

In order to offer responsive nursing care, nurses require a relational inquiry approach to learn about what is important and meaningful for individuals and families and to acknowledge people's experiences of discrimination (Varcoe et al., 2019). Nurses can provide appropriate care by asking all people they serve about their religious affiliations and how their beliefs affect their values and beliefs about healing. Nurses should also try to learn families' expectations regarding how health care professionals can incorporate religious beliefs into their treatment plan when appropriate and possible. Nurses cannot be knowledgeable about all religions; therefore, it is essential to follow the lead of the families and individuals served. For example, in some hospital settings, health care providers have repeatedly shaved off the facial hair of Sikh men, against their will and against their beliefs and practices (Kaur Kang-Dhillon et al., 2020). This could have been avoided had the providers inquired about what was important to the people involved and held their well-being as being of greater importance than the preferences of providers.

HOW FAMILY IS UNDERSTOOD IN CANADA

Given this incredible geographical, economic, ethnic, and religious diversity, what constitutes family in Canada and how family is lived and experienced varies greatly. Despite this diversity, however, age-old assumptions about family continue to dominate. These ideas shape our expectations about families, such as that families are "normally" nuclear and are composed of a mother, father, and two children. They shape policies, such as the idea that people receiving social assistance should turn to extended family and exhaust family resources before accepting social assistance. And they also shape health care providers' expectations and practices, such as the belief that families should (and are able to) provide care to elderly members. Exploring and critically scrutinizing these dominant ideas in light of the diverse contextual elements that shape any particular family assists nurses to understand their own and families' expectations, the differences between those expectations, and tensions that might arise among different stakeholders.

Three general assumptions or expectations about family are especially useful for nurses to explore in order to understand families in Canada and similar industrialized Western countries. First, families are generally assumed to be nuclear, that is, to consist of two generations, including parents (generally assumed to be heterosexual) and children. Second, women generally are expected to do the majority of parenting and caregiving. Third, family is generally held to be a safe and nurturing experience. In reality, however, people's experiences vary greatly and differ from these assumptions.

Heterosexual Nuclear Family as the So-Called Norm

The dominance of the idea that the heterosexual nuclear family is the norm is belied by statistics and slowly shifting with challenges to simplistic understandings of gender as a binary (male/female) and greater awareness of gender diversity. For instance, the number of same-sex couples increased steadily in Canada from 2006 to 2016, at about six times the rate of opposite-sex couples. Similarly, the number of same-sex couples who resided with children increased during this time. As of 2016, same-sex couples comprised almost 1% of all couples, 12% of whom lived with children (Statistics Canada, 2017d). More generally, according to the 2016 census, approximately 30% of all children were living in families not comprised of two biological or adoptive parents; roughly 10% are living with other relatives or other caregivers, 10% are living with a parent and a stepparent, and 10% are in single-parent families. The number of lone mothers heading families is, in part, a reflection of the prevalence of violence against women and the social expectation for women to leave abusive partners. Nearly one-third of all police-reported violence occurs between intimate partners, which has a disproportionate impact on women, who are approximately 8 in 10 victims, or 79% of all reported intimate partner violence (IPV) (Conroy et al., 2019).

In 2016, the number of father-led single-parent households continued to increase. This decades-long trend is partially explained by the rise of father's rights as a backlash against feminist gains in child custody, particularly in the context of violence against women, courts' growing recognition of a father's capacity to parent, and a corollary increase in court-ordered joint custody to men (Statistics Canada, 2015b; Bohnert et al., 2014). While the social factors influencing increased father-led single-parent families arose from civil rights discourses in the 1960s, Statistics Canada (2015b) helps in avoiding overestimating the novelty of this situation, noting that in the early twentieth century when maternal mortality was higher, more single-parent families were led by fathers. Bohnert et al. (2014) also observed that more orphaned children were raised by relatives in 1901 than in 2011. Hence, while the social factors underlying the rates and numbers of non-nuclear families change, these data show that people in Canada have adapted family structures to meet changing circumstances for more than a century.

Although the number of single-person households is at an all-time high in Canada, multigenerational homes are the fastest growing type of living situation. This is especially true among Indigenous people in Canada's north as well as among newcomers to Canada (Battams, 2017). Although some people construe living in households with larger numbers of people as a cultural preference, the shift toward this structure may have more to do with increased housing prices and downward trends in the labor market (Battams, 2017). In addition, the overcrowded and underhoused conditions in which northern Indigenous people report living signal that economic pressures require the adoption of multigenerational arrangements (Statistics Canada, 2015a).

These trends have important implications for nursing care. For example, nurses should not expect children to have two heterosexual parents in their home. Nurses need to understand the current family structure and avoid assumptions or biases based on stereotypes about expected norms. Each family structure has benefits and risks, and nurses need both to assess these within families and to understand how changes in structure may influence child development. For example, although grandparents raising grandchildren may also be negotiating economic challenges, this arrangement has been shown to increase grandparents' sense of purpose as well as offer children a loving and stable home with natural supports (Sumo et al., 2018). Nurses also need to be familiar with and connect families to appropriate support services to help families do the best they can for their children regardless of the family structure. For example, some provinces provide some financial support, health care, and legal support for grandparents raising their grandchildren.

Ideals of Motherhood and Women

In Canada, prevalent ideas about mothering and women shape families' experiences, their health, and health care provider expectations. These include the idea that women live with male partners and are the primary caretakers for their children. Despite the diversity of family structures and roles, in Canada, the social ideal continues to be that a woman mothers children within a two-parent family (Lam et al., 2020), with the ideal being exclusive mothering, or mothering without work outside the home. Another social expectation for women is primary responsibility for family caregiving for dependent elders or those who are ill or have disabilities, especially in the wake of changes to the health care and social services systems that include deinstitutionalization of care.

These expectations are at odds with other social forces, however, including financial forces and changes to views about women's interests and capabilities. Women, including mothers, are increasingly expected and desire to work outside the home (Statistics Canada, 2017e). In 2014, 69.5% of women with children younger than age 6 were employed, more than double the figure in 1976, when only 32.1% of these women were employed. Women's employment has been shown to increase as their children age; in 2014, 81.4% of women with children 12 to 17 living at home were part of the employed workforce, compared to 51.4% in

1974 (Moyser, 2017). Social policies, such as workfare social assistance policies, increasingly provide financial assistance to women with dependent children only if they seek employment, making many women feel they are forced into waged labor, even when the work available is not adequate to cover the costs of safe child care. At the same time, policies such as minimum wage levels inadequate to meet basic needs have deepened women's poverty, even as they attempt to participate in the wage labor force (Smith-Carrier, 2017). Women are also seeking higher education and more professional careers, and they continue to achieve university and college credentials at a higher rate than men. Beginning at the baccalaureate level, the earnings discrepancy between women and men is narrowing (Ferguson, 2016). This trend has also contributed to women shifting away from full-time caregiving to the more common situation of responsibilities to work, career, and home.

When families are judged against the ideal of exclusive mothering, or against the ideals of family caregiving, they are often found wanting. That is, when women do not devote themselves to mothering exclusively or take up caregiving for a parent, spouse, or other dependent person and forego labor force participation, they are often judged as inadequate. Still, the economic and social conditions do not exist for most women to care for children and other dependents without also participating in wage work. In Canada, as in most Western countries, the typical mother is working outside the home, is often the lone head of a household, and may also be living under or near the poverty line, while at the same time being responsible for mothering and/or caregiving of other family members. These trends, juxtaposed against ideals of good mothering, have contributed to phrases such as "working mother" and "welfare mom" that convey negative judgments.

Family as Safe and Nurturing

In Canada, as in many Western countries, family is portrayed generally as positive, supportive, and safe. But statistics belie this ideal as well. Canada is similar to other Western countries in the levels of violence perpetrated within families and the levels of substance use, both of which counter the notion of families as safe. In 2018, police-reported violent crime statistics included 18,965 child and

youth victimized by a family member; of these, a parent (59%) was the most common perpetrator, followed by another type of family member—such as a grandparent, uncle, or aunt—or a sibling (24% and 16%, respectively) (Conroy et al., 2019). There were 12,202 senior victims (aged 65 and older) of police-reported violence in Canada in 2018 (Conroy et al., 2019). Police-reported crimes represent only a small fraction of violent incidents, underscoring the point that many families are harmful and dangerous.

Problematic substance use within families is another factor that may make the experience of family less than safe and nurturing. Alcohol is by far the substance most commonly used by Canadians; at least 20% of drinkers consume above Canada's Low-Risk Alcohol Drinking Guidelines (Canadian Centre on Substance Abuse and Addiction, 2017). Between 2015 and 2016, there were approximately 77,000 hospitalizations caused by alcohol, compared to 75,000 hospitalizations for heart attacks (Canadian Centre on Substance Abuse and Addiction, 2017). While research suggests that involvement with family is protective against harms related to substance use, particularly among young people (Khan, 2017; Qadeer et al., 2019), it also shows that substance use can have significant negative effects on families (Pearson, 2015). For example, having a parent with a substance use problem is considered an adverse childhood event (ACE). ACEs have been associated with myriad negative outcomes in Canada, including substance use problems among youth (Afifi et al., 2020), and heavy drinking, drug use, depressed affect, and suicide attempts in adulthood (Merrick et al., 2017). Thus, although many families are safe and nurturing, nurses cannot safely assume this is the case given the evidence regarding violence and substance use.

Given what we know about the ubiquity of violence against women, children, and older persons and the levels of substance use, nurses can anticipate that many families they meet are experiencing or have been affected by violence, problematic substance use, or other significant problems. Due to the gravity of harm and the frequency with which people experience IPV, it may seem counterintuitive that universal screening at the point of care is discouraged. Indeed, in Canada, although it is mandatory to report child abuse, it is not recommended to screen for child abuse; because of the high rate of false-positive results in screening for child maltreatment and the potential for incorrectly labeling people as child abusers, the possible harms outweigh the benefits (MacMillan & Canadian Task Force on Preventive Health Care, 2000. Further, a meta-synthesis of 44 articles on 42 studies by McTavish et al. (2017) reported that, although some articles (14%) reported positive experiences associated with mandatory reporting, negative experiences were reported in 73% of the articles, including harm to therapeutic relationships and child death following removal from their family of origin. Similarly, insufficient evidence of benefit has been reported to warrant screening for other forms of violence (McTavish et al., 2107), and there are no legal reporting requirements for other forms of abuse outside child abuse. Rather than screening, it is widely recommended that nurses practice from a trauma-and-violence-informed perspective (Wathen & Varcoe, 2019). Trauma-and-violence-informed care is based on understanding the pervasiveness of interpersonal violence so that nurses assume anyone may have experienced or may be experiencing violence (Wathen & Varcoe, 2019). In relation to IPV, WHO recommends case finding, that is, asking about violence when assessing conditions, for example, depression or chronic pain, that may be caused by or made worse by such violence (WHO, 2013). In short, nurses can best support families by being sensitive to how power and violence operate in intimate relationships and being prepared to respond to indications of misuse of power in intimate relationships through focused assessments and interventions.

THE CANADIAN HEALTH CARE CONTEXT

The funding and structure of the Canadian health care system influence families, health, and family nursing. Although Canada has universal health care and all Canadian citizens have access to what are termed *medically necessary services*, there are considerable inequities in access to health care, and these inequities are deepening as the health care system is increasingly privatized. The privatized portion of health care primarily includes funding for services and products not covered by the public services and not considered medically necessary, such as vision and dental care, cosmetic surgery, most home health services, and

pharmaceuticals. The amount covered and not covered by the public health care system varies from province to province. This means that many important elements of health care are paid for by individuals or by private insurance. Therefore, in most provinces, medications outside the hospital, many types of treatments such as physiotherapy, and services such as home care are paid for privately in whole or in part.

Thus, despite commitment to universal access, access to health care in Canada is inequitable along many dimensions (Kalich et al., 2016; Horrill et al., 2019). Families in rural settings have access to fewer services and must pay for their own transportation, accommodation, and loss of income to access services. Families without private insurance and those with lower incomes face more financial hardship associated with illness. Because some groups of people are more likely to have lower incomes, such as those who are elderly, those with disabilities, and women, families with members from such groups are more likely to face greater barriers.

Although the Canadian health care system has been dominated by hospital care, during the past several decades, fiscal concerns have stimulated shifts to decrease hospital care and increase care provided at home. From mental illness to surgery, to maternity care, to elder care, to end-of-life care, the trend has been to deinstitutionalize care, shorten the length of stay, and shift to care in the community. Care in the community mostly means care by family members, which affects family well-being and health and in turn affects patterns of family nursing (Becque et al., 2019; del Pino Casado et al., 2019). Nurses need to provide added support to all family members in teaching home health care to avoid women in the family suffering from role overload and caregiver burnout. Nurses can also help advocate for families needing hospitalized care longer when family members are unable to care for the individual at home.

As stated earlier, family nursing is not funded or identified as a separate area of practice in Canada, with most nurses still practicing in hospital settings. Because government health care funding covers only what is deemed to be medically necessary, only a very small proportion of nursing care in homes and communities is funded, leaving families to pay directly. In some areas, the shortage of primary-care physicians has increasingly made room for family nurse practitioners to provide primary care and enhance health care access. These trends shape families' experiences of health and affect their health care.

FAMILY NURSING PRACTICE: ATTENDING TO CONTEXT

This chapter has outlined the significance of context and offered details on the specific context in which nurses operate in Canada. As the discussion earlier highlighted, families in Canada live diverse lives that are shaped by the interface of geography, economics, culture, language, and religion. Similarly, their lives and their health and illness experiences are shaped by differing understandings and forms of family and by the imperfect health care system in place in Canada. This health care system, including policies and norms that dominate health care practices, has been built on limited understandings of family and health. For example, understandings of family most often reflect Eurocentric, post–World War II notions of the nuclear two-parent, heterosexual family. This discrepancy between the reality of families' lives and the normative expectations and understandings of family often dominates health care settings and practices and makes attending to context not only important but ethically essential in family nursing practice.

Overall, attending to context requires taking a relational stance of inquiry. It involves listening carefully to families; inquiring into their health and illness situations; paying attention to, observing, and critically considering the ways in which contextual elements are embodied in people and families and shape their experiences; and reflecting on how current contextual aspects might be addressed to promote health. An essential feature of this inquiry process is reflexive consideration of your own contextual location, including your values, norms, and assumptions of family, health, and nursing that inform your practice.

The following case study illustrates the significance of context to families' health experiences and how attending to context enhances nursing care. As you read Morgan's story, stay mindful of the contextual elements that may be shaping the experiences of the two families. Focus on how the elements discussed earlier (e.g., geography, economics, culture, language, religion, understandings of family, health care policies, and normative practices) are shaping the experience and responses of the different family members and of Morgan as a nurse. Also note how Morgan is or is not attending to those elements as they engage with the families. Ask yourself how your own context is similar to or different from Morgan's and from the two families'. Reflect on how those similarities and differences might affect how you would respond as a nurse and how you would provide care.

Case Study: Morgan's Story

After several years of experience on a pediatric medical unit, Morgan has begun to work in a pediatric diabetic teaching clinic. They just completed a 1-week orientation and this morning is about to do an intake on two families new to the clinic. It is clinic policy to have a half-hour appointment for intake and 15 minutes for subsequent appointments. Families usually attend the clinic for about three or four sessions biweekly, depending on their needs. The referral information Morgan has on the two families is as follows:

- *Family 1:* Justin Henderson, 11 years old, is from Stony Lake Reserve.[1] Justin has been newly diagnosed with diabetes. He began an insulin regimen on Tuesday (3 days earlier) that was ordered by the general practitioner in a walk-in clinic

[1]Precursors to the modern reserve system existed in Canada prior to Confederation and the Indian Act as products of the colonial drive to "civilize" Indigenous peoples by introducing them to agriculture, Christianity, and a sedentary way of life based on private property. An Indian Reserve in Canada was created within this assimilation agenda: "The great aim of our legislation has been to do away with the tribal system and assimilate the Indian people in all respects with the other inhabitants of the Dominion as speedily as they are fit to change" (John A Macdonald, 1887). A reserve is a tract of land set aside under the Indian Act in 1867 for First Nations Bands; reserves are not owned by bands but are held in trust for bands by the State to enact power, control, and authority over daily life. More about the Canadian Indian Act and its regulations over reserves can be found here (Government of Canada, 2021): http://laws-lois.justice.gc.ca/eng/acts/i-5/.

(continued)

Case Study: Morgan's Story—cont'd

close to where he lives. Justin was referred to the clinic for diabetic teaching and counseling, and this is his first visit to the clinic.

- *Family 2:* Greg Stanek, 12 years old, is from Belcarra. Greg has been newly diagnosed with diabetes. His insulin regimen was started yesterday by the family's general practitioner, who referred Greg to the clinic for diabetic teaching and counseling. This is his first visit.

Justin's appointment was scheduled for 9:00, but he does not arrive on time. At 9:15, Morgan decides to see the other new client, Greg Stanek, because he and his father arrived early. Greg seems small for his age; he is thin and looks quite pale. He is very quiet and barely looks at Morgan. Greg's father speaks with heavily accented English that Morgan recognizes as Czech, in part because Morgan associates Belcarra with the large community of people who emigrated from the Czech Republic. Morgan does a brief physical assessment, noting that Greg is 4 feet 8 inches (142 cm) tall but weighs only 41 kg (about 90 pounds). Morgan attempts to take the family history as outlined on the intake form, but Greg's father wants to address the fact that he cannot bring his son to clinic. Greg's father tells Morgan that he was just laid off from his job as a carpet layer and is required by unemployment insurance policies to be searching for work. Mr. Stanek says bitterly that when he came to Canada, he had been promised he could find work in his field as a mining engineer. Greg's mother works in a local meat-processing plant, and she cannot take time off to bring Greg to the clinic without risking the loss of her job.

Morgan reinforces with the father how important it is for Greg to learn about his diabetes and how to manage it, and how important supportive family is. Mr. Stanek becomes annoyed and insists that they cannot come to the clinic again. As Greg's father becomes more frustrated, Morgan finds it more difficult to understand what he is saying because of his heavy accent and rapid talking. Morgan tries to engage Greg by asking him how he is feeling and how it is going at school, but Greg answers Morgan's questions by shrugging his shoulders and saying, "Okay." Greg's father attempts to return the conversation back to his own concerns. Eventually, Morgan says, "I'll see what I can do." The half-hour clinic visit ends with little of the intake form completed, all parties feeling frustrated, and no follow-up appointment scheduled. As Morgan walks out of the room, the clinic receptionist lets Morgan know that Justin and a woman, who turns out to be his grandmother, have been waiting for their appointment.

Morgan reviews what is known about Justin from reading his intake information. Morgan remembers that the Stony Lake Reserve is located several hours from the hospital in which the clinic is located, and that Jackson is a small town near the reserve. Morgan wonders how Justin and his grandmother got to the clinic today. Morgan walks into the room apologizing for keeping them waiting and asks if they drove to the appointment. Justin's grandmother says one of her brothers drove them because the appointment was too early to be able to come by bus. She also shares that she had to borrow money to pay her brother for gas.

Morgan does a brief physical assessment on Justin. Justin, similar to Greg, barely looks at Morgan, even when Morgan addresses him directly. Justin appears somewhat overweight, as does his grandmother, and on assessment Morgan notes that he is 4 feet 5 inches tall (134.62 cm) and weighs 55 kg (121 lb). With Justin and his grandmother, who introduces herself as Rose Tarlier, the intake assessment goes more smoothly for Morgan. Mrs. Tarlier tells Morgan that she has had custody of Justin and his two younger sisters since he was 4 years old and the sisters were infants. She shares with Morgan that Justin's mother, her daughter, has had problems with her mental health for many years, is now living in Montréal, and has not seen her children for several years. Mrs. Tarlier makes it a point to tell Morgan that she herself has been "clean and sober" for more than 20 years. As the intake assessment continues, Morgan finds out that Justin's grandmother gives Justin his insulin and helps him check his blood sugar. Morgan listens as the grandmother describes what she has been doing, and Morgan provides positive feedback and encouragement. Although Morgan tries to bring Justin into the conversation, he does not look up and does not answer Morgan's questions. Morgan reviews what subsequent appointments will cover and, thinking about the distance and gas money, asks if they need one longer appointment next week rather than the usual two short ones a week apart, and schedules the next appointment.

Taking a Relational Inquiry Stance

Attending to context begins by taking a relational inquiry stance to understand and inquire into what is meaningful and significant to a particular family, their current experience, and the contextual intricacies shaping everyday life. From this stance, what becomes immediately apparent is the way that contextual forces have contributed to and are shaping each of the families' situations. For example, although Justin's family may want to live in the Indigenous community for cultural and social reasons,

Case Study: Morgan's Story—cont'd

they may have little choice for economic reasons. Justin's grandmother may well be one of many Indigenous women living on low income or in poverty. High rates of poverty among Indigenous people have overwhelming effects on health, with the life expectancy of Indigenous people being 12 years fewer than the overall Canadian population (Kolahdooz et al., 2015). Also, infant mortality and stillbirth rates are higher among Indigenous people than among the rest of the Canadian population (Gilbert et al., 2015). As noted, Indigenous children are much more likely to live in poverty than other Canadian children.

The fact that Justin lives on a reserve may negatively influence his health care access and ability to adhere to recommendations. The matrix of policies related to Indigenous people in Canada has ensured that many reserve communities have been denied access to traditional foods and face food insecurity (fish, game, naturally growing plants) and have substandard housing, poor water supplies, and insufficient income opportunities.

Justin's grandmother had been forced into a residential school in her early life and both his mother and grandmother had experiences with alcohol addiction. Those experiences, combined with the current situation with Justin's grandmother being his primary caregiver, present a clear example of the impact colonization has on family well-being. Historical colonizing policies and practices in Canada included the creation of the Indian Act; displacement of entire communities onto reserves, often with insufficient resources to sustain daily life; government appropriation of Indigenous lands; forced removal of children into residential schools; outlawing of cultural and spiritual practices; and widespread discriminatory attitudes toward Indigenous peoples. The effects of colonization continue to shape people's health, social, and economic status today (Nickel et al., 2018). Colonizing practices continue as Indigenous people are racialized by wider society and governed by race-based policies, including those related to land ownership, education, banking, and health care.

Although Justin and his grandmother's situation may not reflect all these contextual challenges, this historical and current contextual backdrop shapes their situation and responses to health care providers, including their willingness and ability to attend the clinic. The challenges they face accessing the clinic (e.g., appointment times that do not coincide with bus schedules, having younger children to care for, the cost of travel) may make coming to the clinic seem less than positive in terms of the effect on Justin's and the family's overall health.

Similarly, Greg's family experience has been shaped by multiple factors. Both parents are facing significant job insecurity. The family has experienced immigration laws and policies that limit employment opportunities and contribute to the downward mobility experienced by many well-educated immigrants. Children in recent immigrant families and racialized families are most likely to live in poverty because of overrepresentation of racialized groups in low-paying jobs, market failure to recognize international work experience and credentials, and racial discrimination in employment (First Call, 2020).

Canada is a country of considerable ethnic diversity, but despite national commitment to tolerance and multiculturalism, racialized groups experience considerable discrimination in policies, institutions, and the attitudes expressed toward them at an interpersonal level. Was this playing out during the clinic visit? Although it may not have been Morgan's intent to be discriminatory, the way they disregarded the contextual reality of Mr. Stanek's employment and its implications for future clinic visits and the frustration they felt toward him was a form of intolerance. Inquiring into context would have enabled Morgan to be aware of the likelihood of discriminatory experiences that Mr. Stanek has faced and of the potential health effects.

Listening and Paying Attention to Experience and Context

Attending to context involves listening carefully to families and to what is meaningful and significant within the current context of their lives. For Justin and his grandmother, who live in a rural setting, and for Greg's family, where both parents need to work, it becomes apparent that geography, economics, and health are intricately intertwined. For example, what is most significant for Morgan is getting Greg's family to attend the clinic so Greg's diabetes can be monitored and addressed, but for Greg's father, finding and maintaining employment is of greatest concern. The experience of being told that he would be able to work in his profession and then finding that this was not the case may well be influencing his response and willingness to engage with yet another authority and institution that does not seem to be recognizing the importance of his employment or interested in what is most pressing for him. Although Morgan cannot address the employment concern directly within a nursing role (i.e., Morgan cannot help find him a job), it is obvious that those concerns will ultimately affect Greg's experience and management of diabetes. Thus, listening to and recognizing the interrelationship of those concerns regarding how the family will be able and willing to care for Greg and his diabetes is crucial.

(continued)

Case Study: Morgan's Story—cont'd

In fact, the well-intended clinic may be heightening health challenges for families by not considering these contextual elements. Even how clinic appointments have been structured as short, frequent sessions affects both families' ability to attend the clinic and ignores the socioenvironmental elements affecting families' health on a day-to-day basis. Thus, attending to family context involves also attending to the health care context. Depending on the setting of care, the nurse would have to work within that context to support more responsive care. For example, is it possible to have fewer, longer appointments? Can the appointments be done by phone or Zoom? Do the clients have e-mail and internet access? Are there shuttles available to the clinic? Is a longer intake visit possible—not just for Greg's family but for others as well? Can the clinic offer evening appointments? Even within the prescribed time frame, the nurse should acknowledge what is of meaning and significance to the family whether or not the nurse can directly address the immediate concern.

Attending to context involves acknowledging Greg's father's distress about his employment and inviting him to talk about how it has been for different family members as they have sought employment and attempted to build a life with limited resources, support, or both. As part of this process, it would be important to communicate genuine respect, interest, and concern, asking what might be helpful from the client's perspective and how the clinic could assist the father in caring for Greg's diabetes in light of the other challenges the family is experiencing. On the surface, focusing on the father's concerns might not seem to be the top nursing priority (or even relevant to diabetic care), but doing so might reduce frustration for both Morgan and Greg's father, make better use of time, and allow them to attend to Greg's diabetes more effectively. If the family concerns are not addressed, Greg's care is jeopardized because he may not come back to the clinic, which may in turn affect the family's resources and capacities to provide support for Greg's diabetes treatment regime.

Listening and paying attention to experience and context with Justin's family brings attention to the geographical distance between the family's home and the clinic and raises questions about other possibilities for supporting the family in diabetes care. For example, knowing the economic statistics for Indigenous women, the cost of travel to the clinic might have a negative impact on the family. If the family is on a limited income, frequent travel may be impossible and may take money from other essential needs. In response, Morgan might look into resources at the local level, such as a community health representative or local community health nurse, who might be able to provide face-to-face care to the family while liaising with the clinic using telehealth or videoconferencing so that the family does not need to travel such a great distance so frequently.

Overall, attending to context sets one up to be curious, to be interested, and to inquire rather than make judgments and assumptions based on surface characteristics and behaviors. For example, both Greg and Justin were quiet, did not make eye contact, and responded minimally to Morgan. Rather than making assumptions about the children based on their own location and context, Morgan might intentionally reflect on the contexts in which the families have been living recently. Therefore, their responses might be viewed through a range of interpretations and possibilities, including everything from wondering about the physiological effect of diabetes to the immediate effect of the diagnosis of diabetes, to the experience of coming to the clinic for the first time, to the multiple contextual experiences and challenges they and their families have been facing. Part of assessing the context also includes paying attention to how culture shapes families' ways of being and their needs, interactions, and experiences with the health care system. When family members experience discrimination based on gender, racism, classism, ageism, ableism, sizeism, and other forms of isms, it shapes their reactions to health professionals and may deter them from seeking care altogether. For example, avoiding eye contact can signal a person or family member's lack of safety due to unequal power relations. It is quite likely that, for both Justin and Greg, the clinic context felt institutional and authoritative, regardless of Morgan's efforts to connect and inquire. Attending to context can cue nurses to stay open to possibilities, such as reflecting on how welcoming the clinic is through the eyes of youth, and gently and thoughtfully reaching out to connect with people and families as they are experiencing the present moment. Rather than focusing on behavior or lack of response as a problem or frustration, any response is viewed contextually and can signal a nurse's potential action. People and families cannot be measured against any norms; rather, the goal is to use inquiry rather than judgment to understand their reactions contextually and to respond in a meaningful and relevant manner.

Attending to context helps nurses respond to both the immediate situation of particular patients and to question how larger policies and structures governing practice and the clinic are affecting families. That is, the contextual particularities of these families reveal limitations of the policies and structures of the clinic more generally. Clinic policies and structures might have to be changed to be more responsive to families. For example, offering home visits, evening appointments, or both for families who have both

Case Study: Morgan's Story—cont'd

parents working and are unable to make daytime appointments might enhance the clinic's responsiveness. Similarly, seeing the family in context draws attention to the importance of working with the contexts within which the families live. This could include everything from intentionally establishing relationships with government departments and community agencies that are part of the family's context and that might liaise with the clinic in providing services and resources to lobbying for increased access and resources for particular groups or particular services and supplies.

In regard to the families in the case study, first, nurses would want to optimize their ability to provide effective care given the restrictions within the current system. Nurses must prioritize care to both acknowledge the families' circumstances and begin to support Greg and Justin within their families and their circumstances. Beyond a more flexible pattern of appointments, are there other providers who might be involved? A social worker, child and youth care worker, or other resources may be available. Ways to enhance access to health care, such as resources for transportation, may be available. Nurses would want to draw on broader social resources, such as those related to immigration and employment, working parents (i.e., evening hours, weekend hours, online care, etc.), and parents (i.e., counseling; support groups; other forms of diabetic care education such as local classes, online classes, and books; home health services). Acknowledging Greg's father's concerns and supporting him through referrals would allow the nurse to integrate attention to the family while focusing on Greg and his diabetes. In so doing, Morgan will develop approaches and knowledge of resources for a range of other families as well.

Reflexivity

Reflexivity, or intentional and critical reflection on one's own understanding and actions in context, is central to using contextual knowledge. Reflexivity draws attention to a nurse's own contextual background, including taken-for-granted assumptions, stereotypes, and the knowledge one draws on when engaging with families. Examining how each nurse's own context and social location shape and structure her or his nursing is a first step to attending to families' contexts. For example, if Morgan had grown up in a rural setting or in poverty, it would be important to consider reflexively how those experiences influence them when working with families who share that context and social location. Morgan's background might lead them to see themselves as successful despite those constraints and to overlook how the challenges faced and privileges enjoyed might differ from the experiences of the families with whom Morgan is working. In contrast, if Morgan had grown up in a middle-class urban setting, they may be somewhat oblivious to or not think to consider the challenges that poverty and geography raise in accessing health care. Similarly, as a nurse working within a diverse milieu, it is important for Morgan to consider how their own family history might be shaping their attitudes toward immigrants, people whose first language is not English, racialized groups, Indigenous people, and other groups. Perhaps Morgan is an immigrant, a member of a racialized group, or a member of a dominant group—English speaking, Euro-Canadian, middle class. It is important that Morgan reflect on how their own religious affiliations (or lack thereof) shape how they think religion is relevant to health and nursing practice. Although each aspect of Morgan's social location may shape their thinking, it does not reflect one particular perspective.

By reflexively scrutinizing our own social locations, we can examine our understandings and make explicit decisions about how to draw on (or not) various views and assumptions. Examining our own contexts and social locations to see how we are limiting our views of families can be challenging. We can see more easily our own disadvantages than our privileges. For example, Morgan might have to work harder to see how their privilege as a securely employed, fluent English-speaking health care provider gives an advantage that Greg's father does not have. If Morgan has experienced employment disadvantages based on gender, they might see Greg's father as a privileged man and have difficulty recognizing the challenges he faces.

Overall, reflexivity in family nursing involves developing a critical awareness of our own context and social location, scrutinizing how that context and/or location shapes our view of a particular family, and intentionally looking *beyond* that location to consider the family within its own context. In Morgan's situation, this would involve examining how the rural context, economics, language, ethnicity, and religion and Morgan's understandings of these factors shape how they engage with the families. Morgan might ask how their own experiences of family shape their ability to see and accept the differing forms of family—for example, if the family includes parents that are separated, or a family that is led by a grandparent as the primary caregiver. How does Morgan's own location enable or limit their ability to understand how difficult it might be for Greg's father and mother to get him to the clinic appointments given their current family situation?

(continued)

Case Study: Morgan's Story—cont'd

Engaging in such reflexive examination also enables consideration of the wider sociopolitical elements shaping families' experiences, such as contextual factors (e.g., the stress of immigration), that may have contributed to the stability of the family. At the same time, approaching nursing work in this reflexive manner highlights areas where Morgan may need to learn more. For example, how well does Morgan understand the history of the Indigenous people served by the clinic or the relationship between historical trauma and diabetes? How is diabetes cared for in Czechoslovakia versus Indigenous cultures versus the broader Canadian culture? What are the roles of children in understanding and participating in their care across these multiple overlapping cultures?

Case Study: Attending to Context

Mrs. Dickson, a 40-year-old woman admitted with a diagnosis of bowel cancer, is a single parent of four children who is experiencing postoperative complications. Discharged home 3 days prior, Mrs. Dickson has been readmitted via ambulance with undiagnosed pain and extreme nausea. Her eldest daughter Sandra (age 21 years and married) and her third daughter Simone (age 17 years), who are present in the room, describe how their mother collapsed at home after screaming out in pain. Throughout Mrs. Dickson's illness, Simone, who is the eldest child at home (their middle sister lives in another city), has taken on the role of primary caregiver for her mother, her 13-year-old brother, and her 86-year-old grandfather, who lives with them. As you enter the room, the two sisters are sitting beside their sedated mother. They look up with strained expressions and ask whether the doctors have figured out what is wrong with their mom.

What Intervention Strategies Might You Employ?
A relational inquiry approach to family nursing rests on the assumption that what constitutes high-quality nursing care can only be determined in the relational situation. Because the experiences of people and families vary so greatly, as do the realities within which health care occurs, there is no linear sequence or prescribed method. There are no prescriptions for assessment or action because everything depends on the situation. What constitutes contextually responsive care depends on the particularities of specific nursing situations. Because we work with particular people and families in particular situations, it is impossible to present standardized action steps. The same action may be responsive and health promoting in one case, and it may not be in another case. Thus, the question of how to intervene is one that must be asked in and tailored to each and every situation: How might I best relate to this family in a way that is meaningful and significant and promotes their health and healing capacity?

Consider how you might respond as a family nurse in the Dickson family situation. Where would you begin? What would you focus on? For example, it is evident from their facial expressions and the question they pose that the daughters are very worried about their mother. That might be an effective place to start because the question points to their immediate concern, to what is of meaning and significance to them. "Following their lead" (their worried expressions) is a form of both assessment and intervention in a relational inquiry approach. Acknowledging Sandra's and Simone's worry could be a way of joining them in their experience and furthering your understanding of both the immediate family situation and the context of their lives.

As you follow their lead and inquire into their experiences and what is of meaning and significance to them, focus too on picking up contextual cues. For example, you might respond by sharing your observations in a tentative manner by stating, "You look pretty worried," or "It's hard not knowing what is wrong with your mom," to invite them to confirm, expand, or modify your understanding. Making inclusive observations, asking open-ended questions, and being interested in knowing more invites people and families to lead the way. By working in this collaborative manner, you work with the family to make connections between experiences and context and discern the desired and necessary action. This involves recognizing the patterns of capacity and of adversity that are simultaneously part of the person's or family's illness experience. It also enables you to understand how contextual elements are shaping the situation and what their immediate needs might be. For example, as you look contextually, you might be concerned about the caregiving load that Simone is carrying (looking after her mother, brother, and grandfather). If you were working from a relational inquiry approach that nursing concern is not something you know, you inquire into its relevance in terms of capacity and adversity; keep in mind that what might be considered adversity to one person and family

Case Study: Attending to Context—cont'd

may not be adversity to another. Asking, "How has it been for you to be caring for your mom, brother, and grandfather while your mom is ill?" enables you to learn how contextual elements are meaningfully experienced by the person and family. By inquiring, you might find that nothing has changed—that because her mother works long hours, Simone is used to assuming a lot of the domestic chores or that she has a lot of support from friends or relatives. Or you may find that the added responsibility of caring for her mother while her mother is ill is more than she can handle, and she may open up and ask for more assistance in problem solving.

As you listen to and for context, you might learn of other sociocontextual structures and processes (economics, health care policies, values, norms, traditions, history) that are shaping the family's experience. Knowing about the populations you serve (e.g., income levels, employment opportunities, social financial assistance) helps you to listen for a range of possibilities without assuming how this particular family "fits" with population norms. The Dickson family might be fine in terms of managing household and caregiving needs, but they might not have access to money or transportation to get to the hospital. Or the worry for her mother may be affecting Simone's ability to do schoolwork or hold down a part-time job that could contribute to the family's income. Thus, as you listen contextually, you are listening and inquiring into resources—the resources they have, need, and/or can access. You also listen for what has enabled them to live in adversity—that is, what capacities they have within them and/or have accessed or enlisted. Similarly, check your own view and your own capacities. Are your immediate nursing concerns obscuring your understanding of broader contextual issues and/or longer-term concerns? For example, given that you are located in an acute-care setting, is Mrs. Dickson's physical well-being your primary concern? Are you able to extend your view to consider the longer-term health impact of this illness situation? How do you balance your need to care for Mrs. Dickson's acute health needs while simultaneously considering her family's contextual needs?

Evaluating Family Nursing Action

Specifically, relational inquiry involves asking the person and the family for *their* version of the story and purposefully opening the space for *their* decision making. Thus, evaluation of your nursing intervention involves an ongoing reflexive process where you check in with the client, the family, and yourself. Evaluation is centered in continually asking the following questions: How might I be as responsive as possible? How are my actions expanding (or constraining) the choice and capacity of this family? How might I support this family in ways that are meaningful to them and in ways that enable them to address their concerns and realize their aspirations? Relational inquiry helps you to evaluate nursing effectiveness in the longer as well as the shorter term. For example, a quick discharge may result in a readmission for Mrs. Dickson if the context of the family situation is not considered. It also helps nurses provide nursing care to *family,* beyond the immediate individual patient and beyond the immediate acute health care needs.

SUMMARY

- One of the few predictable characteristics of families is diversity. By understanding and intentionally attending to diversity when providing care, nurses in Canada are prepared to consider the contextual nature of families' health and illness experiences and how their lives are shaped by their circumstances.

- All nursing involves families. How nurses provide care to families depends on specific situations, what is relevant and meaningful for people, how individual patients experience family, and the significance of family relationships for health and well-being over the life span.

- Contexts are literally embodied in people; both nurses and families live their contexts and circumstances.

- For nurses in Canada to work responsively with diverse families, they need to use relational inquiry to inquire into the particular experiences and contexts of families' lives.

- Understanding families entails taking a stance of inquiry, listening and paying attention to the experiences of particular families, reflexively attending to one's own understandings and assumptions, and continuously developing new knowledge that is oriented toward the family's well-being.

■ Nurses in Canada must deliver their care through an understanding of the risks facing families, including changing family structures, health disparities, family violence, and families living in poverty, especially in rural communities.

■ Nurses in Canada must provide families with optimal care within a structure that limits out-of-hospital care and limits access to care in rural communities. Nurses need to collaborate with other providers and resources to help families attain optimal health and wellness and long-term health outcomes.

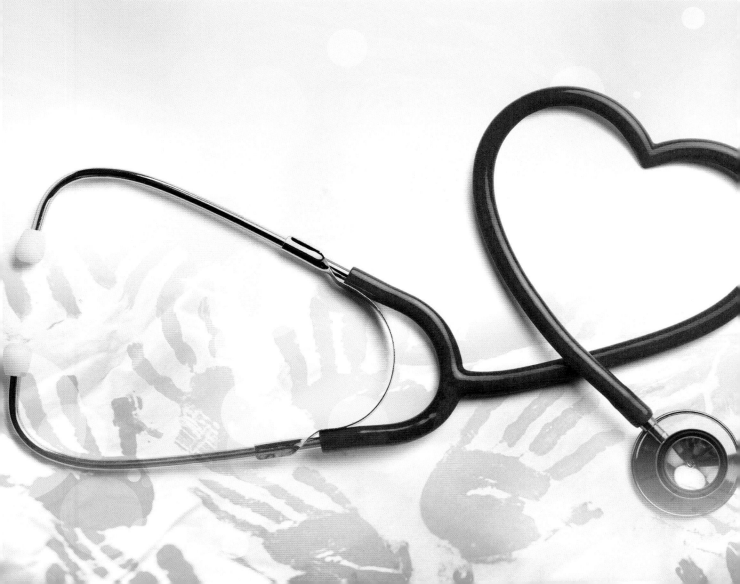

Nursing Care of Families in Clinical Areas

chapter 14

Family Nursing With Childbearing Families

Joyce M. O'Mahony, PhD, RN

Karline Wilson-Mitchell, DNP, MSN, CNM, RN, RM, FACNM

Shahin Kassam, MN, RN, PhD(c)

Critical Concepts

- Childbearing family nursing is not synonymous with obstetrical nursing, which only considers the woman as the client and the family as the context for care. In contrast, childbearing family nursing considers the family as the client, the family as the context for the care of its members, or both. Childbearing family nursing focuses primarily on health and wellness rather than on procedures and medical treatment.

- Nurses must understand and utilize multiple theories to plan and guide nursing care for childbearing families.

- Nurses must understand the impact that social policy, available resources, and geographical location have on childbearing families.

- The holistic care of these families is best provided with an approach that acknowledges the social determinants of health and the integration of all the members of the health care team and community resources.

- Nurses need to be aware of stressors that childbearing families encounter before, during, and after reproductive events so that they can anticipate, identify, and respond to needs appropriately.

- The family constellation and the definition of family depend on the culture, worldview, sexual orientation, and perspective of each family. Consequently, childbearing family nursing necessitates demonstrating respect and cultural competence.

- Nursing care for adoptive families should be provided in a manner similar to what is provided to biological families. Nurses should recognize and meet the unique needs of every family, regardless of the family constellation.

- Nurses caring for childbearing families experiencing infertility must consider, understand, and address the family's emotional and physical needs.

- Understanding the many ways that families experience grief and loss allows nurses to advocate for practices that best facilitate childbearing as a transitional event in the life of the family.

- A process of bereavement should be anticipated with perinatal loss, adverse perinatal outcome, the diagnosis of genetic disorders, palliative care, or the birth of a child with a congenital disability or birth impairment.

(continued)

- When a mother or a newborn has serious threats to health, family nurses act to maintain and promote family relationships. Threats to the health and integrity of the family become a reality when separation from family members occurs (e.g., apprehension of children because of child protection risks or incarceration of the mother).

- Understanding the effect that a new baby has on all family members allows nurses to help parents develop realistic expectations about themselves, each other, and their children, as well as to identify appropriate support and resources.

- Postpartum depression (PPD) is treatable, and patients can recover from it. Therefore, family nurses must work diligently to identify and refer women for appropriate treatment as early as possible to reduce the effects of maternal depression on the woman and her family.

- Family nurses can be leaders in practice, policy development, and research related to childbearing families.

Before the onset of professional nursing in North America during the late 19th century, caregivers for childbearing families were women. Female family members, in-laws, neighbors, friends, and midwives came to the home to encourage, support, and nurture a woman during and after childbirth (King et al., 2018; Linn et al., 2015; Marcellus, 2019). During this time, many of these women midwives were settlers who followed the European colonists and were African slaves or First Nations/Native Americans (Dawley & Walsh, 2016). In Canada, Canadian pioneer and Aboriginal midwives also attended births up through the 1940s. These women caregivers maintained family functions of the household, tended to new babies and mothers' other children, and provided postpartum physical care. Male obstetricians emerged as primary clinical providers of birth management and influenced both maternity education and health care policy in the 1860s. However, male family members, friends, and children were excluded from the childbirth experience until the 1970s. This practice was justified by the belief that nonmedical participants increased the risk of introducing infection into the perinatal setting.

Beginning in the late 1960s, families became increasingly knowledgeable about childbearing and desired a more satisfying birth experience as a family event. Families became savvy health care consumers who found hospital routines and policies too restrictive if they required rigid adherence to newborn feeding and sleeping schedules, kept fathers and siblings out of the delivery room, or separated parents from their newborns. In response, informed families lobbied for changes in childbearing practices; they used evidence to support not separating mothers and babies immediately after delivery, as well as other hallmark findings demonstrating improved parent-child attachment with immediate and frequent contact between mothers, fathers, and siblings and their newborns (de Chateau, 1976, 1977; Johnson, 2013; Klaus et al., 1972; Marcellus, 2019). Families presented compelling arguments for hospitals to support exclusive breastfeeding, skin-to-skin baby carrying (or kangaroo care), and delayed cord clamping (Elarousy & Mostafa, 2019).

In time, nurses, hospitals, and other health care providers for women began to recognize the effect that reproductive events have on all family members, as well as the reciprocal influence of the family on the parents and infants. This recognition has resulted in inclusion of family concepts into nursing care of childbearing families. With the trend for increased family education about reproductive events, increased responsibility for family members to plan for care during pregnancy and delivery, and shorter hospital stays after birth, postpartum care is returning to family care within the context of the home with nursing guidance rather than being medically based in a hospital. This shift in focus from caring for the individual woman as the client toward consideration and inclusion of the family in care from preconception to the postpartum period is known as *childbearing family nursing*. The historical perspective is outlined in Box 14-1.

BOX 14-1

Historical Perspective of Childbearing Family Nursing

Late 1800s: Industrialization

- Families moved to more urban areas; household size and functions diminished.
- Traditional networks of women were not always available, and mothers needed to replace care previously carried out in the home.
- Childbearing still occurred at home for many middle-class families.
- European colonists' enslaved African Americans, First Nations, and Native Americans served as midwives.

First Third of the 20th Century

- The hospital became the place for labor, birth, and early postpartum recovery for middle-class families.
- Many immigrant and working-class urban families continued to have newborns at home with their traditional care providers.
- An impetus to the development of public health nursing was concern for the health of urban mothers and babies.
- Realizing that the health needs of all the family members were intertwined, early public health nurses considered families, not individuals, as their clients.

1930s Through the Baby Boom of the 1950s and 1960s

- In Canada, Canadian settler and Aboriginal midwives attended births up through the 1940s.
- With the dramatic shift of births to hospitals, family involvement with childbearing diminished.
- Concerns about infection control contributed to separation of family members.
- Family members, especially males, were forbidden to be with women in the hospital.
- Babies were segregated into nurseries and brought out to their mothers only for brief feeding sessions.
- Nurses focused on the smooth operation of postpartum wards and nurseries through the use of routine and order.
- Despite these inflexible conditions, families tolerated them because they believed that hospital births were safer for mothers and newborns.

1960s to 1970s

- Families and health care providers questioned the need for heavy sedation and analgesia for childbearing and embraced natural childbirth.

- A feature of natural childbirth was the close relationship between the laboring woman and a supportive person serving as a coach; in North America, husbands often assumed this supportive role.
- Expectant parents actively sought out physicians and hospitals that would best meet their expectations for father involvement, and the control over childbearing began to shift from health care providers to families.
- Some nurses were skeptical about the changes that families demanded, but others were enthusiastic about increased family participation.
- Many hospital-based maternity nurses began to consider themselves to be mother-baby nurses rather than nursery or postpartum nurses, and labor and delivery nurses often collaborated with family members in helping women cope with the discomforts of labor.

1980s to the Present

- Klaus and Kennel's (1976) research served as the impetus for the growth of family-centered care (American College of Obstetricians and Gynecologists and the Interprofessional Task Force on Health Care of Women and Children, 1978).
- Recent studies reveal that the beta-endorphin-mediated fear responses during physiological labor may disrupt oxytocin secretion, adversely interfering with labor, birth, and breastfeeding processes (Sakala et al., 2016).
- Family members are integral to client-centered care that promotes alternative therapies such as hydrotherapy; imagery; and the promotion of agency, cultural safety, and informed decision making, all of which might mitigate fear responses. Respectful maternity-care principles promote freedom of movement; the presence of a supportive family member; and access to high-quality, evidence-based care (Wilson-Mitchell et al., 2018).
- Today, promotion of family contact is the hallmark of childbearing care.
- Many hospitals renamed their obstetrical services, using names such as family birth center, to convey the importance of family members in childbearing health care despite the trend of increasing dependency on obstetrical technology.

The practice of childbearing family nursing is *not* synonymous with obstetrical nursing. Obstetrical nursing considers the woman as the client and views the family as the context for care. Childbearing family nursing, by contrast, considers the family as the client and the family as the context for the care of its members. It is a health and wellness rather than an illness model of care. Childbearing family nurses take a holistic approach to care; they consider the woman and her family's physical, mental, emotional, spiritual, social, and cultural indicators of health. Using this family-centered approach to care requires that childbearing family nurses *assist* families to make informed choices to achieve outcomes desired versus *telling* families what is best for them (Ward et al., 2016).

Family nursing with childbearing families covers the preconception period, pregnancy, labor, birth, and the postpartum period. Childbearing family nursing traditionally begins with a family's decision to start having children and continues until parents have achieved a degree of relative comfort in their roles as parents of infants and/or have ceased the addition of new children to their families. Childbearing family nursing is often expanded to include the periods between pregnancies and includes other aspects of reproductive care such as family planning, infertility, perinatal loss, sexuality, adoption, foster care, and parenting grandchildren. Decisions and changes surrounding childbearing vary for families throughout the reproductive cycle. Factors driving these decisions or changes include prevailing health policies and the family's cultural, socioeconomic, and psychological needs. Therefore, the beginning and end points of the reproductive period may be different for each family.

The focus of childbearing family nurses is centered on family relationships and the health of all family members. Therefore, nurses involved with childbearing families use family concepts and theories as part of developing the plan of nursing care. This chapter starts by presenting theoretical perspectives that guide nursing practice with childbearing families. It continues with an exploration of family nursing with childbearing families before conception through the postpartum period. The chapter concludes with implications for nursing practice, research, and policy, along with two case studies that explore family adaptations to stressors and changing roles related to childbearing.

THEORY-GUIDED, EVIDENCE-BASED CHILDBEARING NURSING

Application of theory to family health situations during childbearing can guide family nurses in making more complete assessments and planning interventions congruent with the pattern of events during childbearing. Several of the theories discussed in Chapter 2 contribute to nurses' understanding of how families grow, develop, function, and change during childbearing. Two theories in particular, Family Systems Theory and Family Developmental and Life Cycle Theory, are especially applicable to childbearing families. A brief summary of these theories and their application to childbearing families follows.

Family Systems Theory

Family Systems Theory provides a framework for viewing the family as a system: as an organized whole and/or as individuals within the family who form interactive and interdependent systems. Four main concepts underlie this theory: (1) all parts of the system are interconnected, (2) the whole is more than the sum of the parts, (3) all systems have some form of boundaries or borders between the system and its environment, and (4) systems can be further organized into subsystems. Family systems are designed primarily to maintain stability, and a change in one member of the family affects all members of the family.

Becoming parents or adding a child brings stress to a family by challenging family stability, not only

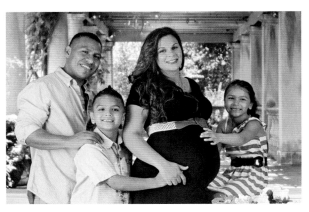

Source: © *LindaYolanda/iStock/Thinkstock*

for the nuclear and extended family systems themselves but also for the individual members and subsystems of the family. As new subsystems are created or modified by pregnancy and childbirth, a sense of disequilibrium exists until a family adapts to its new member and achieves stability again. For example, changes in the husband-wife subsystem occur as a response to development of the new parent-child subsystems.

Imbalance, or disequilibrium, occurs while adjustments are still needed and new roles are being learned. Families with greater flexibility in role expectations and behaviors tend to experience these periods of disequilibrium with less discomfort. The greater the range or number of coping strategies available to the family, the greater the ability to engage in various family roles, and the more support that is available, the more effective the family's response will be to both internal strains and external stress associated with childbearing. External stresses, such as concerns about outside employment, child care, and lack of health insurance, may be important in predicting family disequilibrium. These issues have emerged as significant stressors as new immigrant and refugee families settle and integrate into their new communities (Sangalang & Vang, 2017). Consequently, researchers and policymakers encourage health care providers to employ creative strategies, innovation, and cultural sensitivity in their role as global citizens (Patterson et al., 2017). Internal strains such as an ill or disabled child, or unhealthy habits such as substance abuse may tax family coping mechanisms to the breaking point. Therefore, it is imperative that nurses identify both present and potential family stressors and assess the effect of stressors on family stability.

Family Systems Theory is especially effective for use by childbearing family nurses because, following childbirth, families who are in a state of change and readjustment tend to have more permeable family boundaries. For example, families with flexible or open boundaries have varying degrees of openness to the outside environment, which stems from the need for additional resources beyond what the family can supply for itself. Consequently, a family in transition may be engaged in more interactions with systems outside the family and may become more receptive to interventions such as health teaching than it would be at other times in the family life cycle (Kaakinen, 2018). This openness of family boundaries allows

nurses more access to the family for assessment, diagnosis, and health promotion.

On the other hand, childbearing family nurses should be aware of very closed or enmeshed families who may have nonpermeable or closed boundaries, because they are likely to reject outside influences, including nursing care. Families can become closed because they interpret the outside environment and systems as hostile, threatening, or difficult to cope with. These families are challenging for nurses because they are less readily accessible or responsive to family nurses. Telehealth, mobile health (mHealth), and mobile units are creative ways of positioning the family nurse to provide health care access during narrow windows of opportunity (Demiris et al., 2019).

Nurses working with childbearing families from a systems perspective view the family as the client and aim to assist families to maintain and regain stability. Therefore, assessment questions should be focused on the family as a whole. At the same time, it is important to remember that family nurses also work with the individuals and the subsystems within the family. Interventions have to be directed at the various systems and levels of subsystems within the family. For example, a family ecomap helps the nurse see how individual members and the family as a whole relate to one another and to the community around them. Understanding the family process and functioning through careful assessment of the family as a whole and of the individual family members allows the nurse to offer intervention strategies that help provide stability in the family's everyday functioning.

Family Developmental and Life Cycle Theory

Duvall's (1977) Family Developmental and Life Cycle Theory described a process of developing over time that is predictable and yet individual based on unique life circumstances and family interactions. Although the life cycle of most families around the world follows a universal sequence of family development, it is important for childbearing family nurses to recognize that wide variations exist in the timing and sequencing of family life cycle phases (Berk, 2013; Duvall, 1977). Many present-day childbearing families in North America do not fit into the classic sequence and timing of family developmental stages and tasks originally described by Duvall and Miller (1985). For example, families may be blended, with one or both partners having children from a previous relationship. Other types of nontraditional family structures include adoptive families; communal or multigenerational families; and parents who may be cohabitating, unmarried, single, of the same sex, or have children born later in life (Berk, 2013; McKinney et al., 2018; Stephens, 2013). Therefore, nontraditional and high-risk families—such as those experiencing unusual levels of stress from marital conflict and divorce, violence, substance abuse, having a child with a congenital disability or a birth impairment, infertility, being an adolescent parent, or stressors during refugee migration and settlement—require care that is different from that needed by traditional families (McKinney et al., 2018). In addition, families who are members of vulnerable populations may experience multiple and intersecting stressors from discrimination because of race, socioeconomic level, ethnicity, gender, and/or sexual orientation.

Despite how diverse the family is today, Family Developmental and Life Cycle Theory remains a helpful guide for childbearing family nurses because it addresses the patterns of adaptation to parenthood that are typical for many families. This theory has relevance for family nurses regardless of how families are structured because the essential tasks families must perform to survive as healthy units are generally present to some extent in all families (Silbert-Flagg & Pillitteri, 2017).

According to Duvall's (1977) Family Developmental and Life Cycle Theory, family changes occur in stages during which there is upheaval while adjustments are being made. What occurs during these stages is generally referred to as a developmental task. The Childbearing Family with Infants stage is pertinent to childbearing family nursing practice because during this stage, childbearing families must accomplish nine specific tasks in order to grow and achieve family well-being. These nine tasks for childbearing families and nursing interventions are explained in the following subsections.

Task One: Arranging Space (Territory) for a Child

Arranging space (territory) involves families making space preparations for their infants. Families often accommodate newborns by moving to a new residence during pregnancy or the first year after birth or by modifying their living quarters and furnishings. Families may delay or avoid space preparations for a new baby for several reasons. For example, busy families, those who fear or have experienced prior fetal loss, and families involved with adoption or foster placement may delay or avoid space preparations. The lack of space preparation may also result from the parents not having accepted the reality of the coming baby (denial). It may also emerge from various social risks or health disparities, including expensive health care needs incurred by other family members; inadequate, unsafe housing arrangements or homelessness; underemployment or poverty; recent immigration; and incarceration. Adolescent parents may not make space arrangements because of denial of the pregnancy or fear of repercussions from their families if the pregnancy is revealed.

Family Nursing Interventions

- Inquire about the safety and health of the family's home environment; food; security; including freedom from domestic violence; space arrangements made for the baby; and other child-care resources, community resources, or other support systems.
- Refer refugee and other families who are homeless or live in inadequate or unsafe housing to appropriate resources for obtaining safer housing.
- Inquire about the families' thoughts, values, beliefs, and possible fears about making preparations for the anticipated arrival of the baby.
- Assist families in exploring and managing their fear about survival or loss of the baby and then mobilize resources to help them cope so that family development can continue.
- Assist adolescents to find ways to communicate with their families and make plans for the future placement and well-being of the infant and the well-being of the adolescent parents.
- Work with people who are incarcerated, interested stakeholders, and state and/or federal penal systems to establish units where newborns and mothers can stay together to encourage bonding and breastfeeding while the mother is incarcerated.
- During pandemics, civil unrest, or other complex community contexts, family nurses require flexible, innovative strategies that provide choice to the family for accessing health care, for example, telehealth, mHealth,

virtual visits, or curbside visits (Breslin et al., 2020; Demiris et al., 2019). Pandemics such as SARS or COVID-19 are examples of threats that may challenge the resources of an otherwise resilient family and increase openness to community assistance (World Health Organization [WHO], 2020).

Task Two: Financing Childbearing and Child Rearing

Childbearing results in additional expenses and lower family income. American families, having experienced two major economic downturns since the start of the 21st century, are finding the decision to bear and the ability to raise children increasingly financially difficult (Glavin et al., 2020; Seltzer, 2019). Low-income families and children, especially African Americans and those of Hispanic descent, have been disproportionally burdened by these recessions and continue to struggle just to make ends meet (Kong et al., 2018). Financial stresses can be even harder for mothers without partners, women who provide most of the income for their families, mothers who are fleeing domestic violence, or mothers experiencing unplanned pregnancy. Younger or middle-aged adults, people in low-income families with at least one worker in the family, and families with precarious immigration status (including refugee claimants or migrant workers) may likewise experience severe financial stress because of lack of health insurance coverage (Guruge et al., 2019; Kaiser Family Foundation, 2020). These populations are particularly vulnerable to fiscally restrictive social policies aimed at limiting systemic health care costs. For example, the Canadian Immigration Bill reduced accessibility to Interim Federal Health Program (IFHP) coverage and limited eligibility for immigration and refugee status, thus producing increases in uninsured newcomers as a consequence (Parliament of Canada, 2012). Although the subsequent government enacted legislation to improve the situation, challenges continue to exist.

Health care surrounding childbirth can add another layer of financial stress on a family. Health care providers may not be able to accept patients who are uninsured, are insured by federal or state programs, or cannot pay out of pocket for obstetrical services, further increasing the financial strain on families. A portion of this financial stress, experienced by Canadian childbearing families, is offset by a publicly funded universal health care plan. In the United States, the Affordable Care Act (ACA) has reduced the number of uninsured Americans and thus helped alleviate some of the financial stressors faced by childbearing families (Kaiser Family Foundation, 2020). Under ACA, most health plans are required to cover 10 essential health benefits, including maternity and newborn care (U.S. Department of Health and Human Services, 2019).

Although most employed women miss some employment during childbearing, many return to the labor force or increase the number of hours that they work following childbirth (Lu et al., 2017). Others, especially those of high socioeconomic status or with a college or university education, may choose to delay reentry into the workforce or forego possible career advancement during childbearing (Kuziemko et al., 2018). Adolescent mothers are especially prone to financial difficulties because childbearing may disrupt their education, which increases their risk for future poverty (Lu et al., 2017). Regardless of the reason, missed employment brings many consequences for women beyond loss of earnings during the childbearing years. Other consequences are detailed in Box 14-2.

BOX 14-2

Consequences of Maternal Unemployment During the Childbearing Years

The consequences of maternal unemployment during the childbearing years include the following:

- Loss of status or identity as an employee
- Earnings lost during the times of unemployment
- Loss of on-the-job training opportunities and opportunities for career advancement
- Depreciation of skills and experience, often followed by a loss of confidence about returning to work
- Loss of work-related benefits if job is subsequently lost
- Family medical leave taken before childbirth may reduce the leave time available postpartum
- Reinforcement of traditional roles and responsibilities in two-parent, heterosexual families where the father takes the breadwinner role

Sources: Adapted from Nomaguchi, K., & Milkie, M. (2020). Parenthood and well-being: A decade in review. *Journal of Marriage and Family, 82*(1), 198–223.; Schwartz, D. A., & Engler, C. (2015). Unraveling the mysteries of the Family and Medical Leave Act. *GP Solo, 32*(2), 30; and Weckstrom, S. (2012). Self-assessed consequences of unemployment on individual wellbeing and family relationships: A study of unemployed women and men in Finland. *International Journal of Social Welfare, 21*(4), 372–383.

Family Nursing Interventions

- Assist families with finding high-quality resources, such as nutrition programs; food banks; family shelters; counseling or settlement services; and government-funded prenatal clinics, including midwifery clinics, community health centers, or public health clinics that support families with limited socioeconomic resources.
- Identify barriers to prenatal care, such as cultural differences, lack of transportation or insurance coverage, child care, hours of service that conflict with family employment, and difficulty obtaining or using health care benefits.
- Assist families to find safe and appropriate child care by providing culturally appropriate information and resources in their preferred language.
- Fully inform families about their health care options resulting from reform and redesign of the health care system.
- Educate families about new federal health care coverage and assist them in navigating the enrollment process.
- Advocate for expansion of Medicaid eligibility for adults whose incomes are low in all U.S. states.

Task Three: Assuming Mutual Responsibility for Child Care and Nurturing

The care and nurturing of infants bring sleep disruptions, demands on time and physical and emotional energy, additional household tasks, and personal discomfort for caretakers. New parents spend most of their time caring for children, thus decreasing both leisure and downtime, both of which are important to maintain balance in the family. Parents can experience role strain and role overload from combining the increased work within the family with employment demands, or they may face difficulty arranging and affording child care.

The first decision parents make regarding their infant's nutrition is whether to breastfeed or bottle-feed. With the exception of decreased feeding costs, the benefits of breastfeeding have traditionally been viewed in North America as being primarily for the child. For example, breastfed babies are less likely to develop diarrhea or ear and other infections and have a reduced rate of sudden infant death syndrome (SIDS) (Thompson et al., 2017). Evidence also suggests that one of the long-term impacts of breastfeeding may be better performance in intelligence tests and developmental outcomes (Horta et al., 2018). The consensus around the world is that exclusive breastfeeding until 6 months is best for both mother and child to achieve optimal growth, development, and health (American Academy of Pediatrics, 2020; WHO, 2019). Sufficient evidence confirms that mothers who breastfeed for 1 year or longer experience multiple physiological and emotional benefits. These benefits include reduced risk for breast and ovarian cancer, osteoporosis, type 2 diabetes, cardiovascular disease, rheumatoid arthritis, and postpartum depression (PPD) (WHO, 2019). Nurses must be aware that the father's or partner's role in the newborn feeding decision and the level of support and encouragement are important factors in the success of the breastfeeding relationship (Abbass-Dick et al., 2019; Earle & Hadley, 2018).

In both the United States and Canada, the rate at which women initiate breastfeeding is very high. The rate at which women in North America are exclusively breastfeeding at 6 months following birth falls dramatically (WHO, 2019) Although the rate of breastfeeding has increased in all demographic groups, certain populations are less likely to breastfeed, including lower-income women, first-time mothers, African Americans, women participating in the Special Supplemental Nutrition Program for Women, Infants, and Children (WIC), those with high-school education or less, and those employed full-time outside the home (Kim et al., 2017; Henninger et al., 2017).

In addition, an increasing number of clients identifying as mothers, women, or transgender

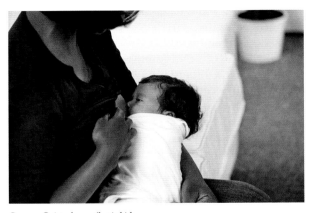

Source: © istock.com/lostinbids

men report concerns surrounding postpartum hypogalactia following breast reduction surgery. These parents derive a more satisfying postpartum experience and their newborns benefit when their lactation efforts are respected and supported, for example, with lactation aids, pumping, and formula supplementation (Thibaudeau et al., 2010; Wolfe-Roubatis & Spatz, 2015). It is crucial for childbearing family nurses to understand the relationship between maternal employment and breastfeeding practices, including the phenomenon of infant feeding with breast milk that has been pumped while the mother is away from the home. Nurses should also strive to provide a culturally safe environment for families by keeping up to date with the changing landscape of evidence-based strategies and concerns of a culturally diverse clientele (Kim et al., 2017).

For both mothers and partners, one of the benefits of having a period of time off from work following childbirth is the increased ability for parents and their newborn to establish a relationship through the process of bonding and attachment. A vast body of research on bonding and attachment, beginning with Bowlby (1952), continued by Ainsworth (1967), and popularized by Klaus and Kennel (1976), supports the premise that optimum child development and well-being is achieved through early and ongoing contact between mothers, fathers (or partners), and their newborn. Mothers may automatically bond with their newborns throughout pregnancy and early contact within minutes of the child's birth. By contrast, fathers must work to establish a bond by being involved in the delivery as well as being available to the infant to strengthen paternal attachment through early contact with the infant in the months following birth (Abbass-Dick et al., 2019)

If an infant must be separated from the parents because of prematurity or for medical or surgical interventions, interruptions in bonding may occur. To promote optimal bonding in these special circumstances, the nurse must allow parents early and frequent access to the baby, encourage parents to be involved in the care of their infant, practice skin-to-skin contact, and speak to and hold their newborn (Govindaswamy et al., 2019). If these actions are not possible, photographs of the infant should be sent to parents as soon as possible and they should be updated frequently with information about the newborn's status. The affectionate bond (or attachment) that develops between

parents and their children may be one of the motivational driving forces for engaging in infant care and nurturing even under difficult circumstances.

Family Nursing Interventions
- Educate parents about the realities of parenting, such as interrupted sleep and changes in time management and family roles.
- Teach the family to alternate who responds to the baby's needs, including feeding, changing, and comforting.
- Assist parents to develop new skills in caregiving and ways of interacting with their babies, such as baby carrying, smiling, talking to their infant, or making eye contact.
- Observe for signs of attachment by listening to what parents say about their babies and by observing parent behaviors. Box 14-3 outlines parental behaviors that facilitate attachment.
- Refer families who do not demonstrate nurturing behaviors to other professionals,

BOX 14-3
Parental Behaviors That Facilitate Attachment

Selected parental behaviors that facilitate attachment between infant and parent include the following:
- Arranges self or the newborn to have face-to-face and eye-to-eye contact with infant.
- Directs attention to the infant; maintains contact with infant physically and emotionally.
- Identifies infant as a separate, unique individual with independent needs.
- Identifies characteristics of family members in infant.
- Names infant; calls infant by name.
- Smiles, coos, talks to, or sings to infant.
- Verbalizes pride in the infant.
- Responds to sounds made by the infant, such as crying, sneezing, or grunting.
- Assigns meaning to the infant's actions; interprets infant's needs sensitively.
- Has a positive view of infant's behaviors and appearance.

Sources: Adapted from Alden, K. R., Lowdermilk, D. L., Cashion, M. C., & Perry, S. E. (2012). *Maternity and women's health care* (10th ed.). St. Louis, MO: Mosby; Davidson, M. R., London, M. L., & Ladewig, P. A. (2016). *Olds' maternal-newborn nursing and women's health across the lifespan* (10th ed.). Upper Saddle River, NJ: Pearson Prentice Hall; and Schenk, L. K., Kelley, J. H., & Schenk, M. P. (2005). Models of maternal-infant attachment: A role for nurses. *Pediatric Nursing, 31*(6), 514–517.

such as local counselors, psychologists, social workers, or childhood development experts, who can provide more intensive intervention.

■ Promote culturally competent perceptions of parenting behavior in underrepresented cultures by building partnerships in the ethnic community of the families in care. Respected elders, doulas, or community members may act as translators and cultural brokers for the health care team (Waller-Wise, 2018).

■ Provide information about and support for breastfeeding, including how to manage lactation problems, feeding expressed breast milk when appropriate, and referral for lactation consultation as necessary (Brown & Jones, 2019; Wambach & Spencer, 2021).

■ Participate in active listening and respect for mothers who decline breastfeeding (or chestfeeding) possibly because of a past history of trauma, body image concerns, or postoperative sequelae of breast reconstruction.

■ Promote maternal and paternal early and frequent contact with their newborn; encourage involvement in newborn care activities.

Task Four: Facilitating Role Learning of Family Members

Learning roles is particularly important for child-bearing families, including those families that depart from traditional heterosexual structures. For many couples, taking on the role of parents is a dramatic shift in their lives. Difficulty adapting to parenthood may be related to the stress of learning new roles. Role learning involves coming to understand the expectations about the role, developing the ability to assume the role, and taking on the role. Another important demand that children create, which affects women in particular, is increased housework. Household chores associated with children (laundry, cleaning, cooking, child care, etc.) can lead to increased levels of distress for women and can affect relationships between partners. The relationship between LGBTQ+(lesbian, gay, bisexual, transgender, queer, and questioning) partners is also affected when the couple takes on the parenting role. For example, parenting can result in differing energy levels between partners, especially if one partner

has assumed primary responsibility for child rearing. The toll parenting has on their ability to be good partners to each other influences their relationship (Giesler, 2012).

The stress of parenting depends in large part on marital status, race and ethnicity, identification as heterosexual or gay, or the presence of a child with chronic illness. For example, Nam et al. (2015) found higher average parenting stress among Hispanics, followed by Blacks, Native Americans, and Whites. LGBTQ+ partners who decided to become parents revealed that sacrificing lifestyle goals and desires—such as travel and changes to the quality of their sex life—was a source of stress in their partner relationship (Giesler, 2012). Cousino and Hazen's (2013) meta-analysis revealed that generic aspects of caregiving, unrelated to a child's chronic illness, increased stress for parents of children with chronic illness. Parents also experience stress related to frequent health care appointments and demanding treatment regimes.

Family Nursing Interventions

■ Encourage expectant women to bring their partners into the experience by sharing their physical sensations and emotions of being pregnant and restating the value of their role as parents.

■ Assist and encourage pregnant couples to explore their attitudes and expectations about the role(s) of their partner within the household and family after the baby arrives.

■ Encourage contact with others who are in the process of taking on the parenting role, especially if the parents are isolated, adolescent, same sex, or culturally diverse and living apart from traditional networks. Respect culturally prescribed roles that resist (or require) change from the prevailing Western cultural worldview.

■ Provide opportunities for fathers and other partners or significant others in the family to become skilled infant caregivers.

■ Empower parents by assisting them to recognize their own strengths.

■ Moderate parenting stress by assisting new mothers, especially mothers from underrepresented groups, to reduce their depression symptoms and develop strong social support networks (Nam et al., 2015).

Task Five: Adjusting to Changed Communication Patterns

Childbearing families experience changes in their overall communication patterns in order for the family to accommodate newborn and young children. The role of new parents also requires changes in communication patterns. As parents and infants learn to interpret and respond to each other's communication cues, they develop effective, reciprocal communication patterns. Nurses can assist parents in correctly interpreting and responding to their infant's communication cues. For example, many babies respond to being held by cuddling and nuzzling, but others respond by back arching and stiffening. Parents may interpret the latter as rejecting and unloving responses, and these negative interpretations may adversely affect the parent-infant relationship. Positive parenting practices, self-esteem, and parenting efficacy have been found to increase with accurate interpretation and response to infants' communicative cues (Tryphonopoulos & Letourneau, 2020).

Abusive head trauma, which includes shaken baby syndrome, is an extreme example of an inability to adapt to changed communication patterns with an infant. Whether intentional or unintentional, shaking a baby as a form of communication in response to anger and frustration with crying or in an attempt to accomplish discipline results in traumatic brain injury. Infants age 2 to 4 months are at the greatest risk for shaken baby syndrome, a form of physical child abuse that occurs among families of any ethnicity, income range, or family composition. Males, mothers, and other female caregivers alike have been found to have shaken babies. However, infants suffer worse injuries from male perpetrators who are more likely than females to be convicted of this crime (Centers for Disease Control and Prevention [CDC], 2020; Cleveland Clinic Children's, 2019).

Communication between parents also changes with the transition to parenthood. During the years of childbearing, many couples devote considerable time to career development. The time demands of work coupled with parenting may affect a couple's relationship. Along with taking on the everyday aspects of rearing children, communication can then either fall to the wayside or be the key way of making the new family structure function effectively.

Family Nursing Interventions

- Educate parents about different infant temperaments so they can interpret their baby's unique style of communication.
- Teach parents how to recognize and respond to their baby's cues.
- Encourage parents to talk to and engage in eye contact with their baby.
- Educate parents on the various reasons for crying and methods of comforting a crying baby.
- Educate parents and infant caretakers that it is never appropriate or safe to shake a baby.
- Support paid family leave workplace policies that would allow working parents to be with their infants between 4 and 20 weeks of age, a period of increased infant crying (CDC, 2020).
- Incorporate couple communication techniques into education of expectant parents.
- Promote effective couple communication by encouraging the partners to listen to each other by actively using "I" phrases instead of blaming one another.
- Encourage couples to set aside a regular time to talk and to enjoy each other as loving partners.

Task Six: Planning for Subsequent Children

After the birth, some couples will have definite, mutually agreed-on plans with each other for additional children, whereas others may have decided against future children or be ambivalent about family plans. Some couples may make plans for subsequent children that might involve surrogacy or adoption. The nurse should be aware that many couples resume sexual intimacy before the routine 6-week postpartum checkup, and therefore pregnancy may occur even if the mother is breastfeeding. Therefore, postpartum teaching should include information about when it is safe to resume intercourse after childbirth and reliable methods of birth control. Childbearing family nurses are valuable resources for those who desire information or demonstrate a willingness to discuss family planning options.

Family Nursing Interventions

- Identify the power structure and locus of decision-making control in the family when discussing reproductive matters.

- Consider a family's cultural and religious background before initiating a discussion about contraceptive choices, because these factors often dictate whether the discussion is appropriate.
- Explore previously used methods of contraception for appropriateness after childbirth.
- Provide current, evidence-based information about family planning options either during pregnancy or in the immediate postpartum period.
- Debunk myths about breastfeeding as a method of family planning.

Task Seven: Realigning Intergenerational Patterns

The first baby adds a new generation in the family lineage that carries the family into the future. Expectant parents change roles from being their parents' children to becoming parents themselves. Childbearing may signify the onset of taking on an adult role for adolescent parents and for some cultural groups. Childbearing changes relationships within extended families as parents' siblings become aunts and uncles, children from previous relationships become stepsiblings, and parents become grandparents.

Siblings typically experience many emotional changes with the arrival of a new family member. Feelings of confusion, hurt, anger, resentment, jealousy, and sibling rivalry are common among younger siblings, as is behavioral regression. Parents should be prepared for these emotional upheavals with strategies that help the sibling(s) adjust to and accept the new baby.

Grandparents often provide the greatest amount of support to families when a child is born. The degree of their involvement may be linked to cultural expectations. The nurse should be aware that in some cultures, grandparents are a strong influence on child-rearing practices and are often intimately involved in daily family dynamics (Hayslip et al., 2019).

Family Nursing Interventions
- Assist new parents to seek support from friends, family members, organized parent groups, and work colleagues as a way to cope with the demands of parenting.

- Work with families to develop strategies that maintain their couple activities, adult interests, and friendships.
- Facilitate partner discussions about perceptions of extended family involvement in the care of the new child.
- Facilitate new parents' participation in the decision-making process when health care decisions, such as infant nutrition decisions, are required for their child.
- Provide learning opportunities to help move new parents from dependence to independence and self-reliance.
- Offer sibling classes during childbirth education for young children (2 to 8 years) and provide parents with information on how to help ease the transition.
- Offer classes for grandparents during childbirth education with topics varying from assistance with household management to current recommendations on infant positioning, feeding, and clothing, as well as positive strategies to help them assume a supportive (nonparenting) role.

Task Eight: Maintaining Family Members' Motivation and Morale

After the initial excitement that often surrounds the arrival of a new baby, families must learn to adjust to and cope with the demands that caring for the baby will have on their time, energy, sexual relationship, and personal resources. Many new mothers experience postpartum fatigue, which is a feeling of exhaustion and decreased ability to engage in physical and mental work (Davidson et al., 2020). Women may be fatigued because of many interrelated factors, including the blood loss associated with birth, breastfeeding, sleep difficulties, and depression. In addition, a relationship exists between maternal fatigue and PPD, both of which affect family processes (Davidson et al., 2020). The first 3 months after childbirth are recognized as the most vulnerable emotional period for mothers (Dennis & Dowswell, 2013; Ward et al., 2016) and, by extension, for their families. During this time and extending past the first year postpartum, mothers' depressive symptoms can continue; therefore, nurses must be alert for cues of depression from the new mother and other family members (Dennis et al., 2012).

In the months following childbirth, families must be realistic about infant sleep patterns and crying behaviors, the potential to experience loneliness, and changes in their sexual relationship. For example, many young families, especially single mothers, experience loneliness in the postpartum period because they live in communities far from their extended families. Some families have recently moved into a new neighborhood and may not have established friendships or a sense of community. Many ethnically diverse groups had special support and recognition of the postpartum period in their countries of origin. For example, by not taking part in traditional childbirth rituals such as the practice of "doing the month" (laying-in period of 40 days), some new immigrant mothers may be more prone to depression. Traditional practices have been recognized as protective factors and have implications in the prevention and treatment of PPD (Han et al., 2020).

Family Nursing Interventions

- Inform family members about ways to promote comfort, rest, and sleep, which will make it easier for them to cope with fatigue.
- Promote parental rest while a baby needs nighttime feedings by encouraging parents to alternate who responds to the baby.
- Teach parents ways to cope with a crying infant, which will boost family morale, increase confidence, and allow family members to get additional sleep.
- Provide information on ways that parents can reduce isolation and loneliness by seeking support from friends, family members, organized parent groups, work colleagues, and community support groups such as La Leche League.
- Encourage parents to articulate their needs and to find help in ways that support their self-esteem as new parents.
- Counsel couples about changes in sexuality after birth and help them develop mutually satisfying sexual expression.
- Help families to develop strategies that maintain their couple activities, adult interests, and friendships.
- Take a proactive approach to prepare and educate women and their families about signs of PPD.

Task Nine: Establishing Family Rituals and Routines

Family rituals and routines consist of activities that the family performs and teaches its members for continuity and stability (Ward et al., 2016). The predictability of rituals helps babies develop trust. Family rituals have been described as celebrations, traditions, religious observances, and other symbolic events. Family rituals include the observance of celebrations such as birthdays, whereas family routines center on meal, bedtime, and bathing; greeting and dismissal routines (a kiss goodbye or goodnight); children's special possessions such as a treasured blanket; and nicknames for body functions. For some families, rituals have special cultural meanings that nurses should respect. When families are disrupted or separated during childbearing, nurses can help them deal with stress by encouraging them to carry out their usual routines and established rituals related to their babies and other children.

Family Nursing Interventions

- Determine the special cultural meaning each ritual has for the family and respect those meanings.
- Assess through observation and/or questioning, or as guided by an assessment survey tool, how families observe or acknowledge important days.
- Encourage families to carry out their usual routines and established rituals related to their babies and other children.
- Create a supportive environment that encourages parental knowledge and confidence in caring for themselves and their infants.
- Facilitate couple discussion of bedtime and bathing routines; a baby's special possessions such as a treasured blanket; nicknames; language for body functions; and welcoming rituals such as announcements, baptisms, circumcision, or other celebrations.

Family Transitions

Although it is not another task, transition is a major concept in the Family Developmental and Life Cycle Theory (Duvall, 1977). Inherent in transition from one developmental stage to the next is a period of upheaval as the family moves from one state to another. Historically, "transition to parenthood" was thought by early family researchers to be a crisis (LeMasters, 1957; Steffensmeier, 1982). The idea of transition to parenthood as a crisis is being abandoned. More recent work focuses on the transition processes associated with a change in families.

Life transitions, including entering pregnancy or parenthood, are peak times for change. Nurse researchers have mostly focused on the transition to motherhood. Even though other family members experience the transition when a newborn joins the family, concepts related to motherhood give nurses insight into family transition. For example, opening of self relates to making a commitment to mothering, experiencing the presence of a child, and caring for the child. The notion of family transition gives a foundation for nursing interventions that promote parenting because opening of self involves the real experience of being with and caring for the child. Nurses who understand the stressors that families experience as they transition from one state to another can use this theoretical concept to realize that a mother or father may be frustrated over not being able to cope in old ways.

Just as no one theory covers all aspects of nursing, no single theory will work for every situation involving childbearing families. Therefore, nurses must understand and utilize multiple theories to plan and guide nursing care for childbearing families. Major concepts from Family Systems Theory and Family Developmental and Life Cycle Theory help nurses organize assessments and manage the predictable and unpredictable experiences encountered by childbearing families.

CHILDBEARING FAMILY STRESSORS

Childbearing family nursing begins when a couple anticipates and plans for pregnancy, has already conceived, or is planning to adopt a child. Any pregnancy-related event such as infertility, adoption, pregnancy loss, or an unplanned pregnancy may be enough to disrupt the delicately formed bonds of the family in this stage. Nurses need to be aware of problems that childbearing families might encounter before, during, and after reproductive events so that they can anticipate, identify, and respond to needs appropriately.

Infertility

The ability to conceive is a major milestone in a couple's life (Wong et al., 2012). Both men and women perceive fertility to be a sign of competence as reproductive human beings. Therefore, the experience of infertility can be a life crisis that disrupts a couple's marital and/or sexual relationship. Infertility is "a disease defined by failure to achieve a successful pregnancy after 12 months or more of appropriate, timed unprotected intercourse or therapeutic donor insemination" (American Society for Reproductive Medicine, 2012, para 1). Infertility is a medical and social problem that is of concern to childbearing family nurses, especially in cultures where the expectation of motherhood is strong and because of the increasing trend of delayed childbearing in all industrialized countries (Gossett et al., 2013; Wong et al., 2012).

Nurses should anticipate that infertile couples will experience several different physical, emotional, and psychological symptoms. Couples dealing with infertility struggle between feelings of hope and hopelessness, and they report feelings of sadness, fatigue, anxiety, and urgency; changes in sleeping patterns (e.g., oversleeping, night waking, insomnia); and headaches (Braverman et al., 2015; Wilson & Leese, 2013). Their level of success with advanced reproductive technology and the level of empathetic responses they receive from caregivers often influences their perceptions of satisfaction and well-being (Wilson & Leese, 2013). Problems with infertility change a couple's social relationships and support, which may result in increased levels of depression and psychological distress (Box 14-4).

The experience of infertility is stressful for both men and women. Yet the way in which men and women respond varies (Galhardo et al., 2016). For example, many men believe their central role during fertility treatment is to be a source of strength and support for their partner (Bai et al., 2019). In contrast, women typically experience a higher risk for emotional distress than men. Feelings of anger, anxiety, shame, loss of self-esteem, grief, and depression are just some emotions that infertile woman report experiencing (Wong et al., 2012). Women want to spend time talking about their infertility experience, whereas men report that talking about it only increases their anxiety. Therefore, men dealing with infertility tend to talk, communicate, and listen less than do women. Men also cope with infertility

BOX 14-4

Common Symptoms and Stressors Infertile Couples May Experience

Some common symptoms and stressors experienced by infertile couples include the following:

- Irritability
- Insomnia
- Tension
- Depression
- Increased anxiety
- Anger toward each other, God, friends, and other fertile women
- Feelings of rejection, alienation, stigmatization, isolation, and estrangement

Sources: Braverman, A. M., Domar, A. D., Brisman, M. B., & Webb, K. J. (2015). ART nurses as the patient's partner in care: Targeting depression, stress, and other barriers. *Contemporary OB/GYN, 60*(6), s1–s12; Peterson, B. D., Sejbaek, C. S., Pirritano, M., & Schmidt, L. (2014). Are severe depressive symptoms associated with infertility-related distress in individuals and their partners? *Human Reproduction, 29*(1), 76–82; and Grunberg, P., Miner, S., & Zelkowitz. P. (2020). Infertility and perceived stress: The role of identity concern in treatment-seeking men and women, *Human Fertility,* 1–11.

through avoidance and by disguising their feelings to protect themselves, their partners, or both (Grunberg et al., 2020; Wong et al., 2012). More recently, men-only online discussion boards have provided opportunities via forum posts for men to emote in relation to infertility. In this venue, men "talk" to each other about the emotional burdens of infertility, personal coping strategies, and their relationships with others (Hanna & Gough, 2016).

Testing and treatment for infertility is expensive. Assisted reproductive therapy services provided in the United States and Canada, for the most part, are not covered under most health insurance plans or by provincial health insurance. Two Canadian provinces, Quebec and Ontario, have made provision for in vitro fertilization, a type of advanced assisted reproductive therapy, to be a covered treatment only under certain conditions.

Infertility testing and treatment is also painful, time consuming, and inconvenient. It can lead to a loss of spontaneity and privacy in sexual activities, which only compounds the stress and strain couples are experiencing. Although every test or treatment is another painful reminder of the inability to reproduce, it is nurses' lack of knowledge and understanding of the emotional aspects of infertility that

really frustrates infertile couples. Therefore, couples interpret nursing care to be insensitive and uncompassionate when nurses focus primarily on physiological or technical aspects of infertility rather than on emotional needs (Bedi et al., 2019; Grunberg et al., 2020). Therefore, it is vital that nurses caring for childbearing families experiencing infertility understand, consider, and address the emotional needs of couples undergoing assessment, diagnosis, and treatment for infertility. Families experiencing the crisis of infertility are in as much need of a personal touch as they are of technical competence and accurate, evidence-based information about testing and treatment options. See Box 14-5 for specific nursing interventions to help couples deal with infertility.

Adoption

Adoption is one of the ways people may become parents (Giesler, 2012; Foli et al., 2017). Many different types of families adopt (U.S. Department of Health and Human Services, n.d.), including single parents; families formed by second parents or with stepparents; and transracial, transcultural, relative, and LGBTQ+ families. Although adoptive mothers and families may not experience the physical context of pregnancy, they may have many of the same feelings and fears as biological families (Cao et al., 2016). Childbearing family nurses must be aware that all parents react to the intense feelings and emotions, ranging from happiness to distress, in the first moments they meet their child, regardless of the way in which a family is formed. Even though the child is not biological or the parental relationship may not be established immediately at birth, bonding can be just as strong and immediate for adoptive parents and children (Hockenberry & Wilson, 2018; Wrobel et al., 2020). Therefore, nurses caring for women in the preadoption and early postadoption period must recognize and provide care that is respectful and family-centered according to the needs of the individual family. Although many of the clinical assessment and physical needs might differ, educational, parenting, and feeding concerns may be similar to those of biological mothers in the prenatal and postpartum periods (Cao et al., 2016; Wrobel et al., 2020).

Once families decide to adopt a child, they may pursue several routes, such as international adoption (also known as intercountry adoption), public domestic adoption, or private domestic adoption.

BOX 14-5

Nursing Interventions That Are Helpful to Couples Dealing With Infertility

Helpful nursing interventions for couples dealing with infertility include the following:

- Avoid assigning blame to one partner or the other.
- Encourage social support from friends, spouse, or significant other.
- Assess couples' coping strategies, encourage open discussion between couples, suggest different coping strategies.
- Facilitate communication between couples in order to give men, in particular, the opportunity to acknowledge and express their feelings and process their response to the infertility experience.
- Provide information related to cost and insurance coverage for treatment.
- Suggest appropriate stress-relieving activities, such as acupuncture.
- Refer the couple to support groups and/or other professionals for counseling.

Sources: Adapted from Bai, C. F., Sun, J. W., Li, J., Jing, W. H., Zhang, X. K., Zhang, X., Li Li, M., Yue, R., & Cao, F. L. (2019). Gender differences in factors associated with depression in infertility patients. *Journal of Advanced Nursing, 75*(12), 3515–3524; Grant, L.-E., & Cochrane, S. (2014). Acupuncture for the mental and emotional health of women undergoing IVF treatment. A comprehensive review. *Australian Journal of Acupuncture and Chinese Medicine, 9*(1), 5–12; Bedi, S., Ferrell, S., & Harris, J. Y. (2019). Experiences of adults participating in infertility support groups: A qualitative systematic review protocol. *JBI Database Systematic Reviews and Implement Reports, 17*(8),1552–1557; and Wong, C., Pang, J., Tan, G., Soh, W., & Lim, J. (2012). The impact of fertility on women's psychological health: A literature review. *Singapore Nursing Journal, 39*(3), 11–17.

In the United States, domestic adoption can be a difficult, lengthy, bureaucratic, and costly process that takes anywhere from 2 to 7 years for a healthy infant (National Adoption Center, n.d.). The laws favoring birth mothers also complicate domestic adoption. This long waiting period and fear of the court system result in many families turning to intercountry adoptions, which generally take 1 to 4 years before a child can enter the United States. The length of time it takes to complete intercountry adoptions depends on many factors, including procedures in the child's country of origin, the adoption service provider's process, the U.S. immigration process, and the specific circumstance of the adoption (Intercountry Adoption, 2018). One drawback to an international adoption is that little to no information about the child's

birth parents' background, prenatal health care, or medical history may be available to the adopting family (Hilferty & Katz, 2019). The lack of birth history places families at risk for adopting a child who may have experienced a significant number of threats to physical health as well as brain and behavioral development, which can contribute to future struggles as families cope with the consequences of these problems (Wrobel et al., 2020). Box 14-6 lists other issues and challenges related to international and also transracial adoption.

In Canada, approximately 20% of families are affected by adoption, either through the public child welfare (foster care) system or private adoption agencies. A prerequisite for all Canadian adoption is successful completion of the Parent Resource for Information Development and Education (PRIDE) course. In addition, private Canadian adoption agencies are required to provide birth parents with counseling before the birth, to offer emotional support for adoptive parents, and to organize the court and legal services involved.

Private adoption is another alternative for families considering adoption. Private adoptions can range from being strictly anonymous to very open, where the adopting couple and birth mother get to know each other extremely well. Often, the internet is a place where women wanting to place babies for adoption and families seeking to adopt connect. Canadian families wishing to adopt should be aware that some provinces do not allow for direct advertising on the internet or in newspaper classifieds (Canada Adopts!, 2014). Regardless of how North American families connect or interact with the birth mother, it is paramount that families pursuing private adoption retain professional legal advice and counsel to ensure that everyone involved, including the birth father, understands the legal ramifications and to work out all aspects related to the adoption before the baby's birth. In Canada, adoption falls under provincial jurisdiction, and laws are highly variable between provinces. For example, some provinces allow families themselves to find a child to adopt rather than having an agency choose one for them. Nurses should encourage Canadian families working with private agencies to understand any adoption restrictions or limitations set by the province in which they reside (Canada Adopts!, 2014).

Nurses should be aware that when a private adoption has been negotiated, one of the important points is whether the adopting family will be

BOX 14-6

The Issues and Challenges of International and Transracial Adoption

Issues and Challenges to Families Before International and Transracial Adoption

- Ability to travel on short notice to pick up a child
- Changing political conditions, which may stop the adoption process at any time
- Ways family will maintain the adopted child's natural heritage
- Ways family will deal with racial and other types of prejudice
- The many rules and conditions that sometimes prevent families from adopting a child from a particular country

Issues and Challenges to Families After International Adoption

- Limited postadoption resources are available, such as pediatricians trained in international adoption, or international adoption clinics for families seeking help for a child's developmental and behavioral problems.
- The child's emotional and developmental issues can be exhausting and can tax the family financially.
- Limited or no information about the child's maternal or paternal medical history can be a source of uncertainty and adoptive parental stress.

Issues and Challenges to Families After Transracial Adoption

- There is a need to redefine the family as multiracial and multiethnic.
- Extra attention and comments about the child's looks may occur from strangers in public places.
- Neighbors, family members, and others may express prejudice toward the child.

Sources: Adapted from Gunnar, M., & Pollak, S. D. (2007). Supporting parents so that they can support their internationally adopted children: The larger challenge lurking behind the fatality statistics. *Child Maltreatment, 12*(4), 381–382; Pillitteri, A. (2014). *Maternal and child health nursing: Care of the childbearing and childbearing family* (7th ed.). Philadelphia, PA: Lippincott Williams & Wilkins; Rykkje, L. (2007). Intercountry adoption and nursing care. *Scandinavian Journal of Caring Sciences, 21*(4), 507–514; and Smit, E. (2010). International adoption families: A unique health care journey. *Pediatric Nursing, 36*(5), 253–258.

BOX 14-7

Nursing Interventions for Adoptive Families

The following are selected nursing interventions for adoptive families:

- Encourage families to seek help from adoption experts and agencies.
- Encourage families to understand and follow any legal and provincial limitations or restrictions related to adoption.
- Refer families to adoption specialists, such as social workers, counselors, and lawyers.
- Recommend that families speak with and secure pediatric providers during the preadoption process.
- Recommend that adoptive parents attend parenting classes and include them in prenatal and infant care classes.
- Incorporate adoption-sensitive material into classes and other educational resources.
- Keep lines of communication open between nurses and adoptive families as a way to alleviate fears about being judged or undermined.
- Address other siblings' response to the adopted child because a biological child's feelings of inferiority or superiority to an adopted child can interfere with relationships within the family.
- Address family concerns about attachment issues.

Sources: Adapted from Canada Adopts! (2014). Adopting in Canada. Retrieved from www.canadaadopts.com/canada/domestic_private.shtml; Fontenot, H. (2007). Transition and adaptation to adoptive motherhood. *Journal of Obstetrics, Gynecologic and Neonatal Nursing, 36*(2), 175–182; Pillitteri, A. (2014). *Maternal and child health nursing: Care of the childbearing and childbearing family* (7th ed.). Philadelphia, PA: Lippincott Williams & Wilkins; and Smit, E. (2010). International adoption families: A unique health care journey. *Pediatric Nursing, 36*(5), 253–258.

2017). See Box 14-7 for appropriate nursing interventions when caring for adoptive families.

Perinatal Loss

Perinatal loss is not uncommon, and it is a traumatic event for families around the globe (Callister, 2014; Umphrey & Cacciatore, 2014; Willis, 2019). Losing a child during pregnancy, after birth, or in the early postpartum period is one of the hardest things a family can experience. The loss may be anticipated and voluntary, such as with abortion or relinquishing parental rights for adoption, or unanticipated, such as death or loss of custody to the state. An adoptive family may lose their intended child if a birth mother changes her mind about giving up a baby for adoption. Box 14-8

present at the child's birth. Nurses must also be prepared and ready to intervene should a birth mother reverse her decision to give up the baby for adoption or a birth father who has not relinquished his legal right to the baby asserts his rights (McKinney et al., 2018; Silbert-Flagg & Pillitteri,

BOX 14-8

Types of Perinatal Loss Families May Experience

Families may experience the following types of perinatal loss:

- Miscarriage
- Elective abortion
- Ectopic pregnancy
- Selective reduction after in vitro implantation of multiple fertilized eggs
- Stillbirth
- Death of a child after a live birth
- Recurrent pregnancy loss
- Death of a twin during pregnancy, labor, birth, or after birth
- Termination of pregnancy for identified fetal anomalies, which is increasing because of technological advances in prenatal diagnosis of such anomalies
- Loss of what was believed to be the anticipated "perfect" child because of anomalies or malformations

lists other types of perinatal loss that families may experience.

Loss of a child is a unique and profound experience for parents. When parents lose a child, they lose part of their hoped-for identity, including all hopes and dreams held for the child they anticipated and loved; they also often experience a lack of social recognition regarding the significance of their loss (Heazell et al., 2016; Willis, 2019). Societal invisibility of infant loss contributes to parental frustration, especially when they are denied time to mourn or are asked why they are not yet over their loss (Umphrey & Cacciatore, 2014). One mother put it this way when describing her loss experience, "Oh God, please help me. I need someone to help me pass through this pain" (Callister, 2014, p. 207). Therefore, nurses caring for childbearing families must engage in ongoing assessment and interventions related to potential, previous, or current loss. Grief and a process of bereavement should also be anticipated secondary to perinatal loss, an adverse perinatal outcome, diagnosis of congenital or genetic disorders, palliative care, or the birth of a child with special health needs.

Nurses providing care to childbearing families should anticipate that each family member will experience loss differently. For example, research shows that mothers are more apt to grieve visibly by emotional expression, sharing of feelings, and participation in grief support groups. Fathers, in contrast, tend to feel a sense of loneliness and isolation and have feelings of helplessness. Fathers, who often see their role as primarily supportive of their partner, may feel the need to "act as men" by being strong and may hold back their own feelings of grief and pain (Koopmans et al., 2013; Umphrey & Cacciatore, 2014). Siblings may describe their grief experience as "hurting inside," which is a way to express feelings of sadness, frustration, loneliness, fear, and anger (Heazell et al., 2016). Grandparents experience a triple measure of grief and sorrow when a grandchild dies: their own personal grief as a human being suffering the death of a loved one; the pain over the loss of a grandchild, which carries with it the loss of their dreams and expectations for their relationship with that child; and seeing their own children suffer (Heazell et al., 2016).

Demonstrations of grief and rituals tied to bereavement and loss vary across personality types, cultural mores, and societal expectations globally. Despite the differences, researchers have noted that there may be a similar sense of loss across all cultures that represents the loss of a cherished or valuable family member. The role of the grieving individual, whether an infant, child or adult, may be accompanied by strong emotions and passionate behaviors, or it might be accompanied by solitude, anger, or changes to normal routines. Most loss and bereavement researchers describe behaviors that signify a continued attachment to the conceived individual, their role in the family, and the identities of those left behind. Feelings of loss and bereavement might follow perinatal loss after any planned or unplanned pregnancy loss at any gestational age, infant loss, or loss of a child or older family members (Charrois et al., 2020; Davidson et al., 2020; Fernandez-Basanta et al., 2020a).

Considering the effect of perinatal loss on all family members, nurses must work to support and strengthen the familial bond in the face of such loss (Heazell et al., 2016; Koopmans et al., 2013). Nurses can support families' experience of perinatal loss by being present and listening attentively, expressing emotions, gathering memorabilia, and helping the family make meaning of the experience. Referral to support groups or provision of a list of available resources may be helpful depending on the needs of the grieving couple or family (Koopmans et al., 2013; McKinney et al., 2018). Compassionate Friends is one of many groups to which nurses might refer grieving parents, siblings, and grandparents for support.

Culture influences how families respond to perinatal loss. Therefore, it is essential for nurses to understand several different culturally diverse practices and rituals associated with loss, as well as provide culturally competent care. In Western cultures, holding and touching the stillborn infant and mementos are commonly used support strategies. However, mothers from certain countries may avoid touching and holding their stillborn babies because these behaviors are considered unacceptable in their countries of origin (Callister, 2014; Heazell et al., 2016). Patients may also have specific burial requirements depending on culture or religion. Families from Indigenous and Muslim cultures may request early burial and accommodation in the hospital room for respected religious elders to perform rituals (Cacciatore & Flint, 2012; Fernández-Basanta et al., 2020b). Nurses demonstrate cultural sensitivity when they validate what families perceive to be the "right way" to grieve (Boyle et al., 2020).

Pregnancy Following Perinatal Loss

Psychological distress is higher in parents who have experienced a prior perinatal loss, with maternal anxiety about a child's well-being extending a year or more after the birth of another child (Smorti et al., 2020). Women may not perceive pregnancy as normal after experiencing perinatal loss but rather may be plagued with a sense of anxiety, insecurity, ambivalence, doubt, and concern that another loss may occur (Davidson et al., 2020; Umphrey & Cacciatore, 2014; Wool, 2013). They also experience higher levels of anxiety than fathers. Fathers may shut down their feelings when pregnancy occurs after loss because of unresolved feelings related to prior pregnancy loss. They may even be too frightened to share or may not be conscious of their feelings.

Nurses caring for childbearing families during pregnancy after perinatal loss are in a prime position to help mothers and fathers open doors of communication that may have been closed because of fear (Jones et al., 2019). One strategy that nurses could use to encourage communication is to ask fathers, "How are you doing?" in front of the mothers, which provides an opportunity to share what they are feeling (Davidson et al., 2020; Koopmans et al., 2013; Umphrey & Cacciatore, 2014). In addition, nurses need to be caring, sensitive, and patient. They need to offer clear specific information about prenatal care and opportunities for both parents to ask questions. If anxiety or unresolved grief issues are present, a referral to a grief counselor may be supportive and beneficial for the parents (Davidson et al., 2020; Wool, 2013).

THREATS TO HEALTH DURING CHILDBEARING

For the majority of families, childbearing is a physically healthy experience. For some families, however, health during childbearing is threatened and the childbearing experience becomes an illness experience. In such cases, concern for the physical health of the mother and the fetus tends to outweigh other aspects of pregnancy; rather than eagerly anticipating the birth and baby, family members experience fear and apprehension. In addition, the family's functioning and developmental tasks are disrupted as the family focuses its attention on the health of the mother and survival of the fetus or baby. Childbearing nurses must be aware that families with threats to health have additional needs for maintaining and preserving family health.

Acute and Chronic Illness During Childbearing

This chapter defines *acute* as health threats that arise suddenly and may have life-threatening implications. Examples of acute health threats that childbearing families may encounter are fetal distress during labor and pulmonary embolism for postpartum women. In contrast, the word *chronic* comprises conditions occurring during pregnancy that persist, linger, need control, or have no cure and that require careful monitoring and treatment to avoid becoming an acute threat to maternal or infant health. Gestational hypertension, preexisting and gestational diabetes, and PPD are some examples of chronic health threats. Some threats to health during childbearing vacillate between acute and chronic. For example, preterm labor can be an acute health threat that results in a preterm birth. If preterm labor contractions are suppressed, it becomes a chronic health threat requiring adherence to prescribed regimens to keep contractions from recurring.

Effect of Threats to Health on Childbearing Families

Chronic threats to childbearing health are disruptive to childbearing families. Knowledge of the family as a dynamic system explains why the effects of these chronic conditions extend to the entire family and result in the upset of family functioning, communication, and roles (Arestedt et al., 2014). When childbearing health is threatened, all family members experience stress as families strive to regain balance. For example, three sources of stress that alter family processes when the mother or infant experiences a chronic health threat are (1) assuming household tasks, (2) managing changes in income and resources, and (3) facing uncertainty and separation or loss.

Assuming Household Tasks

When women experience chronic threats to childbearing health, other members of the family must assume responsibility for household tasks and functioning, regardless of whether the condition is managed at the hospital or at home. Assumption of household tasks by others creates family stress, especially for partners who must take on the role of caring for the family as well as caring for the expectant mother and/or infant (Cava-Tadik et al., 2020). Expectant partners especially may find that all their time and energy are consumed by employment and household management, tasks that previously were shared or done solely by their partners. Children's lives change when mothers have to limit activities. Toddlers do not understand why their mothers cannot pick them up or run after them. The resulting frustration for children can manifest itself in behavioral changes, such as tantrums and regression in developmental tasks (e.g., toilet training).

Managing Changes in Income and Resources

An at-risk pregnancy is stressful in terms of the family's finances and other resources. For example, if a mother is placed on bedrest to manage antepartum bleeding from a placenta previa, she may miss time away from paid employment. Or a mother may not have the ability to seek employment, which also results in loss of income. At the same time, medical expenses may increase because of the need for increased care, including possible neonatal intensive care and maintaining multiple health care provider visits or hospital stays. Personal expenses associated with the cost of specialized diets, medications, and hiring personnel to assist with household tasks may also increase; such costs are not usually covered by health care systems in Canada or the United States. For families already in debt or struggling with unemployment or other financial challenges, these threats to health serve to increase the burden of debt.

Although resources, such as energy and social networks, cannot be measured as easily as money, family nurses are in a position to help families consider and manage changes in their nonmonetary resources. Some of the nonmonetary changes that family nurses should anticipate families will encounter include the following: others outside the nuclear family may need to assume various household tasks, such as meal preparation, laundry, and cleaning; all families may not have social networks or extended families in the immediate vicinity; changes in employment may cause separation from persons and activities that were stimulating; and isolation, regardless of the cause, can increase a family's burden.

Facing Uncertainty and Separation or Loss

The unpredictable nature of high-risk childbearing makes planning for the future difficult for childbearing families because it leaves them facing uncertainty and possible separation. For example, expectant parents, especially employed women, face uncertainty with pending preterm birth; they may not be able to determine accurately when to begin and end parental leave because of the need to cope with sudden hospitalization. Separation can occur when mothers are suddenly hospitalized or when families living in remote rural areas are transferred to a distant perinatal center for days or weeks. When families are separated, it becomes difficult for them to maintain and develop family relationships. Separation from the family and concerns about family status are two of the greatest stressors experienced by women hospitalized for chronic threats to childbearing health (Finlayson et al., 2020). In addition, small children experience extreme anxiety over the sudden departure of their mother, especially if they are unprepared or unable to comprehend what is happening to their mother and the new baby.

Even if the logistical problems related to separation are solved and a family can be together, coping with basic tasks of living is challenging in new settings. For instance, a family may not know where to stay, how to find reasonably priced meals, how to obtain transportation, or where to park a car.

Box 14-9 presents nursing interventions related to childbearing families who are experiencing chronic threats to health.

FAMILY NURSING OF POSTPARTUM FAMILIES

All family members experience household upheaval during the first few days and weeks that a newborn is in the home. Throughout the childbearing cycle, nurses assist families to understand, prepare, and respond to the effect of a new baby on the family. Assisting parents to be realistic in their expectations about themselves, each other, and their children helps them to plan ahead by identifying appropriate support and resources. This section discusses appropriate nursing assessments and interventions that family nurses should

---

BOX 14-9

Family Nursing Interventions for Childbearing Families Experiencing Chronic Threats to Health

Assuming Household Tasks

- Help families find ways to streamline and prioritize household tasks to reduce stress and increase adherence to medical regimens.
- Assist adults to list household management tasks and determine who does what and when so that the family can be more efficient and effective in managing these tasks.
- Educate families about the impact of parents' health difficulties on children.
- Provide practical, age-appropriate suggestions for managing children, such as hiring a teenager after school for active play with young children.
- Encourage parents to provide ways for young children to have some quiet one-on-one time with their mothers as a way to reduce stress for both mothers and children.

Managing Changes in Income and Resources

- Refer families to an appropriate counselor who can explore with family members ways to manage financial problems.
- Assist families to identify others outside the nuclear family who can assume various household tasks, such as meal preparation, laundry, and cleaning.
- Help families identify and use resources, such as home-health agencies and parents' groups in the community, to assist with household management.
- Encourage families with necessary resources to use a computer to connect with each other, friends, coworkers, and other at-risk families to prevent or decrease feelings of isolation.
- Direct families to appropriate internet sites.

Facing Uncertainty, Separation, and Loss

- Acknowledge the stresses of uncertainties associated with difficult perinatal situations.
- Be honest and informative about the condition and prognosis of both the mother and fetus.
- Use terms understood by all family members to provide accurate and thorough explanations tailored to families' anxiety levels.
- Assist families to cope with the basic tasks of living in high-tech settings such as the neonatal intensive care unit.
- Investigate and reduce the barriers that families may encounter at a distant perinatal center, such as lack of transportation, disruptions in employment, and the threatening environment of a strange setting.
- Provide families with information on where to stay, how to find reasonably priced meals, how to obtain transportation, and where to park a car.
- Encourage use of electronic communication, such as e-mail, to facilitate contact between family members and health care professionals.
- Encourage calling families about their members' progress and sending photographs as a way to help families cope with uncertainty and enhance relationships of physically separated family members.
- Encourage family members to participate in care of their infants to promote development of parenting skills.

incorporate into their practice when caring for families during the postpartum period.

Feeding Management

Success in feeding their babies induces feelings of competency in mothers. A family's comfort with its infant feeding method is as crucial for physical, emotional, and social well-being of the infant as is the food itself. Regardless of the parents' choice of feeding method, nurses' instructions should emphasize the development of relationships between infant and parent through feeding. Being held during feeding enhances social development whether a baby is being breastfed or bottle-fed. Parents should take the time during feedings to enjoy interacting with their babies. When the infant is adopted, social interaction with feeding is a special opportunity for developing attachment.

Even though the act of breastfeeding is associated with the mother, fathers and partners need not be excluded from the feeding experience. Nurses can promote parent-infant attachment by encouraging fathers and partners to be involved with feeding. For example, the father can burp the baby during or after feedings, hold and comfort the infant once feeding has been completed, and feed the baby a bottle of expressed breast milk once breastfeeding is well established (McKinney et al., 2018). Early involvement of fathers and partners in feeding is beneficial later when infants are being weaned from the breast or mothers are preparing to return to employment.

Many people assume that breastfeeding is natural and so should not present any difficulties. Nevertheless, many women initially may experience breastfeeding difficulties, especially if the baby has difficulty latching or milk takes longer than expected to come in. It is important that nurses assess a mother's breastfeeding technique early and provide hands-on teaching so mothers can learn how to breastfeed successfully. Referral to a lactation consultant may be necessary before the new family leaves the hospital. Most hospitals have lactation specialists in the hospital and some also provide postdischarge services in the community. Nurses should also ensure that the family is given resource information about breastfeeding, including how to obtain assistance at postdischarge clinics when breastfeeding challenges arise.

Attachment

Positive parent-infant attachment must take place to foster optimal growth and development of infants as well as to encourage the parent-infant love relationship. The attachment process requires early involvement and physical contact between parents and their infant for a strong link to develop (Barlow et al., 2015). Extreme stress, health risk factors, and illness can interfere with the physical contact and early parent-infant involvement needed for the development of attachment. Stressful conditions that pull parents' energies and attention away from their newborns can be detrimental to attachment. Adoption can be another factor influencing attachment, especially if the child had multiple caretakers or frequently changed living locations. Children who were adopted from more stable environments may also have attachment difficulties if they struggle to transfer their attachment from a previous caretaker to their adoptive parents (Wrobel et al., 2020).

Nurses should be alert for families who are likely to have difficulty with attachment, especially if family history indicates a parent has suffered abuse, neglect, or abandonment during childhood. In addition, nurses may identify families at risk for poor attachment through listening to what parents say about their babies and by observing parent behaviors. Families at risk for poor attachment may have misconceptions about infant behavior, such as believing that infants cry just to annoy their parents. Hence, family nurses must address verbal expressions of dissatisfaction with the infant, comparison of the infant with disliked family members, failure to respond to the infant's crying, lack of spontaneity in touching the infant, and stiffness or discomfort in holding the infant after the first week. Although isolated incidences of these behaviors are probably not detrimental to attachment, persistent trends and patterns could be an indicator of future relationship difficulties.

Another signal of attachment difficulty is inconsistent maternal behaviors, such as a mother who exhibits intense concern at times interspersed with apathy at other times without any predictable cause or pattern. Therefore, an important step when assessing attachment behaviors is to evaluate whether the parent-infant relationship is progressing positively and if the enjoyment and love of the child is growing over time. If the parents' enjoyment of the baby as a unique individual and their commitment to the baby are not progressing, the nurse needs to help the family understand what attachment is and also needs to identify factors that might be interfering with attachment to the infant. For example, mothers struggling with PPD need treatment for their depression before they can address attachment to the infant. Nurses can assess, support, and positively affect mothers and their families through postpartum home visits (Aston et al., 2015). Childbearing family nurses may need to refer families who do not demonstrate nurturing behaviors to other professionals such as social workers, psychotherapists, and developmental specialists who can provide more intensive interventions that will help parents care for and nurture their children.

Siblings

No matter what the age of the siblings, the addition of a new baby affects the position, role, and power of older children, thereby creating stress for both parents and children. Teaching parents to emphasize the positive aspects of adding a family member helps them focus on sibling relationships rather than rivalry. Parents need help to address *all* the children's needs, not just those of the new baby. Parents may be concerned about whether they have enough energy, time, and love for additional children. Practical ideas for time and task management can alleviate some of their concerns, as can helping parents delegate nonparenting tasks, such as housecleaning and meal preparation, to friends and relatives when possible.

PPD

The period after childbirth can be a stressful time for women because of their need to face the new tasks of the maternal role. Changes in relationships, economic demands, and social support also take place during this time and can result in postpartum stress (Kassam, 2019). Beck (2006, 2020) described PPD as a "thief." In other words, PPD metaphorically robs women of happiness and the experience of loving their infants during the first several weeks to months of the postpartum period (Beck, 2020).

PPD, or "baby blues," is common, with up to 80% of mothers experiencing this temporary emotional distress during the first 3 to 5 days after delivery. These changes in mood may be caused by the quick hormonal changes after delivery, fatigue, emotional letdown, and the stresses of being a new mother. Depressive symptoms that persist during the first year are of concern to family nurses because they can adversely affect infant health, maternal health, and the ability of mothers to function in their new role (Beck, 2020; Kassam, 2019). PPD is a treatable disorder; prompt intervention improves long-term outcomes. The optimal treatment plan for a woman with PPD involves a coordinated interdisciplinary team and a holistic, family-centered approach.

PPD and perinatal mood disorders were included in the *Diagnostic and Statistical Manual of Mental Disorders* (*DSM–5*) for the first time in 2013 (American Psychiatric Association [APA], 2013; Smith-Nielsen et al., 2018). Pundits have argued that this development marked the continuing pathologizing of normal variations in the expected adaptations to significant changes to the life of an individual or family. Consequently, the emotions and behaviors such as sadness, frequent crying, insomnia, or excessive sleeping; lack of interest or pleasure in usual activities, including sexual relations; difficulty thinking, concentrating, or making decisions; lack of concern about personal appearance; and fatigue or loss of energy might all be expected for mothers following stressful life experiences such as immigration to a new country, family violence, or racism (Brown-Bowers et al., 2015). Instead, the persistent experience of feelings of worthlessness, depressed mood, thoughts of death, suicidal ideation without a plan, or suicide plan or attempt might be the only reliable indications of pathology requiring pharmaceutical and/or psychotherapeutic intervention (Brown-Bowers et al., 2015; Davidson et al., 2020; Smith-Nielsen, 2018).

Left unidentified and untreated, PPD leads to serious consequences for families, such as maternal suicide, poor attachment to the infant, altered family dynamics, and lowered cognitive development in children. Considering these consequences, it becomes imperative that all health care providers educate women and their families about potential causes and symptoms of PPD, as well as immediately identify and appropriately refer women experiencing this mood disorder so that early treatment can begin (O'Mahony, 2017;

BOX 14-10

Signs of PPD

The following are signs of PPD:

- Sadness
- Frequent crying
- Insomnia or excessive sleeping
- Lack of interest or pleasure in usual activities, including sexual relations
- Difficulty thinking, concentrating, or making decisions
- Lack of concern about personal appearance
- Feelings of worthlessness
- Fatigue or loss of energy
- Depressed mood
- Thoughts of death: suicidal ideation without a plan; suicide plan or attempt

Stewart & Vigod, 2019; Van Lieshout et al., 2019). Box 14-10 lists signs of PPD.

Women do not usually volunteer information about their depression out of shame, fear, cultural stigma, lack of understanding about the seriousness of their illness, or lack of available access to appropriate health care services (Kassam, 2019; O'Mahony, 2017; Stewart & Vigod, 2019). Therefore, it is incumbent on nurses to identify its existence by understanding and recognizing the signs and symptoms, even if they are subtle. If the new mother is making negative comments about herself, the baby, or her partner; if she is ignoring her other children's needs; if her physical appearance shows signs of neglect; or if family members report a change in the woman's mood or behavior, it is time to screen for PPD. Childbearing family nurses might consider incorporating brief screening tool measures such as the Patient Health Questionnaire-2 (PHQ-2) and the Pregnancy Risk Assessment Monitoring System Questionnaire (PRAMS) developed as a rapid way to begin the identification of women at risk for PPD (Davis et al., 2013). However, such tools have to be used with the understanding that women who are at risk for depression may be missed (Slavin et al., 2020). Drawing on Slavin et al.'s (2020) recommendations, nurses using brief screening tools are advised to heighten scoring sensitivity. For example, after scoring positively to one out of the two PHQ-2 questions, the Edinburgh Postnatal Depression Scale (EPDS) should be applied to ensure accuracy (Slavin et al., 2020). In addition, it is important to move beyond quantifying specific indicators toward understanding the interplay of a woman's contextual health determinants with her postpartum symptoms.

Family nurses caring for childbearing families might also consider using one of many readily available and easy-to-use depression scales, such as EPDS or the Postpartum Depression Predictors Inventory–Revised, as a routine screening tool for PPD (Davidson et al., 2020; McKinney et al., 2018). In particular, EPDS has been found to be valid for several cultures, has been translated into several different languages, and has been used with men (Carlberg et al., 2018; Slavin et al., 2020). Regardless of which screening tool is used to identify women at risk for PPD, childbearing family nurses have a professional responsibility to assess for the disorder, recommend women be referred for treatment, and provide self-care strategies and support to the woman and her family (Bina et al., 2019).

Although much attention has been given to maternal PPD, shifting gender roles and paternal involvement in child care require adjustments for men as well, which puts them at risk for experiencing depression after the birth of a child, especially if the mother is depressed. This consequence makes sense to nurses who understand Family Systems Theory because anything that affects one family member directly or indirectly affects other family members. Viewed from this theoretical perspective, it is easy to see how maternal or paternal depression affects all family members and relationships within the family and results in serious implications for family health and well-being. Therefore, family nurses must recognize PPD in fathers or other partners just as in mothers because, when both parents are depressed, the risk to infants and children increases. As with mothers, referral for fathers to mental health care providers should be made in an effort to initiate early treatment and reduce negative effects on the family system (Carlberg et al., 2018; Sethna et al., 2015). Box 14-11 lists additional nursing interventions for PPD.

POLICY IMPLICATIONS FOR FAMILY NURSING

The concerns of childbearing family nursing go beyond care of the individual family. Nurses are participants in understanding, developing, and

BOX 14-11

Nursing Interventions for PPD

Nursing interventions for PPD include the following:

- Help women differentiate between myths of the mother role—which imply that at 6 weeks after birth, women are ready to resume all their previous activities—and the reality of motherhood.
- Assist women to re-create, restructure, and integrate changes that new motherhood brings into their daily lives.
- Encourage women with PPD to share feelings as they grieve the loss of who they were and begin to build on who they are becoming.
- Solicit input from family members about changes in mood or behavior.
- Offer information about PPD at various times to perinatal women through outreach support.
- Encourage women to seek help with symptoms of anxiety, anger, obsessive thinking, fear, guilt, and/or suicidal thoughts.
- Ensure that regular PPD screening is a shared responsibility between obstetrics, primary-care community health, and family health care providers.
- Develop standard protocols for screening men whose partners are depressed after childbirth.
- Ensure that education for PPD includes family members.
- Work with women to establish connections within community-based services for new mothers and their families.

Sources: Adapted from Bina, R., Glasser, S., Honovich, M., Levinson, D., & Ferber, Y. (2019). Nurses' perceived preparedness to screen, intervene, and refer women with suspected postpartum depression. *Midwifery, 76*, 132–141; O'Mahony, J. M., Donnelly, T. T., Este, D., & Raffin Bouchal, S. (2012). Using critical ethnography to explore issues among immigrant and refugee women seeking help for postpartum depression. *Issues in Mental Health Nursing, 33*(11), 735–742; and Sethna, V., Murray, L., Netsi, E., Psychogiou, L., & Ramchandani, P.G. (2015). Paternal depression in the postnatal period and early father–infant interactions. *Journal of Parenting, Science and Practice, 15*(1), 1–8.

implementing policy as it relates to childbearing families. Much of Chapter 4 addresses important social policy issues relevant for childbearing families. The legal definitions of family, official recognition of the diversity of families, access to health care, alternatives to traditional childbearing such as cross-cultural adoption, and the growing needs of poverty-stricken and other disenfranchised families are just a few of the policy areas vital to childbearing family nursing.

Nurses need to be aware of the effect of legislation on childbearing families. One example is family leave for childbirth, which can profoundly affect the health and development of childbearing families. In the United States, the Family and Medical Leave Act (FMLA), a federal law enacted in 1993, entitles family members to take up to 12 weeks of *unpaid* time away from employment for certain medical or family reasons and ensures that employees can return to their same position. Birth, adoption, foster placement of a child, and caring for a child or spouse with a serious condition are permissible reasons for mothers and fathers to take leave under the FMLA. Unfortunately, many families cannot take advantage of FMLA benefits because the act only applies to those who worked for their current employer for a certain number of months and hours, for certain size businesses, and for a covered employer (Schwartz & Engler, 2015). Unlike the citizens of many developed nations, parents in the United States are not entitled to government benefits for childbearing except for tax deductions and other incentives. Many European countries, by contrast, offer paid parental leave.

In Canada, some social policies have been put into place in an effort to assist both parents to balance work-life issues and manage the care of newborns. All families in every Canadian province and territory are entitled to maternity leave or parental leave following childbirth and adoption. A federally funded Employment Insurance (EI) program provides, except in Quebec, 15 weeks of paid maternity/parental leave at 55% of the mother's usual salary (to a maximum amount, which in 2021 was $595) providing she worked 600 hours in the 52 weeks before the onset of maternity leave. In the event of a premature birth, this benefit may be extended anywhere from 17 to 52 weeks. Families residing in the province of Quebec receive maternity, paternity, parental, and adoption benefits under the Quebec Parental Insurance Program (Government of Canada, 2021).

All types of policies affect family nursing every day. Health policy has far-reaching ethical and practical implications for childbearing family nursing. For instance, certain genetic screenings during pregnancy and hearing screens for the newborn have become compulsory for health care providers in some Canadian provinces. Cystic fibrosis screening in pregnancy and newborn screening for metabolic and genetic diseases are mandatory for maternity providers in many American states. The informed decision-making models that are the impetus for these policies are not replicated in European health care systems; by contrast, they are often viewed negatively as eugenic solutions (i.e., with the goal of producing genetically improved offspring) to reduce the incidence of disability. European systems, unlike in North America, heavily fund services for disabled children and their families.

Hospitals also have policies affecting families that should be of concern to family nurses, especially considering how varied the family of today is. For example, increasing numbers of nontraditional families, such as lesbian couples, are having children through donor insemination or adoption (Malmquist & Nieminen, 2021; Tzur-Peled et al., 2019). Yet policies that guide perinatal practices—from the visual images hanging on the wall to if or how well partners are welcomed in prenatal groups, the delivery room, or other hospital environments—may be a barrier to these particular families' welfare and relationships (Snyder, 2018; Tzur-Peled et al., 2019). In these situations, family nurses have an obligation to speak out on behalf of families. Often, nurses think of policies as entities beyond their control. In actuality, nurses have a voice and power in forming and changing policies. Beginning steps include close scrutiny of their practice settings for issues related to the welfare of families and their members.

FAMILY CASE STUDIES

This section illustrates the art and science of nursing with childbearing families. The Spencer family case study demonstrates family nursing care when unexpected health problems occur during pregnancy. The Amari-Issa family case study reveals how a nurse provides culturally sensitive care to young parents who are quite new in the country.

Case Study: Spencer Family

David and Doris Spencer are both university graduates who have been married to each other for 6 years. David, a Scottish Canadian, age 34, and Doris, a Grenadian Canadian, age 34, have a blended family that includes David's 8-year-old daughter Megan and Doris's 14-year-old daughter Marcia, both children of previous relationships. This biracial couple is now pregnant with their first child together, their first son. Doris, of African descent, did not experience any health problems with her first pregnancy. At that time, she lived in a large urban part of Canada, near her parents, siblings, and childhood friends, as well as cultural and employment networks within the African Canadian community; that is, she was close to social capital (Alvarez et al., 2017; Hernandez et al., 2019; Rodgers et al., 2019). Shortly after their fifth anniversary, the Spencers moved across the country, two time zones away. The promise of a lucrative job in western Canada, a higher standard of living, and safe school districts were motivating factors. Families like the Spencers often experience internal migration to pursue better professional opportunities and hope that the improved living conditions will outweigh any potential loss in social capital. A month after the move, they discovered that Doris was about 3 months pregnant. Although David's new job provided medical insurance for the family, Doris was concerned about finding and obtaining obstetrical care in their new community. Fortunately, Doris was able to secure a position as a hospital dietician, and her benefits supplemented her provincial insurance to cover the family's dental care and Megan's asthma medications. After her son was born, Doris expected to begin a 6-month maternity leave that provided 50% of her normal earnings. However, this pregnancy left her much more tired than her previous pregnancy and too distracted to engage in the work of preparing her son's nursery. Fortunately, Megan and Marcia were highly motivated to help with preparing their brother's nursery. Their Aunt Cora, David's older sister, was also very supportive and instrumental in organizing her baby showers. Figure 14-1 presents a Spencer family genogram.

Despite their small family's enthusiasm and support, Doris felt lonely and insecure about her new job, this unplanned pregnancy, and navigating the challenges of moving to a new city. Doris was used to the complexities of interpersonal relationships at work, the social responsibility of earning peoples' trust, and gaining a sense of belonging as a racialized Canadian. She had been navigating these complexities since secondary school. However, she noted that she was often the only Black woman in many of the team meetings and seemed to be the only one to offer intersectional, decolonized approaches to the analysis and diagnosis

Case Study: Spencer Family—cont'd

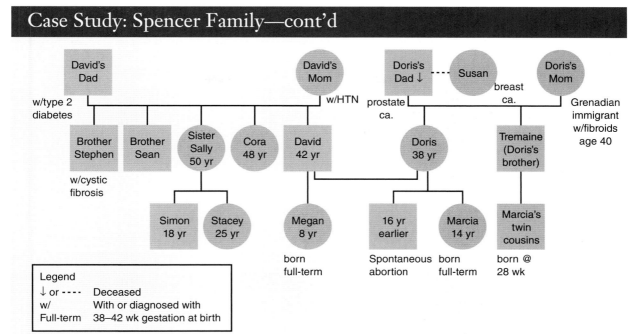

FIGURE 14-1 Spencer Family Genogram

of their diabetic patients. This was particularly the case when she tried to recommend modifications to culturally recognized foods to achieved recommended daily nutritional requirements for Indigenous clients. It became clear that the institutional changes would require more long-term systematic activities that were beyond her energy level or patience. The result was that she remained silent or agreed to come to consensus while often feeling guilty and coopted by the status quo. In many WhatsApp calls to friends and calls to her mother on the east coast, she lamented about her powerlessness and conflicted feelings. Instead of her large, comfortable home providing comfort at the end of a long day, she felt guilty for her privilege and access. Both her mother and David reminded her that it wasn't her job to "fix everyone and everything." Doris accepted this explanation gratefully, buried her feelings, and plowed on.

Doris had unexpected health problems with this pregnancy. At 20 weeks gestation, her midwife diagnosed multiple anterior and fundal, myometrial fibroids, the largest of which was 17 cm in diameter. One 7-cm fibroid was pedunculated at the right horn of the uterus. These complicated fibroids required an obstetrical consultation that led to serial ultrasounds at monthly intervals. By 34 weeks, Doris's fundal height was 40 cm, the anterior lower segment fibroid measured 15 cm, and the fundal fibroid measured 20 cm. Doris had one episode of painful bleeding at 28 weeks that required hospitalization and transfer to obstetrical care. It was anticipated that the location and size of the fibroids might adversely affect labor progress. Doris and David were provided with preterm labor precautions and instructions about when to page for emergencies, such as vaginal bleeding, decreased fetal movement, or severe abdominal pain that might signal torsion of the right ovary. Doris experienced severe abdominal pain and a short episode of vaginal bleeding at 28 weeks. She was placed on bedrest for one week, during which David, Megan, and Marcia took turns with meal preparation, housecleaning, and caring for Doris. Because he had not yet accrued vacation or sick time, David could not take time off from his job to help Doris without sacrificing pay. Doris was frustrated because she had to stop her house renovation projects on doctor's orders. David and the girls tried their best, but she tended to follow up with remediation of their cooking and housecleaning efforts when they were not up to her standards. Doris resumed modified work at 29.5 weeks and continued biweekly prenatal visits with the obstetrician. But even at 32 weeks, she was tempted to run the vacuum cleaner and wash dishes after work, which seemed to relieve some of her anxiety.

Doris's anxiety was heightened after she noticed that 14-year-old Marcia was finding it a challenge to make new friends. She was the only Black Canadian student in classes and was becoming more moody and irritable. Tensions peaked during an outing to buy baby clothes with Aunt Cora, when Marcia was mistakenly accused of shoplifting and the clerk refused to believe that Cora

(continued)

Case Study: Spencer Family—cont'd

was actually her aunt. Cora was embarrassed and incredulous that she would need to prove that they were in fact shopping for baby clothes together. She felt inadequate in her advocacy, deescalation, and attempts to exonerate her niece. Doris considered how to provide Marcia with more opportunities to debrief after this.

At 33 weeks of pregnancy, Doris experienced strong regular contractions and a return of the vaginal bleeding. Fortunately, her obstetrician was on call at the level two community hospital in which the neonatal intensive care unit (NICU) accepted newborns of 32 weeks and higher. A transport to the level three hospital 50 km (31 miles) away was unnecessary. Deshawn was born by emergency cesarean section 2 hours after the Spencer family arrived at the hospital. He was intubated for respiratory distress syndrome. Following administration of surfactant by endotracheal tube, he was gradually weaned from intubation and intravenous fluids, and began nasogastric tube feedings.

Doris was discharged from the postpartum floor within 48 hours after Deshawn's birth and transferred to the mother-baby room adjacent to the NICU. Her hemoglobin was 100 mg/dL, but she was treated with iron supplementation because she was asymptomatic. She had received an ilioinguinal nerve block from the anesthesiologist that almost completely eliminated her postop cesarean and involutory pain for 24 hours. Afterward, her incisional pain was treated with nonsteroidal anti-inflammatories (Naprosyn) every 8 to 12 hours. Doris pumped colostrum and then breastmilk. She was aware that narcotics could be expressed in breastmilk, so she decided to forgo narcotics at the recommendation of the lactation specialist. Skin-to-skin contact was encouraged in the NICU, and she was assisted to use the lactation aid while assisting Deshawn to latch. He initially had an underdeveloped and weak sucking reflex, but after his oxygen saturation improved, he was weaned off the nasal cannula, and sucking continued to improve. By 36 weeks, he had regained the 5% weight he had lost and was sucking vigorously every two hours. From her experience pumping and from the cyclical fullness and softness she felt, Doris was reassured that Deshawn was receiving at least 60 to 90 ml every feed. The prefeed and postfeed weights performed by the NICU nurse confirmed this because he appeared to gain between 60 and 90 gm after each feed. Doris was pleased that she did not require any Domperidone (metoclopramide) and that the fenugreek and blessed thistle teas were enough to maintain her milk supply.

Doris and David struggled to determine how best to manage the stairs to the second-floor bedroom and the daily trip to the main floor so that Doris could participate in family activities with Megan and Marcia. They finally decided to create a temporary sleeping arrangement on the main floor for Doris so that she could avoid climbing the stairs for the first two weeks postpartum. After the staples were removed and Steri-Strips™ replaced, Doris found it more comfortable to breastfeed the baby using the cross-cradle hold, and she felt more at ease about navigating the stairs to assist with food preparation and homework. David took 2 weeks of vacation for the baby's first two weeks. When he returned to work, Doris found it helpful that he and Cora were only a phone call away. However, it was her midwife and her mother that Doris relied on the most for support related to caring for her first preterm child. They never made her feel insecure or embarrassed about asking questions, even though this was her second child.

When the public health nurse completed the Edinburgh Postnatal Depression Scale, Doris's score was 4. Doris was relieved that the conflicting feelings she experienced were baby blues but not depression. She received the current evidence about circumcision and decided that Deshawn would not be circumcised like his father. Instead, he would make that decision for himself for social reasons when the time came. The public health home visits met Doris's needs for information and validation. She received some referrals to community groups for racialized adolescent girls for Marcia. At her 6-week midwifery postpartum checkup, Doris was provided with her annual Pap smear and education about her contraceptive options while breastfeeding, and she was discharged from care. Figure 14-2 presents the Spencer family ecomap and how the nurse mobilized resources to help this family.

Questions for reflection on the nursing care of the Spencer family:

1. Identify some of the values and beliefs that you have developed based on your past experiences or interactions with patients or families of a different race than yourself. How do those experiences affect your perceptions and assumptions about how you might communicate with Doris and David about their choices for care, hospital routines and policies, and the plan of care?

Case Study: Spencer Family—cont'd

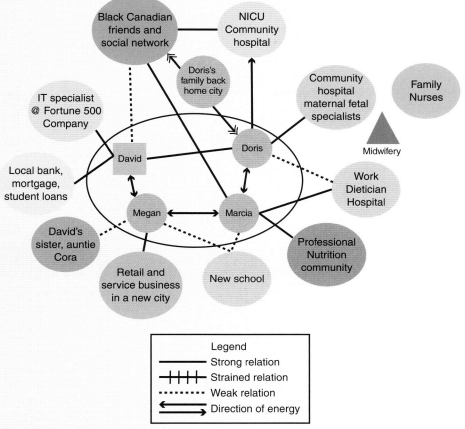

FIGURE 14-2 Spencer Family Ecomap

2. The Spencer family was traumatized by Marcia's experience with racism and stigmatization while shopping. Families often carry traumas that are unknown to the nurse. Family nurses who keep abreast of current events (e.g., police profiling or Black Lives Matter [BLM] activism) tend to be better prepared to screen for stress and trauma in marginalized populations. These families become even more vulnerable during a pandemic (e.g., COVID-19 or H1N1), when new infection control and prevention hospital policies can pose a barrier to family-centered care. How might you mitigate feelings of exclusion when a hospital policy limits family visitation with Doris and her newborn?

3. When an infant is born prematurely or a family experiences unexpected, stressful complications, there is a tendency to feel helpless but also have a strong desire to help the family. What type of measures might help you to advocate for David, Megan, Marcia, or Aunt Cora to be with Doris and the newborn or to participate in their care? How would you engage them in meaningful activities to help them cope with the feeling of helplessness after the baby is born prematurely?

4. According to systems theory, families function to facilitate adaptation to change and thus find a new equilibrium or a new normal. Nonetheless, the changes often strain family reserves and resources. What are some of the Spencer family weaknesses and strengths? What are the implications for how they might take bad news? How will you break the news to David, Megan, and Marcia that Deshawn will not be discharged within 48 hours as a full-term infant might?

5. Doris had a birth plan for a normal, spontaneous, low-intervention birth at term; skin-to-skin contact with Deshawn; and exclusive breast-/chestfeeding. She was unable to realize that dream birth plan due to the diagnosis of antepartum

(continued)

Case Study: Spencer Family—cont'd

hemorrhage, emergency cesarean section, and a premature infant with a weak sucking reflex. Doris is a multiparous woman who previously breastfed successfully, and she is a highly skilled dietician who works in your hospital. But what might cause her to commit one of two common mistakes or assumptions when it's time to decide on infant feeding? Can you anticipate what incorrect assumptions you might make that have to do with discrimination based on race, incorrect assumptions based on her parity, or value judgments you might hold about the level of knowledge that health workers hold?

6. Research shows that Black patients often experience disparate management of pain, underprescribing of analgesia, and suboptimal pain relief (Campbell & Edwards, 2012; Lee et al., 2019). How would you assess Doris's level of pain and the effectiveness of her analgesia? How might you enlist the family members to help in managing pain effectively?

7. Every jurisdiction (U.S. and Canadian) provides community support for parents with premature infants, siblings of newborns, or parents who are new to the community with little social support. The hospital or community social worker provides a good resource for nurses to locate these resources and contacts. List the resources for community nurses and other allied health professionals and support groups that would be appropriate for the Spencer family if they were being discharged from your community hospital.

Case Study: Amari-Issa Family

Aram Amari, age 25, and Hassan Issa, age 29, have been married for 5 years. Aram and Hassan are Kurdish and were born and raised in northern Syria. They moved to Iraq 2 years after getting married and lived in a refugee camp with Hassan's older brother, Rivin, and his family. Aram and Hassan have three children ages 1, 3, and 5 years. A year after moving to Canada, Hassan started working in a factory operating heavy machinery in a large urban city. He attended English classes in the evenings, while Aram cared for the children at home.

Aram's parents continue to live in northern Syria along with her two younger sisters. Aram also has three older sisters and an older brother; however, the brother went missing several years ago and has been presumed deceased. Two of Aram's oldest sisters live in Turkey with their families in a refugee camp, and the third oldest sister lives in Germany with her husband, two children, and father in-law. Aram keeps in touch with all her siblings through texting. She has not seen her mother in 2 years and worries about her health and survival in Syria as the economy continues to worsen.

Also living in northern Syria is Hassan's elderly father. Hassan's mother died after he was born due to birth complications. In addition to Rivin, Hassan has four more older brothers. Two live in Turkey with their families, and two joined the Kurdish military forces stationed in northern Syria. Although Hassan is very close to his father and did not want to leave him, his father urged him and Rivin to escape the dangers of the Syrian war and Turkish regimes to protect their families before it became too dangerous. Figure 14-3 presents a family genogram for Aram and Hassan's family.

Hassan's brother, Rivin, and his family recently arrived from an Iraqi refugee camp and live in a hotel with his family while they await placement. Although Hassan does not have a close relationship with Rivin, he hopes he is located in the same urban city so that both have a sense of family support. Aram shares her husband's sentiment because she is close to her sister-in-law. While living in the Iraqi refugee camp, Aram and her sister-in-law shared personal stories of their experiences during their journeys to the refugee camp. Within these stories, Aram hesitantly revealed her experience of being raped by an unknown male. She has not told anyone else, including her husband. Shamed and fearful of being left alone, Aram has suppressed her experience and has only talked to her sister-in-law about it.

While Hassan is at work during the day, Aram attends a mother's group at a local mosque. Fortunately, many of the women from the local Muslim community center have offered her friendship. They are teaching her how to take the bus and how to find ethnic foods in the local markets. She is grateful because in Syria, only the men run errands for food and basic necessities. Feeling a new sense of what women do in Canada has shed light on her own changing views of self-identity, which raises the urge to pursue her own ambitions. However, Aram has recently discovered that she is pregnant with her fourth child. Feeling mixed emotions, Hassan and Aram wonder how they will accommodate this new child in their one-bedroom basement suite. Hassan

Case Study: Amari-Issa Family—cont'd

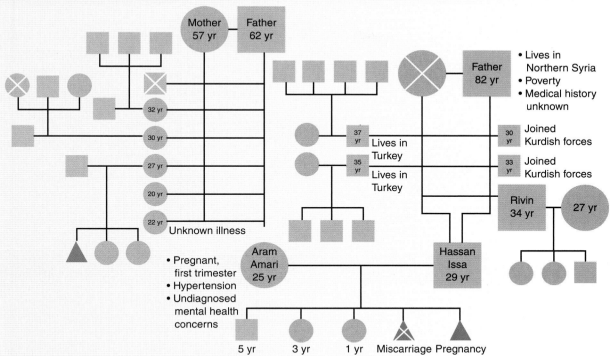

FIGURE 14-3 Amari-Issa Family Genogram

quickly approaches friends at the mosque to start looking at affordable housing options. Disappointed that she will need to wait to pursue English classes and to attend a college, Aram texts her mother to share the news. Excited for her daughter, Aram's mother shares news that her younger sister is quite ill and that they are unable to afford the medication needed, with most of their money going toward food and shelter. Aram's sadness is overwhelming.

Hassan takes Aram and their three children to Aram's first prenatal checkup at her family doctor's clinic. The nurse notes Aram's flat affect and notes her disconnected mood with her children. After taking her blood pressure, the nurse asks how she is doing. Hassan jumps in to answer, knowing that Aram understands some English but is unable to respond. Hassan reads the pamphlets given to him by the nurse, as Aram cannot yet read English, and translates the material on bodily changes expected while being pregnant and the meaning of hypertension. Seeing that Aram is unable to read or speak English, the nurse recommends bringing an interpreter to their next visit. Figure 14-4 presents the Amari-Issa family ecomap.

Questions for reflection on the nursing care of the Amari-Issa family:

1. Reflect on the assumptions you carry about Aram and her circumstances. How would your assumptions shape care provision?
2. As a nurse in a primary health care setting, what health issues would you prioritize in caring for Aram and her family?
3. What approaches can nurses assume within providing care to Aram?
4. What facilitators and barriers could this family be facing?
5. What knowledge is missing from this case study that would be useful in providing care to Aram?
6. Social exclusion is a prevalent experience among migrant families and is further exacerbated among forced migrant populations. What are some strategies that nurses can use to address social exclusion within the primary-care clinic setting?
7. How do you define *inequity*? What inequities within the current migrant system influence how health is experienced among families like the Amari-Issa family?

(continued)

Case Study: Amari-Issa Family—cont'd

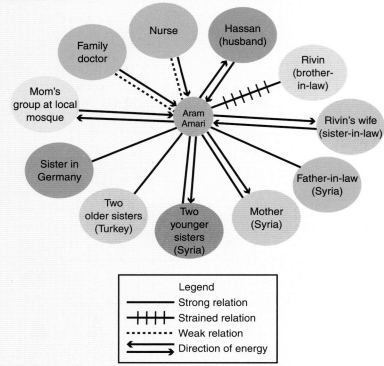

FIGURE 14-4 Amari-Issa Family Ecomap

SUMMARY

Childbearing family nursing focuses on family relationships and the health of all members of the childbearing family, even during times of extreme threats to maternal health. Several different theories available to nurses encountering families during childbearing can help guide their assessment of the family, their plan of care, and interventions for the family. Nurses are also in a position to have a powerful influence on the development of family-friendly policies at both the federal and practice setting levels.

■ Several theories, including Family Systems Theory and Family Developmental and Life Cycle Theory, are helpful to guide nurses' understanding of childbearing families and to structure nursing care.
■ Stress-producing, pregnancy-related events disrupt family functioning regardless of how the family is structured (traditional or nontraditional).

■ While giving direct physical care, teaching patients, or performing other traditional modes of childbearing nursing, family nurses focus on family relationships and the health of all members of the childbearing family.
■ Acute and chronic health conditions can develop during pregnancy and thus disrupt family functioning, development, and structure. When health threats arise, all family members experience stress as they strive to regain balance.
■ Childbearing family nurses can assist families to understand, prepare for, and respond to the effect each newborn has on the family.
■ Nurses must participate in policy development and implementation as it relates to childbearing families.
■ Nurses need to be aware of the effect of legislation on childbearing families.

chapter 15

Family Child Health Nursing

Deborah Padgett Coehlo, PhD, C-PNP, PMHS, CFLE

Elizabeth Straus, MN, RN, COI, PhD(c)

Critical Concepts

- A major task of families is to nurture children to become healthy, responsible, creative adults.
- Families are the major determinant of children's health and well-being.
- Most parents learn the parenting role on the job, so to speak, relying on experiences from their own childhood in their families of origin to guide them.
- Parents are charged with keeping children healthy as well as caring for them during illness.
- Common health promotion challenges of children and their families are experienced during transitions as individual members and their families grow and change.
- Because the leading causes of morbidity and mortality among youth are substance use, sexual activity, and violence (both suicidal and homicidal), there is a need for increased attention to health promotion and prevention in these areas.
- Abuse and neglect may be defined differently from one culture to the next, but nurses must be alert to helping families understand when child-rearing practices harm rather than nurture children.
- Families with children experience challenges and stressors related to congenital and chronic health conditions and stressors related to acute, chronic, and end-of-life transitions.
- Family members and the family as a whole are affected when a child is ill, and the ways a family reacts to a child's illness affect the course of that child's illness.
- The family-centered care (FCC) model can be used by family child health nurses to facilitate and teach healthful activities for growth, prevention of injury and disease, and management of illness conditions in families.
- A primary role for nurses is to assist families while they undergo transitions, including health and illness and developmental and socioeconomic transitions.
- The aim of nurses is to help families develop appropriate ways to carry out family tasks necessary to promote health and to prevent or positively cope with illness and disease.
- Although most child-rearing families experience acute illnesses and become familiar with managing these crises, families do not anticipate that their children may have chronic illness.
- With their knowledge of family and child development, nurses can collaborate with families with chronically ill children to help them strive toward developmental landmarks.
- Family child health nursing must be practiced in collaboration and cooperation with families, as well as other health care providers, according to the principles of FCC.

INTRODUCTION

A major task of families is to nurture children to become healthy, responsible, creative adults who can develop meaningful relationships across the life span. An important job of all parents is to keep children healthy and care for them during illness. Yet most mothers and fathers have little formal education for the health care of children. In fact, most parents learn the role on the job, relying on their childhood experiences in their families of origin to help guide them. Advice from other parents and professionals augment information from families of origin, but this advice is generally implemented only when questions or problems arise.

Family nurses help families promote health, prevent disease, and cope with illness. The importance of family life for children's health and illness care is often invisible because families' everyday routines are commonplace and lie below the level of awareness of health care providers. Family daily life, however, influences many aspects of children's health, including the promotion of health and the experience of illness in children. In turn, family daily life is influenced by the children's health and illness.

Families are groups with unique characteristics, including specific family experiences, memories, and related intergenerational relationships; structure and membership; family rules and routines; aspirations and achievements; and ethnic or cultural patterns (Burr et al., 1988). Family structure and function interact with and are influenced by these family characteristics. Healthy outcomes for children—such as tripling their birthweight by 1 year of age, or successfully completing high school—are partially attributable to the intangible, invisible daily interactions among family members. Nurses, in partnership with families, examine how the characteristics of families influence the health of families and children.

This chapter provides a review of child- and family-centered care (CFCC) and presents foundational concepts that will guide nursing practice with families with children. The chapter goes on to describe the nursing care of well children and families, with an emphasis on health promotion; nursing care of children and families in acute-care settings; nursing care of children with chronic illness and their families; and nursing care of children and their families during end of life. The case study illustrates the application of CFCC across settings.

ELEMENTS OF CFCC

CFCC is a systemwide approach to child health care. This model assumes that families are children's primary source of nurturance, education, and health care. CFCC has emerged as part of the expansion of care from professional-driven care to patient-centered care over the past several decades. Advocates for children and families advanced principles of patient-centered care to family-centered care, using the following guides:

1. Recognizing families as the constants in children's lives, whereas the personnel in other systems, including the health care system, fluctuate and are temporary.
2. Openly sharing information about alternative treatments, ethical concerns, and uncertainties with families helps guide decision-making processes.
3. Forming partnerships between families and health care providers to decide jointly what is important for families improves health outcomes.
4. Respecting the racial, ethnic, cultural, and socioeconomic diversity of families and their ways of coping is an important element of FCC.
5. Supporting and strengthening families' abilities to grow and develop across time strengthens a family's ability to support and nurture their children (Lewandowski & Tesler, 2003; Center for the Study of Social Health Policy, 2021).

See Table 15-1 for more details on the elements of FCC.

The FCC model emphasizes that families are the key health care providers for children. Families determine the culture of health care, including establishing healthy living patterns, care for acute illnesses, and care for chronic illnesses. Health care providers acknowledge the importance of families in developing a comprehensive and holistic treatment plan for those children who need health care services. Families communicated that the uncertainty that surrounds their child's health was lessened if they were included in decision making, and thus they wanted to be informed partners of the health care team's decision making as well as valued collaborators in the care of their child (Chadwick & Miller, 2019).

Table 15-1	Elements of FCC
ELEMENTS	**DEFINITION**
1. The family is at the center.	The family is the constant in the child's life.
2. Family-professional collaboration	Collaboration includes the care of the individual child, program development, and policy formation at all levels of care—hospital, home, and community.
3. Family-professional communication	Information exchange is complete and unbiased, and occurs in a supportive manner at all times.
4. Cultural diversity of families	Honors diversity (ethnic, racial, spiritual, social, economic, educational, and geographic), strengths, and individuality within and across all families.
5. Coping differences and support	Recognizes and respects family coping, supporting families with developmental, educational, emotional, spiritual, environmental, and financial resources to meet diverse needs.
6. Family-centered peer support	Families are encouraged to network and support each other.
7. Specialized service and support systems	Support systems for children with special health and developmental needs in the hospital, home, and community are accessible, flexible, and comprehensive.
8. Holistic perspective of FCC	Families are viewed as families, and children are viewed as children, recognizing their strengths, concerns, emotions, and aspirations beyond their specific health needs.

Source: Lewandowski, L., & Tesler, M. (Eds.). (2003). *Family-centered care: Putting it into action. The SPN/ANA guide to family-centered care.* Society of Pediatric Nurses/American Nurses Association.

The Association for the Care of Children's Health further defined the specific key elements of FCC in 1994 (Shelton & Stepanek, 1994):

1. Recognize that the family is the constant in the child's life, whereas the service systems and personnel within those systems fluctuate.
2. Share complete and unbiased information with parents about their child's health on an ongoing basis. Understand that information may have to be repeated, especially during times of stress (i.e., at the time of diagnosis of an illness or chronic condition).
3. Recognize family strengths and individuality. Respect different methods of coping.
4. Encourage and make referrals for parent-to-parent support, such as parent support groups.
5. Facilitate parent and professional collaboration at all levels of health care—care of an individual child, family care, program development, implementation of child and family policies, and evaluation of policies.
6. Ensure that the design of health care delivery systems is flexible, accessible, and responsive to diverse families.
7. Implement appropriate policies and programs that provide physical, emotional, spiritual, and financial support to children and their families.
8. Understand and incorporate the developmental needs of children and families into the health care delivery systems.

Although the ideas presented were initiated with children with special health care needs (CSHCN), the elements apply to all families with children. These elements are now widely accepted and used by health care providers and families with children with health care needs (Chadwick & Miller, 2019). Studies have shown that parents want to be involved in decision making; however, parents' perceptions of whether other family members should be involved varied greatly (Dadlez et al., 2018) based on the culture of the family and age of the parents. It also seemed that the more significant the decision, the more likely the family wanted to be involved in decision making.

The awareness of the benefits of FCC spread throughout international nursing research, education, and practice, with increasing awareness that, while this model improved family involvement in the care of children, it did not address the children's involvement in and influence on the recommended care. Due to this gap, recent efforts have been made to identify and research the benefits of adding the child to FCC (Gerlach, & Varcoe, 2020). This addition follows the belief that children have the right to participate in their health care and decision making (Gerlach & Varcoe, 2020). Children can understand their health and illness through play, storytelling, and discussion. If they have a better developmentally appropriate understanding of health and illness, then they can contribute to decisions regarding their health care. Because of children's limitations in fully understanding complex health care needs, decision making and collaboration are often left to the parents. By including the child in FCC, culturally and developmentally appropriate interventions are added when the child is included in decision making about health interventions (Coyne et al., 2018; Gerlach & Varcoe, 2020).

Outcomes improved when organizations supported consistency in staffing, coordinated services across disciplines, had a clear model that was communicated to staff and provided clear roles and responsibilities, and were willing to give up past entrenched practices (Coyne et al., 2018). Other researchers have also found the value of FCC in improving collaboration with families, communication and decision making, negotiation on sharing roles and responsibilities, and families' report of support.

An ongoing concern regarding both FCC and CFCC is the difficulty in providing equitable care while accounting for racism, poverty, access concerns due to rural geographic locations with poor health care resources, and other causes of oppression (Garlach & Varcoe, 2020). While CFCC is widely promoted, barriers to universal implementation remain, especially for marginalized populations. This is in direct contrast to the World Health Organization's (WHO's) directive in its publication from the Commission on Social Determinants of Health (2008) calling for equity for every child as a fundamental aspect of addressing health inequities with and between countries. Without success in remediating health inequities, these individuals, families, and populations will continue to be at higher risk for poor health outcomes due to continued racism, material deprivation, and "historically entrenched power imbalances" (Gerlach & Varcoe, 2020, p. 650). Ford-Gilboe et al. (2018) addressed this need with adult populations by developing an evidence-informed program called EQUIP. The outcomes of this program included improved mental health, fewer trauma symptoms, and decreased chronic pain. The approach

to equity-oriented care exhibited in the EQUIP program has great potential for promoting equity-oriented CFCC in family child health nursing (Gerlach & Varcoe, 2020).

CONCEPTS OF FAMILY CHILD HEALTH NURSING

Several foundational concepts guide nursing care of families with children: family development or career, including tasks, communication, development of support, transitions, and understanding and working together with family routines; individual development; and transitions (e.g., health and illness, developmental, and socioeconomic). Family developmental theories assume that families and individuals change over time. Families experience the various developmental stages of each member, and they also progress through a series of family developmental stages. Some are socially constructed and considered on-time events. Those that are off-time leave families feeling vulnerable and alone. By comparing their observations of individual families to socially expected family and individual developmental stages, nurses can plan appropriate and individualized care (Table 15-2).

Family Career

Family career is the dynamic process of change that occurs during the life span of the unique group called the family. Family career incorporates stages, tasks, and transitions, and is similar to family development theory in that it considers family tasks including raising children. These two concepts differ, however, because family development theory views the family in standard sequential steps, progressing from the birth of the first child to raising and launching that child, to experiencing the death of a parent figure in old age (Duvall & Miller, 1985). By contrast, family career considers the diverse experiences of families (Aldous, 1996). Family career includes both the expected developmental changes of the family life cycle and the unexpected changes of situational crises, such as divorce, remarriage, chronic illness and disabilities, and death.

The notion of family career involves the many paths that families can take during their life span. Changes do not necessarily occur in a linear

Table 15-2   Social-Emotional, Cognitive, and Physical Dimensions of Individual Development

PERIOD	SOCIAL-EMOTIONAL STAGES/ SIGNIFICANT RELATIONSHIPS	STAGE-SENSITIVE FAMILY DEVELOPMENT TASKS	VALUES ORIENTATION	COGNITIVE STAGES OF DEVELOPMENT	DEVELOPMENTAL LANDMARKS	PHYSICAL MATURATION	DEVELOPMENTAL STEPS
Infancy birth to 1 yr	Trust versus mistrust (I am what I am given.) Primary parent	Having, adjusting to, and encouraging the development of infants. Establishing a satisfying home for both parents and infant(s). Establishing well-child health care.	Undifferentiated	*Sensory-motor (ages birth to 2 years)* Infants move from neonatal reflex level of complete self/world undifferentiation to relatively coherent organization of sensory-motor actions. They learn that certain actions have specific effects on the environment.	Gazes at complete patterns Social smile (2 mo) 180° visual pursuit (2 mo) Rolls over (5 mo) Ranking grasp (7 mo) Crude purposeful release (9 mo) Inferior pincer grasp Walks unassisted (10–14 mo)	*Rapid (skeletal)* Transitory reflexes present (3 mo) (i.e., Moro reflex, sucking, grasp, tonic neck reflex) Muscle constitutes 25% of total body weight Birthweight doubles (6 mo) Eruption of deciduous central incisors (5 to 10 mo) Birthweight triples (1 yr) Anterior fontanel closes (10 to 14 mo) Transitory reflexes disappear (10 mo) Eruption of deciduous first molars (11 to 18 mo)	Anticipation of feeding Symbiosis (4 to 18 mo) Stranger anxiety (6 to 10 mo) Separation anxiety (8 to 24 mo) Self-feeding
Toddlerhood (1 to 3 yrs)	Autonomy versus shame or doubt (I am what I "will.") Parental persons	Parenting role development. Learning to parent toddler. Developing approaches to discipline. Understanding child's increasing autonomy. Family planning. Providing safe environment. Maintaining well-child health care.	Punishment and obedience	Recognition of the constancy of external objects and primitive internal representation of the world begins. Uses memory to act. Can solve basic problems.	Words: 3 to 4 (13 mo) Builds tower of 2 cubes (15 mo) Scribbles with crayon (18 mo) Words: 10 (18 mo) Builds tower of 5 to 6 cubes (21 mo) Uses 3-word sentences (24 mo)	Babinski reflex extinguished (18 mo) Bowel and bladder nerves myelinated (18 mo) Increase in lymphoid tissue Weight gain 2 kg per year (12 to 36 mo)	Oppositional behavior Messiness Exploratory behavior Parallel play Pleasure in looking at or being looked at Beginning self-concept Orderliness Curiosity

(Continued)

Table 15-2	Social-Emotional, Cognitive, and Physical Dimensions of Individual Development—cont'd						
PERIOD	SOCIAL-EMOTIONAL STAGES/SIGNIFICANT RELATIONSHIPS	STAGE-SENSITIVE FAMILY DEVELOPMENT TASKS	VALUES ORIENTATION	COGNITIVE STAGES OF DEVELOPMENT	DEVELOPMENTAL LANDMARKS	PHYSICAL MATURATION	DEVELOPMENTAL STEPS
					Names 6 body parts (30 mo) Uses appropriate personal pronouns, i.e., *I, you, me* (30 mo) Rides tricycle (36 mo) Copies circle (36 mo) Matches 4 colors (36 mo) Talks to self and others (42 mo) Takes turns (42 mo)		
Preschool age (3 to 5 yrs)	Initiative versus guilt (I am what I imagine I can be.) Basic family	Adapting to the critical needs and interests of preschoolchildren in stimulating, growth-promoting ways. Monitoring child development. Seek developmental screening as needed. Coping with energy depletion and lack of privacy as parents. Socializing children. Providing safe environment/accident prevention. Maintenance of couple relationship. Fostering sibling relationships.	Punishment and obedience moves to meeting own needs and doing for others if that person will do something for the child.	*Preoperational thought (prelogical)—ages 2 to 7 yrs* Begins to use symbols. Thinking tends to be egocentric and intuitive. Conclusions are based on what they feel or what they would like to believe.	Uses 4-word sentences (48 mo) Copies cross (48 mo) Throws ball overhand (48 mo) Copies square (54 mo) Copies triangle (60 mo) Prints name Rides 2-wheel bike	Weight gain 2 kg per year (4 to 6 yrs) Eruption of permanent teeth (5.5 to 8 yrs) Body image solidifying	Cooperative play Fantasy play Imaginary companions Masturbation Task completion Rivalry with parents of same sex Games and rules Problem solving Achievement Voluntary hygiene Competes with partners Hobbies Ritualistic play Rational attitudes about food Companionship (same sex) Invests in community leaders, teachers, impersonal ideals

Stage	Psychosocial	Family Tasks	Moral	Cognitive		Physical	Developmental Skills
School-Age (6 to 12 yrs)	Industry versus inferiority (I am what I learn.) Neighborhood and school	Fitting into the community of school-age families in constructive ways. Letting children go as they become increasingly independent. Encouraging child's education achievement. Balancing parental needs with children's needs.	Moves from instrumental exchange ("If you scratch my back, I'll scratch yours") into wanting to follow rules to be "good," then to rule orientation for maintenance of social order.	*Concrete operational thought—* ages 7 to 12 yrs Conceptual organization increasingly stable. Children begin to seem rational and well organized. Increasingly systematic in approach to the world. Weight and volume are now viewed as constant despite changes in shape and size.	As child moves through stage, he or she copies diamond; knows simple opposite analogies; names days of the week; repeats 5 digits forward; defines *brave* and *nonsense*; knows seasons of the year; able to rhyme words; repeats 5 digits in reverse; understands pity, grief, surprise; knows where sun sets; can define *nitrogen* and *microscope*	Weight gain 2 to 4 kg per year (7 to 11 yrs) Uterus begins to grow Budding of nipples in girls Increased vascularity of penis and scrotum Pubic hair appears in girls Menarche (9 to 11 yrs)	Task completion Rivalry with parents of the same sex Games and rules Problem solving Achievement Voluntary hygiene Competes with partners Has hobbies Ritualistic play Rational attitudes about food Values companionship Invest in community leaders, teachers, impersonal ideals
Adolescence (13 to 20 yrs)	Identity versus role confusion (I know who I am.) Peer in-groups and out-groups Adult models of leadership	Balancing freedom with responsibility as adolescents mature and emancipate themselves. Maintaining communication with teen. Establishing postparental interests and careers as growing parents.	Increasing internalization of ethical standards; can use to make decisions.	*Formal operational thought* Abstract thought and awareness of the world of possibility develop. Adolescents use deductive reasoning and can evaluate the logic and quality of their own thinking. Increased abstract power allows them to work with laws and principles.	Knows why oil floats on water. Can divide 72 by 4 without pencil or paper. Understands "espionage." Can repeat 6 digits forward and 5 digits in reverse.	*Spurt* (skeletal) Girls 1.5 years ahead of boys. Pubic hair appears in boys. Rapid growth of testes and penis. Axillary hair starts to grow. Down on upper lip appears. Voice changes. Mature spermatozoa (11 to 17 yrs). Acne may appear.	"Revolt" Loosens tie to family Cliques Responsible independence Work habits solidifying Personal interests Recreational activities

(Continued)

Table 15-2	Social-Emotional, Cognitive, and Physical Dimensions of Individual Development—cont'd						
PERIOD	SOCIAL-EMOTIONAL STAGES/SIGNIFICANT RELATIONSHIPS	STAGE-SENSITIVE FAMILY DEVELOPMENT TASKS	VALUES ORIENTATION	COGNITIVE STAGES OF DEVELOPMENT	DEVELOPMENTAL LANDMARKS	PHYSICAL MATURATION	DEVELOPMENTAL STEPS
Early adulthood	Intimacy versus isolation Partners in friendship, sex, completion	Releasing young adults into work, military service, college, marriage, and so on, with appropriate rituals and assistance. Maintaining a supportive home base.	Principled social contract			Cessation of skeletal growth Involution of lymphoid tissue Muscle constitutes 43% total body weight Permanent teeth calcified Eruption of permanent third molars (17 to 30 yrs)	Preparation for occupational choice Occupational commitment Elaboration of recreational outlets Marriage readiness Parenthood readiness
Middle adulthood	Generativity versus self-absorption or stagnation Divided labor and shared household	Refocusing on the marriage relationship. Maintaining kin ties with older and younger generations.	Self-actualization—doing what one is capable of.				
Late adulthood	Integrity versus despair, disgust "Humankind" "My kind"	Coping with bereavement and living alone. Closing the family home in adapting to aging. Adjusting to retirement.	Universal ethical principles				

Sources: Adapted from Duvall, E. M., & Miller, B. C. (1985). Developmental tasks: Individual and family. In E. M. Duvall & B. C. Miller (Eds.), *Marriage and family development* (6th ed., p. 62). New York, NY: Harper & Row; Prugh, D. (1983). *The psychological aspects of pediatrics.* Philadelphia, PA: Lea & Febiger; Thomas, R. M. (2005). *Comparing theories of child development* (6th ed.). Belmont, CA: Wadsworth.

Table 15-3	Definitions of Family Career, Individual Development, and Patterns of Health, Disease, and Illness
TERM	**DEFINITION**
Family career	The dynamic process of change that occurs during the life span of the unique group called the family. Whereas family development views the family in standard sequential steps or stages, family career considers the diverse experiences of American families that do not occur in anticipated stages.
Individual development	Physical and maturational change of the individual over time. Some theories perceive change as stages, and others as interactional change.
Health and illness	Health is behavior that promotes optimal dimensions of well-being. Family and individual health are multidimensional; therefore, a family and/or member can have a disease and be healthy in another dimension of health.
Families and their members experience dimensions of health while managing illness among members	Illness is a disease (and family management of the disease) that may be acute (time-limited), chronic (live with over time), or terminal (end-of-life).

fashion. For example, family career considers the possibility that a person without children may have a partner who already has adolescent children, resulting in that person starting parenting with adolescent children. The new parent does not build on parenting skills experienced across time but rather starts the parenting career at the end of the child's childhood career. Family career is a useful concept because it reminds us that families are dynamic and thus require flexibility. Nurses working with child-rearing families need to know that family careers are inclusive of family development stages, transitions, and diversity because these dynamics affect family health. Table 15-3 includes definitions of family career; individual development; and patterns of health, disease, and illness.

Family Stages

Duvall's eight stages of family development, derived from information about the oldest child, describes expected developmental changes in families that are raising children (Duvall & Miller, 1985). According to Duvall and Miller, family careers start with (1) marriage without children, then proceed to (2) childbearing, (3) preschoolchildren, (4) schoolchildren, (5) adolescents, (6) the launching of young adults (i.e., first child gone to last child leaving home), (7) middle age of parents (i.e., empty nest to retirement), and (8) aging of family members (i.e., retirement to death of both parents). This theory has been critiqued because it is becoming increasingly understood that families may experience several developmental stages at one time and consist of different structures. While

stages of family development may vary from the aforementioned normative trajectory, the concept is useful as a sensitizing concept to help nurses consider how family structure and development influence family life and well-being. Nurses can serve families better if they understand and work with families at different stages of family development. Nurses can also help families understand competing developmental tasks and transitions across family members and across time.

Family Transitions

Family transitions are central to nursing practice because they have profound health-related effects on families and family members (Meleis et al., 2000). Family transitions are events that signal a reorganization of family roles and tasks, and include transitions in health and illness, developmental stages, and socioeconomic status. Support from health care providers and other sources has a positive impact on transitions through time, from early infancy to transition to adulthood and beyond (Department of Health and Human Services, 2017). Developmental transitions are typically predictable changes that occur in an expected trajectory. Sometimes families may not make the transition to an expected family stage. For example, families with children who have disabilities and are not able to live independently have difficulty launching their children because of lack of residential living facilities and caregivers.

Socioeconomic transitions, also known as non-normative or situational transitions, include changes in personal relationships, roles and status, the environment, physical and mental capabilities, and changes in material possessions (Meleis, 2010). Not all families experience each of these transitions, and they can occur at any time. For example, changes occur in personal relationships when a stepchild is integrated into the family group or when one becomes a new stepparent after divorce and remarriage. Changes in the environment occur, for example, when working parents move to a new city and a new job and family members adjust to a new house, school, friends, and community.

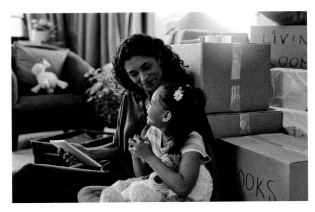
Source: © istock.com/LumiNola

Health and illness transitions are changes in the meaning and behavior of families as they experience an acute or chronic condition or disability over time. The trajectory of these conditions often consists of different phases, including prediagnosis, crisis of the diagnosis or change in condition, daily management of the condition, and a resolved or terminal phase. Families often experience transitions between these phases over time. For example, a family that has learned to manage its child's asthma requires new coping strategies when hospitalization occurs after the child's asthma symptoms are complicated by an upper respiratory illness and become too severe to manage at home. The family will need to reorganize itself to deal with the child's hospitalization and possibly learn to implement different asthma management approaches after hospitalization.

The experiences and outcomes of transitions in families are often mediated by the environment (Meleis, 2010). For example, if a woman experiences pregnancy within a supportive environment and in a community that provides appropriate and accessible resources, her experience is different from that of a woman who experiences pregnancy

alone and in an impoverished community with limited resources.

Transition events are signals to nurses that families may be at risk for health problems. Although families work to create and implement strategies to promote their child's well-being and safety, they may experience challenges during times of transition as parents find themselves coping with the stress of transition while continuing to cope with parenting stress. For example, when an infant transitions from crawling to pulling up, to standing, and to walking, the family needs to allow the child to expand her environment by allowing her out of the security of the playpen and to modify the environment to make it safe for that child. Similarly, when a child is diagnosed with type 1 diabetes mellitus, family members need to adjust family life and tasks to integrate their child's new nutritional and health management needs into their routines. By assessing families for anticipated changes related to family and child developmental transitions as well as situational and health and illness transitions, nurses can help families plan for changes. Meleis's (2010) transition theory can serve as a useful tool for nurses to improve their therapeutic processes to support families during different types of transitions. Figure 15-1 provides a visual depiction of this theory.

NURSING INTERVENTIONS TO SUPPORT CARE OF WELL CHILDREN AND FAMILIES

Families are the context for health promotion and illness care for all family members, including children. Family beliefs, rituals, and routines affect the health of all family members, including, for instance, traditional health practices around food, eating, and types of food served at meals; physical activity and rest; use of alcohol and other substances; and providing care and connection for family members. Barnes et al. (2020) summarized several decades of research on health promotions, offering six areas of focus to improve the health of individuals, families, and communities by promoting family involvement in health promotion. These six areas of focus include the following:

- Considering the larger context for health promotions, including funding priorities in the area of education, the minimum wage,

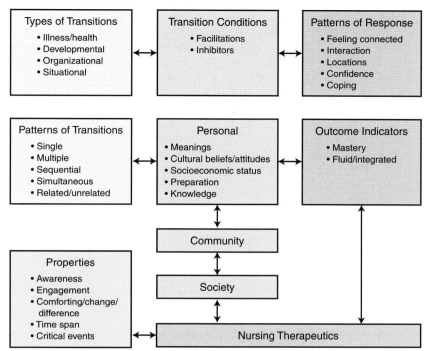

FIGURE 15-1 Transitional Model   *Source: Adapted from Meleis, A. I. (2010).* Transitions Theory Middle-Range and Situational Specific Theories in Nursing Research and Practice. *New York: Springer Publishers.*

promotion of safe and healthy communities, Medicaid services and funding, family leave policies, and family ties during a family member's incarceration

- Emphasizing the importance of family health on societal health. For example, by funding education, intergenerational poverty can be interrupted
- Partnering with families with an optimistic view that family involvement improves health outcomes
- Strengthening family mentors within the community
- Strengthening families' abilities to model and reflect on positive health practices
- Empowering families in their ability to assess their needs, identify strengths and weaknesses, and participate in problem-solving practices

These authors emphasized the need to acknowledge that prenatal and early childhood experiences clearly affect the future health and well-being not only of a child but also of future generations. Because of our changing demographics, with more

older adults caring for children, more single parents living without a partner, and more families living together across generations, the need for families to be the forerunners in health promotion for children has never been greater.

During well-child care, families are considered the care environment for their children. Proposed nursing outcomes of current well-child care focus on family functioning and capacity and the ability to care for and nurture children while providing a safe and developmentally stimulating environment. Specific outcomes include that parents (1) are knowledgeable about their children's physical health status and needs; (2) feel valued and supported as their children's primary caregiver and teacher, and they function in partnership with their children's health care providers and teachers; (3) are screened for maternal depression, family violence, and family substance abuse and are referred to specialists when needed; (4) understand and are able to use well-child care services; (5) understand and can implement developmental monitoring, stimulation, and regulation such as reading regularly to their children; (6) are skilled in anticipating and meeting their children's developmental needs; and

(7) have access to consistent sources of emotional support and are linked to appropriate community services (Kilgore, 2017). Parents strongly influence children's healthy lifestyle choices through modeling healthy lifestyle behaviors. For example, Allen et al. (2016), in their study of 57 adolescents, discussed that the eating patterns of adults had more influence on adolescent eating patterns than any punitive approaches (i.e., restricting unhealthy foods within the environment). In promoting child and family well-being, nurses support families in the care of their children using the following skills and interventions:

- Communicating with families
- Supporting the development of parenting skills and healthy family functioning
- Understanding and working with family routines
- Identifying health risks and teaching prevention strategies
- Supporting health promotion in families with children

Communication With Families

Therapeutic communication with family groups is the foundation of nursing care of families with children. One important feature of communication with families with children is including all the family members in a discussion or interaction (Wright & Leahey, 2016). Cooklin (2001) was one of the early researchers on developing strategies to include all family members in a family assessment. He recommended that each new assessment start with each family member being asked to introduce him- or herself, beginning with the parent or adults of the family and proceeding with each family member in order of age from oldest to youngest. North American children, in particular, are often valued as autonomous beings. A meta-analysis of 14 studies to evaluate the effectiveness of patient, family, and children supported this approach and the idea that children want to be consulted about decisions concerning their education and health care and want their opinions to be respected (Coyne et al., 2018). Nurses can assure children that they have a real voice by inviting them to speak, conveying that their opinion really matters, and demonstrating genuine interest in their point of view. Because the role of children in social situations is influenced by family culture, it

is important to confirm that the children feel that they have permission to choose how they want to participate and that the parents confirm that they will allow the children to participate freely in the discussion (Cooklin, 2001; Didier et al., 2018).

Another important feature of communication with families is considering and adjusting communication style, the content of the message, and vocabulary for developmental appropriateness for each family member (Cooklin, 2001; Kennedy, 2015). During their qualitative study of 10 children and adolescents, Didier et al. (2018) found that use of open-ended and caring questions increased interaction between the health care providers and the patients. Playfulness may assist in establishing communication with children. Children's temperament influences how they engage with new experiences and new people. A quiet, shy child, for example, often wants to watch and see what others are doing before interacting with new people. Instead of asking questions, a nurse may elicit more conversation by inviting the child to color together, or to play together with preferred toys and chat during an activity, instead of putting the focus on what the child is saying. "Draw and tell" or "play and tell" helps nurses learn what children are thinking and feeling through their actions rather than relying only on words (Driessnack, 2005). Asking children to draw their family and then to tell the nurse about the picture starts a meaningful conversation. As a child becomes more comfortable with the nurse, the nurse can ask the child to draw the clinic or hospital and talk about the picture.

In cognition development, children move from concrete to abstract thought. Careful explanation of abstract concepts using real objects or developmentally appropriate stories is especially important when working with children younger than middle-school-age. If a nurse is explaining surgery, for example, children will understand more if they are shown how the incision and bandage will appear on a doll or a stuffed animal, with a drawn incision and bandage on the appropriate body part, rather than just hearing a verbal explanation of the process (Yahya Al-Sagarat et al., 2017). Telling a story about a child going to surgery helps the child understand the event more easily than just telling about the procedure. (See Box 15-1 for examples of discussing surgery with children.) It is important to validate or confirm with all family members that the message

BOX 15-1

Preparing Children and Their Families for Surgery Using Hospital Play

Children learn by doing and playing. Using dolls and real equipment helps children know what to expect and act out their fears. Having parents observe helps them learn how to help their child using play.

Before starting, consult with the physician and parent to learn what information the child has been given. Decide the appropriate explanation for the child's age and emotional maturity. For young children, use neutral words such as *opening, drainage,* and *oozing* instead of *cut* and *bleed.* Gather the visual aids (e.g., pictures, doll) and equipment to be used. Do not give too much information because the child may be overwhelmed. Plan for three sessions: why the child needs surgery, what to expect in the operating room, and what the child will feel and do after surgery.

If a child has never been in the hospital, have toys familiar to the child such as blocks, dollhouses, and stuffed animals available, along with "real" equipment, such as a doll with bandages similar to what the child will have, operating room masks, scrubs that nurses and doctors wear, and intravenous poles. The child may play with the familiar toys. As the child observes the nurse, tell the story of what will happen to the doll using the "real" equipment on the doll so that the child will learn that the equipment is safe.

Session 1: Discuss How the Surgery Will Make the Child Better

- Ask the child what she or he thinks is going to happen. A child may be silent or say, "I do not know," when talking to a stranger. You can repeat a simple explanation reinforcing what the child knows.
- Reassure the child that no one is to blame for her or his condition; make it clear that nothing the child did is responsible.
- Using the doll, show where the surgery will take place and what the surgery will do to make the child better.

Session 2: Teach the Patient What to Expect in the Operating Room and What Will Happen Before the Surgery

- Review why surgery will make the child better.
- Talk about the steps of getting ready for surgery, such as not eating or drinking the night before and how the operation room will smell (alcohol), feel (cold), and look (big lights, a clock, people in special clothes).
- Indicate that the child will wear special clothes (hospital gown). *Note:* Toddlers' body image includes keeping on their underwear because they have just finished learning toilet training.
- Put a mask on the face and talk about a "funny smell." Use a real anesthesia mask on the doll and have the child do this too. This gives the child some control.
- Play with the thermometer, blood pressure cuff, and stethoscope for taking temperatures and listening to heartbeats and breathing on the doll, nurse, and parent.
- Show pictures of an operating room. Point out the "big lights," the clock, the nurses, and doctors dressed in blue (or whatever color your hospital personnel wear in the operating room suites) clothes and wearing "masks." Talk about the ride on a bed with wheels and doors that open in a similar way as the doors in grocery stores. These are things the child is familiar with and will notice.
- Reaffirm that parents will walk with the child to the operating room and be with him or her when the child wakes up from the surgery. Play with a mommy doll walking with the toy doll going to the operating room. The child needs to know that his or her parents know where the child is and will be there for him or her.

Session 3: Review Postoperative Expectations

Using dolls, act out what will happen after surgery:

- Soreness at the site of surgery
- Pain and medication
- Positioning (how to turn after surgery, deep breathe, and cough)
- Bandages (the word *dressing* may be understood as "turkey dressing" at Thanksgiving, or playing "dress-up")
- No eating and drinking right away

---

conveyed is understood and to explain medical words fully. Use of clichés, such as "This won't hurt" or "It will be over before you know it," are rarely appropriate when communicating with children and adolescents. The amount of information given also varies across cultures and from one individual to the next. Some families may want as much information as possible; others may place their trust in health care providers for decision making and may become overwhelmed with too much information. Nurses should assess family information needs and take care not to overwhelm family members, including children, with information they do not want or understand.

Supporting Development of Parenting Skills and Healthy Family Functioning

Providing support for the development of parenting skills is an important nursing intervention. Beginning at birth, children need warm, affectionate relationships with parents. One of the earliest parenting skills found to establish healthy caregiving behavior is a parent's responsiveness to the infant's cues. Responsiveness is noticing and interpreting the infant's cues, then acting promptly in response to those cues. For example, if an infant looks away from a parent, a responsive parent will decrease stimulation until the infant turns back and reestablishes eye contact. Parental responsiveness in early childhood has been associated with improved cognition, language abilities, and emotional outcomes (O'Neal et al., 2017; Wade et al., 2018). The trend of developing programs to support mothers with high-risk stressors on attachment and interaction skills have been replicated across the last two decades (Anis et al., 2020). For example, Anis et al. (2020) found that mothers who were taught interaction and attachment skills through a parent training program demonstrated improved parent-child interaction and can foster cognitive growth. This study emphasizes the importance of nurses teaching and supporting high-risk parents as they learn important parenting skills.

Parenting Styles

After the infancy period, parents generally begin to develop a style of nurturing and caring for their children. We present categorizations of parenting styles here as sensitizing concepts to aid nurses in understanding parenting approaches and providing education and support for parenting.

Authoritative Parenting Style

An authoritative parenting style is characterized by reciprocity, mutual understanding, shared decision making, and flexibility (Kuppens & Coulemans, 2019). Although parents using this style convey clear expectations and demands of their children, those expectations and demands take into consideration their children's developmental level and individual strengths, weaknesses, and personality traits, and parents provide rationales for and support to meet those characteristics as well as warmth in their relationship with the children (Baumrind, 2005). This parenting style promotes feelings of competence in the children, with the ultimate goal of promoting positive self-esteem and autonomy in their children. Authoritative parenting styles influence health by providing the ongoing message that the children have some control over good health and healthy lifestyle choices and have a positive responsibility to care for their own health through these life choices (Kuppens & Coulemans, 2019; Radcliff et al., 2018). The outcomes of this parenting style are generally positive in both Western and non-Western cultures on variables such as self-reliance, self-competence, academic performance, socially accepted behavior, and social acceptance (Kuppens & Coulemans, 2019; Sahithya et al., 2019).

Authoritarian Parenting Style

An authoritarian parenting style, in contrast, is described as parents having more psychological control over their children, with an attempt to control their children's thoughts and behavior (Kuppens & Coulemans, 2019). The authoritarian style promotes the belief that children should not control their own behavior and cannot contribute to the family and for themselves because they do not have the knowledge or experience needed to make good decisions (Kuppen & Coulemans, 2019). Children in such families have also been found to be more depressed and have more external problem behaviors (Kuppens & Coulemans, 2019). It is important to note, however, that this taxonomy of parenting styles was developed based on a White Eurocentric model and that outcomes of this parenting style may vary across cultures and contexts (Sahithya et al., 2019). Overall, however, the long-held consensus is that children fare better when they are praised and supported rather than when they are criticized, controlled, and punished (Kuppens & Coulemans, 2019).

Permissive Parenting Style

A permissive parenting style allows children to pursue child-determined goals with little guidance from the parents. Parents using this style may ignore behavior problems and may not provide the organizational support needed to assist children in reaching goals (Kuppens & Coulemans, 2019). Children raised in the permissive style are less assertive and achievement-oriented and are more likely to develop ineffective coping strategies compared with authoritative and authoritarian parenting styles (Kuppens & Coulemans, 2019). Permissive parents can be nurturing and warm, but they are passive, which means that it can be challenging to establish healthy boundaries. This passive, but often negative, parenting style is also often associated with poor academic and social-emotional outcomes (Kuppens & Coulemans, 2019; Pinquart & Kauser, 2018).

Uninvolved Parenting Style

The fourth parenting style studied is the uninvolved parent. This parenting style is similar to the permissive parenting style except that the parent(s) not only lacks clear boundaries and expectations but also lacks any nurturing, warmth, and responsiveness (Kuppens & Coulemans, 2019). The outcomes of these children are considered worse than the first three parenting styles, with children being at risk for negative coping strategies, including poor academic performance, drug use, criminal behavior, and poor social acceptance (Kuppens & Coulemans, 2019; Pinquart, 2017; Sahithya et al., 2019).

Specific Nursing Interventions Regarding Parenting Styles

Nurses can teach about parenting styles and help parents adopt authoritative parenting strategies that align with their cultural beliefs and practices when doing health promotion and illness care with child rearing. Numerous studies have revealed that increasing knowledge about parenting increases authoritative parenting practices. Early interest in parenting can lead to early positive attachment practices and later warm and involved parenting strategies. Differing parenting styles between the two parents in one family can cause conflict in both stable and divorced families. Using counseling and education with parents can help them recognize and reflect on their differences, which can lead to a united change toward more authoritative practices (Kuppens & Coulemans, 2019).

Nursing interventions for family-focused well-child care include identification of teachable moments to discuss child development, explore parental feelings, model positive interactions with children, and reframe parents' negative attributions about their children's behavior. For example, a nurse may help a parent to see that a child's temper tantrum may be a sign of independence and a need to communicate new thoughts, opinions, and feelings without having the language or emotional regulation skills to do so rather than the child deliberately attempting to embarrass or disobey the parent. The positive health benefits from parents learning more appropriate parenting may include the use of less physical and harsh discipline approaches, increased use of safety strategies such as placing newborns on their backs to sleep, increased likelihood that children will have up-to-date vaccines, and increased family time spent in pleasurable interactions and shared experiences. Nursing actions to reduce negative outcomes in child-rearing families are to identify parental risk factors associated with abuse and/or neglect, such as depression, family violence, poverty, high stress, lack of support, and drug and alcohol use, and use this knowledge to support parents in learning interactive and responsive skills along with attachment skills (Anis et al., 2020). Children's developmental progress has been found to be related to identifying and supporting parental strengths, promoting strong parent-child relationships, teaching parents about child development, and involving parents in activities that encourage learning (Anis et al., 2020).

Understanding and Working With Family Routines

Establishing daily routines and family rituals is an important health promotion strategy. These predictable patterns influence the physical, mental, and social health of children as well as the health of the family itself (Mindell & Williamson, 2018). During their extensive review of research across time and across cultures, Mindell and Williamson (2018) concluded that if parents were supported in developing healthy and adaptive bedtime routines versus maladaptive routines, then children and parents would benefit beyond improved sleep. Healthy bedtime rituals typically include other important routines, including hygiene; dental care; positive parent-child interactions, such as reading stories together, singing songs, reciting prayers, and telling stories; nurturing touch such as rocking or cuddling; and healthy bedtime snacks. When families implement a healthy bedtime routine, children have better emotional regulation during the day, have improved sleep quality and duration during the night, and are more likely to participate in other important routines throughout the day. These children benefit with improved development, academic skills, and social-emotional well-being. Parents report feeling more confident and have less conflict about routines and less family stress. By discussing adaptive bedtime routines at visits, both inpatient and outpatient, nurses can help families change maladaptive practices into healthy behaviors that benefit children well beyond childhood (Mindell & Williamson, 2018).

Child Care, After-School Activities, and Children's Health Promotion

Child-rearing families nurture children through partnerships with siblings, extended family members, nonrelated child-care providers, teachers, and other adults within the community. These relationships help to establish and maintain the family routines that are so important to health and child development. It is now common to see both parents participating in the workforce and therefore requiring assistance with child care. In 2019, close to 77% of mothers with children age 6 to 17 years were in the labor force, and 94% of fathers with children under the age of 18 years were in the labor force (U.S. Department of Labor, Bureau of Labor Statistics, 2020).

Another important issue concerns the length of time that new parents take parental leave from work. How quickly a new parent returns to the workplace often depends in part on access to paid leave. In the United States, the Family Medical Leave Act (FMLA) entitles some workers to 12 weeks of unpaid leave, with recent legislation providing 12 weeks paid leave for federal workers (U.S. Office of Human Resources Management, 2020). In Canada, most new parents are eligible for some level of paid maternity and parental leave benefits for 15 to 50 weeks through the Employment Insurance program (Government of Canada, 2021).

Many families search for the best routines to balance family and work. Care for children is often divided between parents, grandparents, other relatives, friends, neighbors, other nonpaid care, lay professional care (e.g., nannies and unlicensed providers), licensed home-care providers, or licensed and certified center care providers. The trend for care while parent(s) work continues to be split between relatives and paid nonrelative employees. For example, it is estimated that more than 7 million grandparents in the United States live with their own grandchildren; of those, it is estimated that 34% are responsible for caring for their own grandchildren U.S. Census Bureau, 2019). Some parents

strive to work nontraditional hours and/or flexible hours and to work while caring for their children to avoid the risks and costs of formal child care. Studies reveal, however, that single parents or parents working nontraditional hours struggle to find consistent and high-quality care for their children during nontraditional hours (Henley & Adams, 2018; Hepburn, 2018). This trend is likely to continue as the cost of child care continues to increase and parents are often faced with the prospect of employment insecurity as they consider who will provide quality care for their children.

The quality of early childhood education and support for children is an ongoing concern for parents and societies. Multiple studies have documented the importance of education and training of early childhood teachers; developmentally appropriate environments, activities, and equipment; and a recommended safe and effective teacher. Nevertheless, families may be forced to choose child care based on cost rather than quality. Nurses can assist with this concern by educating families about employers providing stipends or pretax payments of child care or about use of government stipends and tax credits for child care, such as those supported through Child Care Resource and Referral Services (Child Care Resource and Referral Network, 2017) in the United States, and by exploring various child-care options together.

For school-age children, it is increasingly common to see them attending before- and after-school care programs; however, some children still spend at least some time home alone. As children get older, they begin to acquire the knowledge and skills that support them to stay safe while home alone. Many states and provinces also have laws governing at what age children can be left alone. Regardless of age, it is important that families whose children care for themselves understand safety measures, such as what to do in an emergency; concealing the house key; and setting rules about safety, especially related to visitors and internet access. Nurses can educate parents on the risks for children being alone at home during afternoon and early evening hours and strategies to promote their child's safety.

Nurses, parents, teachers, government agencies, and other invested community members must work together to continue to develop before- and after-school programs and community center programs during times when school is not in session and parents need to continue to work. This has been a particular concern for families during the COVID-19 pandemic, and research is needed to explore the impacts of these challenges. Overall, nurses can help families review the types of child care and after-school options available and examine the site for health protection features. They can also serve on community boards that advocate for and regulate these programs and services.

By supporting working parents and care of children during working hours, healthy and predictable family routines are better maintained. Lack of reliable, predictable, and safe care for children after school hours is a significant threat to family health. Structure and positive adult contact are important for children throughout their childhood, including the hours after school and the end of their parents' workday (Iachini, 2017).

Identifying Health Risks and Teaching Prevention Strategies

Because of the relationship between health behaviors and illness or death, increased attention to unhealthy social-emotional behaviors is an important part of nursing practice in families with children. Specifically, nurses assess for, identify, and provide interventions to reduce risk factors associated with morbidity (sickness) and mortality (death). Specific risk factors include:

- Safety concerns for unintentional and intentional injuries and death
- Patterns leading to overweight and obese children and adolescents
- Lack of parenting knowledge and support associated with family violence and child maltreatment
- Health concerns more common to families living in poverty, including higher rates of violence, drug use, and teen pregnancy

Unintentional and Intentional Injuries

The leading cause of death among children and youth from age 1 to 24 years is unintentional injuries (Centers for Disease Control and Prevention [CDC], 2020e). The factor that most contributes to deaths caused by motor vehicle crashes is the lack of use of seat belts by children and adolescents and the lack of use of car seats for infants (CDC, 2021). Traumatic brain injury and concussion have also received increased attention in the child health field over the last decade, with increasing numbers of children and youth athletes suffering sports-related concussions. Nurses working with children who have experienced concussion and their families should assess for ongoing concussion symptoms and educate families on appropriate return-to-school and return-to-sports strategies (Society of Pediatric Nurses, 2019).

Family child health care nurses can teach and support families in the prevention of unintentional and intentional injuries. For example, nurses can teach about appropriate car seat restraints and water safety. They can educate parents of toddlers on childproofing the home to prevent poisoning from household supplies and electrical burns from uncovered electrical outlets. Teaching the importance of bicycle helmet use and helping families locate resources when they have limited financial means for purchasing helmets can help to minimize head trauma from bike accidents. Nurses can help parents understand the importance of using approved safety devices, such as car seats, helmets, and door and cabinet locks. Nurses can do this either in an informal role as a next-door neighbor or in a formal role through working at community or clinic programs,

Obesity and Overweight in Families With Children

Nurses help families recognize the harm that can result from obesity and offer methods to intervene in this leading public health problem. Although obesity rates in children have reached a plateau during the past decade, the rates continue to be a major concern for children's health. The incidence of obesity in children ages 2 to 5 years has dropped from 27% in 2010 (Ogden et al., 2012) to 14% in 2018 (CDC, 2018). Between 1980 and 2018, the percentage of children ages 6 to 11 years who were obese increased from 7% to 18.4%; for adolescents, it increased from 5% to 20.6% (CDC, 2018). Prevention and treatment are crucial to the child and family's well-being.

The causes of childhood obesity and overweight are complex, involving the environment (e.g., home and society), genetics, family attitudes and beliefs, cultural practices, nutritional practices, and family activities (Allen et al., 2016; Kumar & Kelly, 2017). The causes of childhood obesity can be broken down into environmental (high calorie intake, especially high levels of high-fat and high-sugar foods, and low activity levels), neurological (e.g., brain injury), monogenetic (e.g., leptin deficiency), endocrine (e.g., Cushing's syndrome), syndromes (e.g., Prader Willi syndrome), psychological (e.g., depression, binge eating disorder), medication-induced (e.g., antipsychotic medications or prolonged antibiotic use), poor sleep (e.g., sleep apnea), and adverse life events (e.g., poverty, low education, trauma). While physical causes of obesity do exist, most children struggling with obesity do not have a single genetic or physical cause for their obesity (less than 1% can list a single cause). Therefore, interventions are centered around changing the family culture of eating and activity, limiting screen time to no more than 2 hours per day, taking screens out of the child's bedroom, and providing support through motivational interviewing techniques (Kumar & Kelly, 2017; Mayo Clinic, 2018). Teaching parents to minimize eating out, increasing fruits and vegetables to five servings per day, and modeling healthy use of screens and outdoor activity helps children develop healthy lifestyles. The psychological impact of obesity is also a risk factor, with high levels of social stigma and shaming that can lead to depression, social isolation, and poor self-esteem (Kumar & Kelly, 2017).

Child Maltreatment

Nurses recognize situations in which children are in danger because of child maltreatment. In 2018, an estimated 9.2 per 1,000 children in the United States experienced child abuse and/or neglect (U.S. Department of Health and Human Services [USDHHS], Administration for Children and Families, 2020). Children from birth to 1 year of age had the highest rate of victimization caused by maltreatment, at 26.7 per 1,000 children of the same age, with 25% of cases of child abuse and neglect occurring in children under the age of 3 years. USDHHS, Administration for Children and Families (2020) identifies child neglect as failing to provide necessary care when financially able or offered financial means to do so; neglect accounts for over 60% of cases of child maltreatment in the United States in 2018, while just over 15% experienced more than one type of maltreatment. In one incidence study in Ontario, Canada, in 2018, there were approximately 16 substantiated investigations of child maltreatment per 1,000 children, almost half of which were identified as exposure to intimate partner violence (Fallon et al., 2020). Parents tend to make up the vast majority of the

perpetrators of child maltreatment: over 90% in the United States in 2018 (USDHHS, Administration for Children and Families, 2020).

Child maltreatment represents a problem in family behavior that demands immediate assessment and action or intervention. Nurses are mandatory reporters and are required by law to report to authorities when they suspect that a child is being maltreated. It is important for nurses who work with children and families to understand their legal and ethical responsibilities. Nurses should explore their provincial or state and federal laws and resources to ensure that they are familiar with their responsibilities as mandatory reporters.

Nurses can screen families for domestic violence and/or child maltreatment by asking questions regarding the safety of the home and the incidence of family violence within the home. See Box 15-2 (Chamberlain, 2016; Stanford Medicine, 2021) for examples of pertinent questions regarding family violence and child maltreatment for nurses assessing families and children. Inquiring about family violence can be uncomfortable for nurses and other health professionals. The standard of practice is to ask all families these questions so that the stigma becomes standardized. By screening for family violence, nurses can assess families and children for dangerous situations, teach safety, and make a referral as necessary.

Prevention is the preferred approach for intervening with families regarding child maltreatment. Nurses identify situations that might foster child maltreatment and intervene accordingly. Risk factors thought to contribute to abuse are categorized into four domains: parent or caregiver factors, family factors, child factors, and community/environmental factors (CDC, 2020a). Parent or caregiver factors include personal characteristics (e.g., age, education, income), a history of abuse in the parent's own childhood, substance abuse, attitudes about child behavior, and inaccurate knowledge or parenting skills (CDC, 2020a; USDHHS, Administration for Children and Families, 2020). Family factors include family conflict or violence, single parenthood, and family or parent stress (CDC, 2020a). Child factors include age, with younger children and infants being the most vulnerable, and the presence of disabilities or chronic illness (CDC, 2020a). Finally, community and environmental factors such as socioeconomic disadvantage and social isolation have been associated with increased rates of child maltreatment (CDC, 2020a). In all cases, it is important to remember that the presence of risk factors is not an indication that the parents or family members are, in fact, abusive. Rather, when the nurse identifies the presence of various stressors and risks, it may be appropriate to evaluate and implement interventions that may decrease the potential for maltreatment.

Nurses should also keep in mind the following protective factors against child abuse and neglect: parental resilience, social connections, knowledge of child development, concrete support in times of need, increased social and emotional competence of children, and nonacceptance of abuse by the community and larger society (CDC, 2020a; Sprague-Jones et al., 2019). Strategies thought to help families are those that facilitate friendships and mutual support, strengthen parenting by teaching and modeling appropriate behavior with children, respond to family crises, link families to services, facilitate children's social and emotional development, and value supporting parents (Sprague-Jones et al., 2019).

Specific Adolescent Risks

Adolescents as a group are especially vulnerable to high-risk behaviors that can lead to illness and death. Data on the prevalence of risk behaviors among adolescents are collected by the Youth Risk Behavior Surveillance System (YRBSS) using a national probability sample of 9th to 12th graders, state and local school-based surveys, and a national household-based survey (CDC, 2020f). In 2019, in the United States, the top four leading causes of death among persons age 15 to 24 years were unintentional injuries or accidents (27.5 per 100,000), suicide (13.9 per 100,000), homicide (11.2 per 100,000),

and cancer (3.3 per 100,000) (CDC, 2020e). Health behaviors that contributed to unintentional injury or to violence were the use of alcohol and other substances, nonuse of seat belts, and distractions during driving such as texting (CDC, 2020b).

The 2019 YRBSS report revealed that adolescents often engaged in behaviors associated with significant morbidity and mortality. Nationwide, 29% reported drinking alcohol in the past 30 days (a decrease from 38% in 2011) and 17% had ridden with a driver who had been drinking alcohol (CDC, 2020d). The 2019 YRBSS report also noted that illicit drug use has decreased over the last decade; however, one in seven still reported ever using illicit drugs (CDC, 2020f). While the use of cigarettes has declined significantly over the last decade, over 32% reported using electronic vapor products in the last 30 days (CDC, 2020c). This is a particularly concerning trend given the risks associated with vaping. The percentage of youth who were sexually active has declined over the last decade (CDC, 2020f).

Violence is a significant risk factor for morbidity and mortality among adolescents. In 2019, the second and third leading causes of death for young people ages 15 to 24 were suicide and homicide (CDC, 2020e). In 2019, 7% were threatened or injured by a weapon (e.g., gun, knife, or club) on school property and 9% missed school due to safety concerns (CDC, 2020f). Bullying is also a significant issue for youth, with 20% of youth in the YRBSS survey reporting experiences of being bullied at school and 16% reporting experience of cyberbullying (CDC, 2020f).

With regard to firearms, child and youth access to firearms is part of the problem. During a national survey on gun ownership and care, Azrael

---

BOX 15-2

Examples of Screening Questions for Family Violence and Child Maltreatment

Examples of interviews and screening questions may include the following (Chamberlain, 2016; Stanford Medicine, 2021):

Questions to Address to Parents
- How are things at home?
- Do you feel that your child is safe (at home, school, child care, and so on)?
- Has your child's behavior changed at all recently?

Questions to Address to Children
- What is your typical day like?
- What happens in your home, day care, and so on, when people get angry?
- Are you scared of anyone?
- Are you hurting anywhere?

et al. (2018) found that only three in 10 households with children stored firearms in the safest manner: locked and unloaded, while two in 10 households stored guns in the least safe manner: loaded and unlocked. The American Academy of Pediatrics (AAP) (2021, 2012) takes a public health position to prevent firearm injuries by removal of guns from families' homes and communities; however, it is crucial that education in gun use also occur. Nurses should include screening for guns in the home and incorporate a discussion and information about gun safety with parents.

Youth mental health and suicide rates are also of significant concern. In the 2019 YRBSS, approximately 37% of youth reported experiencing persistent feelings of sadness or hopelessness, and almost 20% had seriously contemplated attempting suicide, and these trends have been increasing over the last decade (CDC, 2020f). This is particularly concerning and highlights the importance of supporting families in relation to youth mental health. Nurses can be key educators in recognizing signs and symptoms of suicide in adolescents and can support friends and family members in getting help when these signs and symptoms are identified. Many communities are adopting suicide prevention strategies to reduce suicide rates, including decreasing risk factors (e.g., bullying, exposure to violence) and increasing protective factors (e.g., cultural connectedness, improved access and awareness of mental health care, support for diverse sexual and gender identities, decreasing access to firearms, increasing mental health identification and treatment, prevention and treatment for substance abuse, and development of crisis response teams for major family and community traumas) (Suicide Prevention Resource Center, 2016). Nurses are important in these efforts, from both the individual and family level of education and support to the community level of advocacy and participation in identifying and supporting needed change.

An alternate approach to risk assessment is to support what young people need to facilitate positive development. The America's Promise Alliance (2017) program lists the assets believed to be protective for children and predictive of positive outcomes and behaviors: violence avoidance, thriving (i.e., having a special talent or interest that gives them joy), good school grades, and volunteering. The program's five "promises," or goals for positive outcomes, are (1) presence of caring adults, (2) safe places and constructive use of time, (3) a healthy start, (4) effective education, and (5) opportunities to make a difference. One large study demonstrated that the presence of four to five promises resulted in positive adolescent development outcomes. Still, the same study found that only a minority of youth experienced enough of the promises that were related to positive outcomes.

The Influence of Poverty

Socioeconomic factors, such as poverty, lack of education, little or no health insurance, and immigrant status, are strong risk factors related to poor health. There is evidence that behavioral symptoms of child psychiatric disorders are associated with poverty and that those symptoms can be reduced as the family moves out of poverty (Hodgkinson et al., 2017). Programs that provide families with employment, adequate income, day care, and health insurance may have positive effects on academic achievement, classroom behavior, and aspirations.

Families with limited financial resources and those who do not have health insurance have more difficulty with health promotion than families with insurance or other methods of payment. In the United States, in 2018, 16.2% of children (11.9 million) were living in households where the annual income was below $25,701 for a family of four (Children's Defense Fund, 2020). The federal government has stepped up to decrease health disparities for all children, and especially CSHCN, by implementing the Children's Health Insurance Program (CHIP). These state-run programs are designed to ensure that all children have health insurance. The criteria expanded health insurance to low-income families with children who would not qualify for state-funded health insurance (e.g., MediCal, Oregon Health Plan).

The Affordable Care Act of 2010 maintained CHIP funding and increased the percentage of federal matching dollars from a range of 50% to 65% up to an average of 93% per state, maintained until 2015. Each state has the option of operating a separate CHIP program to provide federally funded child health assistance to uninsured, low-income children, to provide federally funded expansion of Medicaid eligibility to targeted low-income children, or to provide a combination of Medicaid expansion and a separate CHIP (Centers for Medicare and Medicaid Services, n.d.). The differences in design determine whether all children are entitled to

CHIP benefits or only those who qualify for Medicaid. The cost of the program has been debated, with many states concerned about the increased cost based on enrollment. The cost of health care is actually reduced, however, when children have a medical home and receive routine well-child care. When investigating barriers to children enrolling in state and federal programs, the most likely reason given by parents is that, if the parents cannot obtain insurance, they are less likely to enroll their children. Although uninsured children pose a major risk to the health of any nation, adults who are not eligible for Medicare are four times more likely not to have insurance than children.

Strategies to Support Health Promotion in Families With Children

Families are the major determinant of children's well-being. Nurses and other health care providers collaborate with parents and do not view parents as secondary and apart from nurses. Health promotion and illness prevention can occur using a variety of strategies across settings, including the following:

- Writing or providing health information for school or community newsletters, e-mail, or online messaging.
- Demonstrating and teaching health promotion activities, such as games or physical activities that promote health.
- Cultivating attributes of healthy families that include accountability, self-reliance, informed decision making, access to supportive social networks, and nurturing relationships.
- Encouraging family councils or family nights that provide venues for communications among all the family members.
- Providing anticipatory guidance about high-risk periods in child and youth development, such as childproofing the home before the infant begins to crawl or walk or providing assistance with appropriate limit setting when an adolescent gets her or his driver's license.
- Providing connections with school and community services; for example, children learn meanings, responses to, and values about health through their interactions in their school communities. Nurses can refer families to community resources, such as the federally funded Head Start programs that serve families of children who are economically disadvantaged and children who have disabilities.

CARE OF CHILDREN WITH CHRONIC CONDITIONS AND/OR DISABILITIES

Although most families raising children experience acute illnesses and become familiar with managing these crises, families do not anticipate that their children may have a chronic illness. They are often unprepared for the unknowns and uncertainties of the course of the disease, the effect on their children's development and adulthood, or the effect on each family member and family life.

Defining Chronic Conditions and Disability in Children

Families of children with chronic conditions and/or disabilities are diverse and represent all racial and ethnic groups and income levels. *Chronic health problems, long-term conditions, life-limiting conditions, impairments, disability,* and *children with special health care needs* are other terms used to describe children with an ongoing condition that cannot be cured. These ongoing conditions may include, but are not limited to, medical conditions, congenital and genetic syndromes, intellectual and developmental disabilities, socioemotional and mental health conditions, and long-term consequences of unintended injury or acute illness. These categories are not mutually exclusive, however. For example, those with genetic conditions may or may not experience developmental disabilities. In addition, many children have more than one medical diagnosis or health care need. Table 15-4 lists examples of chronic conditions and/or disabilities that pediatric nurses working with families may encounter.

According to the 2017 to 2018 National Survey of Children's Health, it is estimated that approximately 18.5% of children under 18 years of age in the United States have a special health care need (Data Resource Center for Child and Adolescent Health [DRCCAH], 2018). Of those, it is estimated that approximately 72% have complex health care needs that require treatment beyond a

Table 15-4	Examples of Chronic Conditions and/or Disabilities	
Medical problems	Allergies
	Asthma
	Diabetes
	Congenital heart disease
	Joint problems (e.g., juvenile rheumatoid arthritis)
Congenital and genetic syndromes	Down's syndrome
	Cerebral palsy
	Spina bifida
	Muscular dystrophy (e.g., Duchenne's muscular dystrophy, spinal muscular atrophy)
	Mitochondrial diseases
Intellectual and developmental disabilities and behavioral health conditions	Global developmental delay
	Learning disabilities
	Autism spectrum disorder
	Attention deficit-hyperactivity disorder (ADHD)
Social-emotional and mental health conditions	Depression
	Anxiety
	Eating disorders
Consequences of injuries or acute illness	Traumatic brain injury
	Stroke
	Paralysis (e.g., from spinal cord injury, acute flaccid myelitis)
	Cancer-related long-term conditions

medication prescription. In Canada, limited data is available for children under 12 years of age. In 2017, approximately 22.3% of young people ages 15 to 24 years experienced a disability (Statistics Canada, 2018).

While the term *CSHCN* is common in the literature, some families prefer not to use the term *special* to describe their child and their care needs. Other terms are also used to describe children with chronic conditions and/or disabilities, including *life-limiting conditions, chronic health problems, long-term conditions, impairments,* and *disability.* Another term that is becoming increasingly used is *children with medical complexity (CMC).* Cohen et al. (2011, p. s203) defined *medical complexity* as: "chronic conditions associated with medical fragility, substantial functional limitations, increased health and other service needs, and increased health care costs." There has been a particularly significant increase in focus on CMC and their families in research, practice, and policy, especially in Canada, over the last decade (Cohen et al., 2018). Nurses working with families should consider the terms they use to describe children with chronic conditions and/or disabilities and check with the family about which term the family prefers.

Families often fare better when they know the trajectory and management of the specific disease or chronic condition. Families often require different levels and types of support and information at different points along the life trajectory. Nurses and other health care providers tend to reteach the disease and medicine management aspects repeatedly, but families may be more concerned with social-emotional and behavioral responses. If nurses spend time with the family members carefully assessing their knowledge and their social and emotional responses to their child's illness, the plan of care will be more appropriate and effective.

Families with children with chronic conditions and/or disabilities vary greatly in their needs, ranging from families who are rarely affected by their children's condition, such as mild asthma, to those who are significantly affected, such as children who depend on a ventilator. To varying degrees, however, all families of children with chronic conditions bear the consequences of their children's conditions. A noncategorical approach, or the understanding by health care providers and parents that care across different diagnoses has similar needs and qualities, directs attention to the consequences that several different chronic conditions have on the children, their families, their communities, and the health care systems. The intent is to focus on overall well-being and move toward each member's and the family's goals.

Parenting a Child With Chronic Conditions and/or Disabilities

Parenting is the nurturance of children to become healthy, responsible, and creative adults. In considering parenting a child with chronic conditions and/or disabilities, an ecological perspective, such as bioecological theory discussed in Chapter 2, enables us to account for the interdependencies among children, parents, and the whole family within their community environments, which can be compared with a set of nesting dolls. Children with chronic conditions and/or disabilities are most often cared for by their families, who share a household and family history; are nested in communities; and use local and national health care, social services, and education systems. The complex, changing interactions among child, family, community, and systems influence the experiences of parenting children with chronic conditions and/or disabilities into adulthood. Tasks specific to health care are integrated with nurturance during their caregiving. Sullivan-Bolyai et al. (2003) described parenting responsibilities as taking care of the illness, nurturing and caring for their child, maintaining family life, and taking care of oneself.

Taking Care of the Child's Medical, Functional, and/or Behavioral Needs

Direct care of children's conditions involves the time, knowledge, and skills for technical and nontechnical management while simultaneously caring for the child's developmental and emotional needs (Currie & Szabo, 2019). The types and amount of technical and nontechnical management that parents may undertake varies based on their child's condition and its trajectory. Technical care involves doing procedures and monitoring for changes in their child's condition. This may include specialized medical care, such as administering medications and caring for indwelling tubes, or other specialized care, such as physical therapy, speech therapy, or behavior management techniques such as Applied Behavioral Analysis (ABA). It accounts for crisis care (e.g., unanticipated seizure, elevated temperature), which may involve complex first aid,

management, or emergent transportation to the hospital (Currie & Szabo, 2019). Nontechnical care includes the time and skills needed for feeding, bathing, dressing, grooming, bowel and bladder care, transferring from the bed to a chair, and toileting, along with the necessary extra laundry and house cleaning.

Complex care, such as suctioning tracheotomy tubes or diet and insulin regulation, may be a further challenge for relatives who may normally help with child care. Finding qualified caregivers that parents trust is more difficult than finding care for healthy children. Parents may cut back or quit work in order to provide care (Schuster & Chung, 2014) or decide against taking a new job or promotion if the health insurance benefits will not cover their children's health care needs or the responsibilities take a parent away from the child in terms of time or distance.

Parents also coordinate resources for their child. Children with chronic conditions and/or disabilities often require clinic visits, specialized therapy, community pharmacy stocking medications, and medical equipment delivered to the home. In addition, these children also need wellness care. AAP (2020) recommends a "medical home" in pediatric offices in order to provide disease prevention through immunizations, promote wellness through anticipatory guidance, address illness questions, and ideally serve as a coordination center for families of CSHCN (White et al., 2018). Yet not all pediatrician offices have the resources or training to provide coordination of care and specialized consideration of wellness child care for these children. Many offices are not equipped with wheelchair accessibility, appropriate exam tables for disabled individuals, or adapted reading material for those with visual or learning impairments.

Besides health care, parents may also advocate for special educational services. The Individuals with Disabilities Education Act (IDEA) requires free public education to all eligible children in the United States. For children with disabilities, this involves an individual family service plan (IFSP) for children from birth to 5 years of age, and an individual education program (IEP) for children age 5 to 21 years. In the United States and Canada, children with health impairments often access accommodations and adaptations to curriculum and daily instruction and test taking. Many children with disabilities also receive physical, occupational, and/or speech therapy through the school system. Families are often tasked with advocating for access to these supports in school systems; those living in rural areas seem to struggle the most with finding appropriate and available services for their children. Families add time to an already stretched schedule to advocate for their child's educational needs.

Nurturing the Child

The care of children with chronic conditions and/or disabilities does not exclude nurturing the child as the foundation to care. Parents often feel overwhelmed with the tasks involved with medical care and management and may need support and encouragement to maintain optimum nurturing. The common aspects of positive nurturing—including regular touch and rocking; encouragement of social connections; shared positive experiences, discoveries, and communication; and response to physical, emotional, and spiritual needs—can be pushed aside as medical treatments, procedures, and appointments take precedence (McCann et al., 2016; Wilkinson et al., 2020). Nurses can play a key role in helping parents optimize nurturing their child by explaining the importance of nurturing activities to health and optimum brain development and working with families to explore strategies to integrate nurturing actions into their daily lives, such as when providing medical care. Nurses can also help to alleviate parents' guilt of wanting to nurture and play with their child rather than provide medical care and help parents access supports to delegate medical care to professionals when possible.

Supporting Family Life

Nurturing the family as a whole and keeping each member moving toward family and individual goals are as important as care management (Sullivan-Bolyai et al., 2003). As the leaders of the family, parents help the family find meaning in the situation and find ways to include caregiving into daily life. The meaning that families ascribe to the child's condition and the family's identity can change over time based on a variety of factors, such as patterns of symptoms or behavior or how the family is coping. These meanings and identities for families should be an important part of nursing assessments with these families.

Parents maintain the household and financial security (Sullivan-Bolyai et al., 2003). The diversity of family structures and family member involvement has significantly increased over the past several decades; however, gendered roles may continue to be the norm in some families. Single-parent and split-parent households may be faced with the demands of caregiving, household management, and maintaining financial security that may require some additional consideration from nurses working to support these families (Allshouse et al., 2018). Financial security may also be a challenge as costs of caring for their child frequently exceed what insurance will cover, and many parents are left to cover large costs out of pocket (Allshouse et al., 2018).

A common concern for parents of children with chronic conditions and/or disabilities is the healthy development and care of siblings. Parents want the siblings not to be forgotten or overshadowed by the child with the chronic illness (Batchelor & Duke, 2019; Nabors et al., 2019). Siblings may assume the responsibilities of the parent, such as the 5-year-old who shares a bedroom with her or his sibling and alerts the parents that the sibling needs suctioning (Nabors et al., 2019). Siblings may also crave more of their parent's attention and, at the same time, worry about their parents as they see their parents working so hard to care for their sibling (Gorjy et al., 2017; Woodgate et al., 2016). They often take pride in being able to help their sibling, simultaneously complaining of doing more than their share of chores and noticing differential treatment from their parents and other relatives. Siblings can be supported by establishing open communication between the parent and sibling, finding parent support and social opportunities for siblings outside the home, establishing positive experiences and interests, and supporting positive meaning for challenging experiences (Fullerton et al., 2016).

Parents also have to manage social stigma, which is most common for families of children who have visible disabilities; are technology dependent; have developmental/behavioral disabilities; or have been diagnosed with a condition that has been historically stigmatized, such as HIV infection. Managing the effects of stigma often involves finding safe environments where families can relax and participate, such as Special Olympics or organizations designed to bring similar families together (e.g., National Autism Association). Without a feeling of trust and safety, families may limit social activities or split the family so that the child with the disability is cared for while other family members participate in social events (Alsharaydeh et al., 2019; Eaton et al., 2016). A major risk for families with children with chronic conditions and/or disabilities is social isolation and lack of social support (Alsharaydeh et al., 2019).

Parent Support

It is difficult for parents to take care of themselves when they are balancing caring for their child with a chronic condition and/or disability and the ongoing demands of family life. Parents experience numerous transitions throughout their child's life course that influence parent well-being, coping, and support needs. One common concept described in the literature is "chronic sorrow," which describes what many refer to as the normal grief response parents experience at the "loss of the idealized child" (Batchelor & Duke, 2019, p. 164). When the child is first diagnosed or at key normative milestones, parents may experience feelings of loss and challenges adjusting to a new reality of having a child with a chronic condition and/or disability (Batchelor & Duke, 2019; Coughlin & Sethares, 2017). The busy-ness of daily care can distract parents from thinking that their child is not normal. The differences become more evident, however, when the condition worsens, or at family events when their child is compared to other family members. Health care providers should become familiar with the concept of chronic sorrow and the impact on the daily lives of families as families and the primary parent caregiver have the expertise in the management of the child's care (Batchelor & Duke, 2019). By considering needs and aspirations alongside concerns and challenges, family nurses can better consider the myriad of ways that families experience life with a child with a chronic condition and/or disability and how best to support them.

"Living worried" has been found to be part of the day-to-day parenting of many children with chronic conditions (Currie & Szabo, 2019). Parents may worry about their judgment on when to seek care. They may worry that the neighbors would report them for child abuse if their toddler screams during treatments or as a form of communication. They may worry that their child was taking care of them. Nurses can help families to decrease their worry by connecting parents to support groups to discuss their worries. Connecting a family with another similarly situated family is an important nursing intervention to decrease the chronic anxiety felt by parents and to decrease isolation (Currie & Szabo, 2019).

With survival rates for many acute and chronic conditions improving drastically over the last several decades, most children with chronic conditions and/or disabilities live and are cared for at home with their family, and their conditions are managed in the home and community. *Caregiver burden* is a term often used to describe the strain or overload that caregivers experience across physical, psychological, social, and/or financial domains as a result of caregiving responsibilities (Liu et al., 2020; Wightman, 2019). Many parents may object to the word *burden* to describe the care they willingly give to their children. It is essential for family nurses to assess caregiver well-being across these four domains. Interventions such as respite, financial support, and support groups have been suggested across numerous studies (Society of Pediatric Nurses, 2018). Finding safe and appropriate respite care for families is often a barrier for partners and marital couples, especially in rural areas. Coordinated care between health clinics, specialty clinics, educational services, and social services can increase the resources for parents and increase the chances of finding appropriate respite care.

It is possible, however, that parents may struggle and not be able to care for their child, especially if needs are complex or behavior is so difficult that injury to the child or other family members is a risk. These parents may seek out-of-home placement but at the same time feel guilty about doing so. Yet it is important to understand out-of-home placement as a valuable option to support child and family well-being in some cases. Finding appropriate community resources for specialized care is often particularly difficult, especially for school-age and adolescent children, and often respite services and home care are fragmented. This fragmentation can place further stress on parents. Nurses have a key role in assessing the family's ability to maintain care, the need for increased support or home care, and the need for out-of-home support or placement when needed.

Developmental and Situational Transitions

Transition-of-care issues have been discussed in the health care industry for decades and can be particularly important for families of children with chronic conditions and/or disabilities. As discussed earlier in this chapter, children with chronic conditions and/or disabilities and families may experience many transitions throughout childhood and adolescence. Health-illness transitions such as a new diagnosis or sudden changes in the child's condition were discussed earlier in how parents experience and adapt to their child's diagnosis and changes across the life span. Situational transitions, such as moving to a new school or being discharged from hospital, are also common across childhood and adolescence and require ongoing attention by family nurses. Hospital-to-home transitions will be discussed further later in this chapter.

One of arguably the most challenging transitions encountered by families of children with chronic conditions and/or disabilities is that of the transition to adulthood and adult-oriented services. These transitions, also commonly known in the literature as health care transition, have frequently been framed as a global and public health problem (Office of Disease Prevention and Health Promotion, 2020). During this time, adolescents and young adults experience a multitude of transitions simultaneously. They experience developmental transitions; for example, many will be working on developing the knowledge and skills to manage their conditions and care. Some will also be starting postsecondary education, while others transition into day programs or the workplace. All will be preparing for, transferring into, and becoming situated in the adult care health and social services systems. In this way, addressing health care transition must attend not only to ensuring transfer from pediatric to adult services but also to broader developmental, psychosocial, educational, and vocational needs across these numerous transitions (Joly, 2016).

Health care transition has been described as a process or journey that consists of three main phases related to the transfer from pediatric to adult-oriented services: preparing for transition, change/transfer of care, and postchange/transfer of care and becoming situated in the adult world (Betz, 2017; Joly, 2016). Transition experts have suggested several overarching principles to guide clinical recommendations for health care transition research, practice, and policy (Children's Healthcare Canada, 2018; Betz, 2017; White et al., 2018). The principles, included in Box 15-3, are informed by transition theory and social ecological models relevant to transitions.

Families play important roles throughout the health care transition process. Many families, and especially parents, feel challenged with making sense of the transition process and letting go when responsibility for day-to-day management is transferred to the adolescent (Kerr et al., 2018; Li et al., 2020). Families are integral to supporting the development of self-management skills with their adolescent child. Some parents or guardians, however, will continue to manage their young

---

BOX 15-3

Key Principles for Supporting the Transition to Adulthood for Youth and Families

- Transition care should be youth- and family-centered and adopt a strengths-based approach.
- Family and/or caregiver management is essential to the transition process.
- Transition care should attend to the variability and complexity of youth and family lives.
- An emphasis on equity and culturally safe spaces can further enhance the transition process.
- Transition is multidimensional and should address the physical, developmental, psychosocial, mental health, educational, and financial needs of the youth and family.
- Transition care should be built on a foundation of communication and collaboration between

providers and youth and their families and on shared accountability between pediatric and adult services, with an emphasis on ongoing coordination.
- Planning for transition and transfer should start early and be ongoing and individualized.
- Planning should attend to assessment of readiness, building knowledge and skills for the adult world, including self-management skills as applicable, in collaboration with youth and their families.
- Outcomes indicating successful transition should emphasize health equity alongside health, well-being, quality of life, and connectedness to adult services.

Sources: Children's Healthcare Canada, 2018; Society of Pediatric Nurses, 2018; White et al., 2018.

adult child's care well into adulthood. In these situations, family nurses must also consider family knowledge and skills required to transition successfully to adult-oriented services with their adolescent.

Nurses who work with families and their adolescents with chronic conditions and/or disabilities should begin discussing the health care transition process early; some suggest as early as age 12 or 13. Plans for transfer to adult providers and services should be discussed at least a year or more in advance of transfer, and nurses should work with the family to design a well-thought-out, purposeful plan of transition. One difficult part of this care process is working with the family and the health care team to determine when is the best time for the transition to occur. Typically, the transition occurs sometime between years 18 and 21, often based on eligibility criteria for children's hospital services. For many adolescents, their readiness to demonstrate responsibility and to participate as much as possible in self-care management are better predictors than age (White et al., 2018). Other factors nurses need to consider and address besides self-efficacy and age in this transition plan are the adolescent's attitude toward transition and the complexity of the illness and treatment plan.

Various nursing and health care organizations have developed useful resources, including transition guidelines, checklists, and assessment tools, to support adolescents and their families throughout the transition process (Betz, 2017). For example, Got Transition provides many resources for families as well as those who support families through the health care transition process, including a Family Toolkit (Got Transition, 2020). Several readiness assessment tools that focus on parents' knowledge and perceptions of youth's self-management skills are available (Hart et al., 2021; Nazareth et al., 2018).

Partnering With Families of Children With Chronic Conditions and/or Disabilities

An essential component of CFCC for nurses working with families of children with chronic conditions and/or disabilities is collaboration and partnership. Families often want to be in control in decision-making processes and for their expertise to be taken seriously (Lin et al., 2020). Mendes (2016) has suggested that partnerships with families of children with chronic conditions and/or disabilities should be characterized by respect, flexibility, caring professionalism, communication, acknowledgment of parental control, and parent support.

Respect should be the cornerstone of partnerships with families. Information and knowledge should flow bidirectionally between nurses and families. Nurses can support families by providing information about new diagnoses, treatments, technologies, or procedures and help families integrate this new knowledge into their everyday lives. At the same time, nurses must also recognize and respect families' often intimate and specific expertise of their child and their child's care needs (Rafferty et al., 2019; Rafferty & Sullivan, 2017). Parents often play key roles in coordinating their child's care across various systems, so nurses and other health care providers across the continuum of care should share information and collaborate with parents to promote empowerment and support the child's well-being.

With the patient engagement and patient-oriented research movements in health research, families are also increasingly being involved in child health and family nursing research. Family engagement in research moves beyond research *on* or *about* children and families to research *with* them. Family engagement in research can make research more meaningful to children and families and improve the quality and appropriateness of outcomes (Shannon & Mardell, 2018). Promoting family engagement in research requires a deep commitment to collaboration beyond just informing or consulting (Bartlett et al., 2017). Family and child health researchers have engaged families as co-researchers on the research team and through family advisory councils that are involved at each stage of the research process, from priority setting to conducting the research, to knowledge translation (Bartlett et al., 2017; Woodgate et al., 2015). Many articles and resources are available to support family nurse researchers in engaging families in their research (Bartlett et al., 2017; Patient-Centered Outcomes Research Institute, 2018; Shannon & Mardell, 2018). For example, CanChild, which is based on Ontario, Canada, offers a 10-week online certificate course on family engagement in research for researchers, students, and family members (CanChild, 2020).

CONSENT IN FAMILY CHILD HEALTH NURSING

Families with children experiencing acute or chronic illness or injury may be asked to make difficult decisions regarding health care. In most instances, when young children are involved, health care providers collaborate with parents to obtain informed consent, except in emergency situations when parents are absent. As children grow and develop, it is important for them to take on more responsibility as primary guardians of personal health and decision making. Children, especially adolescents, want to be involved in decision making regarding their health care. Some family members and health care providers may feel uncomfortable with the inclusion of children in health care decision making (Carnevale et al., 2017; Wangmo, 2017). Some authorities believe that children may not make rational decisions; however, many studies have shown how children can be viewed as active agents who often have the ability to participate in and contribute to conversations about their care (Carnevale et al., 2017). Carnevale et al. (2017) suggest that viewing children's voices relationally—that is, viewing children as both agential and dependent and their relations with parents as interdependent—directs health care providers to inquire about what they consider right (or wrong) or good (or bad) in their everyday lives and asking directly what is important to the child as well as each family member. While younger children can sometimes have a difficult time visualizing the future, it is important that their voices are accounted for in decision-making processes with families.

Laws regarding informed consent of minors vary from state to state or province to province. It is important that health care providers know individual state or provincial statutes. In addition, some states consider some minors "emancipated" and give these individuals the authority to make personal health care decisions. These minors may be self-supporting; live outside the parental home; or be married, pregnant, a parent, or in the military. They may also be declared emancipated by the courts. Some states and provinces also have statutes related to "mature minors": these persons are not emancipated but still have the authority to make health care decisions in certain situations (Patton & Dobson, 2020; Weithorn, 2020).

On occasion, the wishes of children, families, and health care providers may differ. It is assumed that all parties will act in the best interest of the child, but best interests are in the eye of the beholder when it comes down to personally held values, such as answers to questions like "What makes a life worth living?" (Carnevale et al., 2017). Although it is uncommon for parents to be overruled, the courts sometimes invoke the Child Abuse Prevention and Treatment Act, which gives the state's interest in protecting minors greater weight than the rights of parents in decision making. In these situations, health care providers should respect the fact that some patients may need time to understand the situation or come to terms with concerns regarding proposed care. Legal intervention should be the last resort and should occur only when there is a substantial risk to the child, because state intervention can cause serious harm itself to the family and child.

CARE OF CHILDREN AND FAMILIES IN THE HOSPITAL

Another issue that family nurses experience when caring for families with children is the admission of a child to the hospital. Hospital admission is a stressful event for families. Nurses and health care providers have the opportunity to take this crisis situation and make it the best it can be for the child and family by decreasing stressors whenever possible. Applying the principles of partnering, shared decision making, setting mutual goals with the family, enhancing family connectedness to the child, valuing the family's areas of expertise, and assisting the family to understand health care processes and procedures and options for treatment are all ways to help alleviate some of the stress of a hospital stay (Franck et al., 2015). Family and child attendance at interdisciplinary team rounds is an ideal place to set mutual goals, and such rounds have been shown to increase patient and family satisfaction and provide essential comfort and support for families (Kelly et al., 2019; American Association for Respiratory Care, 2018). In fact, positive feelings from the family can improve health outcomes.

Nurses often take on the role of coordinating and maintaining communication with family members throughout a hospitalization. Identifying one or two key family members to provide communication to other family members and friends helps build trust and decreases the risk for communication errors and related conflict. Having a designated number of health care providers, including assigning primary nurses following relationship-based care models, improves safety, care, and family satisfaction (Nadeau et al., 2016).

Families should be considered more than just visitors when their child is in the hospital. Referring to family members as visitors diminishes the significance of the family relationship and may even be perceived as insulting; it is the health care providers who are the visitors or temporary caregivers for the hospitalized child. Ensuring that *family* is broadly defined can make available a wide base of support from loved ones. The family, rather than hospital administrators, should determine individuals allowed to be part of the care of the child. While most parents embrace being an active and respected part of the care team, others may feel intimidated and fearful, especially if providing unfamiliar technical care. Therefore, while acknowledging that most parents want and expect to be active team members, it is important to continually assess the parents' comfort level in providing care.

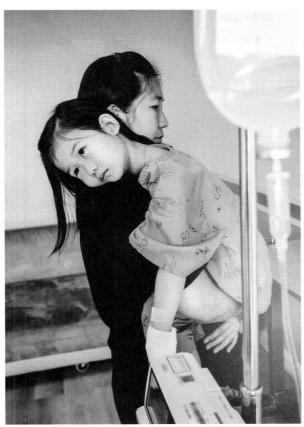

Source: © istock.com/kdshutterman

Health care providers, especially those working with critically ill children, need to be aware that parents may struggle with stress responses related to their ability to cope with the hospitalization of their child. During their study of 107 parents experiencing hospitalization within an intensive care unit (ICU) of their children, Franck et al. (2015) found that 32.7% of parents had symptoms of post-traumatic stress disorder (PTSD) 3 months after their child was discharged and had enough symptoms to qualify for a diagnosis of PTSD. When nurses recognize the stress experienced by parents when their child is hospitalized, nurses are more able to assist parents in coping with hospitalization of their child. Offering parents resources, such as support groups or working with a social worker or in-hospital counselor, provides options to improve parents' ability to cope positively with the stress of having a critically ill child.

The needs of siblings should also be addressed during a child's hospitalization. Younger siblings have vivid imaginations and may believe that they caused their sibling to become ill or injured, or they may fear that the hospitalized child may die. Nurses are equipped to provide parents with information, guidance, and reassurance about the appropriateness of sibling visitation for individual situations and to support these visits with appropriate preparation and support that is developmentally appropriate. If a child cannot visit their sibling, other strategies can help decrease distress, including having healthy siblings write a letter to their sibling, or for younger children, draw a picture. Another common concern is protecting the ill child from community infections. During the COVID-19 pandemic, visits from family members, relatives, and friends has been severely limited, generally to one person at a time. These policies often place the burden of limiting time with a critically ill and possibly dying child in the hands of one parent, something that the parents have to decide on in a state of fear. This policy of restricting parental time with a critically ill child prevents nurses from providing humane CFCC (Andrist et al., 2020). As hospitals decide on difficult policies aimed at preventing the spread of a dangerous contagion, the debate on essential services will continue. Many may argue that family presence during the hospitalization of a critically ill child is an essential service (Andrist et al., 2020).

Avoiding family separation from the hospitalized child remains a high priority. Separation increases stress for children and families and does not encourage a partnership philosophy. Since 2003, the Society of Pediatric Nurses and the American Nurses Association (Lewandowski & Tesler, 2003) have supported 24-hour parental access to hospitalized children. This access includes giving families the option to remain with their children during procedures, treatments, and resuscitation attempts, including in the emergency department (McAlvin & Carew-Lyons, 2014). Nurses can assist families by supporting the decision to be present or not; assessing family reactions as needed; answering questions; helping family members to find a comfortable spot in the room; providing instructions of what they can and cannot do; contacting spiritual support as requested; and providing comfort items such as tissues, beverages, and seating. See Box 15-4, which describes a family's experience during their child's resuscitation.

Although families are glad to have their children discharged from the hospital, stressors can accompany this transition as well. This is especially true for parents of children who have been in the ICU or for CMC. Families and children do better when family members are part of the discharge team (Leyenaar et al., 2017). Nurses are in a unique position to continue CFCC through the transition from hospital to home. Nurses are often found in the case management role because of their education and experience working with families.

BOX 15-4

Family Experiences During Resuscitation at a Children's Hospital Emergency Department

Introduction: Family presence during cardiopulmonary resuscitation has been recommended by national professional organizations, which include the American Emergency Nurses Association and AAP.

Purpose of study: In an effort to improve the care of families during resuscitation events, the authors of this study examined the experiences of family members whose children underwent resuscitation and their health and mental health following the episode.

Methodology: Ten family members participated in a 1-hour audiotaped interview in this descriptive, retrospective study. Data collection included both quantitative and qualitative instruments, which contained previously validated and investigator-developed items. Seven family members were present during resuscitation and three were not.

Results: Analysis of interview data revealed that families felt that: (1) they had the right to be present during resuscitation, (2) their child wanted them present during resuscitation and that they were sources of strength for the child, (3) they were reassured by seeing that all possible options to help their child were exhausted, and (4) a facilitator for information giving would be helpful during the event because no one was prepared to face resuscitation.

Nursing implications: Whether present or not, all family members in this study expressed the importance of the option to be present during resuscitation. There was no indication of post-traumatic stress to family members following the event.

Source: McGahey-Oakland, P. R., Lieder, H. S., Young, A., & Jefferson, L. S. (2007). Family experiences during resuscitation at a children's hospital emergency department. *Journal of Pediatric Health Care, 21*(4), 217–225.

Case Study: Comantan Family

This case study of the Comantan family demonstrates family nursing approaches to providing health care to a family with children. The primary patient is Carl, although other family members have health care issues as well. The focus of this case study is Carl's health and the health of his family. See the genogram and environmental ecomap of the Comantan family in Figures 15-2 and 15-3, respectively.

Setting

Carl Comantan is a 9-year-old boy who lives with his family in a wood-frame house in a coastal, rural area of the northwest region of Alaska. He has chronic respiratory illnesses and has been diagnosed by his physician as having asthma.

Case Study: Comantan Family—cont'd

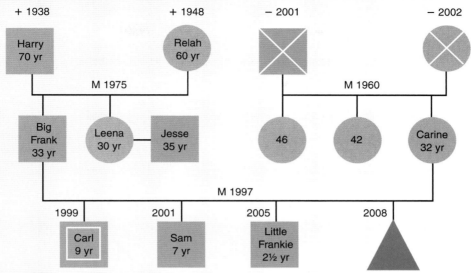

FIGURE 15-2 Comantan Family Genogram

Family Members

Carl's ethnicity is Alaskan Native, or Inuit. His father and mother, as well as his maternal and paternal grandfathers and grandmothers, are also Alaskan Native. His maternal grandfather and grandmother both passed away several years ago from pneumonia. The remaining family members have light brown skin and dark brown or black hair. The family speaks English and the elders also speak their native language, Inuktitut.

Carl's family consists of his mother, Carine, age 32; his father, Big Frank, age 33; and his two brothers, Sam, age 7, and little Frankie, age 2½. Carine is approximately 4 months pregnant. Big Frank's sister, Leena, age 30, helps with child care. Grandfather Harry and Grandmother Relah are very involved with their children and grandchildren.

The Family Story

Big Frank and Carine have been married for more than 11 years. The children are their biological children from this marriage. Neither has been married before. They went to high school together and met when Big Frank did business at the gas station where Carine worked. They both attend the same church.

Big Frank works part-time as a professional truck driver for a trucking corporation in the region. He is often gone from home for 2 to 3 days at a time for his work. The company offers limited major medical insurance for Big Frank and his family. Office visits and care under $800 are not covered. Carine's pregnancy care and births are covered at 60% of the cost. She receives no paid maternity leave benefit from her employer.

Carine works at a local gas station that has a small grocery store attached. She manages the grocery store. The store is 5 miles from their home in the nearby village of Anokiviac. Big Frank and Carine are worried that they cannot make enough money to save, let alone pay the ongoing bills for electricity, gasoline for their vehicles, heating oil for their home, and clothing. They feel fortunate to be members of a cohesive community of family and friends and to have jobs. Many people in their area do not have full-time employment. There are no family aid programs in the area. They travel each month to the town an hour's drive away to go to the local food bank. They get a box of staples that includes flour, rice, canned vegetables, and dried milk. The food bank requires that they show bills and pay statements to prove that they qualify for the food. Sometimes the food bank has a very limited number of items.

Big Frank and Carine strongly believe in making and keeping strong relationships with the people in their family and community circles. They talk about how people have helped each other in the past and how they are always on the lookout for someone who needs help. From one conversation with a teacher, Carine learned about a summer program for first-graders. She

(continued)

Case Study: Comantan Family—cont'd

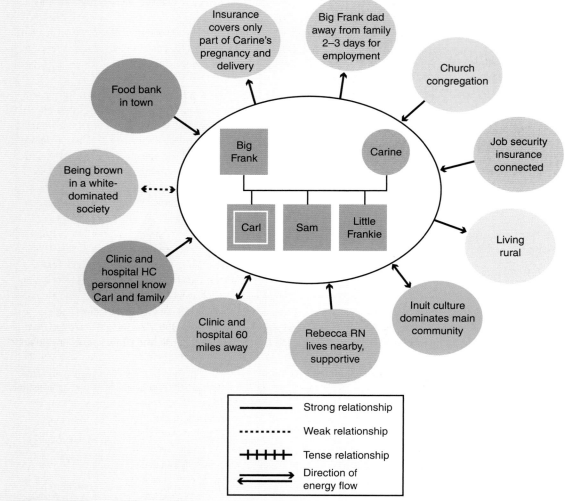

FIGURE 15-3 Comantan Family Ecomap

was able to enroll Sam in that 2-week-long program in the town, where he stayed with a cousin's family. In exchange for the cost of the program, she helped several evenings in their local school program during the school year.

These evening programs during the school year were also helpful for Carl, who missed several days during the school year because of his coughing and respiratory illnesses. Because of the extra time and attention, he has been able to keep up with his classmates at his school. Carine and Big Frank help the children's Aunt Leena understand how to help Carl with his studies because she cares for the children while the parents are working. Carine and Big Frank believe that if they and a few other people, such as Aunt Leena and the schoolteachers, know Carl well, they will notice when he starts to become ill. They believe that they have been able to avert many serious illnesses for Carl because they and the adults around him know him well. They do not get overly worried if he wheezes a little, which they consider normal for Carl. If he gets shorter of breath, however, or if his appetite wanes, then they know he is getting sick. Even his brother Sam knows about Carl being "fever hot," as he calls it, and worries openly about his brother when he is ill. Sam and little Frankie bring Carl water and crackers when he is sick. The younger children also know about Carl's inhaler and bring it to him when he is wheezing.

Case Study: Comantan Family—cont'd

The physicians and nurses at the clinic in the town know that when Carine, Big Frank, Aunt Leena, or other family members call saying Carl is ill, the situation is serious. They listen with high regard.

Big Frank is a partially disabled veteran of the U.S. army. He served in an international war overseas and was injured in a tank attack. His disability involves his left leg and left arm, both of which are severely scarred from burns. He has decreased range of motion and sensation in both of these limbs. His left chest and face are also scarred; however, he did not lose vision or function of his shoulder or face. He is not overweight and is physically strong and fit.

Carine is in good health but knows there is a family history of coughing spells. She is not overweight and is physically strong and fit. Both Carine and Big Frank work hard to eat well and feed their children healthy food. They eat frozen vegetables and fruits, and bread made by various family members. Their protein sources include fish that they catch and either elk or caribou from the annual fall family hunt. Occasionally they have seal, obtained courtesy of traditional hunts by Big Frank and the extended family.

Carine and Big Frank drink an occasional beer, but they do not drink any other alcoholic beverages. Many of their extended family members and folks in their community drink beer, sometimes to excess, resulting in drunken behavior. Carine and Big Frank worry that their children may drink excessively as adolescents and adults. They do not allow their children to drink any beer or other alcoholic beverage. The extended family members and the folks in the community practice the same behavior. Group disapproval occurs when drunken behavior occurs, and those persons are taken home.

Carl is generally healthy except for his asthma and frequent episodes of upper respiratory infections. These often progress into lengthy bouts of wheezing and coughing. He frequently wheezes in the morning on awakening and when he plays outside. He misses all or parts of days from school because of his illnesses approximately 25% of the time. He has an inhaler, but he occasionally forgets to bring it with him to school and church or out to play. He takes his antibiotics and other medications well. He says out loud, "This is for my breathing!" He also says to little Frankie, "This is not for you, this is my medicine! It is icky, you should never eat it!" Carl knows that his mother, Aunt Leena, schoolteacher, and Sunday schoolteacher know about each of his medicines. Carine and Big Frank are considering sending Carl to asthma camp for 2 weeks in the city during the summer. The physician at the hospital has recommended that Carl receive a foundation-funded scholarship at the camp because they note that he learns quickly and likes to be with other children. Also, the physician told Carine and Frank that they think Carl could benefit from the time to focus on learning more about managing his own condition.

Sam and little Frankie are both healthy. They have had occasional respiratory illnesses. Sam and Carl both had the chickenpox (the varicella vaccine was not available in their area at the time). Carine and the children are up-to-date on their vaccines. Big Frank has not had an influenza vaccine and does not recall when he had other immunizations since he left the military.

While Carine is at work, all three children go to their Aunt Leena's home either all day or after school, depending on their age. Aunt Leena's home is a 5-minute walk from the school. Aunt Leena has a car and has driven Carl to the emergency department several times during the last year when he has had severe bouts of wheezing and a fever. Aunt Leena lives with her husband, Uncle Jesse, who works as a truck driver and bush plane pilot in the area. Aunt Leena does not work outside her home. She is involved in the care of her brother's children and is looking forward to the next child. She occasionally takes a little gas money when her brother, Big Frank, offers. She is committed to helping her brother and his family in any way she can. She and her husband want children but have been unable to conceive.

Grandparents Harry and Relah are a 5-minute walk from Big Frank and his family, and they are also involved in watching, guiding, and helping their three grandchildren. Grandmother Relah has learned many treatments for illnesses over her lifetime. She studied for a while with one of the tribal shamans many years ago and maintains contact with the shaman. She makes mint and berry teas for Carl, makes steam for him in the kitchen, and feeds him dried fish for strength and healing. She talks to Carl and his brothers about the herbs she makes from various berries, bark, and leaves in their environment. She also encourages them to think about being strong and quick, wise and caring in their world. She talks to Big Frank about taking Carl to visit the shaman. They have not yet decided if they will follow through with this recommendation.

Big Frank and Carine consult extended family members, particularly older adult parents and other elders in the area, regarding health and family matters of all kinds, including seeking advice regarding Carl's respiratory infections and wheezing. The nearest clinic, hospital, or health care facility is more than 60 miles away, so they are careful about taking the time and gasoline to drive there. Big Frank and Carine consider themselves equal decision makers with regard to family health matters and consult providers

(continued)

Case Study: Comantan Family—cont'd

and family members. Both are held in high esteem in their family and surrounding community. They are supported through congregational prayer in their church, particularly when Carl is ill. Church members, especially direct relatives, often bring food to the Comantan family home when Carl is ill or when Big Frank is gone for several days on his job.

One of the Comantan family's neighbors, Rebecca, is a registered nurse who lives about 5 miles away. She works at one of the clinics associated with the hospital that is in the town 60 miles away. One time she took Carl with her to the clinic so that he could see his physician and get a renewal on an anti-inflammatory medication. She often laughs and says she is another auntie for Carl and his siblings. She says she is, at least, their cousin, even though she is Salish and not Inuit.

Health Care Goals for the Comantan Family

- Reduce the frequency and severity of Carl's respiratory illnesses.
- Reduce the number of Carl's missed school days to ensure age-appropriate academic success.
- Increase the number of developmentally appropriate responsibilities and decision-making processes for Carl as he learns to manage his own illness.
- Prevent Carl's daily wheezing by improving management of his asthma.
- Promote Carine's health during her pregnancy.
- Promote Big Frank's healthy coping with the pain and discomfort of his injuries.
- Enhance health resources for the family in its community.
- Reduce the family's barriers to health and increase its strengths for health.

Goals for Nurses Working With the Comantan Family Across Health Care Settings

- Build a therapeutic and collaborative, health-focused relationship with Carl and the Comantan family.
- Explore ways to reduce the frequency and severity of Carl's respiratory symptoms.
- Explore with Carl and his family ways to mediate and adapt to the overall impact of his illness on him and his family.
- Explore the health care resources for the Comantan family.
- Explore the main strengths and stressors for Carl and his family.
- Commend the Comantan family for its current health efforts and outcomes.
- Focus on maintaining stability in the Comantan family.

Family Systems Theory in Relation to the Comantan Family

The use of Family Systems Theory addresses the complex needs of each individual within the family and the family as a whole. The individual concepts from the Family Systems Theory apply as follows.

Concept 1—All Parts of the System Are Connected

Carl and his family are deeply and actively embedded in their family life and their community. Each family and community member contributes to the health of Carl and his family. When Carl is ill, supportive connections are activated in a focused manner, according to the needs identified.

One assumption of family systems is that the features of the system are designed to maintain its stability, using both adaptive and maladaptive means. The Comantan family is adaptive to Carl's illnesses in its frequent, focused interactions with family and friends. The family members realize that their situation may change quickly, for example, with finances, and that they may suddenly find themselves in financial stress. Family members also recognize that Carl's health may change quickly, and they are aware that several people should know how to monitor Carl's health and know what to do if he shows signs of respiratory distress. Their connections with Aunt Leena are part of that adaptation. They realize that, with an intentional increase in the number of people who know Carl well, there is a greater likelihood that he can be assessed quickly and accurately for severity and risk no matter where he is.

Each family member has many roles, each affecting one another. Big Frank, for instance, is a provider of financial resources, a responsible adult in his social community, a caring son to his parents, a guardian of the culture, and a caring father. These roles influence many aspects of his family. Carine is a provider of financial resources; a responsible adult in her social community, including the school; and a caring mother. These roles influence many aspects of her family.

Case Study: Comantan Family—cont'd

Concept 2—The Whole Is More Than the Sum of Its Parts

The family members support each other consistently, recognizing the strength of the whole. The Comantan family believes individuals doing their part contribute to the overall health of all and the ability of each to help at various times. The Comantan family adults focus on maintaining the health of all members in the long term while adapting to Carl's illness. For example, because illness sometimes forces Carl to miss school, they plan for Aunt Leena to help him. They also arrange for Sam and Carl to be in summer programs. The family adapts to the health needs of one member while taking care not to compromise the health of the other members.

The Comantan family is an interdependent and cohesive unit. This is consistent with its societal beliefs of helping each other survive and thrive. Family members believe that each person has value, yet each has responsibilities to the others in the group. They take great pride in teaching each other necessary and helpful things. This is especially true of the elders in their relation to the younger members. The elders do listen to the new ideas of the younger members, however, realizing that all ideas are worth consideration.

The entire family is happily anticipating the arrival of the new baby. They hope it is a girl, but they will be happy whether the baby is a boy or a girl. This normative, expected event may require the three boys, Carl, Sam, and little Frankie, to stay with Aunt Leena and Uncle Jesse during the birth and early postpartum stage. This will depend on the circumstances, and the aunt and uncle are prepared.

Concept 3—All Systems Have Some Form of Boundaries or Border Between the System and Its Environment

The Comantan family stays close to family and friends yet is mindful of the amount and types of contributions made between families. For example, if Carl needs to go to the hospital, Aunt Leena strives to be the one who takes him rather than asking Rebecca to do so.

The family has fairly open boundaries within its local community and does reach out to a few resources in the town 60 miles away. The family likes the idea of Sam going to the summer program and staying with his cousins because they know the teacher and the supervisors.

The grandparents help Carl and his brothers find the boundaries of their heritage within the larger white American culture. They are teaching Carl about these boundaries and expect Carl to model these for his two younger brothers as well as for other children in the community.

Rebecca, the nurse, who is Salish (not Inuit), is trusted and the family is open with her. The family is also open with the members of their church's congregation.

Concept 4—Systems Can Be Further Organized Into Subsystems

The Comantan family and the family of Aunt Leena and Uncle Jesse are an important subsystem in the Comantan family's overall functioning. Aunt Leena and Uncle Jesse contribute a lot while gaining contact with their beloved nephews. The grandparents, Harry and Relah, are also an important subsystem of the Comantan family, as are the children versus the adults.

Nursing Plan Using the Family Systems Approach

The nursing plan for this family is more holistic if the Family Systems Approach is used.

Nurse Assessment—Noticing/Data Gathering and Interpretation

- Explore in detail the expectations the family—including parents, grandparents, and aunt and uncle—has for Carl in relation to managing his health. Use affirmations, clarifications, respect, salutations, and honesty.
- Ask the family to share details of its health practices, including any herbal or practice treatments used by Carl's grandparents Harry and Relah.
- Learn the history and what the family expects about the future of Carl's chronic illness.
- Explore triggers and factors that worsen Carl's condition.

(continued)

Case Study: Comantan Family—cont'd

- Assess Carl's overall growth and development, his medications, what substances he has used or been given for his health, his health-related behaviors, and his interpretations of all these items. For example, determine the level of growth and development impairment the family has noticed because of his respiratory illnesses and treatment.
- Discuss the concept of illness trajectory for the Comantan family.
- Explore what the family thinks is helpful, what might be helpful, and what is not helpful.
- Explore the main adaptive features the family identifies.
- Explore additional health and health cost resources for the family, particularly for Carl's potential future hospitalizations, for Carine's pregnancy and delivery, and for Big Frank's pain management.
- Explore any health care disparities the family has experienced or perceived.
- Assess the entire family's immunization status.
- Explore the impact of Big Frank's absence for 3 days at a time when he is driving his truck for work.
- Ensure that various family members have Carl's medications handy at their homes.
- Assess the boundaries of care and involvement for Aunt Leena and Carl's grandparents Harry and Relah.
- Look for trends, health patterns, illness patterns, and disease patterns for Carl's management behaviors and outcomes.

Interpretations

- The Comantan family's strengths include their health behaviors, health actions, and beliefs. They reportedly practice health behaviors that help all members without the expense of hurting another family member.
- The Comantan family has coordinated care for Carl within its family and community. They are strong advocates for his health and well-being.
- Many members of the extended family are integral to Carl's health and the health of the entire Comantan family.
- Realize that the data so far do not support any major stressors when Big Frank is gone for 3 days at a time. This may change with Carine's advancing pregnancy and the birth of the child.
- The Comantan family career has multiple concurrent developmental needs, tasks, and transitions. For example, consider the dynamics of the transition of the new baby coming via Carine's pregnancy, Carl's chronic illness, and developmental needs of all the family's children.

Nursing Interventions

- After assessing parents' interest and ability to read written material, bring appropriate written materials to Carl and his family about treatment and management of asthma.
- Review with Carl how to use an inhaler and talk with Carl and his family about recognizing and reducing respiratory triggers.
- Counsel and educate family members on appropriate treatment and management of asthma and review treatment goals and objectives.
- Commend the family on its management of each illness episode and its overall management of family members' health.
- Explore with the family members what they believe will be risky times for Carl's health, such as spring, when plants are blooming and his asthma symptoms increase.
- Support the various roles of family members and subsystems within the family, such as Carl interacting with his uncle and grandfather as adult male role models when his father is away on the road.
- Recognize the principle of honoring cultural diversity and incorporate the roles of Aunt Leena and Uncle Jesse.
- Recognize the role of the grandparents in Carl's cultural upbringing, especially learning about his Inuit culture and history.
- Recognize the strengths in the family, for example, its efforts to keep Carl successful at his grade level in school.
- Work collaboratively with the family in identifying and evaluating sources of help and support they already use.
- Discuss with the Comantan family the advantages and disadvantages of sending Carl to a 2-week residential camp for children with asthma.

Case Study: Comantan Family—cont'd

Evaluation

- Notice how the family has coordinated the help of many people for Carl's care: the nurse, Rebecca; Aunt Leena; and the grandparents.
- Assess how the family is doing with regard to reducing triggers for Carl's asthma as well as helping him when he wheezes.
- Monitor for the presence or absence of wheezing, number and duration of respiratory infections, and number of school days attended.
- Consider the impact on the family if Carl is hospitalized for a severe attack, infection, or both.
- Consider the projected impact of Carl's illnesses on the new baby (for example, the risks of Carl's infections on a newborn infant).
- Consider types and potential impact of health-illness transitions for the Comantan family.
- Consider additional developmental challenges that the family may face in the future, such as the increased mobility of little Frankie and the increased activity needs of Sam.
- Ask if there are any additional foci for the family that have not been addressed.
- Consider asking the family about their plans for financial resources during Carine's maternity leave.
- Ask what additional family strengths could be engaged to assist the Comantan family m in the future.

  Questions for reflections on the nursing care of the Comantan family:

1. The Comantan family is one of many families that has insurance, but it includes limited coverage. How does this affect the health of the children in this family?
2. How does the Comantan family use family and community relationships to enhance the children's well-being?
3. What risk factors do the Comantan children have that may affect their future health?
4. What barriers does the Comantan family face in obtaining health care for the children?
5. Using the Family Systems Theory, assess how has the Comantan family opened their boundaries to improve the health of their children.

SUMMARY

In this chapter, family child health nursing care covered the following:

- Family child health nurses focus on the relationships between family life and children's health and illness, and they assist families and family members to achieve and maintain well-being.
- Through FCC, family child health nurses enhance family life and the development of family members to their fullest potential.
- The family child health concepts incorporate relevant components of family life and interaction, family careers, family development and transitions, family tasks, family communication, family routines, and family health and illness, and help nurses take a comprehensive and collaborative approach to families.

- The family child health concepts enable nurses to screen for potentially harmful situations (e.g., risk for unintentional and intentional injury and death); instruct families about health issues and healthy lifestyles; and help families to cope with acute illness, chronic illness, and life-threatening conditions.
- The family child nurse addresses the needs of individuals within the family and the family as a whole to reach developmental and health potential. For example, siblings of children with special needs can fare well if given the guidance and support they need to develop understanding and empathy, and if they are included in the care of their sibling.

chapter 16

Family Nursing in Acute-Care Adult Settings

Julie S. Fitzwater, PhD, RN, CNRN, CNE

Paul S. Smith, PhD, RN, CNE

Jordan Ferris, MSN, RN

Critical Concepts

- Family nursing is the provision of care to the entire family unit and is an integral aspect of care provided by nurses in adult acute-care settings.

- Families who are viewed as part of the health care team are empowered to deal with the stressors of a family member's hospitalization and are prepared to provide support, aid in recovery, or facilitate a comfortable death.

- Supportive actions by family members, as well as conflict and criticism, have an effect on patients' health behaviors, emotional well-being, immune function, and illness exacerbations.

- During the acute illness phase, nursing interventions should focus on patients and their families by providing physical care and emotional support, facilitating family communication, providing timely information, and establishing a collaborative, trusting partnership.

- Unit and hospital policies should include patient-identified family members. Restricted, nonflexible visitation policies add stress and trauma for both the patient and the patient's loved ones.

- Transferring loved ones from critical-care units (CCUs) to the medical-surgical units is stressful for families because it creates a sense of conflict. On one hand, families are glad their loved ones are better, but they also worry that their family members may not be ready to be moved out of such intensive nurse watchfulness.

- The family member who advocates for a loved one in the hospital assumes a difficult, time-consuming, and fatiguing role: this family member often travels long distances to get to the hospital, takes time off work, may stay all night in the hospital, manages the informational needs of the patient and the family, and works through a complex health care system.

- Effective communication with patients, families, and interdisciplinary health care providers improves client satisfaction, promotes positive response to care, reduces the length of stay in care settings, and results in decreased overall cost and resource utilization.

- Compassionate communication provides crucial care to families while they are asked to make multiple decisions as their loved one dies in the hospital.

The concept of family can be complex and moves beyond the nuclear family to include any loving, supportive persons that the patient identifies as having an important role in her or his life, without regard to social and legal boundaries (Davidson et al., 2017; Institute for Patient-and Family-Centered Care [IPFCC], n.d.; Tracy, 2019). *Family nursing* is the provision of care to the entire family unit and is an integral aspect of care provided by nurses in adult acute-care settings. Hospitalization for an acute or critical illness, acute or critical injury, or exacerbation of a chronic illness is not only stressful for patients and their families but can also have long-term effects. Patients and families often feel alone and unsure of their role in an acute-care setting, and it is important for the health care team to engage families in this environment. The ill adult enters the hospital, usually in a physiological crisis, and the family most often accompanies the ill or injured person to the hospital. During this acute-care admission, family caregivers may focus attention on the critically ill family member and pay little attention to their own health needs. Simultaneously, family members continue to cope with external demands such as occupational and household responsibilities, navigate complex and often difficult financial decisions, and provide care for and maintain the needs of other family members. Nurses and other health care providers should place emphasis on supporting family members during acute hospitalization.

When nurses provide care for and develop personal relationships with the whole family, families are included as part of the health care team, which can improve communication and care planning, prevent errors, and reduce nursing time spent on hygiene activities (Davidson et al., 2017; Heydari et al., 2020). Involving family members in intervention strategies not only strengthens family relationships and enhances the effects of the interventions, it also allows family members to be more than passive bystanders by contributing to both the physiological and psychological well-being of their hospitalized relative (Davidson et al., 2017; Heydari et al., 2020). Close social relationships, especially family relationships, affect physical and psychological well-being, and promote adherence to disease management plans that involve changes in health behavior. When families are involved in the care of the loved one in the hospital, the patient experiences increased ability to cope with and

recover from a critical illness and increased likelihood of positive health outcomes (Tracy, 2019).

Families with members who are acutely or critically ill are seen in adult medical-surgical units, intensive-care units (ICUs) or critical-care units (CCUs), or emergency departments. The acute phase of illness or injury refers to the period immediately after the onset of the illness or the injury. During this time, family members want to be able to ask the following questions about the person who is ill or injured: Is he or she doing as well as can be expected? Is he or she getting any better? Is he or she in any pain? Has there been any change? What can I expect in the future? What can I do to help? These questions may be expressed in thousands of different ways, but they arise from common concern and/or fear for the loved one's well-being. Having loved ones in an acute-care hospital can be an upsetting experience at any time, but when a stay in an adult CCU unit occurs, it can be especially traumatic. Family members and significant others of critically ill patients are integral to the recovery of their loved ones. Patient- and family-centered care is an approach that establishes a partnership between the care team, patients, and family (IPFCC, n.d.). Being involved in providing care brings people together and helps the patient feel comfortable in an unaccustomed setting, such as an acute-care setting.

The purpose of this chapter is to describe family nursing in acute-care settings, including families in CCUs and medical-surgical units. A review of the literature reported the major stressors that families face during hospitalization of an adult family member, including the transfer from one unit to another, being discharged home, participation in cardiopulmonary resuscitation (CPR), withdrawing life support therapy, and organ donation. This chapter concludes with a family case study that (1) highlights the issues families experience and adapt to when an adult member is ill, and (2) applies Family Systems Theory to demonstrate one theoretical approach for working with families.

FAMILIES IN CRITICAL-CARE UNITS

In the United States, more than 5.7 million patients are admitted annually to CCUs for treatment and intensive or invasive monitoring, as well as for the restoration of a stable health status or palliative care (comfort while dying) (Society of Critical Care Medicine, 2017). Approximately 20% of acute-care hospital admissions are to a CCU; of the patients who are seen in the emergency department, approximately 58% are admitted to a CCU (Society of Critical Care Medicine, 2017).

The American College of Critical Care Medicine (ACCM) published multidisciplinary guidelines for family-centered care in the neonatal, pediatric, and adult ICU (Davidson et al., 2017). The guidelines address topics to build an optimal program of family-centered care, including communication, clinician and family training, family presence, involvement and engagement, provision of resources and organizational processes. This section presents evidence-based practice on family nursing in CCUs, specifically addressing family needs when a member is in the ICU; visiting policies, waiting rooms, family interventions in the ICU; and ways to work with families to decrease family relocation stress and transfer anxiety.

Family Needs in the ICU

Family members of patients in the ICU may experience anxiety, depression, post-traumatic stress disorder (PTSD), and complicated grief, referred to as post-intensive-care syndrome–family (PICS-F) (Twibell et al., 2018; Zante et al., 2020). Between 14% and 50% of family members may develop PICS-F, but nursing interventions to prevent it and support family members may help to decrease incidence of the syndrome (Twibell et al., 2018).

The needs of family members with loved ones in the ICU have long been studied. The classic work of Molter (1979) first identified the following 10 family needs in the ICU, listed in descending order:

1. Hope
2. Health care provider caring about the patient
3. Having a waiting room near the patient
4. Being called at home for a change in the patient's condition
5. Knowing about the prognosis
6. Having questions answered honestly
7. Knowing specific facts about prognosis
8. Receiving information about the patient once a day
9. Receiving explanations in understandable terms
10. Seeing the patient frequently

The Critical Care Family Needs Inventory (CCFNI) is a self-report questionnaire, first developed by Molter (1979) and then revised by Leske (1986), that provides a list of 45 need statements developed for family assessment and report of self-perceived needs of families in the ICU. The CCFNI is known to be a valid and reliable instrument to assess family needs and has been used in many studies in a variety of countries (Redley et al., 2019). The CCFNI organized family needs into five dimensions: (1) assurance, (2) information, (3) proximity, (4) comfort, and (5) support (Leske, 1986).

To determine the most valued aspects of care for patients and families during an ICU experience, Auriemma and colleagues (2021) completed a qualitative study. Both patients and their families prioritized communication, patient comfort, and feeling that the team was providing exhaustive care. Families appreciated clear and direct communication, feeling heard and understood, being included in rounds, and being able to ask questions (Auriemma et al., 2021). Families indicated feeling less alone and afraid with good communication, and they had a sense of peace if the patient received all necessary care with an emphasis on pain control and comfort, even if the patient eventually died (Auriemma et al., 2021).

Redley and colleagues (2019) found that family member needs may be different between cultures, making it important to tailor communication and interventions to the family and patient. Communication and participation are key elements in family-centered care (IPFCC, n.d.), and studies with the CCFNI reinforce these elements as important to families globally (Redley et al., 2019).

The Society for Critical Care Medicine included a sample of survivors and family members to make recommendations about the importance of outcomes in a systematic review of the literature to develop guidelines for family-centered care in the ICU (Davidson et al., 2017). The following is a summary of the guidelines:

- Use open and flexible communication, including therapeutic presence, with the family at the bedside.
- Provide family members with options to participate in interdisciplinary rounds and routine family conferences.
- Provide family members with options to participate in care of their loved one.

- Provide peer-to-peer support groups, informational leaflets, and ICU diaries.
- When patients have a poor prognosis, clinicians can use a validated communication approach during family conferences by using the following mnemonic: VALUE = Value family statements, Acknowledge emotions, Listen, Understand the patient as a person, Elicit questions.
- Provide written bereavement brochures for families whose member is dying. See Chapter 11 for a detailed discussion of end-of-life and palliative care.
- Use proactive palliative care consultations.
- Use ethics consultation for any value-related conflicts between clinicians and family members.
- Use family navigators, spiritual support, social workers, and psychologists for specific needs of families.
- Use protocols and trainings for clinicians to implement family-centered care.
- Use private rooms, noise reduction, and support of family sleep strategies.

Families are not only the primary support for loved ones in the ICU, but they do have a positive impact on the ability of patients to cope and recover from a critical illness (Tracy, 2019). The American Association of Critical-Care Nurses' (AACN) *Essentials of Critical Care Nursing* (Tracy, 2019) identified evidence-based practice areas to assess the family's needs and resources in order to develop interventions that optimize the family's impact on the patient and the interactions with the health care team. Areas for family interventions include the following:

- Offer realistic hope.
- Give honest answers and information.
- Give reassurance.
- Use open-ended communication and assess the family's communication style.
- Assess family members' level of anxiety.
- Assess perceptions of the situation (knowledge, comprehension, expectations of staff, expected outcomes).
- Assess family roles and dynamics (cultural and religious practices, values, family spokesperson).
- Assess coping mechanisms and resources (what do family members use for a social network and for support?).

Studies show that an increased number of family visits can have a positive effect on patient outcomes (Akbari et al., 2020). Families experience cognitive, emotional, and social stress when family members are in the ICU, which can include:

- Information ambiguity
- Uncertain prognosis
- Fear of death
- Role changes
- Financial concerns
- Disruption of normal routines

Nursing Roles in Family-Centered Care

ICU nurses are in the best position to support families because they see them often, know the patient intimately, and are called to practice holistically instead of based on a biomedical model. Nurses are an important part of team efforts to implement successful family-centered care strategies, but they may have competing priorities in their daily routines that create barriers to using evidence-based strategies. A survey of ICU nurses about visitation policies resulted in more than half of the nurses opposing the implementation of flexible visitation policies (Akbari et al., 2020). With increased visitation hours, nurses would devote more time to talking to family members, which results in less time to do their routine tasks.

In a qualitative study of ICU nurses, the nurses supported the policy changes for families, but they encountered challenges implementing family-centered care (Coats et al., 2018). Nurses reported feeling stretched to include the needs of families, such as addressing their stress and grief, while also attending to the needs of critically ill patients. The family members sometimes prioritized the small acts of kindness nurses performed over the complex medical care with technology that the nurses were managing. Family reliance on the nurse to interpret communications from other team members and explain the big picture can be challenging because the nurse may need to navigate disagreements about priorities and expected outcomes. Physical changes such as private rooms for ICU patients meet patient-centered care needs, but nurses cannot hear and see patients and alarms in multiple rooms at the same time and must seek other nurses for assistance when patients are isolated in private rooms (Coats et al., 2018).

Another qualitative study reported nurses' lived experiences that highlighted differences in the ideal of family-centered care in ICUs compared to actual implementation (Mirlashari et al., 2019). Nurses discussed challenges with family members and their expectations of nurses and interrupting routine work, plus the multiple roles of educating family and monitoring care given to patients by family. Additional themes included the positive effects on the patient of family presence and moments when family members were learning and successful in assisting with care.

In order for family-centered care in the ICU to be implemented effectively, nurses' input and support are important. Nurses' work, in concert with organizational and interdisciplinary support of family-centered care, is necessary to overcome barriers to implemented strategies (Coats et al., 2018; Mirlashari et al., 2019).

One hospital used simulation scenarios to assist nurses and staff members to become comfortable and confident in supporting families in an open visitation policy (Winkelman et al., 2020). The scenarios included actors portraying family members who demonstrated a variety of challenging behaviors and reactions to patient emergencies and cardiac resuscitation. Practice in simulations with answering family member questions and learning to perform nursing care with visitors in patient rooms at any time was successful in supporting an important element of family-centered care in one hospital (Winkelman et al., 2020).

Visiting Policy

While 78% of ICU nurses in adult critical-care units prefer unrestricted visitation policies, most ICUs (70%) have visitation policies that restrict visitors (AACN Practice Alerts, 2016). Yet the evidence is clear that unrestricted visitation decreases patient anxiety, confusion, and agitation; reduces cardiovascular complications; decreases ICU lengths of stay; makes patients feel more secure; increases patient satisfaction; and enhances quality and safety (AACN Practice Alerts, 2016). Evidence also suggests that unrestricted visitation increases family satisfaction, decreases family members' anxiety, promotes better communication, contributes to better understanding of the patient, allows more opportunities for patient and family teaching because the family becomes more involved in

care, and is not associated with longer family visits (AACN Practice Alerts, 2016). AACN suggests that sometimes family visits should be restricted, for example, for documented legal reasons, when a visitor has a communicable disease, or if the behavior of a visitor is a direct risk to the patient. AACN also recommends that children supervised by an adult family member should be welcome in the ICU and should not be restricted by age alone. Open visitation, as recommended by AACN, is defined as visitor access 24 hours a day, 7 days a week, with no limits on visiting hours or the number, type, or age of visitors.

Evidence in the literature shows that increasing the hours for family visitation leads to physiological improvements in patients' conditions, improved family and patient satisfaction, and decreased anxiety and depression in family members (Akbari et al., 2020; Ning & Cope, 2020). A literature review of open visitation in adult ICUs indicated that the benefits to patients and families are evident, but challenges include negative staff member attitudes and a lack of consistent implementation (Ning & Cope, 2020). A follow-up study of implementation of open visitation in ICUs across the United States found that only 18.5% followed the AACN recommendations (Milner et al., 2020). The limitations to open visitation policies included not allowing children to visit family in ICUs, allowing only two family members to visit at a time, and limiting visitation during shift changes (Milner et al., 2020).

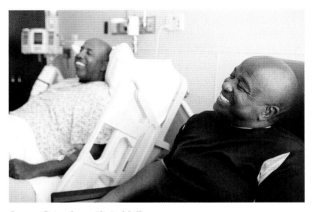

Source: © *istock.com/digitalskillet*

Professional nursing organizations, such as AACN (mentioned earlier) and the American Nurses Association (ANA), have supported the position that, despite patients' being in critical condition, care will be enhanced by the presence of their families. The Joint Commission on Accreditation of Healthcare Organizations recognizes the importance of visitation. In 2011, the commission added an element to the Patient Rights Standard, which states that hospitals should permit family members and friends to be present during hospitalization in order to provide emotional support to the patient (Joint Commission on Accreditation of Healthcare Organizations, 2010).

Waiting Rooms and Family Spaces

When families of critically ill patients are not at the bedside with their loved ones, they are likely spending time in the hospital's waiting areas. Environmental considerations for families visiting and staying in the hospital include noise reduction, private spaces, areas for sleeping, access to Wi-Fi, accessible bathrooms, healthy food and drinks, and natural areas to reduce stress. Improving the family experience can increase satisfaction with care and reduce psychological and physical stress responses. Recommendations from IPFCC (2017) include asking questions, based on the following list, about the environment and design of hospitals. The design of the hospital should do the following:

- Create positive and welcoming impressions throughout for patients and families.
- Display messages that communicate to patients and families that they are essential members of the health care team.
- Reflect the diversity of patients and families served and address their unique needs.
- Provide for the privacy and comfort of patients and families.
- Support the presence and participation of families.
- Support the collaboration of physicians and staff members across disciplines.

The American College of Critical Care Medicine (2017) recommendations for reducing stress and anxiety for family members include providing a sleep surface to prevent the effects of sleep deprivation and providing private rooms with natural lighting and noise control. Hospitals can evaluate the environment provided for families and work on improvements.

A study of hospital environments for visitors found that an available garden space close to an ICU can decrease stress somewhat more effectively than indoor relaxation spaces (Ulrich et al., 2020). Although the indoor waiting rooms in the study provided movable seating, Wi-Fi access, free coffee and tea, water service, adjustable lighting, noise-control elements, and live plants, the outdoor garden space was more therapeutic in reducing visitor survey responses indicating sadness (Ulrich et al., 2020). Natural garden spaces incorporated into hospital design may result in stress reduction and encourage healing (Ulrich et al., 2020).

Nurses can reduce some of the strain that family members experience by providing and seeking information for the family members, asking how they are doing, providing a quiet place for them to rest or sleep, and determining each day how much they wish to be involved in the patient's care. Family interventions are frequently advocated for and sustained by nurses.

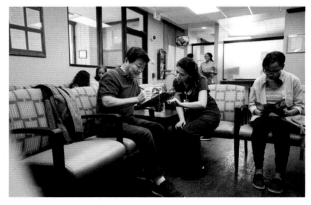

Source: © istock.com/SDI Productions

Family Interventions

Family members may find the fast-paced and noisy environment of the ICU overwhelming. ICU nurses who practice from a family perspective realize how their everyday world in this fast-paced, emotionally charged setting is stressful for families. After the patient is initially stabilized on admission to the ICU, nurses should spend time explaining the equipment and the immediate goals of nursing care, and role-modeling how family members can support their loved one, including how to touch the person. Nurses should address fear of all the equipment used in this setting. This approach is helpful to decrease family stress and builds on the knowledge that family members have a strong desire to be by their loved one's side, particularly when there is a change in the patient's condition. They want to be an integral part of the patient's care.

The categories identified as prerequisites to family participation in care of loved ones in the ICU are (1) staff and family members' preferences and attitudes, (2) preparation and education, (3) establishing positive communication, (4) family contextual characteristics, and (5) hospital policy (Heydari et al., 2020). A scoping review of family participation in the care of older adult patients in the ICU reported that family members' involvement has the potential to improve the physical, emotional, and psychological outcomes of patients and families (Heydari et al., 2020). Guidelines based on systematic review of the literature also recommend that family members be supported in learning to assist in the care of neonates in ICUs as a way to improve parental psychological health and confidence in the caregiving role (Davidson et al., 2017).

Family members can be encouraged to assist with personal hygiene activities such as cleaning face and hands, brushing hair, shaving, and other grooming activities. Families can assist with cognitive activities such as orienting to date, time, and place; providing family pictures; and telling stories, as well as providing in-bed exercises. These bedside activities can help families feel included in their loved one's recovery, improve satisfaction with care, and build rapport with the care team (Davidson et al., 2017; Yoo & Shim, 2020).

In a survey of ICU nurses concerning family engagement in personal-care activities, nurses agreed this involvement could help with symptom assessment and improve patient safety, decision making, and overall quality of care (Hetland et al., 2017). Nurses indicated that family involvement decreased levels of stress, anxiety, and fear, but they also indicated being less likely to involve family in patient high-acuity activities or intimate care (Hetland et al., 2017).

Supporting the family is another important nursing intervention. Because nurses provide 24-hour care, they are in the best position to identify and support families. Although the nurses' priority is the patient, families also need support. Emotional stress arises when a family member is acutely ill and families suffer with the patient during illness and treatment. They attempt to control these emotions in order to be supportive to the patient and other members of the family. It is important that the nurse support the family members by connecting with them. Nurses should spend time, provide information (good and bad), be honest, share themselves, involve families in care, and acknowledge the emotional stress that family members are undergoing.

Including family members in multidisciplinary daily rounds can increase family satisfaction with communication (Simon et al., 2021). Careful and consistent information can help mitigate fears. A positive outcome of family members participating in rounds was providing information about patient history and discharge challenges that the care team did not know about previously (Kydonaki et al., 2021; Simon et al., 2021).

An integrative review of family rounds in adult ICUs in the United States and Canada suggests that scheduled communication with family can help with decision making and care of their family member (Kydonaki et al., 2021). Patients and families gain a better understanding of the plan of care when they have the opportunity to verify information, ask questions, and share concerns. When away from the bedside and the stimulation of the ICU environment, family members are able to hear more clearly and accurately the explanations and answers to their questions and concerns. Therefore, nurses should plan to spend time (e.g., a short 10-minute conference) with families away from the patient's bedside on every shift. Plans for language interpreters should be made in advance. Periodic planned family conferences with the care team is another way to support understanding and shared decision making.

Shared decision making is a collaborative process in which patients and providers make health care decisions together, weighing the medical evidence of various options and considering the patient's values. Shared decision making is crucial in the ICU because patients often cannot speak for themselves, and many of the treatment options are highly invasive and may have a high mortality or morbidity component. Refer to Chapter 5 for detailed information on family shared decision making. A systematic review of the literature to determine the effectiveness of interventions to increase the use of shared decision making in health care with patients indicated low evidence and the need for more research (Legare et al., 2018). Interventions highlighted in the reviewed studies include training programs for health care professionals to learn to implement shared decision making and providing brochures to educate patients and families about choices and how to communicate preferences and values (Legare et al., 2018). Family education and varied methods of communication are recommended as vital areas of family support (Davidson et al., 2017).

Encouraging families to keep a family progress journal, ICU diary, or a computer family blog for extended family and friends can reduce anxiety and depression (Davidson et al., 2017). Another recommendation to meet family needs and assist with a diary or journal development is a specific nursing position, such as a clinical nurse specialist, to work with families in the ICU. This approach allows the ICU nurses to focus on providing care to the ill person and relieves some stress of providing care to the family client. Having this clinical nurse specialist in the ICU resulted in increased family satisfaction (Davidson et al., 2017). The feasibility of a dedicated nursing position to work with families is one that shows promise and one that could have a direct impact on family resilience and satisfaction.

Family Relocation Stress and Transfer Anxiety

As a patient's condition becomes stable, transfer out of the ICU to another hospital unit can lead to family relocation stress and transfer anxiety. Excellent communication and planning can help with these stressors.

Moving ill family members from the ICU to the medical-surgical unit is stressful for families. Even though families report relief that their loved ones are able to transfer out of the ICU, they can also experience worries about decreased nursing presence (Op 't Hoog et al., 2020). Providing pretransfer information and involving families in the transfer process can relieve anxiety. Families in a qualitative study report their experiences as wanting to communicate their involvement in their loved one's care and in decision making (Op 't Hoog et al., 2020).

Chaboyer et al. (2005) classified families' emotions related to relocation stress into four categories of emotions or feelings: abandonment, vulnerability, unimportance, and ambivalence. Families felt *abandonment* when the transfer was abrupt and not planned. Families described experiencing *vulnerability* when they had to accept their new responsibility as a different kind of family caregiver within the hospital setting. For example, rather than being supportive family members working from the background, they now had to provide more actual physical care for their loved one as her or his physical status improved. Their sense of vulnerability was found to be the most intense of these family emotions. The families reported having a feeling of *unimportance* because of the different staffing ratio on the medical-surgical unit. The last feeling identified was *ambivalence*. The families expressed being caught between the extremes of feeling relieved and happy their loved ones were better and feeling fear and doubt that their loved ones were well enough to leave the ICU.

Family conferences scheduled with the health care team are a perfect opportunity for family members to express concerns about transfer out of the ICU and for team members to respond to all concerns with factual, straightforward information. Ideally, both the nurse manager and supervisor of the sending and receiving hospital units should participate in this transition. Using effective communication techniques, a daily care plan with family input, and tours of the new unit are methods to support the family and patient before the transfer.

FAMILIES IN MEDICAL-SURGICAL UNITS

Families who have adult members in acute medical-surgical units are stressed by hospitalization, yet this is one of the least studied areas of family nursing. In this section, family visitation, family communication needs, and family needs are explored. Family interventions relative to discharge are discussed.

Families in acute-care settings reported numerous stressors and changes in their family environment, and they are often desperately in need of support. Nurses can provide support through building relationships and establishing rapport. Some of the ways that nurses can build relationships and rapport include the following:

- Use effective communication. Listen to the family's concerns, feelings, and questions; answer all questions or assist the family in finding the answers.

- Respect and support family coping mechanisms and caregiving behaviors.
- Recognize the uniqueness of each family.
- Assist the family in decision making by providing information about options.
- Permit the family to make decisions about patient care when appropriate.
- Provide adequate time to visit privately, when possible.
- Facilitate family conferences to allow open sharing of family feelings.
- Clarify information and sharing resources regarding support groups.
- Foster positive nurse-family relationships through all phases of care.

Family Visitation and Caregiving in the Hospital

Visitation helps to promote family cohesion, resilience, and unity (Hurst et al., 2019; Wong et al., 2019). Many of the same issues about family visitation in the ICU described previously in this chapter hold true for family visitation on a medical-surgical inpatient setting.

Many families enact a bedside vigil to stay close and protect their loved one while hospitalized. Families displayed both *directive* behaviors and *supportive* behaviors as family caregivers in the hospital, especially when the hospitalized family member was older (Jacelon, 2006). Family *directive* behaviors were described as follows:

- Acting in place of the ill family member by making decisions about care without consulting the ill family member, talking to health care providers, and being the organizer of care.
- Acting as an adviser to the ill family member by working collaboratively with the family member on decisions.
- Not acting in some cases; some family members were found to be available but did not become involved in any decision making.

Family *supportive* behaviors identified by Jacelon (2006) were as follows:

- Keeping the older family members going and active: families brought items from home, visited daily, and sometimes brought the family pet in for a visit.

- Keeping the older family member's life going: they did many things behind the scenes, such as running errands, paying bills, keeping up homes, and keeping friends informed.
- Staying in the background: some family members were available but not actively involved in daily caregiving.

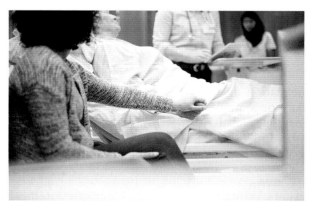

Source: © istock.com/sturti

More specifically, families helped their loved ones in the hospital in many ways that improved patient outcomes, decreased recovery time, increased reports of comfort, and decreased the length of the hospital stay (Glose, 2020; Agency for Healthcare Research and Quality [AHRQ], 2017).

In contrast, health care providers on medical-surgical units did not always see families as partners in patient care (Mackie et al., 2019). Therefore, families reported feeling unwelcome. Families have stated that gaining access to see their loved ones was a privilege, which was extended to them by the nurses, and that they were careful not to abuse the visiting rules. While in the patient's room, they were fearful of annoying the nurses by their constant presence (Alshahrani et al., 2018). Families saw themselves as guests of the patient, not partners in the care of the patient.

The work environment can be an obstacle to allowing medical-surgical nurses to provide family-centered care. The floor nurses often carry a heavy nurse-patient caseload. Many of these patients are of high acuity, which challenges these nurses with the same role conflict mentioned earlier: balancing the technical needs of their patients and practicing holistic family-centered care. These work challenges set the stage for nurses to convey their stress inadvertently to families and patients in unintended ways. Nurses may convey messages in casual conversation about how busy they are, move quickly and be in a hurry when they enter and exit the room, and not address the family when they enter the room but instead focus on procedures (Afriyie, 2020). Nurses can strive to ensure that nonverbal and inadvertent communications match their concern and caring for the client so that a disconnection is not perceived by patients or family members. Taking a few moments to center oneself before entering the client's room allows the nurse to slow down and focus on the client and family in the room and not on what has to be done in the busy day.

Communication with the family is crucial for the nurses, the patients, and the families in order to improve the patients' health outcomes. AHRQ (2017) reports that communication breakdowns among caregivers and between caregivers and patients account for more than 70% of adverse events. Whiteboards in patient rooms are routinely used in hospital settings to improve communication. These boards, typically placed on a wall near a patient's hospital bed, allow any number of providers to communicate a wide range of information such as the date; the names of the nurse, aide, and doctors on that shift; notes from loved ones to the ill person; phone numbers of the family to call in case of condition changes; patient-identified outcome goals for that specific day; questions for providers; and expected date of discharge (Goyal et al., 2019). Including families in patient rounds with physicians and in bedside handoffs with nurses helps to keep communication clear between providers and family members. In addition, limiting the number of interruptions to the nurse while working with the patient and family can improve communication and send messages of importance to the family and patient (McCloskey et al., 2019). Proactively providing information to patients' families can reduce the number of interruptions for nurses.

Family Communication Needs

Effective communication between and with patients, families, and interdisciplinary health care providers improves client satisfaction, promotes positive response to care, reduces length of stay in care settings, and results in decreased overall cost

and resource utilization (Goldfarb et al., 2017). Assessment of patient needs is integral to nursing and providing optimal care at the bedside. It is essential to complete a thorough psychosocial, emotional, and communication needs evaluation to interact with patients and their families effectively while paying close attention to feelings around the uncertainty of hospitalization, anxieties, and fears. Additional attention should be focused on how the patient and family want to be involved in care and how they prefer to have communication provided to them.

Conveying information to families is essential when caring for both acute and chronically ill patients. Nurses frequently underestimate the needs of families, particularly the need for information and the need of family members to be close to the patient (Greenway et al., 2019). Nurses identified additional barriers to family communication that included feeling like they were already communicating information effectively to patients and family; a lack of knowledge on how to incorporate new communication approaches into care; and that the nursing profession, while changing, has traditionally emphasized technical skills over communication skills (AHRQ, 2017). Patients share the disappointment with nurses when communication is lacking (Kirca & Bademli, 2019). Nurse-patient relationships are built on a foundation of communication that is bidirectional. Nurses need to talk with patients and families as much as they need to listen to patients and families. Nurses need to be provided with enough time to have meaningful conversations with patients in their care.

Nurses must advocate more readily for sharing information with families. One way for nurses to advocate is to be present in the patient's room and participate in physician-family conferences and interdisciplinary rounds. Nurses are in a position to help families understand what the physician means, and they serve as a sounding board for the family. In facilitating patient-family interactions and patient-family communication, nurses can increase family support of hospitalized patients. Offering systematic, integrated, relevant information provides guidance to family members. Relevant information includes the daily plan and schedule, overview of the patient's situation, comfort of the patient, how the family can participate in care, and descriptions of the patient (Rodriguez-Huerta et al., 2019). Clear, concise, timely information has been found to reduce family anxiety and have a calming effect (AHRQ, 2017; Goldfarb et al., 2017; Rodriguez-Huerta et al., 2019).

Communication from a variety of providers is best when health care providers are sensitive, unhurried, and honest, and use plain, nonmedical language. Assessment of a patient's and families' health literacy is an important component of communication. Access to information that was shared verbally at patient-care conferences has also been found to be effective in promoting family coping and understanding (Benham-Hutchins et al., 2017; Fritz et al., 2019).

Family-nurse communication is crucial during the hospital stay. Families are key members of the health care team and will be the primary providers of care once the patient leaves the acute-care setting. Thus, addressing the family's educational and information needs is a critical part of the discharge process.

Family Needs During Discharge

Families and patients are excited about leaving the hospital. For some, however, it is a time when anxieties and uncertainties are high; families worry about their loved one not receiving the round-the-clock care available in the hospital. Adverse and poor outcomes are associated with poor transitions, specifically with problems in continuity of care and caregiver burden (Benham-Hutchins et al., 2017; Gadbois et al., 2018). From 2010 to 2016, the 30-day readmission rates to hospitals in the United States for all payers decreased slightly, from 14.2% to 13.9%, with Medicare readmissions falling the most, from 18.3% to 17.1%. Medicaid readmissions remained steady at 13.7%, and individuals who were uninsured had an increase in readmissions, from 10.4% to 11.8% (Agency for Healthcare Research and Quality, 2019). It is likely that many of these readmissions could have been avoided. Clearly, involving family in discharge planning is crucial for a smooth transition of care.

Families worry about adding the home caregiver role to their already overburdened load of family responsibilities. In fact, many families of discharged patients reported forgetting what they were taught about what to expect and what resources were available to them, and experienced confusion in the home setting (Sheikh et al., 2018;

Schenhals et al., 2019). Families often participate in extensive discharge planning and teaching, yet their severe anxiety inhibits their learning. Families of individuals with ongoing illness needs told of not being able to hear the conversations during the care conferences because they were so worried about how they were going to manage at home. Other families shared that they were so overwhelmed with the complexity of the situation and the health care system that they could not pay attention in the conferences (Smith et al., 2018).

In order to make discharge more streamlined and readmission less likely, nurses can begin facilitating discharge earlier in the care process—much earlier than the typical "day of" discharge teaching. Using care conferences can help families transition smoothly to providing care in the home environment. Families are providing nursing care at home that is traditionally done by nurses in the hospital, such as assisting with ambulation, transfer, wound care, and medication administration, and, in some cases, operating high-tech equipment. When families are involved in discharge planning, there is increased patient adherence to treatment recommendations (Smith et al., 2018).

The importance of providing a comprehensive discharge plan cannot be overemphasized. Discharge planning should begin when the person is admitted to the acute-care setting by anticipating and identifying the patient's continuing needs. A comprehensive plan should include, at a minimum, the following: what to do when the person gets home, how to do it, and what to look for and do when a problem develops. In addition, the plan should include instructions about who will follow the care of the client in the outpatient setting and a follow-up appointment, if possible. The plan should also contain referrals to other care providers in advance of discharge. Review client management plans with the family daily and update progress toward discharge with the family. Discuss possible resources that the family will need to address in the home once the family members arrive there. If there is concern about the safety or complexity of the discharge, additional disciplines, such as case management and social work, should be involved for additional needs assessments.

As the coordinators of care, nurses can facilitate the planning of care before the patient is discharged. Establishing guidelines so that every patient has a medical appointment before discharge is essential. Nurses can make sure that patients have the correct discharge medications and receive a sufficient amount to last them for a few days; many facilities are now involving the pharmacist in discharges to ensure understanding of medication regimens. Comparing discharge medications to those medications that the patients normally take at home should be part of discharge planning. It is not unusual for a patient's medication list at discharge to be different from the medication list before admission. Unfortunately, these changes often are not conveyed to the patient's primary doctors, resulting in confusion over medication and possible readmission.

Recently, hospitals have been using transition coaches who help reduce hospital readmission by targeting population groups that have a higher hospital readmission rate. These programs vary, but the central tenet is to begin discharge planning while the patient is hospitalized and continue with intensive postdischarge care. Often, nurses assume the role of the transition coach. Research has demonstrated that a multicomponent intervention program—which includes early assessment of the patient's discharge needs, enhanced patient education and counseling, and early postdischarge follow-up care—is associated with reduced readmissions (Coffey et al., 2019).

Family Interventions at Discharge

Discharge planning for patients and families is crucial for success after a patient leaves the hospital. The time of transition between hospital and home is one of the more vulnerable times in a patient's life (Facchinetti et al., 2019). It is imperative that nurses work with patients and families not only to address the medical discharge regimen but also to include education or resources for how to manage the new or existing needs, such as dressing, cooking, toileting, transportation, eating, or mobility. Follow-up after discharge has been shown to decrease readmission rates and posthospitalization complications (Oh et al., 2019).

Patient discharge is an area that has been studied for decades. The current focus in the United States on reducing health care costs and client morbidity and mortality rates by reducing hospital readmission rates has placed patient discharge in the spotlight. Health care systems are creating transition care programs and seeing success. One intervention that is part of these programs includes family care transition conferences, which entail discussion on the physical care of the patient, ways to assist the family to adjust to having an ill or recuperating family member at home, and barriers to providing care at home. Concepts to include in this discharge family conference are listed in Box 16-1. Other interventions include interprofessional follow-up teams, nurse navigators, and less formalized telephone and e-mail tracking. Oh et al. (2019) used a combination of individual discharge planning by case managers and home visits by home-care nurses, followed by telephone calls during the month following discharge. Their research resulted in a significant decrease in caregiver burden and improvement in the quality of life both physically and mentally for their patients.

In a concerted effort to reduce hospital readmission rates, hospitals are delivering discharge education that begins before discharge and includes a follow-up with an interprofessional team after discharge. While the patient is still in the hospital, the team discusses the case, and different

---

BOX 16-1

Addressing Family Needs During the Final Discharge Conference

It is important to talk about the physical care of the family member who is being discharged home and to work with the family on its specific needs. The following points are examples of items to cover with family during a the final discharge conference:

- Discuss when the family member can be left alone and for how long.
- Help the family set up an emergency call system.
- Discuss concerns about modifying the home environment.
- Facilitate setting up a family routine of care.
- Be sure the family knows when to call for help.
- Help the family learn to handle visitors, especially children.
- Talk about the balance of sleep and rest for the family caregivers.
- Provide names and numbers for personnel in the billing department for the family members to call when they start to receive insurance forms and hospital bills.

members work to ensure that, by discharge, clients and family members understand the medications, have follow-up appointments, and order any post-acute-care services. The team makes follow-up phone calls to discuss care and any concerns for up to 30 days after discharge. Outcomes of these types of programs are positive and a step in helping families care for loved ones in the home.

Nurse who conduct a follow-up care phone call should address the following information while thoroughly documenting the call:

- The client's health status since discharge and any changes that may have occurred
- Whether or not the client is taking medications correctly or following the recommendations for care correctly
- The need for, or the status of, follow-up visits
- What to do when or if a problem arises

Another intervention to help adults and families in the acute-care setting is the use of a position termed *nurse navigator*. Nurse navigators are educated in a specific area of nursing and in the hospital system, such as working with clients who have heart failure or working with clients who have cancer. They meet with patients and families; conduct client and family education; advocate on their behalf by helping ensure clear communication between the client/family and their health care team; conduct medication reconciliation; and help clients and families transition from one setting to another, such as arranging for home visits with community health nurses (Fowler et al., 2019). Nurse navigators often work as the point of primary contact for patients and families, reducing the fractured nature of medicine and medical communication.

Regardless of the interventions used, all patients should have routine follow-up from nurses after discharge. Nurses are uniquely educated to assess and intervene when questions or complications arise after discharge. The involvement of nurses during and after discharge reduces readmissions, increases patient and family confidence and satisfaction, and reduces burdens placed on health care systems. Follow-up phone calls or e-mails to clients after discharge should include knowledge about the illness, new medications, potential complications, behavioral and lifestyle changes, and emotional support.

END-OF-LIFE FAMILY CARE IN THE HOSPITAL

An important transition of care in acute-care settings includes supporting the patient and family at the end of the patient's life. Goals of care in the hospital can transition from providing life-saving or curative measures to providing comfort care at the end of life. For a detailed discussion of how to work with families in palliative and end-of-life care, including those being cared for in home and community-based settings, please refer to Chapter 11. The next section addresses working with patients and families during end-of-life experiences in acute-care settings. The topics include advance care planning, family presence during CPR, family involvement in do not resuscitate (DNR) orders, family involvement in decisions to withhold or withdraw life-sustaining treatments, and organ donation.

When the condition of a loved one becomes terminal or death occurs unexpectedly, nurses may be challenged to support the needs of the family. Strategies to facilitate support of the family include clear communication with explanations about death and dying. When it comes to language, using interpreters effectively to communicate with patients and family is vital so that end-of-life wishes can be understood and questions addressed (Coombs et al., 2017). Nurses can make a difference by advocating for patients and families, facilitating decision making, ensuring optimum pain and symptom control, and communicating consistent information with families that includes information about the patient's impending death.

Nurses work in close proximity to patients and families. Therefore, nurses can initiate discussions about family and patient wishes as transitions caused by advancing illness or disease develop. Advance care planning offers patients and families the opportunity to participate fully in care by identifying goals and preferences before the end of life. Identifying the needs of the patient and the family helps nurses facilitate decision making to support choices made by patients and families, increase the quality of care, and provide comfort during a stressful experience.

Although efforts toward advance care planning have increased in recent years, the majority of individuals do not have their wishes documented in writing. A systematic review of studies in the United States between 2011 and 2016 indicate that about only one in three adults has completed any type of advance directive (Yadav et al., 2017). This review reported that the people more likely to complete an advance directive include those 65 years or older, those in hospice or palliative care, and nursing home residents (Yadav et al., 2017). People may be reluctant to complete a document about end-of-life preferences due to fears of not being able to change their preferences. Some patients felt that completing an advance directive was helpful to organize their thoughts about end-of-life topics.

Advance Directives

The 1990 Patient Self-Determination Act (PSDA) encourages everyone to make their own decisions about the medical care that they would choose if they became unable to make decisions because of illness. PSDA requires all health care providers and organizations to recognize the living will and durable power of attorney for health care (American Cancer Society [ACS], 2016).

The legislation stimulated a host of documents related to end-of-life choices, such as advance directives, living wills, durable power of attorney for health care, DNR orders, and physician orders for life-sustaining treatment (POLST), all of which are described in Box 16-2.

Advance directives can be general or very specific, depending on the wishes of the patient. The directive can involve identifying a certain individual, such as a family member or legal representative, to serve as a decision maker who will carry out the wishes of the patient if the patient is no longer able to participate in her or his own health care decisions. Specific instructions about various life-sustaining therapies (LSTs) that the patient would accept or refuse may be included. Some types of advance directives, such as the living will, specify what to do in certain situations or specify the patient's choices for organ or tissue donation, or what actions the patient wants taken if his or her heart or breathing stops (ACS, 2016). The ANA code of ethics supports nursing care that protects patient autonomy, dignity, and rights, and includes supporting patient choices for family and surrogate decision makers (ANA, 2015).

BOX 16-2
Documents Related to End-of-Life Choices

Advance Directive

An advance directive is a legal document that a competent person completes. It specifies instructions and medical care preferences regarding interventions or medical treatments, such as termination of life support or organ donation, that the individual would like in the event he or she is incompetent to make such decisions. The purpose of an advance directive is to reduce confusion and disagreement. Typically, the advance directive includes the name of the person who holds the durable power of attorney for health care.

Living Will

A living will is a legal document that specifically outlines medical treatments and interventions that the person does or does not want administered when the person is terminally ill or in a coma and is unable to communicate personal desires.

Durable Power of Attorney for Health Care

A durable power of attorney for health care is a legal document that designates an individual to act as a health care proxy or agent to make medical decisions in the event that a person cannot communicate her or his own choices or make her or his own decisions.

Do Not Resuscitate (DNR) Order

A DNR order is a request not to have CPR in the event one's heart stops. This order may or may not be part of an advance directive or living will. A physician can put this order in a client's chart for that person.

Physician Orders for Life-Sustaining Treatment (POLST)

POLST is a form (not a legal document) that states what kind of medical treatment patients want toward the end of life. It is signed by both the patient and the doctor or nurse practitioner. This form documents the end-of-life conversation between the patient and her or his health care provider. POLST gives seriously ill patients more control over their end-of-life care. It is typically written on bright-colored (pink) paper.

The nurse is often involved in conveying the patient's preferences to the family and other health care providers in order to facilitate the development of the advance directive. To elicit specific information about a patient's preferences and choices for his or her care, the nurse could ask the following:

1. Where would you prefer to be toward the end of your life?
2. What kinds of treatment would you want or not want if you become sicker?
3. If your health condition changed, when would you like to discuss shifting from curing an illness to trying to enjoy the end of life as much as possible?

To ensure the patient's wishes are carried out, it is important that the nurse document the patient's wishes and communicate this information with providers and families.

Family Involvement in DNR Orders

The family member or appointed decision maker may be in the position of making the decision for her or his loved one to transition to a DNR order for care. Handy et al. (2008) investigated the experience of surrogate decision makers—durable power of attorney or next of legal kin—who are involved in authorizing DNR orders. These individuals described this experience as a process, as a cascade of decisions and negotiations, not just a single decision not to resuscitate. One of the essential elements of this process was honest, sensitive, ongoing communication with the health care team. The surrogates reported a feeling guilty if they authorized the order and guilty if they did not. In the end, the surrogates reported that knowing they were alleviating their loved one's pain was crucial in their decision making.

A study of 122 women with gynecological cancers uncovered preferences for end-of-life choices. The study indicated that the women would like end-of-life discussions to occur as a routine part of their care, but they would like the discussion to be initiated by their providers (Díaz-Montes et al., 2013). Patients report that they would like these discussions because they want the opportunity to prepare for the end of their lives. The end-of-life preparations included assigning someone to make decisions, arranging financial matters, knowing what to expect as their health status declines, and preparing written preferences for management of their end-of-life care. The most important factors regarding end-of-life care for patients included trust in the treating physician, avoidance of unwanted life support, effective communication from the physician regarding disease status, and the ability to prepare for the end of life (Diaz-Montes et al., 2013). The decision-making process of determining whether to authorize a DNR order in an acute-care setting is similar to the family's decision whether to withdraw or withhold LSTs.

Family Experiences of Withdrawing or Withholding LSTs

Families often become intricately involved in decisions to withdraw or withhold LSTs when no advance directive has been completed or when no previous conversations about end-of-life choices have occurred among members of the family. LSTs include, but are not limited to, advanced cardiac life support, CPR, cardiac support devices, renal support services and renal medications, blood products, artificial nutrition and hydration, cancer treatments, and surgery (Hospice and Palliative Care Nurses Association [HPNA], 2016). Withdrawing and withholding LSTs may also be described as forgoing treatment. Forgoing treatment includes making the decision to do without an LST that would extend the patient's life (HPNA, 2016). Withdrawing and withholding treatment are different from euthanasia or physician-assisted suicide, which are discussed in Chapter 11.

The decision to withdraw or withhold LSTs is central to advance care planning and a significant challenge for families. Nurses have a primary role in facilitating the patient's and family's understanding and decision making with regard to forgoing treatment. An important distinction for nurses to make is that the limitation of life-sustaining treatment does not mean limiting care (HPNA, 2016). It is the responsibility of the health care team to honor the decisions and advance directive in place while supporting the appropriate symptom management and personal comfort care. Family members may be affected by stress and grief during the process of making treatment decisions because of the overall poor prognosis and condition of their loved one and the weight of the responsibility. The emotional distress of patients and family members can be reduced by effective communication to help them understand the disease process, prognosis, and various options for the effective management of symptoms at the end of life (Peden-McAlpine et al., 2015).

Wiegand and colleagues (2008) conducted research to describe the different family management styles when faced with making decisions about withdrawing or withholding LSTs. The five family management styles described are progressing, accommodating, maintaining, struggling, and floundering. Table 16-1 illustrates how families differ in their approach to making this crucial family decision. Families were found to vary in the following areas:

- Their level of understanding of the severity of their loved one's illness
- Their level of hope for recovery
- The tense (past, present, or future) with which they talk about their family member
- Their willingness to engage in a discussion about possibly withdrawing LSTs
- The overall family communication
- The prevalence of facts or emotions in making the decision
- The actual decision to withdraw LSTs

Families should be informed well before death is imminent. The final decision to withdraw life support may take time and discussion. Physicians were found to prolong the withdrawal of life support systems to accommodate the needs of the families, which resulted in families' higher level of satisfaction (Gerstel et al., 2008). But in doing so, physicians felt that patients did not benefit from this prolongation because it caused nonbeneficial and sometimes painful therapies. In fact, the lack of communication between physicians and families caused slower decision making by families. If families are alerted to the possibility of the patient's death earlier in the hospital stay, when the indication for withdrawal is finally made by the physician, the families will be better prepared. Given that most deaths in critical care occur within 4 hours of withdrawal of treatment, this short time period does not allow families to prepare for death. This short time frame puts an

enormous demand on nurses as they attempt to transition care to a need for palliative care for the patient and the bereaved family (Efstathiou & Clifford, 2011; Peden-McAlpine et al., 2015). Working collaboratively with the family and the health care team during this time helps the nurse be most effective in supporting the patient's and the family's needs.

Family conferences can be an effective way to understand the primary needs and concerns of family members so that the nurse can prioritize the issues. In a study that examined 51 family conferences with the health care team in the decision-making process to withdraw LSTs, Hsieh et al. (2006) identified five contradictory arguments that families often talked about during these conferences:

- If the family believed a decision to remove LSTs was actually killing the loved one versus allowing them to die a natural death
- If the family's decision was viewed as a benefit by alleviating suffering or by eliminating a burden on the family
- If the family was honoring their loved one's end-of-life choices or following their own personal wishes
- If the ill family member expressed several differing end-of-life choices, the family had to work through which one to follow
- Determining whether one family member would be responsible for making the final decision or the family as a whole would make the decision

No matter which of these contradictions families discussed during the conference, information-seeking strategies used by the health care team members were found to facilitate these difficult emotional discussions. Some of these information-seeking strategies included acknowledging the contradictions; clarifying the views of each person, including the patient who was not present; bringing the conversation back to the point that all family members wanted to help their loved one; and reaffirming their choices even if the health care team did not agree with them (Hsieh et al., 2006).

Once a family has reached a decision to withdraw LSTs, nurses work closely with family members to guide them through this difficult procedure. A trusting nurse-family relationship is crucial to working with families in this type of situation. The

Table 16-1   Family Management Styles for Family Decision to Withhold LSTs

FAMILY MANAGEMENT STYLE	SEVERITY OF CONDITION UNDERSTOOD	HOPE OF RECOVERY	VERB TENSE USED TO TALK ABOUT FAMILY MEMBER	WILLINGNESS TO ENGAGE IN DISCUSSION OF WITHDRAWAL OF LSTs	FAMILY COMMUNICATION	PRIMARY FACTORS USED IN DECISION MAKING	FAMILY MADE THE DECISION TO SUSTAIN TREATMENTS
Progressing family type	Yes	None or minimal	More past tense used	Willing	Good communication with each other and extended family	Mostly used facts and supported wishes of family member	Planned date and time of withdrawal
Accommodating family type	Yes	None or minimal	More past tense used	Somewhat willing	Fairly good communication	Mostly facts used, mixed with some emotions	Yes, with little to moderate conflict
Maintaining family type	Yes	Very hopeful of recovery	Present and past tenses used	Undecided	Varied communication, good at times and not good at other times	Mixed some facts with emotions	Yes, with moderate to extreme difficulty
Struggling family type	Uncertain if understood	Very hopeful of recovery	Present tense used	Not willing	Most family conflict of all styles	Mostly emotions	Some unable to decide, family not in agreement
Floundering family type	No	Believe full recovery was going to happen	Present and future tense used	Not willing	Little family discussion with each other	Emotions only and not following family member's wishes	Decided when dying was active and made with extreme family conflict

Source: Adapted from Wiegand, D. L., Deatrick, J. A., & Knafl, K. (2008). Family management styles related to withdrawal of life-sustaining therapy from adults who are acutely ill or injured. *Journal of Family Nursing, 14*(1), 16–32.

following nursing actions help prepare the family (Kirchhoff & Faas, 2008):

- Telling the family that the exact time of death cannot be anticipated, but that the nurse will monitor the situation and inform them when death appears more imminent
- Assuring the family the nurse will continue to provide compassionate comfort care
- Giving each family member a choice to watch the actual withdrawal of the therapies
- Providing for the physical and emotional intimacy needs of the family
- Informing the family of the expected signs and symptoms that they may see during the active dying process
- Encouraging or giving permission for the family to hold, touch, caress, lie with, talk to, and show emotion to the dying family member

Nurses need to make every effort to keep families involved and informed as death approaches. Providing the ideal level of privacy is not always possible in acute-care settings; however, every effort should be made to allow for families to be with their loved ones in a private, unhurried, and quiet environment. Many families and cultures have rituals or spiritual beliefs and procedures that ought to be honored. Resources such as spiritual support, social services, and palliative care can be implemented to support the patient and family, especially when death is approaching. Nurse managers need to relieve bedside nurses from responsibilities of caring for other patients so that they can remain with families and patients who are dying.

Informing family members about what is most important to the dying patient requires communication between these two groups, and nurses can be instrumental in facilitating these discussions. For example, families sometimes prefer not to tell the patient she or he is dying because they fear that the patient will lose hope. Yet patients and family members have the opportunity to address personal issues and say goodbye to loved ones before they die. Therefore, it is important to assess the personal wishes of the dying patient and to facilitate open discussion between the patient and family members. Compassionate communication provides crucial care to families as they are asked to make multiple decisions during the dying of their loved ones in the hospital. The more the nurse

knows about the family, the better. The way a family deals with death is affected by cultural background, stage in the family life cycle, values and beliefs, and nature of the illness. Whether the loss is sudden or expected, the role played by the dying person in the family, and the emotional functioning of the family before the illness also influence the family's needs and reactions to the situation.

Offering and providing emotional support to families of dying patients is one way of meeting the needs of the family. Being at the bedside, providing comfort, and offering an ear to listen demonstrate that families are not dealing with the grieving process alone (Cronin et al., 2015). Providing for privacy allows families emotional and physical intimacy. Of utmost concern to family members is to be reassured that the nurse is keeping their loved one comfortable and as pain free as possible, and is continuing to provide comfort nursing care. Keeping the family informed through anticipatory guidance of the physical signs and symptoms they are likely to see is important. Giving family members the option to be present or excused during the actual death is compassionate caring. Ask the family members whether they have any special spiritual or religious rituals and ceremonies that should to be conducted at this time. For many families, spirituality provides immense comfort whereas, for the patient, it is an essential element in creating a peaceful death (Kruse et al., 2007). Most hospitals have various religious services available that can be called in to help the dying patient and their family. After the death, it is important to allow enough time for questions, allow the family the opportunity to view the body, and describe the events at the time of death. Offering families the choice to participate in after-life preparations, such as bathing the body, is providing culturally sensitive care.

Caring for families when a member is dying is not easy. It is challenging for nurses to help families cope. Nurses in acute-care settings may not feel comfortable and confident discussing death with patients or families. One component of hospital end-of-life care that many families express dissatisfaction with the management of care before death. Factors contributing to dissatisfaction include patient suffering, pain, and lack of communication with the family (Thompson et al., 2012). Part of the reason for this dissatisfaction is that health care providers, particularly nurses, may be uncomfortable caring for and communicating with dying patients. Depending on their experience, nurses may be uncomfortable or lack the confidence needed to speak to patients and families about death. They also may not feel prepared to lead or coordinate the necessary tasks. Therefore, nurses may distance themselves from the patients and engage only in practical tasks with which they are most comfortable, thereby missing opportunities to facilitate interactions with the family (Ingebretsen & Sagbakken, 2016). Facilities that provide educational opportunities for nurses will help them develop the knowledge and skills to plan and deliver end-of-life nursing care.

Mixed messages pertaining to end-of-life issues commonly arise in the acute-care setting. Patients and families hear and see numerous health care providers. They receive conflicting and divergent information and opinions; thus, it is challenging for them to understand the care plan, which compromises the quality of end-of-life care (Beckstrand & Kirchhoff, 2005). Because nurses spend the most time with the patient, they are instrumental in gathering the team players together to provide clarity for the patient and the family (Puntillo & McAdam, 2006).

Family Presence During CPR

Sudden life-threatening events in acute-care settings can result in the possibility of administering CPR. For many years it was standard practice in CCUs and emergency departments to remove family members from the bedside during periods of cardiac arrest, as well as emergent and invasive procedures. That trend is gradually changing. An increasing number of CCUs and emergency departments allow family members to choose to remain present at the patient's bedside during CPR based on research findings that demonstrate positive outcomes (Toronto & LaRocco, 2019). As a family-centered approach, family presence during resuscitation should be introduced as a policy with education for providers to understand how to support families and patients.

The Emergency Nurses Association (2012) and AACN Practice Alerts (2016) recommend that family presence during resuscitation (FPDR) should be offered as an option to appropriate family members and should be based on written institution policy. FPDR is recommended for family members to say goodbye if needed and supports the grieving process. FPDR also reduces anxiety for the family members because they are able to see the efforts implemented to save the life of their loved one. This is particularly important to help family members with coping. The evidence supports allowing family members to be present during CPR; therefore, FPDR should be included in educational curricula and emergency personnel trained in its implementation. Training should include cultural sensitivity and public awareness of the practice (Tiscar-Gonzalez et al., 2021).

Offering the Option of Organ Donation

The number of people who need organs far exceeds the number of donors. In the United States, there are more than 109,000 men, women, and children on the national organ transplant waiting list (Organ Donor, 2020). Each day, about 95 people receive an organ transplant and 17 people die because an organ was unavailable (Organ Donor, 2020). In 2019, there were 39,719 transplants from nearly 11,900 deceased donors and nearly 7,400 living donors (United Network for Organ Sharing, 2020).

Discussing organ donation with a family whose loved one has suddenly died or with whom the decision has been made to withdraw LSTs is difficult. The discussion about organ donation should take place separately from the notification of the family member's death, and it should be done by someone who has been specifically trained in asking for organ and tissue donation. Federal regulations require hospitals to contact their local organ procurement organization (OPO) concerning any death or impending death (U.S. Centers for Medicare and Medicaid, 2020). Once contacted, the OPO sends a representative, or a local hospital representative approaches the family at the appropriate time about the option of organ donation and answer questions.

If organ donation is viewed as a consoling act, the option to elect organ donation is easier for the family. Organ donation benefits the donor family as well as the recipients and their families. Families reported that knowing that the organ of their loved one helped someone else, that a positive came out of a negative, and that their family member lives on in someone else helped them cope with their loss.

Many families worry that donation is disfiguring or will delay the funeral, but neither of these worries is valid, and nurses should reassure families on these points. The body is not disfigured in the process of removing organs. If the body parts that are removed have the potential to disfigure the person, replacement plastic or wooden parts are inserted in place of those removed so that the person is not disfigured. The organ donation team has a rapid response; therefore, the funeral arrangements are not delayed.

The donor family does not pay for the medical expenses once death has been declared; the costs are paid by the OPO and the recipients. The donor family receives a letter from the OPO informing members of the number of people who received organs from the deceased family member. Once the donor process is completed, the donor family can contact the OPO to find out whether the recipient of the organs is interested in corresponding and meeting.

Case Study: Howe Family

This case study presents a family dealing with an acute exacerbation of a long-standing chronic illness and hospitalization of one of its members. Family Systems Theory is used as the theoretical approach to the Howe family (refer to Chapter 2 for specific details of this family nursing theory and model). The Howe family genogram and ecomap are presented in Figures 16-1 and 16-2, respectively.

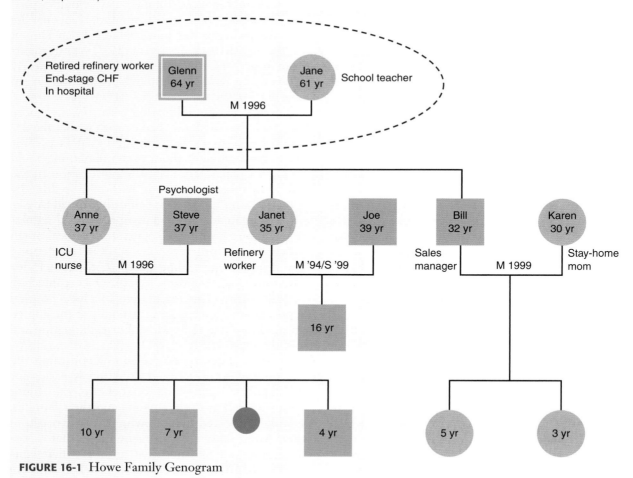

FIGURE 16-1 Howe Family Genogram

Case Study: Howe Family—cont'd

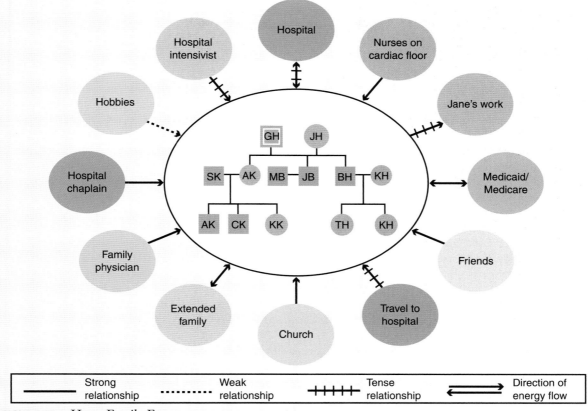

Strong relationship	Weak relationship	Tense relationship	Direction of energy flow

FIGURE 16-2 Howe Family Ecomap

Glenn Howe, a 64-year-old married male, had his first major myocardial infarction at age 41. Since that time, he dutifully embraced numerous lifestyle changes, including smoking cessation, diet modifications, and the establishment of a regular exercise regimen. In addition, he began to take numerous cardiovascular medications to control his blood pressure and enhance his cardiac function. Despite his adherence to his chronic disease management program, Glenn's cardiovascular disease worsened, and he underwent coronary artery bypass surgery 10 years ago. Initial results of the surgery were positive, and Glenn continued to manage his chronic illness well. Recently, however, he experienced another small myocardial infarction, after which his cardiac function declined drastically. Therefore, physicians increased his medications, recommended more severe lifestyle modifications, and dashed his hopes for recovery.

Glenn's immediate family consists of his wife, Jane, three children—Anne, age 37; Janet, age 35; and Bill, age 32—and six young grandchildren. Glenn is currently retired, whereas Jane continues to work as a special education teacher. All family members are upper middle class and attend an Episcopal church regularly. All family members are geographically and emotionally close to Glenn and are quite concerned that he may not survive much longer. Since his first myocardial infarction, the family members lived their lives in a state of anxiety, feeling as if their time with Glenn was likely to be limited, as if they were on borrowed time. This anxiety has resulted in several benefits for the family: numerous family vacations, all holidays together, and the perspective that every chance to be together is special. After Glenn's most recent decline in cardiac function, the family experienced a heightened sense of preciousness, wanting to spend as much time as possible together and wanting every moment with Glenn to be perfect.

(continued)

Case Study: Howe Family—cont'd

Before his first myocardial infarction, Glenn was a healthy, robust, active man with many interests and hobbies. After his cardiac surgery, many of his hobbies, including golf, fell by the wayside. He became increasingly short of breath with exertion and resorted to armchair hobbies, such as coin collecting, crossword puzzles, and world history. Family activities changed as well. Family vacations necessarily became sedate and wheelchair-oriented rather than activity-oriented hiking, fishing, and camping trips. The family endeavored to have at least one very special trip every year, however, the last two being a trip to Disney World with Glenn in a wheelchair and a cruise that required very little exertion.

Glenn became more and more debilitated. His cardiac function was so poor he could not eat without becoming short of breath and tachycardic. His appetite decreased dramatically, and he lost more than 60 pounds. He began to suffer from orthopnea and often tried to sleep upright in his recliner all night. As he and Jane tried to cope with his acute and chronic health care needs, their relationship changed. She became a full-time caretaker, trying anything she could to get him to eat and to make him comfortable. A normally unflappable individual, she found herself expressing her frustration at his refusal to eat more than a few bites at a time. Her outbursts were distressing to her and her children because they were so out of character. Glenn, usually a more demanding individual, became compliant and resigned as his health deteriorated. The children became hypervigilant and attentive to their parents, making frequent visits on weekends and calling every day. Family roles changed as the stressors affecting the family intensified.

Glenn had been hospitalized on numerous occasions, and he approached the impending admission to a medical-surgical unit with his usual calm and trust in his caregivers. He was being admitted for tests because his ventricular function had decreased, his weight had decreased from 200 to 140 pounds, and his urine output was declining. He called his oldest daughter, Anne, a cardiovascular intensive-care nurse, the morning of his scheduled admission and asked her to meet him at the hospital. She replied that she had to travel out of town for an important meeting but would drive up later that night and be with him for the tests the next day. The other children counted on the oldest child to take care of health care needs, and because of her education and experience, it was a role she gladly assumed.

Given the chronic nature of Glenn's cardiovascular disease and the life-threatening potential for acute exacerbations requiring frequent hospitalizations, Jane and Glenn had discussed advance directives openly and honestly. Jane was well aware that Glenn did not wish for any heroic measures, especially CPR. He felt that his two cardiac surgeries were trauma enough and that his heart condition was irreparable. Jane was terrified of losing her husband, best friend, and companion, and was very concerned about having to make the decision that would honor Glenn's wishes.

During this hospital stay, Glenn and Jane renewed their close and trusting relationship with the nurses at their small community hospital. While awaiting his tests and the arrival of their daughters, Glenn experienced a lapse in consciousness with Jane at his bedside. Jane called for help, and two nurses entered the room and quickly assessed the situation. Glenn was in full cardiac arrest. One of the nurses turned to Jane and asked, "Do you want us to bring him back? We can bring him back." Jane hesitated, then shook her head no. The nurse asked again, "Are you sure? Do you want us to bring him back?" Once again, Jane answered no. She immediately realized the consequences of her decision to deny CPR. Glenn, her husband of 45 years, was gone; her children did not expect this hospitalization to result in his death, and she was alone at his bedside.

Jane experienced regret for her decision not to "bring him back." Her decision was so very final. She also regretted the times that she had felt frustrated at his disinterest in eating and his hobbies. Although never an angry person, she had experienced anger at her husband on more than one occasion. The children all felt a measure of guilt as well: Anne for going to a meeting instead of being with her dad at the hospital, and Janet and Bill for being at work instead of at their dad's bedside. Everyone wished they had more time together as a family.

Jane became a grieving widow, very dependent, sad, and indecisive—a person her children barely recognized. At a time when they needed a strong, supportive mother, that person was absent. The individuals best able to provide support to Jane and her children were the grandchildren and spouses. Having never experienced the death of someone so dear to them, all family members struggled with daily life for several weeks after Glenn's death.

Family Systems Theory Applied to the Howe Family

Family Systems Theory will be used to address the complex needs of each individual within the family, and the family as a whole. All members of the Howe family were affected by Glenn's admission to the medical-surgical unit as well as his death. Chapter 2 provides more detailed information about Family Systems Theory.

Case Study: Howe Family—cont'd

Concept 1: All Parts of the System Are Interconnected
For the Howe family, all members of the family are affected by Glenn's declining health and eventual death in the hospital setting. Jane feels immense guilt for not "bringing him back," and all three of Glenn's children feel guilt and remorse for not being at their dad's bedside. Both Janet and Bill verbalized anger toward Anne because she was out of town for a meeting instead of being with their dad. As an ICU nurse, Anne always assumed responsibility for her dad's health care needs.

Concept 2: The Whole Is More Than the Sum of Its Parts
In the Howe case study, it is not just the mother and children who are affected by this hospitalization and death. The spouses of Anne, Janet, and Bill and the six grandchildren are also greatly affected. A nurse working with this family would need to understand that the family is a complex system where significant changes, such as the death of a family member, would have an impact on the entire family system. Jane's overwhelming grief, in addition to the family never having experienced the death of someone so dear to them, all added stressors that could deteriorate the family relationships over time.

Concept 3: All Systems Have Some Form of Boundaries or Borders Between the System and Its Environment
In working with the Howe family, it would be important for the nurse to assess the boundaries within the family. For example, if the Howe family verbalized that they do not want to meet with a grief counselor, they may have a closed boundary. A flexible boundary would be if the family allowed their Episcopal priest to visit but no other members of their church. The nurse might want to help the family understand the value of open boundaries, such as seeking community resources that might assist with the grief process.

Concept 4: Systems Can Be Further Organized Into Subsystems
The nurse would want to think of the Howe family not only as a whole but also as subsystems within the family. This might be Jane to her children, Jane to her grandchildren, Jane's children to their own children, and so forth. The nurse may work with the grief process and the adjustments of the family after the death of Glenn by focusing on the subsystems that are present within the family.

Questions for reflection on the nursing care of the Howe family:

1. How can the nurse support open sharing of family feelings during stressful hospitalizations?
2. Based on the case study, what family management style in deciding to withhold therapies is most evident?
3. Despite honoring Glen's wishes not to have CPR, Jane and the children are grieving and experiencing feelings of guilt. How could the nurse support the family while respecting their boundaries?

SUMMARY

When medical-surgical nurses view families as partners in the care provided to patients, they are providing unfragmented, holistic, humane, and sensitively delivered health care. When nurses practice family-centered care in acute-care settings, families are empowered to manage the stressors of being in the hospital environment, which is foreign territory to most people. Families are better prepared to support their loved ones, aid in their recovery, or facilitate a comfortable death. Families are called on to support their ill family member in the hospital, make important life decisions on behalf of or in partnership with the patient, serve as caregivers, and advocate for the patient in the complex health care system.

- The stress families experience when family members are in the hospital is significant. Family members are at risk for depression, anxiety, and PTSD.
- The role of families in the hospital setting is crucial because patients have been shown to have more positive outcomes when families are involved in their loved one's care while in the hospital.
- The benefits of practicing family nursing or family-centered care in the hospital setting have been well documented. Yet health care providers in the hospital environment

continue to practice patient-centered rather than family-centered care (family nursing).

- Nurses in medical-surgical environments recognize and feel responsible to practice family-centered or family nursing. Yet they struggle with role ambiguity and role conflict because they continue to practice in settings that reward the biomedical model of health care and not a holistic nursing model of care.

- The environment for providing family-centered nursing care (family nursing) in acute-care settings depends on hospital policies and procedures that consider the needs of families.

- Transferring loved ones from CCUs to medical-surgical units is stressful for families because it creates a sense of conflict. On one hand, families are glad their loved ones are better, but on the other hand they also worry that their family members may not be ready to be moved out of such intensive nurse watchfulness.

- The family member who advocates for a loved one in the hospital assumes a potentially difficult, time-consuming, and fatiguing role because they often travel long distances to get to the hospital, take time off work, stay all night in the hospital, manage the informational needs of the patient and the family, and work through a complex health care system.

- Effective communication with patients, families, and interdisciplinary health care providers improves client satisfaction, promotes positive response to care, reduces length of stay in care settings, and results in decreased overall cost and resource utilization.

- Compassionate communication provides crucial care to families as they are asked to make multiple decisions when their loved one dies in the hospital.

chapter 17

Families and Aging

Elizabeth Straus, MN, RN, COI, PhD(c)

Melissa Robinson, PhD, RN

Critical Concepts

- Gerontological nursing takes place in all care settings, although the specific needs of older adults and their families vary.

- Most older adults live and receive care in community settings. Although older adults generally are healthy and independent, the risk of chronic conditions increases with age, causing many older adults to become more limited in activities of daily living (ADLs).

- Older adults have family ties that are generally positive, meaningful, and supportive. It is rare for older adults to be neglected or uncared for by their families.

- As is the case in all families, families of older adults are diverse across numerous categories, including history, race, class, gender, and individual family history and traditions. These factors influence family composition, health status, health beliefs, and capacity to support each other during times of illness or stress.

- All families experience transitions over the life course, both expected and unexpected. Each transition is influenced by health status, culture, financial security, and social supports.

- Older adults can be givers and/or receivers of family care. They may provide more economic, social, and emotional support to adult children than they receive; they often step in to assist family members in crisis, and are often key in providing child care for grandchildren. Most caregivers of older adults with chronic conditions are partners.

- A majority of those receiving care in almost all care settings are older than 65 years. All nurses will work with increasing numbers of older adults simply because the population is aging so rapidly and because of the increased risk of chronic conditions with advancing age that require nursing care. Even nurses who focus on maternal and child or pediatric nursing are more likely now than in the past to encounter grandparents as caregivers or major support persons.

- Families are often responsible for providing complex, technical nursing care, which was once only the purview of nurses. The health care system, however, often provides inadequate preparation and support for families to take on these roles.

- Nursing care is most effective when done in partnership with families. Families provide most of the care to older adults, regardless of care setting. The organization and structure of care vary.

When we think about aging clients and their families, we often think of individuals or couples who are older than 65 years. These individuals, however, are embedded within a larger family system that includes different and intersecting generations. For example, today a 75-year-old couple may be newlyweds and have living parents. They may be completely healthy with no chronic conditions, and they may spend some of their family time supporting themselves and others. In contrast, a 75-year-old person may be widowed and isolated from social support, have multiple chronic conditions, experience several limitations in activities of daily living (ADLs), and require significant help from others. In either case, if the 75-year-olds have children, they are likely to be grandparents and even great-grandparents, and they may be the primary caregivers to one or more of those grandchildren or great-grandchildren.

When people need help, it comes most often from family members. When older adults need care, families participate in that care in most circumstances. Some family members are active leaders in that care, and others require substantial support from nurses and other professionals. Some older adults may have limited social ties and may be isolated from family and friends as they age. These individuals rely heavily on formal services.

LIFE-COURSE PERSPECTIVE

The aging population is diverse, and family systems are complex. Over the last several decades, family gerontologists (those who study aging) have increasingly taken up a life-course perspective as a way to understand this complexity (Settersten, 2017). The life-course perspective recognizes that individuals are embedded in a family system and that individuals and the family as a whole develop and change over time. This perspective further emphasizes the role of other interacting social forces, such as education, work, policies, and social changes, that influence access to opportunities throughout one's life (Settersten, 2017). The life-course perspective is particularly helpful in understanding the complexity and diversity of family life because it provides a dynamic understanding of family life across generations (Settersten, 2017). This outlook is compatible with many family and social science theories and is often used in conjunction with other theories,

including the theories that guide this book. This chapter integrates the life-course perspective with Family Systems Theories, Family Life Cycle Theory, and the Bioecological Systems Theory. This section describes ways that the life-course perspective enhances these family theories and contributes to greater understanding of the diversity of family experiences in mid- and later life.

Family Systems Theories

Family systems theories emphasize connections among family members. When something happens to or is experienced by one family member, other family members are affected in some way. The life-course perspective encourages us to consider family systems broadly. Connidis and Barnett (2019), for example, describe family relationships in terms of "family ties," which helps us think about families that extend beyond households and the nuclear family. Family ties include extended biological relations as well as those who are "like family" but are not connected through blood or marriage. As described throughout this chapter, and was introduced in Chapter 2, the character of family ties varies within and between families. Responses to life events among family members are influenced by a history of family norms, values, and traditions that have developed over time (Council on Foundations, 2020) and the quality and characteristics of family ties within the family system.

Family Life Cycle Theory

The Family Life Cycle Theory has been used historically to help predict when normative changes would occur. For example, this model has emphasized how many middle-aged and older adults experience their children leaving home and establishing their own households, a normative change. Adult children may form partnerships through marriage or cohabitation. They also begin to achieve financial independence through work. Middle-aged adults who are parents can expect to become grandparents. Retirement is an expected and often desired transition for those with an adequate income and retirement savings. These types of transitions have been considered normative and for many represent "on-time" events. At the same time, the life-course perspective focuses on how the types and timing of transitions that families experience are influenced by the social circumstances, historical events, and series of decisions an individual and family experience over time. In this way, the timing and even the occurrence of what have historically been expected milestones are changing and becoming less predictable. Applying a life-course approach helps us understand how the role of Family Life Cycle Theory in informing how family nurses understand and support aging families is changing. Instead of focusing on only normative or "normal" changes and transitions, the life-course perspective helps us consider diversity in family life cycles. This does not mean that normative trajectories should be ignored altogether. While family diversity has increased dramatically over the past few decades and it is essential to remain open to diversity within and between families, it is also important to recognize the ways in which North American societies are constructed around these normative life cycles and the implications for aging families whose life trajectories differ from these norms.

Bioecological Systems Theory

The life-course perspective in conjunction with the Bioecological Systems Theory (Bronfenbrenner & Morris, 2006) places a strong emphasis on interactions between aging individuals and families and their contexts as influential across the life course. For example, the Bioecological Systems Theory helps explore how social contextual influences and societal changes influence the timing and context of transitions within and across families, and how societal changes shape and are shaped by individual and family decisions. For example, it is increasingly common for young adults to leave home and then return, due to reasons related to education, work, or personal factors. Individuals may go to college in midlife to begin new careers either voluntarily (e.g., a desire for more meaningful work or a better work-family balance) or involuntarily (e.g., needing new skills after a layoff). Some individuals or couples in middle age are just starting their families or are assisting with child care for grandchildren or loved ones. This reflects somewhat of a change in family planning norms. Some couples in their fifties adopt young children, sometimes their own grandchildren. Those in their seventies may seek paid employment because of a desire to work or because of financial necessity. Thus, attitudes and expectations about family norms are changing, and there is much greater flexibility and diversity in family experiences.

As with bioecological models, the life-course perspective emphasizes social and historical contexts, including the societal conditions in which individuals and families function as well as the actions individuals take in shaping their relationships and the trajectories of their lives (Settersten, 2017). Individuals and families are influenced by the historical times and spaces in which they live. For example, those who are currently in their late eighties and nineties and lived in the United States experienced the Great Depression as young children, and many men served in World War II. Later, these children of the Great Depression were parents of the baby-boom generation. The postwar baby boom represented a reversal in the trend toward smaller families, resulting in a population bulge that has dominated family life and public policy in the United States and Canada ever since. Baby boomers had a different set of challenges and opportunities than their parents and are now entering old age.

In all phases of history, societal issues related to race, class, gender, abilities, and immigration have influenced the kinds of opportunities and barriers that individuals and families experience throughout their lives. This combination of historical events and social context must be considered when trying to understand how changing environments, cultural norms, economic conditions, and political circumstances affect families in mid- and later life. Such influences can be seen in work and family decisions, access to health care, and educational opportunities. Many advantages and/or disadvantages accumulate over a lifetime and across generations (Ferarro et al., 2017; Settersten, 2017).

Even as we emphasize the importance of social and historical context in shaping individual and family lives, we must remember that individuals are not passive. They are active agents, even as their actions may be constrained or enhanced by broader societal circumstances (Settersten, 2017). There are many examples of individuals following or going against societal norms and how that affected the individuals' lives. For example, in war-torn countries, the decision to leave or stay within that country influences the individual and the family for generations after. The life-course perspective, in conjunction with the aforementioned theories, will be used in this chapter to foster understanding of families with older adults and the family ties that influence their health and well-being. This perspective will be used to think about optimal nursing care for these families, using the nursing process. This approach will also be used to explain current social policies influencing older adults and their families.

PROFILE OF AGING FAMILIES

Family structures and functions are changing at a rapid pace, all of which have implications for the care needs and resources of families in mid- and later life. In this section, we will explore demographic trends that influence families, including family structures and functions. We will also examine different facets of family relationships, from same-generation and intergenerational relationships, including the influence of ambivalence and conflict. Awareness of the complexity and richness of family life is critically important for nurses who help older adults and their families navigate all aspects of health, illness, and disabilities.

As we describe the most recent changes to family structure in the past several decades, it is important to recognize that the makeup of families and the individual roles within families and society has always been changing and evolving. Families are remarkably resilient, even as the form of the family changes. What remains constant in families is the commitment family members, however defined, have for one another (Connidis, 2015a).

Demographic Profile

The aging of the population worldwide is unprecedented historically and has implications for all aspects of society, especially families. Almost 50 countries, including Canada and the United States, have at least 15% of their populations over the age of 65 (United Nations, 2020). Most of these are in Europe and Asia: Japan leads with 28%, followed by numerous European countries over 20%. In Canada, nearly 18% of the population is over 65, while the United States is slightly lower, at just over 16% (United Nations, 2020).

Globally, the number of people 65 years or older is expected to more than double by 2050 and triple by 2100, increasing from approximately 700 million in 2019 to 1.55 billion in 2050 and 2.45 billion in 2100 (United Nations, 2020). Eastern and Southeastern Asia and Latin America are the most rapidly aging regions (United Nations, 2020). In Canada, the number of people age 65 and over is expected to increase to 25% (a 42% increase) by 2050 (United Nations, 2020); in the United States, an increase to just over 22% (a 38% increase) is projected (United Nations, 2020). Demographers worldwide project similar increases as the population ages; in the United States, for example, the number of people ages 85 and older is expected to more than double between 2017 and 2040 (Administration for Community Living [ACL] & Administration on Aging [AOA], 2018).

Diversity

In this section, the diversity of the older adult population is discussed using a broad definition of diversity that encompasses multiple axes of difference, including ethnicity, gender identity, ability, and economic status. We acknowledge that, while the profiles and experiences presented in this and other subsequent sections are organized by specific social identities or statuses, such as ethnicity, gender, economic status, and ability, we have endeavored where possible to take up an intersectional lens (Hankivsky, 2014) that draws attention to the multiple social identities of older adults and how these interact to affect their lives. In doing so, we draw attention to some of the health and social inequities experienced by older adults to help nurses understand the variety of circumstances of older adults and their families that they may encounter in their care interactions. It is also important to remember, however, that nurses should not limit their assessment to the identification of health and social inequities. To achieve broader understanding of the implications of and how to begin to address these inequities, nurses should further examine how such inequities are produced and sustained. Such an analysis of the production of these inequities, however, is beyond the scope of this chapter.

In the United States, 23% of older adults were members of racial or ethnic minorities, a more diverse population than in previous generations (ACL & AOA, 2018). By 2050, it is estimated that those with an African American, Latinx, or Asian or

Pacific Islander background will make up approximately 40% of the U.S. population (ACL & AOA, 2018). Populations of older adults from African American and Asian backgrounds are expected to at least double by 2060. In Canada, 12.6% of older adults identified as visible minorities, of which 31% are first-generation immigrants (Statistics Canada, 2016).

Immigration is an additional factor contributing to growing diversity in both the United States and Canada. In the United States, about 20% of the immigrant population is 60 years or older. The number of immigrants arriving in the United States each year increased from 37,000 in 2000 to 113,000 in 2017 (Camarota & Zeigler, 2019). In Canada, 22.3% of immigrants are over 65 years old (Statistics Canada, 2016). While only 4.6% of immigrants arriving in Canada between 2011 and 2016 were over 65 years old, this number has been steadily increasing. The factors contributing to increased age at arrival include aging populations in other countries, more parents coming to join their adult children, and decreases in illegal immigration (Camarota & Zeigler, 2019).

Sexual Orientation and Gender Diversity

It is estimated that more than 2.4 million adults over 50 years old in the United States identify as LGBTQ+ and that this number could double by 2030 (Fredriksen-Goldsen, 2014). These numbers could be underestimates: historical contexts of stigma and concerns about discrimination may lead older adults not to want to come out openly or be included in LGBTQ+ communities (Employment and Social Development Canada, 2018; Robinson-Wood & Weber, 2016). As with other younger LGBTQ+ populations, LGBTQ+ older adults and their families may also experience health and social inequities (S. K. Choi & Meyer, 2016). Refer to Chapter 8 for further discussion of nursing implications for the care of LGBTQ+ individuals and their families.

Economic Status

Globalization and various public policies have contributed to growing income inequality worldwide. In 2017, just over 9% of older adults in the United States lived in poverty, although the percentage increased to nearly 14% when medical out-of-pocket expenses were included in poverty calculations (ACL & AOA, 2018). In Canada, it is estimated that between 4% and 14% of older adults live in poverty depending on how poverty is defined (Statistics Canada, 2019; Waddell et al., 2018). Women and people of color are disproportionately represented in the lower-income groups (Federal Interagency Forum on Aging-Related Statistics [FIFARS], 2016). Women have historically experienced income inequalities, often related to pension policies when their partners die (United Nations, 2016). In addition, while only 7% of non-Hispanic European older Americans lived in poverty in 2017, over 19% of African Americans, almost 11% of Asians, and 17% of Hispanic older Americans lived in poverty (ACL & AOA, 2019a, 2019b, 2019c). At the intersection of gender and ethnicity, about 37% of Hispanic older women who lived alone were living in poverty in 2017 (ACL & AOA, 2019c).

Health Status, Impairment, and Disability

As a group, older adults are healthier, better educated, and more financially secure than in previous generations. People throughout the world are living longer than ever before. In Canada, life expectancy at birth is 82 years (Statistics Canada, 2020c). When Canadian women reach age 65, they can expect to live another 22 years; men at age 65 can expect to live another 20 years (Statistics Canada, 2020c). In the United States, 65-year-old women can expect to live 20.6 more years and men another 18 years (ACL & AOA, 2018). Most older adults live independently and in good health. Approximately three quarters of those older than 65 years in the United States report having good, very good, or excellent health (Centers for Disease Prevention and Control [CDC], 2020). This is especially true for non-Hispanic European Americans; over 80% report being in good to excellent health compared with about 65% and 66% for older adults who identify as African American and Hispanic/Latinx, respectively (FIFARS, 2016). These differences reflect health inequities and economic disadvantages in the United States, which are mirrored in other societies as well.

Older adults are disproportionately affected by chronic conditions, including diabetes, arthritis, and heart disease (National Council on Aging, 2018). Approximately 80% of older adults experience at least one chronic condition, and nearly 70% of Medicare beneficiaries experience two or more (National Council on Aging, 2018). The prevalence of many chronic conditions in older adults (e.g., hypertension, asthma, cancer, diabetes) has also increased in recent years (FIFARS, 2016). Six of the top seven causes of death in 2017 in Canada and the United States were chronic illnesses: heart disease, cancer, chronic lower respiratory diseases, stroke, Alzheimer's disease (United States) or liver disease (Canada), and diabetes (Heron, 2019; Statistics Canada, 2020b).

Older adults may also experience sensory impairments with age, which may interfere with abilities to function or to interact socially. Nearly 75% of those over the age of 70 experience hearing loss in at least one ear; hearing loss is more prevalent in men than in women (Goman & Lin, 2016). In Canada, an ongoing longitudinal study has found that 63.5% of older adults age 60 to 79 years in its sample had moderate to profound hearing loss (Ramage-Morin et al., 2019). Hearing loss can be particularly challenging, leading to social isolation, depression, or mistaken perceptions by others that the older adult is cognitively impaired. Recent research indicates that hearing loss can contribute to cognitive decline (Deal et al., 2017). Vision loss also increases with age, increasing risk for falls and limiting activities, such as driving, which can increase isolation and reliance on others. In Canada, almost 86% of adults age 45 to 85 years wear some type of corrective lenses, and just over 15% of older adults over age 75 years experienced vision impairment even with corrective lenses (Aljied et al., 2018; Ramage-Morin et al., 2019). In the United States, 25% of those 80 years and older have significant vision impairment (Pelletier et al., 2016). Senses related to smell and taste generally remain stable into old age when one is healthy, but these senses can be negatively affected by disease or medications (Liu et al., 2016). This in turn may lead to poor nutritional status, which can adversely affect overall health and well-being (Baugreet et al., 2017).

It is important to remember, however, that having a diagnosis of a chronic condition or a disability is not an indicator of an individual's quality of life or ability to engage in meaningful activities. Often, the concept of functioning, which is often tied to ADLs or instrumental ADLs (IADLs), is used as an indicator of ability to engage in meaningful activity. ADLs refer to basic self-care tasks such as bathing, eating, toileting, dressing, and mobility. IADLs include basic functions and activities that allow older individuals to live independently, such as using the telephone, managing money, doing laundry, maintaining one's home, shopping, and managing transportation. The concept of function can be useful in determining one's need for support and assistance; however, care should be taken to ensure that function is not universally equated with health, well-being, or quality of life. We will consider needs related to function, and the role of family and the health care system in meeting them, later in this chapter.

Cognitive Status

Cognitive decline is an issue of particular concern to many older adults. Neuronal and synaptic changes do occur with aging, although the range and impact of these changes vary markedly across individuals (Smith & Cotter, 2016). Although it is not unusual for older adults to have difficulty focusing on multiple tasks at once, recalling recent events, or recalling a specific word, these changes typically do not interfere with an individual's ability to live their lives (Smith & Cotter, 2016). However, the risk of marked cognitive decline does increase with each decade, and the prevalence of Alzheimer's disease and related dementias in the United States rises from 10% of people age 65 and older to 36% of people aged 85 and older (Alzheimer's Association, 2019). The number of people with dementia in Canada is projected to double within the next 20 years (Canadian Institute of Health Information, 2018). This highlights the need for nurses to understand and be responsive to the needs of people with dementia and their families.

FAMILY TIES AND AGING

We now turn to the intersection of family life and aging and its implications for nurses. With increasing life expectancy, family relationships now last for decades. It is common to see newspaper photos of couples celebrating their 60th anniversaries, and for "children" in their sixties or seventies to have living parents. We now encounter siblings with relationships of 90 years or longer; even grandparent-grandchild relationships increasingly extend five or more decades. These long-lasting relationships, with their histories of shared experiences, traditions, and exchanges of help, will most often be an asset to the older adult as illnesses or functional declines occur. This portrait of ties will continue to change as society changes.

A prevailing myth in the United States is that older adults, particularly those who are part of the dominant culture, are isolated from and neglected by their younger family members and ultimately are abandoned in nursing homes. Studies have contradicted these historically ingrained assumptions, however, demonstrating that family ties are often strong but also vary greatly (Fingerman et al., 2020). Although the family structure has changed in recent decades, much about family life has remained the same, including valuing families. Individuals continue to travel through life in relations with others. Some people come and go, but many, especially family members, remain constant social relations for decades. Families value exchanges of emotional and practical support throughout the life course (Connidis & Barnett, 2019).

Romantic Relationships

Romantic relationships are important sources of emotional bonding that are characterized by physical intimacy, emotional support, and deep feelings of care and compassion (Gómez-López et al., 2019). The establishment and maintenance of romantic relationships can contribute to individuals' positive self-concept and to their mental and physical health (Gómez-López et al., 2019). Romantic relationships can lead to marriage, intimate partnerships, or cohabitation, which can contribute to the overall sense of security and well-being of the individual.

Marriage

Age at first marriage is on the rise, 28 years for women and 29.8 for men, an increase of 6 to 8 years since the 1960s (U.S. Census Bureau, 2020). Until recently, marriage was an option only for heterosexual partners. In the United States, Canada, and many European countries, marriage is now available to same-sex couples. Before this change, cohabitation was the major option for same-sex partners. The benefits of marriage are less apparent today than a generation ago, although some studies have found that older adults who are married or are in egalitarian relationships have better physical health and psychological well-being compared to those who are single, widowed, divorced, or separated, especially for men and for couples who report high-quality relationships (Bookwala, 2016; Zhang et al., 2016). Differences have also been described across race and gender (Brown & Wright, 2017; Yu & Zhang, 2017). The way one partner responds to a stressor, such as a chronic condition, influences how the other responds, emphasizing the importance of focusing on family and not just individuals when working with older adults.

Cohabitation

We can no longer assume that those who are single are without partners. Cohabitation was often a precursor to marriage in the past, but now more couples of all ages are choosing not to marry, especially those with less education and economic stability (Manning et al., 2014). Cohabitation as an alternative to marriage has increased in middle and later life. Between 2007 and 2017, the number of cohabiting adults over 50 years of age in the United States increased by 85% (Brown & Wright, 2017). Other contributing factors to this increase include a slight increase in those who have never married, an increase in divorce rates in those over 50 years of age, and a decrease in remarriage for those who are divorced or widowed (Brown & Wright, 2017; Schimmele & Wu, 2016).

Cohabiting couples historically had less stable unions than those who marry, but differences between cohabiting and married couples in the nature of the relationship appear to be diminishing. Wright and Brown (2017) found that psychological well-being, as measured by depressive symptoms, perceived stress, and loneliness, was not related to whether older women were unpartnered, dating, cohabiting, or married. In contrast, both cohabiting and married men had more positive well-being than unpartnered or dating men.

Sexuality

Sexuality is important when considering intimate partnerships regardless of gender or partnership status; however, negative stereotypes of sexuality in older adulthood persist. Many older adults continue to desire sexual relationships well into late life, with many reporting increased freedom to explore sexuality because of decreased concern over procreation and decreased family responsibilities. Greater emotional and physical well-being is associated with being sexually active (Bookwala, 2016;

Gómez-López et al., 2019; Schafer et al., 2018). Sexual activity is influenced by physical health, quality and availability of relationships, change in role from procreation to pleasure and validation, attitudes toward sexuality, societal influences, and previous sexual experiences (Gómez-López et al., 2019; Schafer et al., 2018). For example, how intimacy occurs may differ in older adults after a neurological event such as a stroke or spinal cord injury (Sinković & Towler, 2019). Schafer et al. (2018) emphasized the error of viewing sexuality from only a biological or medical perspective, noting that attitude is more salient in predicting continued sexual desire and behavior than presence or absence of chronic illness or age. Nevertheless, advancing age is associated with decline in sexual activity for many people. Drawing on the World Health Organization (WHO) definition of sexual health, Messelis et al. (2019) emphasized that sexuality involves much more than sexual intercourse, highlighting the importance of intimacy, touch, affection, body image, and one's identity as a sexual being. Loss of a partner through widowhood often means the loss of all these different facets of sexuality, facets that often are unrecognized or unacknowledged.

A common model used to inform assessment of sexuality in older adults is the PLISSIT model, which involves asking Permission before asking questions; providing Limited Information once the nurse understands the older adult's concerns; making Specific Suggestions for a tailored plan of care; and, if needed, suggesting Intensive Therapy (Wallace, 2008). Carpenter and DeLamater's (2012) integrated model of assessing sexuality in later life can also aid nurses in understanding the role of sexuality in the lives of older adults. The model includes the following:

- *Biological influences:* physical health (i.e., presence of chronic conditions that affect sexual function or desire, or both), age, hormonal levels, medical treatments that may affect sexual function
- *Psychological:* attitudes toward sexuality, role of sexual relationships, knowledge, past experiences, mental health
- *Social:* availability of partner, including duration and quality of relationship; societal views and influences on sexuality in later life; socioeconomic status

Romantic Relationship Dissolution

Romantic relationships end through divorce, breakups, or widowhood. These are among the most stressful transitions in family life. In the text that follows, we describe some of the characteristics associated with dissolution. It is beyond the scope of this chapter, however, to explore the psychological, social, economic, and health impacts of these transitions fully. This is due in large part to the heterogeneity of experiences. As indicated by the life-course perspective, the impact may be shaped by sex and gender, the nature and duration of the intimate partnership, the roles played by each partner, the specific causes of the dissolution, the availability of social supports and economic resources, and personal agency. The historical, cultural, and societal context in which the dissolution occurs also shapes response.

Divorce rates in the United States have been falling fast in recent years, hitting a record low in 2019 (Institute for Family Studies, 2020) after increasing dramatically in the 20th century. For every 1,000 marriages in 2019, only 14.9% ended in divorce, according to a recent American Community Survey conducted by the U.S. Census Bureau, which is the lowest rate in 50 years (Institute for Family Studies, 2020). Annual marriage and divorce rates have not been collected by Statistics Canada since 2008; however, it seems widely accepted that more than 40% of Canadian marriages are expected to end in divorce before the couple reaches the 50th wedding anniversary. This estimation is limited to marriage and does not account for separations experienced by unmarried partners (common-law or cohabiting couples and other romantic partnerships), which makes separation and divorce a normative life event for many Canadians (Collaborative Divorce Vancouver Society, 2020).

Most divorces still occur in young adulthood, although it has become more common in middle and late adulthood (Lin et al., 2016). In 1990, these so-called gray divorces accounted for 10% of divorces in the United States, rising to more than 25% by 2010 (Lin et al., 2016). A similar increase has been seen in Canada (Margolis et al., 2019). Reasons for divorce in later life are similar to divorce in younger couples, including marital quality, mental health problems, and economic resources (Crowley, 2019; Lin et al., 2018). It has been estimated that 20% to 25% of older adults in the United States may also repartner (Brown et al., 2019), although repartnering patterns have also been shown to vary.

Siblings

Siblings represent important but often overlooked same-generation family relationships (Jensen et al., 2019). They typically are the family tie of the longest duration, and, for the most part, siblings share the same historical and social context. As with all family relationships, identifying siblings can be complex because siblings may include biological and nonbiological relationships. Although often intense during childhood, sibling relationships may vary throughout adulthood as people focus on their partners, children, and career development (Jensen et al., 2019). During middle and late life, sibling ties may change as time to devote to the relationship changes and as their aging parents require increasing assistance. Adults may also become more involved in the care of a sibling with a disability as their parents age (Lee & Burke, 2018). Having positive sibling relationships is associated with less loneliness in old age (Stocker et al., 2020). As the birth rate declines and more people have no or only one sibling, this important family tie in old age is likely to become increasingly rare.

Intergenerational Relationships

Intergenerational relationships include a wide range of family ties, including parent-child; stepparent and stepchildren; grandparents and grandchildren; aunt/uncle and niece/nephew; and a host of intergenerational relationships that are "like family" but not related by blood, marriage, or adoption. Nurses need to be aware of the multiple ways that adult children and parents or stepparents have a shared history and how that might influence mutual affection, exchange, and caregiving. Intergenerational relationships are increasingly taking on a voluntary quality influenced by affection, commitment, and a wide range of contextual factors. Assumptions about the quality of relationships cannot be made based on gender or type of relationship.

Similar to same-generation relationships, the characteristics of intergenerational family relationships are changing because of technological advances, economic and political factors, and trends in family structure. Trends in how families are structured have also affected characteristics for intergenerational relationships. As discussed earlier, family structures have evolved to include biological and nonbiological family ties. In addition, fertility rates have declined worldwide in the past decades, with rates falling at or below replacement levels in Europe, North America, and Eastern Asia (United Nations, 2015). There are also increasing numbers of adults who do not have children (U.S. Census Bureau, 2019), either voluntarily (e.g., active choice not to have children) or involuntarily (e.g., a result of infertility, death of a child). In addition, marriage and the birth of a first child are occurring at older ages. This means that parents and grandparents experience these roles at later ages or perhaps not at all. The number of children born into a family has also declined in the United States, resulting in more families with one or two children. Although parents can provide more individual attention to fewer children, this has implications as parents age and have fewer family members available for support and adult children have fewer siblings to share parent care responsibilities.

Technological advances and economic and political factors have also significantly changed how intergenerational ties are experienced (Fingerman et al., 2020). How people communicate has changed drastically over the last decade. Ten years ago, smartphones were only just becoming popular, and e-mail and phone remained the primary modes of communication. During the COVID-19 pandemic, technologies available to stay connected have expanded drastically. Yet there is significant variability in how older adults use technology to maintain intergenerational ties. Some older adults have adopted the use of video chat during the pandemic to stay connected with family members; others still prefer to use the phone. Financial downturns and recessions in 2008 and 2020, for example, have affected the number of adult children who co-reside with their older parents (Fingerman et al., 2020; Fry, 2016). Migration trends over the last decade have led both to families living apart and to intergenerational cultural differences, such as between first- and second-generation immigrants (Fingerman et al., 2020). These various factors can have significant implications for intergenerational ties.

Parent-Child Relationships

The strongest intergenerational tie is often the parent-child relationship. Based on data from a

2013 U.S. survey, it has been estimated that almost three quarters of adults have at least one parent or adult child living within 30 miles (Choi et al., 2020). This has remained relatively constant despite the often-cited geographic mobility of younger generations; however, it is unclear how this trend will change as the baby-boom generation ages. At the same time, adult children with college degrees are more likely to live farther away (Choi et al., 2020). Contact between generations is common, although it can vary across family contexts. Relationship quality is often seen as more important than contact. Feelings of closeness between generations have been an important focus in research on intergenerational ties, although it is recognized that these connections are complex and varied (Carr & Utz, 2020; Fingerman et al., 2020). Relationship quality has been associated with older adult well-being; for example, for older fathers, positive relationships with their adult children have been associated with better subjective well-being (Polenick et al., 2018). Exchanges of help and support between generations occur throughout the life course and are motivated by affection as well as by a sense of obligation. We explore exchanges of support among generations in our discussion of caregiving later in the chapter.

Parent-child relationships exist in many different family forms, including those headed by same-sex couples. In addition to step relationships, children of same-sex couples are now arriving more frequently through adoption, surrogacy, or artificial insemination. Numerous studies suggest that the well-being of children raised by same-sex couples is similar to those raised by heterosexual couples: children do best in a loving, stable, and supportive environment regardless of the sexual orientation of the parents (Connidis, 2015a; Knight et al., 2017).

The impact of divorce on parent-child relationships varies, including cause and timing of a parent's divorce; the parents' ability to provide stable, loving, and supportive environments to young children; and financial and educational resources. All of these factors influence the long-term consequences for adult children and their parents. Divorce often results in strained relationships with adult children, placing them at greater risk of isolation as they age (Brown & Wright, 2017). Although relationships with divorced parents may be strained, adult children may maintain relationships with one or both parents and provide support as needed (Carr & Utz, 2020).

Blended Families

Those now entering old age are likely to have complex family systems that include stepchildren because of divorce and remarriage, or cohabitation. As in much of family life, the nature of stepparent-stepchild relationships varies widely (Ganong et al., 2018). Similar findings have been described in relation to step-grandparents (Chapman et al., 2018). In the context of blended families formed in later life, stepparents and stepchildren may experience both obstacles and opportunities in the process of forming new family relationships (Mikucki-Enyart & Heisdorf, 2020). While adult stepchildren may face obstacles with balancing membership with multiple families and feeling caught in the middle, many also experience positive impacts of these new relationships on other family member relationships (Mikucki-Enyart & Heisdorf, 2020).

Grandparent-Grandchild Relationships

Significant intergenerational family relationships include grandparents and grandchildren. As with parenthood, becoming a grandparent is occurring later in the life course. In Canada, for example, more than 60% of women were grandmothers in their fifties in 1985, but only 29% were in 2011 (Margolis, 2016). Although grandchildren are expected to have many years of relationship with grandparents because of increased longevity, there will be a much greater age gap than in the past, with implications for the nature of those relationships. With the aging of both grandparents and grandchildren, the nature of relationships will change.

As in other family relationships, the ways that grandparents relate to grandchildren vary widely among families (von Humboldt et al., 2018). While sometimes called a "roleless role," grandparents can play a variety of roles in families and may even create their role within the family based on the family's stage in the life course and the family history of grandparenting roles (Dolbin-MacNab & Yancura, 2018). Most older adults find grandparenting meaningful and experience the role with both satisfaction and pleasure (Mansson, 2016). Grandparents are often an important resource for their adult children. For example, grandparents may be a major provider of child care when grandchildren are young. There has also been an increasing trend of grandparents acting as primary caregivers for their grandchildren (Glaser et al., 2018), which will be revisited later in this chapter.

Negotiating Tensions and Conflict in Families

Family gerontology researchers have increasingly focused on the complexity of family life. Family members simultaneously hold positive and negative feelings about one another, often because of contradictory roles (Pine & Steffen, 2019; Rojas et al., 2016). For example, family members may want to act as a caregiver for their partner or parents to help them; at the same time, they may also feel like they are limited in achieving their own career aspirations as a result. Connidis (2015b) stresses the importance of thinking about this notion of mixed feelings, often known as ambivalence in the literature, beyond individual feelings and emphasizes how societal-level conditions and expectations affect individual and family life in contradictory ways. For example, Igarashi et al. (2013) noted that those in midlife may experience tensions as they seek to support both younger and older family members within a culture that values independence and autonomy and a society that provides limited supports.

Although less common than the aforementioned tensions and mixed feelings, family conflict or negative social interactions can have serious consequences for family relationships. Several author teams have reported how negative social exchanges can have a negative impact on physical and psychological health and well-being compared to positive social exchanges (Birditt et al., 2018). Widmer et al. (2017) also explored family conflict structures in family networks of older adults and found that the number of conflicts was associated with scores on health-related quality-of-life measures and that these associations were mediated by individual stress. Families experiencing conflict may be less likely to be resources for older family members in need.

Elder Mistreatment

Elder mistreatment (often referred to as elder abuse) includes physical pain or injury, psychological anguish, neglect or abandonment, and financial exploitation. Estimates of the prevalence of all types of mistreatment range from 1.3% to 10% of older adults (Friedman et al., 2015; Lachs & Pillemer, 2015; McDonald, 2018). Types of abuse that are reported most frequently are neglect, emotional abuse, and financial exploitation (McDonald, 2018; Roberto et al., 2015). Most perpetrators are adult children, although other family members, paid caregivers, and predatory acquaintances may be abusers (Lachs & Pillemer, 2015; McDonald, 2018). Causes of mistreatment remain poorly understood, but risk factors include unhealthy dependency of the perpetrator on the victim; disturbed psychological state of the perpetrator; frailty, disability, or impairment of the victim; and low income, lack of social support, and isolation of the family (Lachs & Pillemer, 2015; McDonald, 2018; Pillemer et al., 2016). People with dementia are especially vulnerable to psychological abuse and neglect (Pillemer et al., 2016). Mistreatment is often associated with dementia-related behaviors coupled with limited emotional and psychological abilities of caregivers to provide support. Older adults may have been perpetrators of abuse earlier in their lives, which can make it difficult for adult children, who were their victims, to provide support. Nevertheless, there is evidence that adult children do provide instrumental if not emotional support to their abusive mothers in old age (Kong & Moorman, 2016).

Nurses and other health care providers have a responsibility to screen and assess older adults for abuse. Gallione et al. (2017) reviewed and evaluated several assessment tools. One of the recommended tools is the Elder Mistreatment Assessment Instrument, which can be found on the Try This section of the Hartford Institute for Geriatric Nursing (HIGN) website.

Overall, many family relationships are complex, and the strengths of association may vary considerably over time. Mixed feelings and/or conflict may be apparent for nurses and other health care providers when an older adult needs care. Nurses should be aware that families vary considerably with respect to the quality of relationships and the availability of family resources in times of crisis and health decline. Nurses must be sensitive to underlying tensions and be able to provide support in nonjudgmental ways, remembering that the current family dynamics are embedded in a lifetime of relationships and actions.

FAMILY CAREGIVING

Family life is characterized by exchanges of aid and support throughout the life course. If they are in a position to assist the younger generation, older adults may be primary sources of support. They may provide financial assistance to younger adults in college or starting their careers or even assist those who are making major purchases such as cars or homes (Connidis, 2015a). Older adults may also provide care for their adult children or provide care for their grandchildren.

Regardless of the type of care provided, family caregiving grows out of ongoing, caring family relationships. Specific definitions of what constitutes family caregiving that are used in research, practice, or policy often vary. Similarly, the caregiving role may also take on different meanings in different families. For example, caregiving may simply mean "keeping an eye on" or checking in with an older adult, or it may mean that the older adult requires support to self-monitor and/or maintain well-being (Messecar, 2020). Some adults who provide care to family members may not describe what they do as caregiving. Rather, they may consider it a neutral progression of the work they already do as part of their ongoing family roles and responsibilities.

The transition from mutual aid to support that is defined as caregiving is often a gradual process. As dependency increases and more time is spent on providing support, the family member and now caregiver recognizes that the care recipient is no longer able to perform tasks without help. In contrast, transitions to caregiving and care receiving can happen suddenly if an otherwise healthy older adult has a traumatic injury or experiences a stroke or cardiac arrest. For many older adults, a health crisis may signal a sudden end to independence or ability to live alone. In this case, a variety of decisions are made regarding family care and formal care services.

Estimates of the prevalence of caregiving range widely depending on how caregiving is defined. The definition of providing "unpaid care to a relative or friend 18 years or in order to help them take care of themselves" was used in the recent *Caregiving in the U.S.* report (National Alliance for Caregiving [NAC] & AARP Public Policy Institute [AARP PPI], 2020), which further specified that caregiving included helping with personal needs or household chores, managing finances, arranging outside services, or visiting regularly (p. 1). Using this definition, more than 53 million caregivers were identified in 2019, with about 48 million providing care to an adult older than age 50. Over 60% of care recipients had a long-term physical condition, and 32% had a memory problem (NAC & AARP PPI, 2020). In a recent Canadian study, in which family caregiving was defined as care or help provided to a family member or friend with long-term health condition, disability, or age-related needs, caregiving roles included helping with transportation, housework, home maintenance, and health management (Statistics Canada, 2020a). One-half to two-thirds of caregivers are middle-aged or older and more than 50% (54% in Canada in 2018 and 61% in the United States in 2019) identify as women (NAC & AARP PPI, 2020; Statistics Canada, 2020a).

Duration of caregiving may last for days or decades, with the average length of time being 4.5 years. Yet 29% of caregivers have been providing care for 5 years or longer. Studies that have explored time spent on caregiving vary in their estimates, likely due to how caregiving is defined. In the United States, for example, in the NAC and AARP PPI (2020) report, it was estimated that caregivers spend an average of 24 hours a week with caregiving tasks. In Canada in 2018, where the definition of caregiving was much broader, 41% of caregivers spent 1 to 3 hours a week on caregiving tasks, and 46% spent more than 10 hours a week (Statistics Canada, 2020a). Caregivers often provide assistance to more than one older adult at a time, balancing caregiving tasks with other family responsibilities such as supporting children through school or filling their own grandparenting roles (Igarashi et al., 2013). The Hooper family case study that appears later in this chapter illustrates such multiple caregiving demands, as Maria provides care to her parents while also staying connected with her mother-in-law.

Estimates of the value of unpaid family care are difficult to determine but have been estimated to approach $400 billion in the United States (National Academies of Sciences, Engineering, and Medicine, 2016). Costs include out-of-pocket medical expenses and lost income and retirement benefits, including Social Security income, if partners and adult children leave the workforce early to care for older family members. Those who maintain their jobs often lose time, which negatively affects wages, promotions, or other job opportunities. The loss of income may be particularly difficult for those with low incomes at the start.

Caring for Older Adults

Partners are generally the first line of caregivers for older adults. Partners who are caregivers, in particular, may have their own health concerns that are exacerbated by strains related to caregiving. It is not unusual for partners to support each other; they are both caregivers and care recipients. These situations are often tenuous but can work for a while. Because partners who also act as caregivers typically live with the care recipient, they are at risk for not getting enough rest, not having time to recuperate from illnesses, and experiencing health declines. This may particularly be an issue if the person they are caring for experiences dementia (National Academies of Sciences, Engineering, and Medicine, 2016).

Adult children experience the stresses of care in other ways. Many adults balance work outside the home while providing care for a parent and have to make a range of adjustments to be successful in both roles. This may include going to work late or leaving early, or cutting down on hours worked (National Academies of Sciences, Engineering, and Medicine, 2016). Grandchildren may participate in providing care to their grandparents as they age, especially if their parents are primary caregivers (National Academies of Sciences, Engineering, and Medicine, 2016; Statistics Canada, 2020a). Grandchildren may demonstrate varying ways of coping with the caregiving role based on their previous relationships with their grandparents and the support they are receiving from other members of their family or community.

Caregiving is also influenced by culture. Yet it is important not to stereotype or make assumptions based on race or ethnicity. Nurses should be aware of and sensitive to possible differences in caregiving experiences and resources. Individual and cultural values may influence who takes on the leadership role of caregiving within a family. These values are affected by a sense of filial obligation and a sense of responsibility, cultural norms regarding who provides care (e.g., daughter or daughter-in-law), values of giving back, culturally based illness meanings (e.g., a view that disease is normal or that there is a stigma), and larger belief systems such as religion.

Grandparents Caring for Grandchildren

Many older adults are primary caregivers of younger members of their families. Unlike caregiving for older adults, which often evolves over time, grandparents may suddenly find themselves in the role of raising their grandchildren. This may occur when teenagers have children or because of traumatic circumstances surrounding the parent generation, including divorce, substance abuse, incarceration, child abuse or neglect, or death (Glaser et al., 2018). The number of grandparents who were raising their grandchildren increased dramatically by the end of the 20th century (Glaser et al., 2018). It has been estimated that up to 3 million grandparents have assumed parenting roles (Hayslip et al., 2019). As with many family relations, culture and context greatly influence the role of grandparents caring for their grandchildren (Dolbin-MacNab & Yancura, 2018; Lewis et al., 2018), and it is essential for nurses to consider cultural and contextual influences as they conduct their assessments and interventions in a culturally safe way.

As with other caregiving roles, grandparent-grandchild families may experience financial hardships; some grandparents may leave the workforce to care for grandchildren, and others may postpone retirement for financial reasons (Dolbin-MacNab & Yancura, 2018; Glaser et al., 2018). Older adults raising their grandchildren may also experience role confusion, isolation from peers, or stigma related to having custody of their grandchildren (Hayslip et al., 2019). Ongoing conflict with adult children (parents of their grandchildren) is possible, with accompanying feelings of disappointment, resentment, feeling taken advantage of, and grief. The impact on children and on the custodial grandparent's relationship with the parent can be significant. Depending on the situation, grandparents may suffer additional stress, anxiety, or difficulty coping.

Grandparents and their grandchildren may also experience many benefits when a grandparent is raising a grandchild. Grandparents report benefits such as realizing their inner strength, close relationships with their grandchildren, and a sense of accomplishment and purpose (Hayslip et al., 2019; Lewis et al., 2018). Other studies have found that grandmothers had a close relationship with their grandchildren and did not experience many of the reported negative consequences described earlier, suggesting that interventions to support these relationships are particularly important.

Older Adults Caring for Adult Children

While a less common form of family caregiving than caring for an older adult, some older adults provide care for adult children with chronic conditions and/or disabilities. Sometimes this reflects a lifelong role. For example, with increasing numbers of children with complex chronic conditions and disabilities surviving well into adulthood, more parents continue to care for their adult children. Other times, younger adults, including veterans, may acquire a chronic condition or disability as an adult and may receive caregiving support from their parents. Gilligan et al. (2017) found that mothers well into their eighties provided both instrumental (e.g., help with regular chores) and emotional support to their adult children with a serious health condition. It is not uncommon for aging parents of adult children with intellectual and/or developmental disabilities (IDDs) to provide a significant amount of care and support. An example of this is illustrated in the James family case study that appears later in this chapter.

The consequences of a lifetime of caring for an adult child with IDDs or complex care needs are well documented in the literature. Many adults with IDDs live at home, and about 25% have a parent caregiver who is older than 60 years (Heller et al., 2015). Studies have reported that older parents caring for adults with disabilities experience challenges and restrictions in their lives, such as lower employment levels, less social opportunities, and the physical impacts of care tasks (Baumbusch et al., 2017; Byram, 2018; Pryce et al., 2017; Vanier Institute, 2017). Parents of adult children with IDDs also often experience transitions in caregiving responsibilities and, over time, a potential relinquishing of care tasks as they age (Baumbusch et al., 2017; Byram, 2018; Pryce et al., 2017). They are also vulnerable to the effects of caregiver burden, which can have an impact on depression symptoms (Piazza et al., 2014). Supportive interventions such as strategies to reduce stress and build resilience are needed both for adults with complex care needs and for family caregivers as they age.

Nursing Role in Assessing and Supporting Family Caregivers

Because many family caregivers are unprepared for their roles, they are at risk for negative outcomes. The degree of risk is influenced by the context of caregiving that includes family history and dynamics, nature and extent of the care recipient's limitations (e.g., physical care needs, behavioral expressions), and personal and financial resources. Supporting family caregivers requires thorough assessment and tailored intervention in collaboration with the family caregiver (Messecar, 2020). Yet the support needs of family caregivers are not always assessed routinely.

Messecar (2020) recommends a partnership-based approach to care management that fully acknowledges the family caregiver as well as the care recipient. This approach is based on respectful two-way communication among providers, patients, and families in an environment where families and patients are comfortable asking questions and expressing different perspectives or opinions on treatments or goals of care. Nurses can engage in partnership-based care through active listening, advocating for family and patient participation in care discussions, and being transparent.

While assessment of family caregiving should be an ongoing process, it is particularly important for nurses to assess family both as client and as caregiver in relation to needs for education and support during times of change and transition across the life course. These transitions may be the result of changes in health, cognitive status or mobility, financial status, family or social support, or other situational changes. For example, family caregivers of persons with dementia may be in particular need of education and support at the time of initial diagnosis, when the intensity of care increases, and if residential-care placement is being considered (Budson & Solomon, 2016), as well as at the end of life. In the case of health- or illness-related changes, families are often the first to notice these changes and encourage their family member to seek assessment and care.

When nurses assess family caregiving situations, they tend to focus on tasks related to ADLs (bathing, dressing, eating, toileting, hygiene, and mobility) and IADLs (shopping, managing finances, meal preparation, driving, and managing medications). ADLs are useful for determining how much physical assistance a care recipient may need from the caregiver. IADLs may determine whether an individual can live independently in the community. For example, a person may have significant mobility problems, but if she or he has the ability to plan and direct care through execution of IADLs, it may be possible to remain at home. As Pusey-Murray and Miller (2013) report, assessments must go beyond a list of care recipient needs related to ADLs and IADLs because:

> [t]hose concepts do not adequately capture the complexity and stressfulness of caregiving. Assistance with bathing does not capture bathing a person who is resisting a bath. Helping with medications does not adequately capture the hassles of medication administration, especially when the care recipient is receiving multiple medications several times a day, including injections, inhalers, eye drops, and crushed tablets (p. 115).

Families are often very involved in helping older adults manage multiple and chronic illnesses. A recent report from NAC and AARP PPI (2018) estimated that 58% of family caregivers of adults over the age of 18 in the United States assist with "medical/nursing" tasks such as managing or administering multiple medications, including administering intravenous fluids, providing wound care and other treatments, or using medical devices or monitors. These activities were in addition to providing support with ADLs and IADLs. Nurses and other care providers must consider how families are supporting older adults and should initiate systematic and periodic assessments and interventions that address specific caregiver roles and tasks.

Domains to be included in assessments are context; caregiver perception of health and functional status of the care recipient; caregiver values and principles; well-being of the caregiver; consequences of caregiving, skills, abilities, and knowledge to provide care; and potential resources that the caregiver could choose to use (Messecar, 2020). A variety of caregiver assessment screening tools exist. The Preparedness for Caregiving Scale (Archbold et al., 1990; Zwicker, 2018) is a caregiver self-assessment instrument that asks caregivers to identify how well prepared they believe they are for multiple domains of caregiving. It provides a starting point for understanding caregiver needs related to both their care activities and their own health. The tool supports a relational approach to nursing care that can assist the nurse to prioritize communication with caregivers based on their unique needs (Mazenec et al., 2018). The Informal Caregivers of Older Adults at Home: Let's PREPARE! is often used on admission to home care by nurses performing a comprehensive, holistic assessment of the patient and her or his caregiver's ability to meet her or his needs safely in the home (Atkins et al., 2010). The nurse uses a checklist to identify tasks commonly required when caring for an older adult with a range of medical conditions. The checklist could be used to evaluate caregiver competence to monitor changes in condition or perform specific tasks such as wound care or medication administration. However, this tool does not address long-term consequences of caring for the caregiver. The Modified Caregiver Strain Index (Onega, 2008) facilitates screening for adverse effects of caregiving in multiple domains, including financial, physical, and psychological strain. Screening assessments should be applied periodically along the care trajectory. A summary of screening tools is presented in Table 17-1.

An additional and often overlooked domain of family caregiving assessment and support is

Table 17-1　Caregiver Assessment Tools	
ASSESSMENT TOOLS	**DESCRIPTION**
Preparedness for Caregiving Tool (Archbold et al., 1990; Zwicker, 2018)	Addresses the domains recommended by the family caregiver assessment and provides a starting point for understanding caregiver needs related to both their care activities and their own health.
Informal Caregivers of Older Adults at Home: Let's PREPARE! (Atkins et al., 2010)	Used to identify tasks commonly required when caring for an older adult with a range of medical conditions; could be used periodically to assess and monitor decline in condition. Limited to assessment of caregiving ability and patient condition rather than the impact on the caregiver such as strain or burnout.
The Modified Caregiver Strain Index (Onega, 2008)	Facilitates screening for adverse effects of caregiving in multiple domains, including financial, physical, and psychological strain.

planning for the future. As family caregivers age or their lives change in some way, they may need to relinquish some caregiving responsibilities to others (Byram, 2018). For example, in many cases, adults with complex chronic conditions (CCC's) and disabilities outlive their parents, who often act as primary caregivers, or at minimum as decision-making partners, long after the child reaches adulthood. Studies with family caregivers of adults with IDDs have demonstrated significant variation in the extent to which family caregivers planned for the future (Baumbusch et al., 2017; Pryce et al., 2017). For some, the future was at the forefront of their thoughts and anxieties as they considered the what-ifs; for others, the focus was on living in the present, or the topic was avoided as a coping mechanism. Yet, for many, the future was brought into sharp focus by acute events. While discussions of future planning appear to be more prevalent in research with adults with IDDs, such planning is equally important for all family caregiving roles. Therefore, it is imperative that nurses working with family caregivers assess the family's plans for the future and provide resources to support future planning.

In line with a life-course perspective and the Bioecological Systems Theory, interventions to support family caregivers should be considered at the individual, organizational, and systems levels (National Academies of Sciences, Engineering, and Medicine, 2016). Multiple individual-level interventions have been developed and tested to address the needs of family caregivers, both as clients and as providers of care. Types of interventions to support family caregivers are summarized in Table 17-2. Nurses, particularly in specialty and primary-care settings, are well positioned to integrate some of these individual-level interventions, such as coordinating services delivery, and providing anticipatory guidance, education, and resources to support families, into their practice. For example, families of persons with dementia often want to know what to anticipate and how to maximize their family member's physical and cognitive function and dignity as well as strategies for preventing and/or managing challenging behaviors. Families may also benefit from education and support in attending to environmental modifications to enhance safety and independence and how to manage their family

Table 17-2 Individual-Level Interventions to Support Family Caregivers	
TYPE OF INTERVENTION	**DESCRIPTION**
Education (Abrahams et al., 2018; Messecar, 2020; National Academies of Sciences, Engineering, and Medicine, 2016)	Interventions providing information about the family member's diagnosis and/or resources available for support.
Psychological/counseling (e.g., cognitive-behavioral therapy) (Abrahams et al., 2018; Messecar, 2020; National Academies of Sciences, Engineering, and Medicine, 2016)	Interventions focused on helping caregivers identify and modify beliefs related to the situation and develop new behaviors to cope with caregiving demands.
Support groups (Abrahams et al., 2018; Messecar, 2020; National Academies of Sciences, Engineering, and Medicine, 2016)	Group interventions led by a health care professional or family caregivers (peers) that create a space for sharing of concerns and successes and providing mutual support.
Self-care activities (Abrahams et al., 2018; National Academies of Sciences, Engineering, and Medicine, 2016)	Activities in which family caregivers participate with the aim of reducing stress and caring for their own body and mind. Some activities that show some promise in reducing stress include moderate-intensity exercise programs, yoga, and meditation.
Skill building (Abrahams et al., 2018; Messecar, 2020; National Academies of Sciences, Engineering, and Medicine, 2016)	Interventions aimed at building family caregivers' capacity in skills required to take care of their family member, including those related to ADLs and IADLs, nursing and medical tasks, and system navigation.
Respite (Messecar, 2020; National Academies of Sciences, Engineering, and Medicine, 2016)	In-home or day program services that provide activities and care for the family member to give the family caregiver a break.
Case/care management (Messecar, 2020)	Interventions that support family caregivers with coordination and management of their family member's care.
Multicomponent interventions (Abrahams et al., 2018; Messecar, 2020)	Interventions that involve two or more components, such as education and training, counseling, support groups, stress management, exercise, and environment modification.

member's care as needed. For more information on multicomponent interventions to support family caregivers, see the National Academies of Sciences, Engineering, and Medicine (2016) report.

In addition to individual-level assessments and interventions, it is essential that organizational and system-level programs, practices, and policies exist to support family caregivers (National Academies of Sciences, Engineering, and Medicine, 2016). For example, nurses can advocate at the organizational level for embedding programs and services to support family caregivers into organizational structures. This may include partnerships with organizations such as the Alzheimer's Association, which has chapters in many countries, as resources and to build programs to support family caregivers of persons with dementia. In addition, many interventions are not covered by health insurance (National Academies of Sciences, Engineering, and Medicine, 2016). Nurses are in an excellent position to connect caregivers to support resources and to advocate for policy changes that cover the needs of caregivers.

PUBLIC POLICIES RELATED TO AGING FAMILIES

In both the United States and Canada, family caregiving is a need that is largely unmet by public policies that support families and aging. The U.S. 1993 Family and Medical Leave Act (FMLA) enables some caregivers to take time off from work for their care responsibilities; the details of how this act is implemented vary by state. In Canada, employment insurance compassionate care benefits (Government of Canada, n.d.) guarantee unpaid, job-protected leave for up to 26 weeks to provide physical, emotional, or coordinating care to an older adult relative. Provinces vary in their implementation of this benefit (Government of Canada, n.d.). Under certain conditions in both the United States and Canada, family caregivers may be able to deduct care expenses from their income taxes.

Health Policy and Health Insurance

In the United States, older adults are eligible for Medicare at age 65. Medicare is the federal government's health insurance program for older adults and some younger people meeting specific disability criteria. Medicare coverage focuses on primary, acute, intensive, rehabilitative, and hospice services. Medicare does not cover custodial or nonskilled services, which are critical for families with aging adults who may no longer be able to care for themselves or those who may be experiencing cognitive decline, physical challenges, or medical instability.

Medicare coverage is complicated and does not cover all costs. It does cover portions of hospital and rehabilitation services, outpatient services, and prescription drugs. Some older adults have to purchase additional, supplemental insurance to address gaps in coverage. For assistance with navigating the complexities of Medicare, older adults and families have access to free Medicare counseling services through a federally funded state health insurance program (SHIP). The Affordable Care Act (ACA) provides several benefits to Medicare enrollees including no-copay screenings (e.g., mammography), annual wellness checks, and reduced prescription costs.

Medicaid is the shared federal-state government health insurance plan for eligible low-income adults, children, pregnant women, elderly adults, and adults with disabilities. Approximately 68.8 million people in the United States have Medicaid coverage (Medicaid, 2020). Older adults in need of long-term Medicaid services often have to "spend down" their resources and then qualify. Medicaid is a primary payer for long-term care for older adults. Some states have Medicaid waivers that allow older adults to use this benefit to pay for care in assisted-living, adult care homes, and other home- and community-based care programs.

Older adults who qualify for both Medicare and Medicaid are considered dual eligible. An innovative program for dual-eligible older adults is the Program of All Inclusive Care for the Elderly (PACE) (Centers for Medicare and Medicaid Services, 2020). PACE programs provide and coordinate all care services for enrollees through interdisciplinary care teams and close monitoring of each enrollee's health. PACE strives to keep enrollees living independently in their community despite often advanced comorbidities. Nurses have leadership roles in PACE as care and/or case managers; they run clinics, visit enrollees at home, and supervise other staff members in providing direct care to enrollees (Madden et al., 2014).

In Canada, the federal government's role in health care and health insurance involves setting and administering principles of the Canada Health Act, providing financial support to provinces and territories, and funding supplementary services (Government of Canada, 2019). The Canada Health Act establishes criteria such as provision of medically necessary hospital and physician services (although *medically necessary* is not defined in the Canada Health Act) that provinces and territories must follow in developing their health insurance plans in order to receive federal funding. The federal government is also responsible for direct service delivery for and with First Nations and Inuit populations and veterans for whom services are not available through their province or territory.

In contrast with the U.S. model of care, each province or territory in Canada is responsible for administering health services and insurance for their own residents, including older adults (Government of Canada, 2019). Basic provincial health insurance is provided to all residents who meet physical presence requirements regardless of income. This insurance typically covers only what that province defines as medically necessary, such as hospital stays, doctor's visits, and medically necessary tests, and generally does not cover pharmaceuticals, ambulance costs, rehabilitation, and hearing and vision care. Working adults often obtain supplemental health insurance through their employer or private insurance to cover services not covered by the basic provincial insurance. Most governments offer and fund some kind of supplementary benefits for older adults after retirement (Government of Canada, 2019).

ACUTE AND LONG-TERM SERVICES AND SUPPORTS FOR AGING FAMILIES

Acute Care

Although most nurses who work in acute care do not consider themselves gerontological nurses, a high proportion of acute-and critical-care patients are over age 65 (Balas et al., 2016). Older adults vary greatly in terms of their general health, cognitive abilities, and functional status; however, they are at risk for complex health conditions often referred to as geriatric syndromes. Some of those risks include frailty, incontinence, falls, cognitive impairment, functional impairment, diabetes, depression, delirium, and pressure ulcers (Chiu & Cheng, 2019). These conditions are not normal with aging and should not be considered a normal part of the aging process (Parke & Hunter, 2014). It is important for hospital-based nurses to be current in best practices to prevent, recognize, and manage geriatric conditions. These particular conditions are costly in terms of the impact on quality of life and functioning, care resources, complicating sequelae that lead to increased mortality and morbidity rates, and rehospitalization after discharge. In addition, older adults may present atypically, making it difficult to recognize early signs of infection or heart failure. Families and caregivers can help the nurse to identify the older adult patient's baseline condition, including any assistive devices (e.g., glasses, hearing aid, walker) or routines (e.g., sleeping) that are normal for the patient. Chapter 16 includes a more detailed discussion on family nursing in acute-care adult settings.

Models of Care

Models of care exist in some hospitals to prevent or minimize geriatric syndromes and facilitate a successful posthospital transition. Common features of these models include interdisciplinary communication, care planning that considers evidence-based gerontological practices, environmental modifications that enhance safety (e.g., lighting, sounds, layout of rooms), early and ongoing assessments that screen for risk factors, and patient and family-centered support for making treatment decisions that consider quality of life (Capezuti et al., 2016). Interdisciplinary discharge planning that represents collaboration among the members of the health care team, the patient, and the family strengthens the experience for patients as they experience transitions in care. The Acute Care for Elders unit (ACE unit) is a continuous quality improvement model of care that utilizes an interdisciplinary team educated in evidence-based care for older adults to work closely with patients and their families. Units are designed to accommodate age-related changes and support cognitive orientation as well as functional independence and mobility by the patient, along with family involvement. A body of research on ACE units demonstrates positive patient outcomes and reduced costs compared with non-ACE units (Palmer, 2018).

Another approach uses a geriatric-care consultation program to maximize health outcomes and minimize risks of geriatric syndromes and their sequela. With this model, an interdisciplinary team with geriatric expertise is available to consult for older adult patients and to make recommendations regarding hospital-based care as well as discharge plans (Deschodt et al., 2016). Finally, Nurses Improving Care for Healthsystem Elders (NICHE) is a nurse-led approach that emphasizes systemwide best practices in the care of older adults. NICHE promotes an environment and equipment that are particularly elder-friendly, evidence-based practice protocols in caring for older adults across all disciplines, use of geriatric resource nurses, and unit champions to develop gerontological competency for all staff members (Capezuti et al., 2016). Nurses have a critical role in advocating for elder-friendly and elder-competent care organizations and for educating families on the advantages of seeking out elder-friendly hospitals in their community.

Delayed discharge, also known in Canada as alternative level of care (ALC), is an issue that has grown rapidly in recent years. ALC refers to the situation in which a patient is medically cleared for discharge from acute care but remains in the hospital for reasons ranging from challenges with family care providers to availability of residential-care arrangements (Canadian Institute of Health Information, 2020; Kuluski et al., 2017). Patients whose discharge is delayed and who meet ALC criteria tend to be older adults, and many experience cognitive impairment and/or functional decline (Kuluski et al., 2017). Families of patients whose discharge is delayed and whose status has been designated as ALC may experience uncertainty about where to go for information about the transitional care process and about plans for placement (Everall et al., 2019; Kuluski et al., 2017). They may also express frustration and concern about time, attention, and care given to their loved one during this time and worry about social isolation (Kuluski et al., 2017). Nurses supporting families of patients whose discharge is delayed should encourage family involvement in decision making and promote ongoing collaboration with families to ensure that their concerns and patient-care needs are being met. While ALC has increasingly become a label applied to a patient in the acute-care setting, it is important for nurses to consider delayed discharge

as a systems issue. Additional research and policy work is needed to address the issue of delayed discharge and mitigate its impacts. Nurses working with aging families are well situated to lead and advocate for this work.

In all aspects of care of older adults, including hospitalization, it is important to emphasize that older adults vary significantly in their levels of independence, and family members vary in the nature of their relationship with an older adult. Hospitalization and the associated discharge transition may represent temporary family involvement in the older adult's life, or these events may be part of ongoing caregiving by families. Regardless, families are often asked to give input on treatment decisions and discharge planning. Families spend energy seeking information from myriad providers and struggle to get information on the transitional care plan, whether the plan is for discharge to home or to a care facility, and posthospitalization care needs of the older adult (Digby & Bloomer, 2014; Coleman et al., 2015). In the United States, the Caregiver Advise, Record, and Enable (CARE) Act (Coleman, 2016) acknowledges the significant role of families during hospitalization and transition and will hopefully lead to families feeling empowered and competent to support their older adult after discharge. Nurses are the providers most likely to be responsible for assessing families and providing needed resources, education, and referrals to maximize successful transition on discharge.

Long-Term Services and Supports

Long-term services and supports encompass a wide range of services, both paid and unpaid. Although the term *long-term care (LTC)* is sometimes used interchangeably with *nursing home care,* nursing homes represent only one type of LTC service. A variety of community-based care services are available, including in-home care, supportive housing, adult day care, and a range of residential-care settings. Our exploration of care settings begins with community-based care, where older adults receive care. Particular attention is given to care that is delivered by family members, volunteers, or unpaid caregivers, which occurs mostly in the older adult's or a family member's home. Next is a discussion of LTC in residential settings, such as assisted living, adult foster care, and nursing homes.

Home- and Community-Based Care

Most older adults live in community settings with no or minimal support to manage their personal and health needs. Nurses interact with older adults in a variety of settings, such as where they help them learn to manage chronic health problems or where they receive primary health care. Some older adults may also receive home visits from nurses for chronic-care support. A variety of home- and community-based programs have been developed to support the preference of older adults to remain in their homes. Many older adults and their families, however, have limited knowledge about what might be needed to continue living at home, the range of service options available in their communities, and how to access them. Health care professionals may also have limited knowledge about services outside their own agencies.

One of the major reasons older adults prefer to remain in their own homes is to maintain autonomy and control over their lives. Unfortunately, safety concerns among family members can make it challenging for older adults to remain autonomous. Nurses can play an important role in working with families to identify ways to balance safety and risk related to mobility and cognitive problems. Nurses can also help caregivers understand the normal aging process, including recognition of changes that should prompt an evaluation for potential problems. For example, nurses can teach caregivers and family members to recognize risk factors and early signs of delirium in order to ensure the safety of older adults in the home and community. When caregivers feel more capable and competent, they are more likely to address conditions quickly when they arise.

Technology: The use of technology in the home is a strategy to support autonomy and safety for older adults and to facilitate family caregiving. A range of technological innovations can support older adults to age in place in their home and facilitate family caregiving. Assistive technologies include devices to help older adults with personal ADLs and IADLs, such as programmable pill boxes; utensils that prevent spills by accommodating hand tremors (e.g., Google spoon); smart hearing aids that adjust to external conditions; a wearable, invisible exoskeleton that stabilizes gait even on stairs; online assistants that support bill paying;

and sensors that turn off unused stove burners (Jordan et al., 2016).

Telehealth applications can monitor and generate physiologic trend data and enable providers to adjust treatments accordingly without requiring an office visit. Telecare via phone, Internet, or video interactions uses physiologic data to trigger emergency responders or phone contact by providers through sensors. For example, sensing technology is being increasingly used to detect falls and fall risk for older adults at home (Liu et al., 2016). Phone, videoconferencing, and e-mail communications between providers and older adults already supplement some face-to-face visits. These applications have particular relevance for aging adults in rural and frontier regions.

Technology applications have significant implications for family caregivers, particularly if they do not live with the older adult (Lindeman et al., 2020). Families often use video chat technologies, such as Skype or Facetime, and other technologies for social interactions that provide visual as well as auditory information about the care recipient, and some older adults enjoy ongoing contact with friends to play games or chat via the internet. Interactive technologies may be valuable in reducing social isolation and improving social engagement with family and friends (Hung et al., 2020; Jordan et al., 2016; Lindeman et al., 2020), although further research is needed, especially in light of the COVID-19 pandemic.

Physical, social, and economic challenges exist to integrating technology as a support mechanism for older adults living in the community. Some electronic devices are not user-friendly for people with conditions that impair vision or fine motor dexterity. Older adults with limited internet or smartphone experience may need help envisioning how technologies may have a positive impact on their health or lives. However, there is increasingly strong evidence for technology as a way to improve quality of life and support care for the expanding population of older adults around the world (Centre for Policy on Ageing, 2020). Nurses can assist patients and families to use technologies by educating them on the features that make equipment user-friendly for older adults, how to support older adults and their families in using technologies and interpreting transmitted data, and how to sustain interdisciplinary teams in ways that maximize provider-patient/family caregiving relationships. It is also imperative that nurses consider issues of accessibility and patient privacy in the use of these technologies in home and residential-care settings (Lindeman et al., 2020).

Age-Friendly Communities

Increasingly, communities are considering ways to support aging adults. WHO's (2018) Global Network of Age-friendly Cities and Communities identified eight domains of livability that affect the quality of life for older adults:

- Domain 1: Outdoor Spaces and Buildings
- Domain 2: Transportation
- Domain 3: Housing
- Domain 4: Social Participation
- Domain 5: Respect and Social Inclusion
- Domain 6: Civic Participation and Employment
- Domain 7: Communication and Information
- Domain 8: Community and Health Services

An age-friendly community is one that allows people to engage in activities safely and with respect, regardless of their age (Council on Aging of Central Oregon, 2020). The community prioritizes opportunities for older adults to connect with the people that are important to them while remaining as independent as possible in their local community. In addition, WHO (2020a) describes age-friendly environments as being free from physical and social barriers and supported by policies, systems, services, products, and technologies that promote physical and mental health across the life span and enable people to continue to do the things they value, even as they experience changes in their functional status. Age-friendly practices help people meet their basic needs; allow people to learn, grow, and make decisions; provide accessible transportation to enhance mobility; help people maintain relationships in their community; and contribute to the overall well-being of the community (WHO, 2020a). Key features of age-friendly communities are listed in Table 17-3.

In Canada, several provinces have launched age-friendly initiatives, including the Province of Manitoba's Age-friendly Initiative, Age Friendly Manitoba, which builds on WHO's Healthy Aging Framework. The Manitoba Age-friendly Initiative is a comprehensive, multifaceted approach that prioritizes public policy as a primary approach to addressing the needs of a growing senior population (Age Friendly Manitoba, n.d.). Recent evaluation studies in Canada have demonstrated an association between age-friendliness and life satisfaction and self-perceived health (Davern et al., 2020; Menec & Nowicki, 2014; Orpana et al., 2016). An initial long-term, mixed-methods study was conducted in five communities in Canada, when researchers analyzed the key components of age-friendly communities and assessed their association with positive health outcomes, social participation, and health equity (Levasseur et al., 2017). The current goal is to continue to build on new and existing collaborations while generating evidence to help communities promote age-friendly policies, services, and structures that foster positive health, social participation, and health equity at the population level (Levasseur et al., 2017).

Residential-Care Settings

Residential-care options include assisted living, board and care homes, continuing-care retirement communities, and home-care services. In both the United States and Canada, states or provinces regulate these settings, although nursing homes are also federally regulated in the United States.

Financing for these services is primarily the individual's responsibility in the United States and Canada. In the United States, Medicare provides limited coverage for short-term rehabilitation in a nursing home, and private health insurance may provide no coverage. Long-term care insurance is another option that is available in the United States; however, these policies can be expensive and provide limited coverage. The majority of older adults in the United States do not have a long-term care insurance policy. Continuing-care retirement communities include elements of both independent living and supportive care provided through home care, assisted living, and/or skilled nursing services. Each setting has its own set of eligibility criteria for admission or discharge, minimal educational requirements for the staff members, staff–client ratios, and care service requirements.

Families continue to be integrally involved and nurses play a vital role in assessing residents, managing and coordinating care with an interprofessional team, ensuring that the facility complies with regulations, ensuring ongoing quality improvement, and advocating for older adults and their families.

Table 17-3	**Key Features of Age-Friendly Communities**	
Age-friendly services (AARP, 2020; Council on Aging of Central Oregon, 2020; State of California, Equity in Aging Resource Center, 2021)	Services and resources for aging adults: • Accessible transportation options • Caregiving services and support • Community meals • Dental resources • Educational programs • Engagement and outreach programs • Equity support • Family caregiver support • Home-care services • Housing programs • Legal services • Meals on Wheels (home meal delivery) • Medicare and Medicaid counseling • Nutritional services
Age-friendly communities (WHO, 2007; 2020a)	Policies, services, and structures that support aging actively: • Outdoor spaces and buildings are safe and provide accessibility to community members. • Transportation opportunities are accessible, affordable, and reliable. • Housing is sufficient, affordable, safe, and accessible. • Activities and social participation opportunities are inclusive, affordable, and accessible. • Civic participation and employment opportunities are provided. • Public communication with community members is basic and effective for persons across the life span; information is accessible and relevant. • Community and health services are safe, accessible, and advertised openly; economic and social barriers are minimized; community emergency services consider the vulnerabilities of persons across the life span. • Access to healthy food and recreational activities.

Assisted Living and Adult Foster Homes

Assisted-living facilities were developed to provide a homelike option for older adults that provides a social model of care. The model is supportive because older adults transition between living independently and requiring a higher level of care. Assisted living is often viewed positively by older adults and their families. Designed for aging adults who are no longer able to manage living independently, assisted-living facilities can assist people with daily activities such as bathing or dressing, without the 24-hour care that a long-term care facility would provide (AARP, 2019). The cost of assisted living is lower than nursing home care and thus provides an accessible option for some families.

The services provided by assisted-living facilities vary widely, from simple medication reminders to personal care for activities of daily living, to more supportive care for individuals who may be experiencing dementia. Typically, services are available 24 hours per day and include meal preparation with modified special diets, assistance with personal care, housekeeping and laundry, transportation, and medication management. Each state or province has its own definitions and regulations that influence how assisted living is implemented.

Depending on the unique circumstances of the adult who is aging, the time may come when he or she requires additional care and support beyond what the adult can receive in the assisted-living facility. As their needs change, older adults may be required to transition to a higher level of care in a nursing home or adult foster home. Adult foster homes have become more common in certain states, including Colorado, Hawaii, and Oregon; they provide a higher level of care in a homelike environment (Paying for Senior Care, 2020). Adult foster homes are often managed by caregivers who have committed to caring for seniors in private homes in the community. In most cases, coverage is private pay or Medicaid. When working with older adults and their families, it is critical that they understand the characteristics of assisted living or adult foster homes related to admission and discharge criteria; staffing qualifications, including nursing presence; and available services so they can make informed decisions.

The role of nurses in residential settings is evolving and expanding. It is as variable as are the models of assisted living, in part because residents are generally less disabled and the availability of nursing services is lower than in nursing homes. Some assisted-living communities include full- or part-time registered nurses as part of their staff, some do not employ nurses, and still others contract with nurses to provide assessment of residents' health and self-care needs and other services (Madden et al., 2014). It is quite common for nurses to work with primary-care providers to perform admission assessments to ensure that residents meet the criteria for assisted living related to their functional status and personal-care needs; communicate with residents and families to help them understand what services and care are available; and participate in developing plans of care, including needed medical services. When nurses function in a consultation role, they are not direct supervisors of staff members and need to consider different strategies to encourage staff members to adopt their recommendations for care. Nurses have a primary role for staff education and the delegation of nursing tasks in certain states that permit delegating nursing tasks to unlicensed staff members. They educate staff members on what to expect when caring for residents, the importance of implementing evidence-based practices, their role in advocating for residents and families, and the value of establishing long-term, trusting relationships. Nurses also work in collaboration with staff members to monitor residents for changes in condition, communicate with providers regarding

resident status, and engage in ongoing communication with nurses from home health or hospice agencies who visit specific residents.

Nursing Homes

Although a very small proportion of older adults live in nursing homes, the likelihood that older adults may spend time in a skilled nursing facility has increased in recent years because of shortened hospital stays and the need for support during rehabilitation and recovery from surgery and acute illness. The costs of nursing home care are significant and are paid directly by the resident unless they qualify for Medicaid in the United States. The transition to a nursing home represents considerable losses for an older adult, including loss of health, privacy, independence, choice, quality of life, and autonomy. Depending on their circumstances, they may also be displaced from a partner or other loved ones.

Nurses historically have played major roles in nursing home care, but similar to their counterparts in assisted living, their role is evolving and expanding in these settings. Care is increasingly complex, and residents in skilled and rehabilitation units resemble hospitalized patients of the not-too-distant past. Similar to assisted living, nursing home nurses must be able to work independently, assume leadership roles, and possess strong assessment and prioritizing skills. They must be able to work effectively and collaboratively on interdisciplinary teams consisting of direct-care workers; administrators; other staff members who support residents (e.g., social services, rehabilitation, dietary); and other providers who may not be on staff but are critical to the well-being of residents, such as hospice teams, physicians, pharmacists, options counselors, and other home- and community-based care providers.

Many nurses are participating in efforts to promote culture change care in residential-care settings. Person- and family-centered care is consistent with nursing values because nursing strives to individualize care and put the individual and his or her family ahead of the task. Elements of quality care include individualized care; therapeutic communication; seeking understanding of the person, her or his family, and her or his experience; facilitating autonomy and personal choice; providing comfort care; and including family members in decision making.

Family Involvement in Residential-Care Settings

Contrary to prevailing myths, many families remain connected with their older members once they move into facility-based care and often do not cease providing care, although the nature of that care is typically different (Puurveen et al., 2018). Decades of research in nursing homes reveal that family members continue to visit and provide socioemotional support, and, in some cases, personal care and care management after transition into a nursing facility (Baumbusch & Phinney, 2014; Omori et al., 2019; Puurveen et al., 2018). Families typically desire to work in partnership with facility staff, whether to provide care, make decisions, or provide social support (Puurveen et al., 2018). Nurses, other staff members, and organizational- and system-level policies can inadvertently set up barriers that decrease the ability of family members to participate in the life of the resident, such as by limiting visiting hours, limiting family knowledge or involvement in care, or discounting or discouraging family knowledge or input into care decisions (Omori et al., 2019; Puurveen et al., 2018).

Researchers exploring the experiences of families and nursing home staff members have highlighted numerous tensions in negotiating care relationships in these settings. Such studies have highlighted tensions around blurred boundaries between the roles of families and staff members in terms of monitoring changes in resident status (Puurveen et al., 2018). Families are key resources with respect to individuals' history, likes and dislikes, personality, routines, and what is and has been important to them (Baumbusch & Phinney, 2014; Puurveen et al., 2018). This knowledge is critical, particularly when residents are living with dementia and cannot clearly communicate this information themselves. Family members can provide insight into resident actions, which in turn can help staff members respond more quickly to resident needs as conveyed through their behavior.

While many families hold vast knowledge of their family member and are often able to notice subtle changes in their status, staff members may also feel that they are being observed, or surveilled, by family members and that their care is under constant scrutiny. Staff members may also sometimes feel like they need to provide social and emotional support for residents whose families are less present, which can contribute to conflict and stress

for them. Family involvement in personal care, for example, may be spurred by a desire to help the staff; other times, it may be due to a concern about quality of care (Puurveen et al., 2018). Tensions were also noted in how involvement in decision making was negotiated and how the knowledge of staff members and families was valued. Hierarchical and one-way communication structures can easily leave families feeling disempowered and disconnected from their family member's care, even when staff members felt like they were communicating well (Baumbusch & Phinney, 2014; Omori et al., 2019).

Research has highlighted the importance of fostering inclusive spaces for families in residential-care settings. While there is often little agreement in the literature and in practice on how families should be involved, Puurveen et al. (2018) articulated several key principles for fostering inclusive spaces for families. Family involvement should be founded on a relationship grounded in mutual respect and recognition, not just one-way communication or privileging of one type of knowledge. Nurses working with families in residential care, and arguably all settings, should also recognize the ways in which families are involved in care work or not, and how these care relationships are influenced by relationships that have been developed throughout the life course (Puurveen et al., 2018).

Family nurses can play a key role in fostering these inclusive spaces through micro- and macro-level strategies. Developing a successful relationship begins before a resident is admitted, when a family member makes an initial visit to the facility (Barken & Lowndes, 2018). In addition to evaluating the physical environment, families often consider the quality of care provided and whether they can trust the staff to become partners in caring for their family member (Barken & Lowndes, 2018). During the pretransition phase, nurses are in a unique position to provide guidance and resources on types of residential-care options and how to evaluate prospective facilities. Two resources for families in the United States are the Medicare website, Nursing Home Compare, which uses a five-star system to rate facilities on specific quality indicators, and the Centers for Medicare and Medicaid guide, *Your Guide to Choosing a Nursing Home or Other Long-Term Care Services.* State and provincial offices that regulate regional nursing homes can also provide recent survey information on quality of care. In the United States, each state also has an ombudsman service that can provide information on complaints that have been received about specific facilities. In Canada, some provinces, such as British Columbia, have a seniors advocate office that monitors seniors' care and issues across the province. Nurses and other staff members can strengthen the staff-family partnership through communication, making family members feel comfortable and welcome, and providing assurance that the staff is competent and providing good care (Barken & Lowndes, 2018).

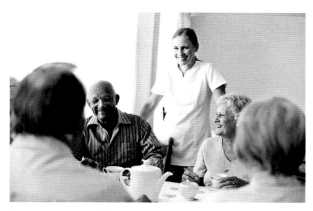

Source: © istock.com/Morsa Images

During the family member's time in residential care, ongoing, adequate, and honest communication and collaborative relationships are a priority. Communication should go beyond sharing information with families to include dialogue that values family knowledge and promotes family involvement in care and decision making (Barken & Lowndes, 2018; Omori et al., 2019). While nurses play a significant role in fostering inclusive environments for families in residential care, their efforts must also be supported by policies at the organizational and system levels. As Puurveen et al. (2018) suggested, organizational policies that formalize the rights and roles of families could go a long way in fostering inclusive environments. This is important to consider in light of the COVID-19 pandemic, which resulted in families being barred from entering facilities for long periods. The full extent of the impact of these pandemic policies is not yet fully understood. At the systems level, family nursing scholars have suggested that the current policy framings of family involvement as

a solution can actually lead to limiting family involvement in nursing home settings. In contrast, reframing policies to view family involvement as a policy challenge rather than a solution has the potential to lead to policies that are more inclusive of families and that promote greater valuing of family care work in these settings (Baumbusch & Phinney, 2014; Puurveen et al., 2018).

Palliative Care and End-of-Life Care for Aging Adults

Palliative care improves the quality of life of aging adults and their families who are experiencing challenges with life-limiting illness. Worldwide, an estimated 40 million people need palliative care, yet only about 14% of people are currently receiving it (WHO, 2020b). The need for palliative care will continue to increase as populations age and as the burden of chronic disease continues to rise. Palliative care is aimed at providing supportive care to patients and their families using a wide range of services delivered by a diverse team of interdisciplinary professionals, including medical providers, nurses, social workers, pharmacists, chaplains, physical therapists, caregivers, and more. Patients receiving palliative care may be receiving curative treatments and therapies concurrently. The goal of palliative care is to relieve suffering through early identification and skilled assessment; ongoing treatment of pain and other symptoms; and a holistic approach to the needs of the aging adult and their family, including physical, psychosocial, and spiritual needs (WHO, 2020b).

Hospice or end-of-life care is often associated with a location or formal model of care; however, it is also a philosophy of care provided at the end of life. It is designed to address the individual's and family's needs during the terminal or advanced phase of illness when curative interventions are no longer appropriate. Hospice care is delivered in the home setting of the individual, including assisted-living, residential-care, and LTC settings. The goal of hospice care is to provide comfort and dignity for the person living with the illness and the best quality of life for the person for the remainder of her or his life, as well as offering support for their family (Canadian Hospice Palliative Care Association, 2020).

Residents in long-term care facilities who are experiencing chronic illness are ideally suited for palliative care; however, it may be not be utilized for a variety of reasons. There may be confusion among providers and within communities about the meaning and availability of palliative-care support. The similarities and differences between palliative care and hospice care may be confusing to providers, facility staff members, and families, which may delay discussions about care until the individual is nearing the end of life. Nurses who work with aging adults and their families can influence the quality of life for people experiencing life-limiting illness and can reduce suffering by performing skilled assessment of symptoms, advocating for palliative care and end-of-life interventions with providers, engaging interdisciplinary team members in resident-care plans, and educating staff and family members as individuals experience changes in condition.

Another critical aspect of palliative care is working with older adults and their families to prepare advance directives, such as a durable power of attorney for health care or a living will. The process of preparing these documents provides an opportunity to discuss and understand values and preferences to guide decisions when the older adult is not able to communicate directly. Advance directives provide guidance regarding what treatments the individual wants and does not want. Besides advance care planning, in the United States there is a trend to endorse use of physician orders for life-sustaining treatments (POLST) or medical orders for life-sustaining treatments (MOLST) with adults who are seriously ill or for whom death would not be unexpected. POLST converts patient wishes to actual medical orders that facilitate these wishes. Physicians and/or nurse practitioners complete POLST after reviewing and discussing the advance care plan with the patient and/or his or her surrogate decision maker. POLST is a legally binding medical order that applies across medical settings to guide care by emergency responders in emergency departments and other settings, including assisted living and nursing homes. Currently, every state has either adopted some form of POLST or has active legislation to finalize a version of POLST, and regulations vary by state (National POLST, 2020). Refer to Chapter 11 for a more in-depth discussion on working with individuals and families in palliative and end-of-life care.

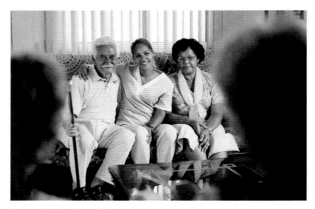

Source: © istock.com/diego_cervo

Case Study: Hooper Family

This case study about the Hooper family uses the life-course perspective to explore transitions that families experience as family members age. Maria Hooper and her family's experience illustrate the intersection of families with the health care system. Figure 17-1 depicts the Hooper family genogram,

Maria, age 60, is the oldest of four siblings. She has two brothers, James and Paul, and a sister, Ruth. Maria always counts Jane as her sister, too. Jane is a year younger than Maria and is the daughter of one of her mother's closest friends. When Jane needed a home as a young teenager, Maria's parents, Sarah and Louis, took her in, and Jane lived with them for 5 years. She and Maria became especially close, and now Jane and her family participate in all Maria's and her extended family's gatherings.

Sarah, age 82, and Louis, age 84, have lived in their community since their marriage 60 years earlier. They enjoy good health, except for Sarah's arthritis and mild hearing loss, and Louis's diabetes and hypertension, which are well controlled. They experience no limitations in ADLs, although both complain that it takes them longer to get things done. Still, they both volunteer for several different organizations and spend time with their friends. Maria lives 40 miles away from her parents, closer than the rest of her siblings. Maria and her parents talk on the phone about twice a week and they get together for dinner every couple of weeks.

Case Study: Hooper Family—cont'd

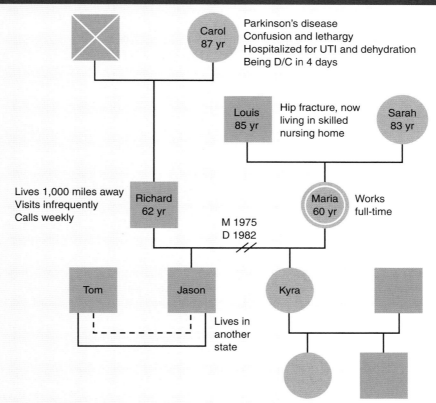

FIGURE 17-1 Hooper Family Genogram

Maria was divorced when her children, Jason and Kyra, were in elementary school. She still maintains connections with her ex-mother-in-law, Carol, who is now 87 years old. Carol has been widowed for 40 years. When Maria and her husband were divorced, Carol was determined that she would not lose contact with her grandchildren because she had seen that happen with some of her friends. Maria had always been on good terms with Carol and felt that it was important that her children know their paternal grandmother, so both Maria and Carol made the effort to maintain contact. Carol lived about an hour away, but Maria and her children would spend at least one Saturday a month with her until the children entered high school and were involved with multiple activities. Their visits became more sporadic, but Carol would come and watch her grandchildren's games and music concerts whenever she could.

When Carol was diagnosed with Parkinson's disease about 10 years ago, Maria became part of a community support system. Her role was to visit every two weeks, purchase groceries, and do some housekeeping. In addition to Parkinson's disease, Carol began to have problems with her memory and could no longer live alone. With some reluctance, she moved into an assisted-living residence in her community. Maria has continued to visit her every two weeks and communicates with the assisted-living staff and Carol at least once per week by phone. Carol usually knows Maria, but she sometimes forgets that Maria is divorced from her son. They mostly reminisce about the grandchildren.

Maria's life is quite busy. She is the office manager of a small business; in addition to her parents and mother-in-law, Maria is also involved in her children's lives. Jason and his partner live several hundred miles away, but Maria talks with him every couple of weeks. Maria often spends her vacations with them. Kyra is married and has two children of her own. Because Kyra lives close, Maria frequently babysits and delights in having each child spend the night about once a month. Maria enjoys being a grandparent, but she feels badly for her sister, Ruth, who has had sole responsibility for raising her own grandchildren for the past 2 years.

(continued)

Case Study: Hooper Family—cont'd

Discussion

Maria's family is reflective of many older families. At 60 years, Maria is part of the postwar baby boom and, similar to many in her generation, she has several siblings who represent potential support systems for both Maria and her parents. This includes Jane, who has a close and family-like relationship with Maria and her parents. Typical for most families, Maria lives relatively close to her parents and is in regular contact with them. Generally, they have a good relationship, characterized by affection, a history of mutual exchanges of help, and many shared values. Maria and her children are especially close to her parents because her parents provided considerable support when Maria was going through her divorce. Support included temporary housing, child care, and some financial assistance. Now, Sarah and Louis (Maria's parents) are close to becoming the older generation, that is, those older than 85 years. They are independent, engaged in their community, and consider themselves in good health. At the same time, both have several chronic illnesses that could cause them problems in the future. Maria's former mother-in-law, Carol, has not been as fortunate. She was widowed in her forties and has lived alone since her son grew up and left home. Her activities have been limited for many years because of Parkinson's disease and more recently because of cognitive impairment. She has resided for several years in an assisted-living facility that accepts Medicaid clients.

Transition 1—Louis From Home to the Hospital

Sarah (now age 83) spent most of the day at a friend's house. When she returned home about 4 p.m., she found her husband, Louis (age 85), on the floor in the garage. He told her that he tripped on the stairs while carrying a chair that needed repair; this occurred about 9:30 a.m. He tried to get up or crawl up the three steps from the attached garage to the kitchen, but he could not move because the pain was too great. Sarah called 911, and Louis was taken to the emergency department. Fortunately, it was a relatively uncomplicated fracture of his hip. He was able to have a surgical repair the next morning. Because he experienced some confusion after surgery, the nurses were reluctant to give him pain medication, believing the medication would cause more confusion. He started physical therapy the day after surgery but could participate only to a limited extent because of the pain. He was also started on insulin to control his diabetes (he previously took an oral medication).

Louis's needs are common. As an older adult, Louis was at a greater risk for falls and related injuries even though he did not have other risk factors. Hospital care by those unfamiliar with the needs of older adults can exacerbate rather than prevent negative outcomes. For example, knowing that untreated pain can increase confusion and delay successful rehabilitation is important for nurses.

Transition 2—Louis From the Hospital to a Skilled Nursing Facility

After 4 days in the hospital, Louis was discharged to the skilled care unit of a nursing home for additional rehabilitation, with the goal of returning to his own home. The timing of the discharge came as a surprise to Sarah and Maria, giving them little time to visit and select a skilled nursing facility or for other siblings to arrive from out of town to provide support. Fortunately, Sarah and Louis had friends who had had a good experience in a skilled nursing facility that was located about 30 minutes away, and it had space available. Maria stopped by to look at it and thought it would work. At the skilled nursing facility, Louis's pain was finally controlled, and he was eager to begin physical and occupational therapy so that he could go home. Although attention was focused on Louis, it was important to pay attention to his caregivers and conduct an assessment to determine their strengths and needs. Sarah needed support to bring Louis home as quickly and successfully as possible. (See Figure 17-2 for the Hooper family ecomap.) One spouse's response to stress affects the way the other spouse experiences stress. During this transitional period, it was important to be cognizant of the stress levels and needs of both Sarah and Louis. For example, nurses and others helped them consider changing their home environment to prevent future falls and provided instruction in managing Louis's pain while his hip healed. Louis's diabetes had to be monitored and assessed to determine whether he would continue to need insulin injections or be able to return to managing the disease through oral medications.

Sarah was not included in the transition planning, and Louis would be likely to spend a longer time in the skilled nursing facility or return home without sufficient support. Without support, Sarah was likely to experience greater levels of stress and caregiver burden in her expanded role as caregiver. Because of her hearing loss, Sarah did not always understand what the physician, nurses, and other staff members told her. Maria noticed that providers tended to treat her mother as if she had dementia and often did not include her in conversations. Therefore, Maria felt the need to be present as much as possible. Caregiver assessment also needed to include Maria because her caregiving responsibilities had also increased. She missed a lot of work, was worried

Case Study: Hooper Family—cont'd

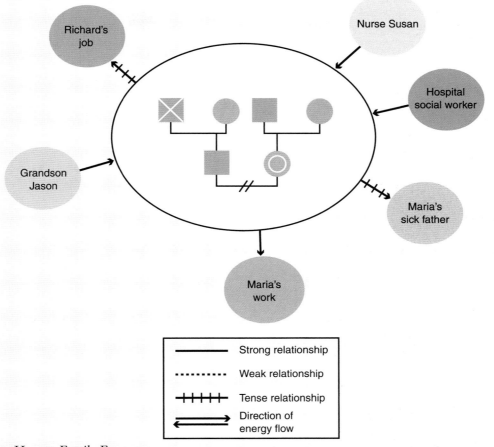

FIGURE 17-2 Hooper Family Ecomap

about losing her job, and could not afford to take more time off. She also felt torn because she still wanted to be available to support Carol as much as she did before. She was able to continue to stay in touch with Carol while Louis was in the hospital and skilled nursing care, but she also realized that Louis needed more support when he returned home. Fortunately, nurses at the skilled nursing facility were aware of these constraints and were able to arrange a care conference with Louis, Sarah, and Maria after regular business hours to begin planning for Louis's discharge home. Maria and her parents were aware that Medicare was funding rehabilitation services, but they were surprised to learn that these benefits would run out sooner if Louis did not keep progressing toward independence.

Transition 3—Louis From the Skilled Nursing Facility to Home
Once again, discharge came quickly, with little time to locate a home health care agency. The discharge coordinator at the skilled nursing facility provided a list of agencies, and Maria selected one. The therapists at the skilled nursing facility gave Sarah and Maria a list of adaptive devices (e.g., raised toilet seat, grabber, elastic shoestrings, a device to help Louis put on his socks, walker) to purchase before Louis's discharge. Because Louis still qualified for Medicare services, he was able to see a physical therapist, an occupational therapist, and a nurse once a week at home. These three providers collaborated to complete a home safety assessment to identify potential risks and strategies to eliminate or reduce the risks. A home health care worker also came to the house to assist with Louis's shower twice a week.

(continued)

Case Study: Hooper Family—cont'd

The social worker at the nursing facility had suggested that the family contact a resource center for seniors' services that was available in their local community. A support specialist from the center met with the family in the nursing facility and again once Louis was home. She was able to provide information about services beyond those provided by the home health agency. Once Medicare benefits ran out, she provided them information about home-care workers. Sarah and Louis hired a worker to continue to help him with showers and to do a little light housekeeping, which they paid for themselves. The support specialist also identified an organization that put a grab bar in the shower and, if needed in the future, could build a ramp into the house. Maria tried to help where she could, although between work, her grandchildren, and trying to still be there for Carol, she was able to help Sarah only on Saturdays. Even with this support, Sarah was exhausted, so the support specialist helped arrange for home-delivered meals. With time, Louis recovered; although he used a cane, he resumed most of his community activities. His diabetes was once again managed through diet and oral medications, and Sarah soon decided that they no longer needed the home-care worker and meals. They kept the phone number of the options counselor on their refrigerator in case they needed assistance in the future.

Questions for reflection on the nursing care of the Hooper family:

1. Reflect on the strengths and challenges that exist for the Hooper family experiencing transitions in care. What concerns do you have for Sarah and Louis now that they are independent in their home again?
2. What strategies can the nurse prioritize for providing a family-centered approach to care in this situation?
3. Now that Louis's condition has stabilized, are there other family members that may be at risk for health issues or support needs?
4. What recommendations can the nurse make for resources in the community that would support the family?

Case Study: James Family

Background

Setting

Raul James is a 46-year-old disabled man who lives with his 75-year-old mother in a small, rural community in Washington State. Raul suffered a severe brain injury due to a choking accident when he was a toddler. He has developmental and physical disabilities that affect his ability to live independently.

Family Members

Raul and his mother identify as Hispanic, speak English, and occasionally attend the Catholic church in their community with extended family members. Raul's father died approximately 5 years ago. He has a 50-year-old sister and two nephews, and a 48-year-old brother and two nieces who live in different states. He was close to both sets of grandparents who are all deceased. He has multiple extended family members, including aunts, uncles, cousins, and a few close family friends. Some of them live in the same community. See the James family genogram depicted in Figure 17-3.

The James Family Story

Raul's parents were married for many years, but they were divorced when he was in his teens. Even after their divorce, Raul's parents spent holidays and family time with Raul, his siblings, and their grandchildren. His father struggled with alcoholism and bipolar disorder but did his best to support and care for Raul whenever he could. Raul's parents struggled for many years following the trauma of his choking accident and subsequent brain injury. They grieved heavily and struggled to cope with the impact on the family.

Raul receives a monthly social security disability payment and has held several volunteer jobs in the community over the years. His favorite job was at a local grocery store that is no longer in business. He currently volunteers at a local library for a few hours a month and occasionally at a local food bank to help with stocking shelves. He is dependent on assistance for transportation. He walks independently but frequently loses his balance and falls when he is out in public; therefore, it is best for him to attend his volunteer position when accompanied by a personal caregiver that is provided by his Medicaid benefit. The caregiver also assists

Case Study: James Family—cont'd

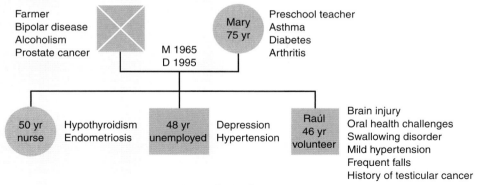

James Family Genogram

FIGURE 17-3 James Family Genogram

with some meal prep, transportation, and stand-by assistance for his daily shower. The caregiver is scheduled a few days a week so his mother can have some respite. See the James family ecomap in Figure 17-4.

Hobbies: Raul

Raul has an active schedule of personal hobbies. He has a passion for movies and TV series. He collects movies, builds model cars on his kitchen table, listens to books on tape, and shops at Walmart and the dollar store. With help from his caregiver, he enjoys baking cookies and banana bread. Raul loves to laugh and has a great sense of humor. He values his privacy, but he also enjoys socializing and going out to the movies. Depending on the weather and transportation, he occasionally complains that he has to stay at home too much. He is at risk for social isolation.

Health Challenges: Raul

Raul was treated for testicular cancer 15 years ago. He had surgery followed by radiation treatment and has been disease-free since that time. For the first 10 years, he saw his oncologist every 6 months for follow-up and monitoring. Raul has challenges with his oral health, which is exacerbated by a sensitive gag reflex (swallowing disorder), possibly a result of his previous choking accident. He often refuses to brush his teeth or allow anyone else to brush them. Every 6 months he has to have general anesthesia to have his teeth cleaned and dental care provided. He has also been diagnosed with mild hypertension but refuses to take medication for this due to challenges with swallowing. He has frequent falls, which often result in broken skin and bruises. A few times, he needed stiches over his eye and on his elbow due to skin lacerations from falls. He has also suffered broken ribs due to falls. He often refuses stand-by assistance for walking, insists on being independent, and does not have the balance needed to use an assistive device. His risk for falls and injury is high.

Health Challenges: Raul's Mother Mary

Raul's mother Mary has chronic health issues including diabetes, hypertension, and asthma. She has recently had mobility challenges due to arthritis in her joints. She has struggled for many years to manage her diabetes and has concerns that she could develop long-term complications from the disease. She is not physically active and struggles to maintain a healthy, balanced diet. She recently retired from her job as a preschool teacher and drives herself and Raul around the community. When they go shopping at Walmart or the grocery store, she waits for Raul in the car and he manages on his own. Mary is reluctant to ask for help from extended family and friends who offer to assist her. They rarely have visitors in the home besides the personal caregiver, who comes to the home approximately three times a week. They often delay asking for assistance with home improvements that will enhance their safety in the home.

Situation

During an outing to the local laundromat, Mary suffered an acute injury and has been hospitalized for treatment. According to Mary, she and Raul have been going out of the house on weekends to do their laundry. Mary reported that the washer and dryer in their home have been out of order for several months. As they were leaving the laundromat and Mary was loading the laundry

(continued)

Case Study: James Family—cont'd

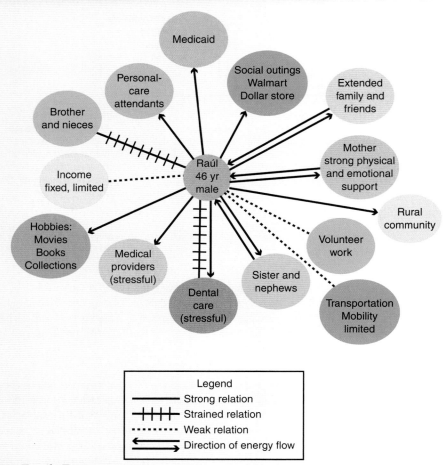

FIGURE 17-4 James Family Ecomap

into the car, Raul took a fall over a curb in the parking lot. When Mary rushed to assist him, she slipped in the rain and also fell to the ground. Raul was able to get to his feet and ask someone in the parking lot for assistance, and this person summoned the clerk at the laundromat. The clerk called 911, and the ambulance arrived within minutes to transport Mary to the hospital. She immediately reported pain and could not stand or tolerate being assisted to her feet. Because Raul was unable to drive himself home, he rode in the ambulance with Mary to the hospital. At the time, Mary declined the offer by the emergency services staff to call a family member or friend to assist with Raul.

Upon arrival to the local emergency room, Mary was having an asthma attack and struggling to breathe, which was possibly exacerbated by anxiety and pain. While she was in the ambulance, she had tried to locate her rescue inhaler, but it was not in her purse or her pockets. Two emergency department nurses got her settled into a room, took her vital signs, and administered oxygen and a nebulizer treatment. The nurses also got Raul settled into the waiting area and began collecting Mary's health and medication history. When Mary was seen by the physician, pain medication, lab work, an electrocardiogram (ECG), and chest x-ray were ordered. Due to the pain in her hips and back, the provider also ordered an x-ray of her hips and pelvis.

- *Vital signs:* 99.0°F, 118, 32, 178/92. SaO_2 on room air, 89%.
- *Pain:* Mary described pain as "not too bad" but winces with any movement; admits that both hips and low back are "sore" and stated, "I just need a few minutes to get my breathing under control."
- *Chief complaint:* Fall with potential injury and asthma attack.

Case Study: James Family—cont'd

Mary rested after diagnostic testing. Her breathing and comfort level improved. Once the diagnostics were completed, the physician discussed the following problem list with Mary.

Problem List
- Pelvis fracture with immobility, pain
- Hyperglycemia (blood glucose 242; A1C 10.2%)
- Elevated White Blood Cell count (urinalysis ordered to rule out infection)
- Mild fluid visible in lungs, lower extremity edema, dyspnea (Mary was advised that this may indicate infection or diminished lung function)

Plan
Mary will be admitted to the hospital to stabilize her medical condition, which will include stabilizing her respiratory status, treating for possible infection, controlling her glucose, and addressing a plan for her diabetes. Once she is stabilized, a plan can be developed to address the fracture of her pelvis. Because she lives alone with Raul, the physician advised Mary that she may need an alternative living situation when she leaves the hospital so that she will have the care that she needs to be safe. They discussed that this could be temporary based on how she does with her recovery. Mary started to cry and told the nurse that she has to get home to take care of Raul.

Questions for reflection on the nursing care of the James family:

1. What priorities exist for the nursing care that Mary will need following the discussion with the physician?
2. What strategies can the nurse use to address Mary's concerns using a family-centered approach?
3. What team members can assist with providing support to the family while Mary is in the hospital?
4. What community resources and long-term planning do you anticipate the family will need to make the upcoming transitions?

SUMMARY

Throughout this chapter, we have examined the complexity of the experiences of older adults and their family members. Aging families vary in structure, size, and a lifetime of experiences and relationships. All will influence how individuals and their families navigate later life and especially caregiving. This chapter has described the aging population in the United States and Canada and provided an overview of family ties of older adults. Family caregiving and the impact of relationships with others, as well as organizational and systems-level policies, were also examined.

- Using the life-course perspective, we discussed the diversity of family structure in later life and how it has been influenced by societal trends.
- Most older adults are embedded in social networks in which families are important sources of emotional and instrumental support. Given the diversity of family life,

many configurations of family exist. In most families, individuals enjoy strong and affectionate relationships and can count on family members to provide care and support when needed. Nonetheless, it is also common for families to have both positive and negative feelings toward one another because they are providing support. In some families, negative feelings may dominate, which will have consequences for health, well-being, and availability of support.

- Older adults have unique health care needs that must be addressed, whether they are in clinics, at home, or in hospitals, or receiving care through a variety of LTC services.
- Nursing and other professions in gerontology have developed evidence-based assessment tools and interventions that are the basis for optimal care of older adults and family caregivers. Nurses must be familiar with these tools and apply them routinely and appropriately.

- Nurses and other professionals must also recognize that older adults, including many care recipients, are also providers of care to their partners, children, grandchildren, or friends. In fact, family members deliver the majority of care.
- As the population ages, it is increasingly important that nurses develop expertise in geriatric care, regardless of setting. Nurses with strong leadership skills are needed, especially in community-based care and nursing home settings.
- In all settings, nurses must partner with older adults and their family members in designing and providing care that addresses unique needs and supports relationships.

chapter 18

Family Mental Health Nursing

Henny Breen, PhD, RN, CNE, COI

Critical Concepts

- Mental health is integral to overall health.

- All parts of the family system are interconnected; therefore, all members are affected when a family member has a mental health condition (MHC).

- The family of a person with an MHC needs to be involved in treatment because it enhances the effectiveness of the health care treatment.

- Comorbidities are frequently present when someone has an MHC (e.g., depression often coexists with eating disorders or anxiety disorders; substance abuse and alcohol and substance use disorders commonly occur with mood disorders; depression often coexists with diabetes and heart disease). Therefore, MHCs typically require integrated and complex treatment.

- Psychoeducation and participating in formal and/or informal support groups are effective interventions for family members who have a member with an MHC.

- People with mental disorders, as well as their families, are stigmatized in many world cultures, including North American societies.

- Nurses must examine their personal attitudes and prejudices toward persons and families who have a member with an MHC and seek additional education and training to challenge the negative stigmas so they can then serve as effective advocates for these families in both community and acute-care settings.

- Nurses must use nonjudgmental and nonblaming communication interactions with families who have a member with an MHC in order to establish a therapeutic professional relationship with the family.

In recent years, mental health has been recognized as integral to overall health. The constitution of the World Health Organization (WHO) states: "Health is a state of complete physical, mental and social well-being and not merely the absence of disease or infirmity" (WHO, n.d., p. 1). The American Psychiatric Nurses Association (APNA), which represents psychiatric mental health nurses at all levels, "asserts that whole health begins with mental health" and that mental health is foundational to physical health (APNA, 2020, p. 1). There is no health without mental health.

The global burden of mental health conditions (MHCs) is so serious that the WHO executive board in 2012 called for a comprehensive and coordinated response to the challenge. Although WHO defined mental health as an integral part of health in 1978 and this has been addressed in many United Nations resolutions, it was only in 2015 that mental health was included as part of the global agenda through Sustainable Development Goals (SDGs) (Dybdahl & Lien, 2017). Mental health is an integral part of almost all SDGs (Table 18-1) given the many biological,

Table 18-1	United Nations Sustainable Development Goals

1. No poverty
2. Zero hunger
3. Good health and well-being
4. Quality education
5. Gender equity
6. Clean water and sanitation
7. Affordable and clean energy
8. Decent work and economic growth
9. Industry innovation and infrastructure
10. Reduced inequities
11. Sustainable cities and communities
12. Responsible consumption and production
13. Climate action
14. Life below water
15. Life on land
16. Peace, justice, and strong institutions
17. Partnerships for the goals

Source: United Nations. (2020). The sustainable development agenda. https://www.un.org/sustainabledevelopment/development-agenda/

socioeconomic, and environment factors that contribute to mental health (Dybdahl & Lien, 2017; Votruba, 2018). SDGs have 17 goals that include a total of 169 targets. Within goal 3, there is a specific target that references mental health and substance abuse. However, many of the social determinants of health, such as poverty, inclusion, human dignity and equality, climate action, economic growth, jobs, hunger, and education, are found within the goals. Promoting factors that enhance mental health can contribute to the overall health and well-being of individuals, families, and communities.

Pandemics bring to light how infection-related poor health outcomes are more of a social problem than a health care problem. In the United States, populations that live in poverty, live in overcrowded neighborhoods, and are part of racial/ethnic groups are disproportionally affected by the COVID-19 pandemic with poor health outcomes (Singu et al., 2020). In a 2012 Canadian study following the H1N1 2009 pandemic, it was found that hospitalization of individuals for the H1N1 illness was associated with several important determinants of health, such as lower education (defined as high school education or less) and living in economically disadvantaged neighborhoods (Lowcock et al., 2012). The Ebola outbreak from 2014 to 2016 in West Africa that spread to European countries and the United States can be attributed to unprecedented spread into crowded urban areas along with weak surveillance systems and poor public health infrastructure. Other factors included increased mobilization across borders and conflicts between key infection control practices and prevailing cultural and traditional practices in West Africa (Centers for Disease Control and Prevention [CDC], 2019). The global context for health is important to understand because mental health is an important indicator of a society's overall well-being and must be understood in the context of the biological, historical, societal, and economic factors that further influence family history and life experiences.

This chapter focuses primarily on mental health family nursing in Canada and the United States; however, studies from other countries will be highlighted when they also inform nursing practice. The chapter begins with an understanding of what constitutes mental health and a brief demographic overview of the pervasiveness of mental health issues in both Canada and the United States. The remainder of the chapter focuses on the impact that MHCs can have on the individual, family members, and the family as a unit and recommends nursing interventions to assist families. The impact and treatment of substance use disorder are addressed within the Johnson family case study.

THE CONCEPT OF MENTAL HEALTH

The concept of mental health has gone through several different iterations as understanding of how integral mental health is to overall health evolved. Mental health has been described in various ways, often including: (1) emotional, psychological, and social well-being; (2) a recognition of one's own abilities; (3) the ability to strengthen one's own physical health and well-being; (4) an ability to cope with the normal stresses of life; (5) the ability to work productively; and (6) the ability to make a contribution to one's community (WHO, 2018a; APNA, 2020; U.S. Department of

Health & Human Services, 2020). Mental health is important at every stage of life, from childhood to older adulthood, and it has an impact on relationships, resiliency, and the ability to make choices (APNA, 2020; U.S. Department of Health & Human Services, 2020).

Mental health problems affect thinking, mood, and behaviors. Mental illness refers collectively to all diagnosable mental disorders that involve a significant change in thinking, emotion, and/or behavior along with distress and/or problems functioning in social, work, or family activities (American Psychiatric Association, 2021). Rather than describe an individual who has been diagnosed with a mental disorder as *mentally ill*, the expression used throughout this chapter will be "*an individual with a mental or behavioral health condition*," or a person with an MHC. Although mental disorders have discrete diagnostic criteria, there are some mental disorders that create a larger burden of care in the community and often have the most negative and intrusive effects on an individual's life and on family members' lives. Individuals with these disorders will be noted as persons with a serious mental illness (SMI). The National Institute of Mental Health (NIMH) (2021) defines SMI as a mental, behavioral, or emotional disorder that results in serious functional impairment and significantly interferes with or limits one or more major life activities. Examples of SMI include schizophrenia, major depression, bipolar disorder (BD), and other mental disorders that cause serious impairment. On the other hand, examples of disorders that typically do not cause significant social, emotional, or behavioral disability include generalized anxiety disorder, adjustment disorder, and dysthymia.

MEDICAL DIAGNOSIS OF A MENTAL DISORDER

The diagnosis of a mental disorder is based on diagnostic criteria from either the American Psychiatric Association's (APA, 2013) *Diagnostic and Statistical Manual of Mental Disorders*, 5th ed. (*DSM-5*), or the *International Classification of Diseases–10* (*ICD-10*), which is endorsed by WHO (2010). New editions are released only after much discussion and typically with many years between editions. For example, there were

13 years between the fourth and fifth editions of the *DSM-5*. The next edition of ICD, *ICD-11*, was released in June 2018, and the World Health Assembly voted unanimously to adopt this updated edition which will take effect in January 2022 (WHO, 2018a). Each set of criteria describes mental disorders as conditions characterized by alterations in a person's thinking, mood, or behavior that (1) cause an individual distress; (2) impair her or his occupational or social functioning; and/or (3) place the individual at significant risk for experiencing death, pain, disability, or a loss of freedom.

NURSING APPROACH TO MENTAL ILLNESS

Although it has long been recognized that mental health is not solely the absence of mental illness, the focus of clinical studies tends to be on the negative aspects of mental health. There is growing recognition, however, that positive factors such as optimism, life satisfaction, resilience, and happiness can be protective factors leading to a decreased incidence of mental disorders and should be taken into consideration (Bieda et al., 2017). The concept of positive mental health, which includes emotional, behavioral, social, and cultural aspects, has to be taken into consideration by nurses when conducting mental health assessments. This is in keeping with a strength-based nursing (SBN) approach that promotes empowerment, self-efficacy, and hope that is guided by eight core interrelated values (Table 18-2) (Gottlieb, 2014). SBN is both a philosophy and a

Table 18-2 The Eight Core Values of SBN
1. Health and healing
2. Uniqueness
3. Holism and embodiment
4. Subjective reality and created meaning
5. Person and environment are integral
6. Self-determination
7. Learning, timing, and readiness
8. Collaborative partnership

Source: Gottlieb, L. (2014). Strengths-based nursing: A holistic approach to care, grounded in eight core values. *The American Journal of Nursing, 114*(8), 24–32.

value-based approach that is grounded in the principles of person- and family-centered care, empowerment, relational care, and innate health and healing (Gottlieb & Gottlieb, 2017). SBN does not negate the devastating impact of SMI; however, it recognizes that deficits coexist with strengths, and it contrasts with the medical model, which places emphasis on deficits and remains the dominant practice model in health care (Gottlieb, 2014).

MHCs IN THE UNITED STATES AND CANADA

This section addresses the prevalence of MHCs in the United States and Canada, comorbidities associated with MHCs, general approaches being taken toward those with MHCs, and the stigma associated with having an MHC.

Prevalence of MHCs

More U.S. and Canadian adults have received mental health and substance use diagnoses than adults in other high-income countries. In 2019, of those 18 or older, 20.6% of Americans suffered from a mental illness (NIMH, 2021), as did 20% of Canadians (Canadian Mental Health Association [CMHA], 2020). However, slightly more Canadians, at 27%, compared to Americans, at 26%, self-reported emotional distress (Tikkanen et al., 2020). As identified earlier, mental health is associated with social and economic needs in all countries. However, nearly half (48%) of adults living in the United States compared to Canadians (36%) reported experiencing emotional distress related to worries about neighborhood safety and not having enough money for food or housing, which is a higher percentage than is seen in other countries (Tikkanen et al., 2020).

The CDC (2018) reported that one in five children in the United States experience a mental illness in a given year, and one in five children have had seriously debilitating mental illness. Mental illness affects all Canadians and Americans either directly or indirectly because those who do not personally have an MHC will be affected through a family member, friend, or colleague. SMI extends to family members across multiple generations and the community (Fedaku et al., 2019).

Mental Health and Comorbidities

It is common for adults and children with an MHC to have another condition, either mental or physical; the coexistence of multiple conditions is termed *comorbidity*. Comorbid mental illness was found to be common in children newly diagnosed with a physical illness and appeared to be chronic according to a study of children ages 6 to 16 who were newly diagnosed with asthma, diabetes, epilepsy, food allergy, or juvenile arthritis (Reaume & Ferro, 2019). Physical illness in this study was found to be more relevant than socioeconomic adversity. However, chronicity was related to parental mental health status (Reaume & Ferro, 2019). Integrating family-centered mental health services soon after the diagnosis of a physical illness should be prioritized in child health settings. Parents of children living with a chronic illness need help in identifying each other's strengths and limitations. They also need to be made aware of the multiple additional roles, such as caregiver, coordinator, teacher, and advocate, that they will need to take on (Reaume & Ferro, 2019).

Among adults, depression and anxiety often coexist with chronic physical illnesses. The relationship is bidirectional, creating challenges in determining the diagnosis and treatment (Parrish, 2018). General medical illnesses may accompany, and even be exacerbated by, an MHC. For example, heart disease, stroke, cancer, HIV/AIDS, diabetes, Parkinson's disease, thyroid problems, and multiple sclerosis are some of the conditions that often coexist with depression. When depression accompanies a serious physical illness, both conditions tend to show more severe symptoms, medical costs increase, quality of life is decreased, and people have more difficulty adapting to the physical condition (Parrish, 2018). Treating the depression along with the coexisting physical illness is imperative. This involves being mindful of the interconnectedness of mental and physical illnesses and having a holistic approach (Parrish, 2018). For nurses, it is also important to be mindful of the social and economic conditions of the patient and her or his family that may also affect their response to treatment.

The coexistence of substance use disorders and mood disorders has long been recognized and often results in a significantly worse course of an MHC. The word *addiction* is no longer used because it also carries a stigma; it promotes marking people who use substances to relieve the symptoms of their mental disorders as bad or of weak character. The National Institute on Drug Abuse (2020) provides a list of terms to use and to avoid, with explanations. The use of alcohol or other substances by people with mental disorders is, in many cases, an attempt to self-medicate the distressing symptoms of mental illness. The term *dual diagnosis* rather than *comorbidity* is used to describe a person with both a substance use disorder and another mental disorder, so it is common in substance use disorder treatment. Given the prevalence of comorbidities, it is important that nurses take a holistic view of the person with an MHC and approach interventions from multiple perspectives, including environmental factors, rather than simply focusing on a single MHC.

Some recent studies have been conducted in both the United States and Canada that examine those with a dual diagnosis and the relationship to social factors. A study in British Columbia, Canada, examined the relationship between substance use, mental health, nutrition, and food insecurity. The findings suggest that substance use and poor mental health are associated with food insecurity. Nutritional status can be undermined by substance use or an MHC. Likewise, substance use or an MHC can undermine nutritional status. Conversely, vulnerability to poor mental health may be triggered by environmental factors such as food insecurity, which is a toxic stressor that can lead to substance use. The outcomes depend on the person's resilience and ability to cope (Davison et al., 2018). An American study found that even mild and moderate to severe forms of food insufficiency were associated with children witnessing physical violence in the home. Although family mental illness and substance misuse are often associated with family violence, food-insecure families were at increased risk. Food insecurity is emotionally taxing for the family and can evolve into toxic stress, resulting in mental health challenges and substance use (Jackson et al., 2019). These findings, along with many other emerging studies, illustrate the need for a more holistic approach that takes into account social and economic factors to facilitate improved coping and resilience. Chapter 12 on trauma-informed care discusses an important approach for nurses and is in keeping with the strength-based approach discussed earlier in this chapter.

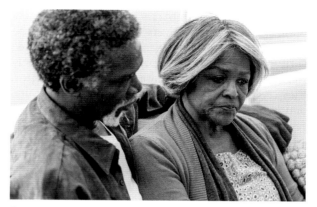

Source: © istock.com/davidf

Mental Health and General Approaches Toward Those With an MHC

Recovery from a mental health disorder is the major goal for mental health care. The Substance Abuse and Mental Health Services Administration (SAMHSA) (2012) has established a set of principles for recovery and has defined recovery as "a process of change through which individuals improve their health and wellness, live a self-directed life, and strive to reach to their full potential" (p. 3). Health, home, purpose, and community have been identified as the four major areas that contribute to maintaining a life in recovery. The 10 guiding principles of the Recovery Model are as follows:

1. Hope
2. Person-driven
3. Many pathways (nonlinear)
4. Holistic
5. Peer support
6. Relational (interactions with others, both formally and informally)
7. Culture
8. Addresses trauma
9. Strengths/responsibilities
10. Respect

Unlike previous views of MHCs—that they are chronic and very difficult if not impossible to manage, especially in relation to the more severe MHCs—part of the Recovery Model is the assertion that there are no limits to the potential for an individual to recover from any MHC. Slade and Longden (2015) proposed seven points that are empirically defensible, more helpful to mental health stakeholders, and in keeping with the recovery model: (1) recovery is best judged by the person living with the experience; (2) many people with mental health problems recover; (3) if a person no longer meets criteria for a mental illness, they are not ill; (4) diagnosis is not a robust foundation; (5) treatment is one route among many to recovery; (6) some people choose not to use mental health services; and (7) the impact of mental health problems is mixed.

Another recovery model with a similar philosophy has been implemented in Canada. Barker's Tidal Model of Mental Health Recovery was developed by Dr. Phil Barker, a professor of psychiatric nursing, and his wife Poppy Buchanan-Barker, a social worker, along with several of their colleagues, to promote recovery (Tidal Model, 2015). This mental health recovery model is the first model to (1) be developed by nurses working in the field of mental health and those who used mental health services, (2) be used for the basis of interdisciplinary mental health care, and (3) focus beginning the recovery journey when the person is experiencing the *most serious* problems in living. It is also recognized internationally as a significant midrange theory of nursing (Tidal Model, 2015).

The Tidal Model emphasizes a shift in how nurses think about the care provided to people with an MHC. Rather than focusing on disease and illness, this model stresses the importance of the individual with an MHC actively participating in decision making related to care and including family in the overall care (Sagna & Walker, 2020). Whereas the Recovery Model has 10 principles, the Tidal Model has 10 commitments which can be found on their website. They include the following commitments, and each has related competencies for mental health practitioners:

1. Value the voice.
2. Respect the language.
3. Become the apprentice.
4. Use the available toolkit.
5. Craft the step beyond.
6. Give the gift of time.
7. Develop genuine curiosity.
8. Know change is constant.
9. Reveal personal wisdom.
10. Be transparent.

At the center of both the Recovery Model and the Tidal Model is the philosophy that nurses recognize the uniqueness of each individual with an MHC and that nurses must collaborate not only with these affected individuals to provide person-centered care but also with their families and the rest of the collaborative care team, including physicians, social workers, community services providers, and mental health care providers. These nursing actions are very much in keeping with the values of SBN. However, it takes nurse advocacy given the trend to focus only on deficits. There are improved outcomes, such as reduced morbidity and mortality rates in persons with MHCs and improved preservation of the psychological and physical health of their family members, when this collaboration takes place (Goodrich et al., 2013). In line with this philosophy, the President's New Freedom Commission on Mental Health (Hogan, 2003) final report (Box 18-1) recommended six national goals to move mental health care in the United States toward a recovery-oriented system, with the overall goal of improving mental health care for Americans. Although the Affordable Care Act of 2010 increased access to mental health services, much more work remains to be done (Baumgartner et al., 2020) to meet the goals of the President's New Freedom Commission on Mental Health (Hogan, 2003).

BOX 18-1

Goals Identified by the President's New Freedom Commission on Mental Health (Hogan, 2003)

The goals identified by the President's New Freedom Commission on Mental Health (Hogan, 2003) were as follows:

- Americans understand that mental health is essential to overall health.
- Mental health care is consumer and family driven.
- Disparities in mental health services are eliminated.
- Early mental health screening, assessment, and referral to services are common practice.
- Excellent mental health care is delivered and research is accelerated.
- Technology is used to access mental health care and information.

Source: President's New Freedom Commission on Mental Health (Hogan, 2003). Recommendations to transform *mental health care in America.* U.S. Department of Health and Human Services. https://doi.org/10.1176/appi.ps.54.11.1467

Also in line with the philosophy of person-centered care is an international trend to provide care to persons with an MHC in the community rather than in an institutional setting. Past practice had been to institutionalize persons with an MHC, often for a lengthy period of time; however, the recovery models shift both the focus and the locus of care provision. Large inpatient, mental health care institutions have been downsized or eliminated in most areas, but many governments have not provided funding for other resources to deliver the care that persons with an MHC might need. This change has resulted in the transfer of care from the institutional level to the family level. The stress and burden of care experienced by these families has been well documented.

Families often suffer financial and social deprivations when providing care to family members with an MHC. Family caregivers may become exhausted by a lack of respite from their affected family member, who requires so much energy for care and supervision, and they often live in fear that the family member with an MHC will cause disruption to family life because of a recurrence or exacerbation of the MHC (Vermeulen et al., 2015). A systematic review conducted by Shiraishi and Reilly (2019) examined the impact of schizophrenia, an SMI, on family caregivers. Negative impacts identified included traumatic experiences, loss of expectation of life and health, lack of personal and social resources, uncertainty and unpredictability, family disruption, conflict in interpersonal relationships, difficulty in understanding, social stigma, and hereditary factors. Positive impacts were also noted, and they included family solidarity, admiration, affirmation, affection, compassion, learning knowledge and skills, self-confidence, personal growth, and appreciation. Common needs for families living with a family member with an MHC are support, including affordable respite care; information; skills training; advocacy; and referral courses (Vermeulen et al., 2015; Hestmark, 2020).

Family involvement for persons with an MHC is often underutilized despite evidence that supported family interventions can improve social function, self-experienced health and adherence to medication, and a reduction of relapse frequency and hospital admissions (Claxton et al., 2017). More than ever, families are integral and instrumental resources for recovery for individuals with an MHC and especially those individuals with an SMI. Families offer more hope in recovery than health care providers. It is evident that nurses and other health care providers must engage the families of individuals with an MHC in their recovery.

Mental Health and Stigma

Stigma has been defined as labeling, stereotyping, separation, status loss, and discrimination. Our culture, not our biology, determines which illnesses are stigmatized. The stigmatization of illness often has the greatest effect on the patient and his or her family members—and also on the kind of care they receive. Mental disorders probably carry the most stigma compared to other illnesses, resulting in significant social disadvantages (Baker, 2020). Psychiatric nurses may also experience the impact of this stigma by working in facilities that are less welcoming or are segregated from other health care areas.

Public perception of mental illness and violence remain intertwined, resulting in much of the stigma associated with mental illness. This perception is reinforced and amplified by the media, which sensationalizes violent crimes. If the person who committed the violent crime has been diagnosed with a mental illness, the focus tends to be on the mental illness in the reporting, ignoring the fact that most of the violence is committed by people without mental illness. In addition, most people with mental health problems are no more likely to be violent than anyone else; those with an SMI are 10 times more likely to be victims of a violent crime than the general population. This stigmatization further contributes to stigma, often resulting in nondisclosure of mental illness and reduced treatment seeking (Varshney et al., 2016).

Western society singles out mental illness as shameful and devalues the person who possesses an MHC (Burke et al., 2016). Society's stigma influences how individuals feel about themselves, which can lead to self-stigma and can both exacerbate MHCs and cause affected individuals to avoid treatment. Hack et al. (2020) found that those with higher levels of education were at greater risk for avoiding treatment due to self-stigma. Providers may even hesitate to include the diagnosis of MHCs in medical records, especially those of children, because of the stigma.

Stigma affects both the individual with the MHC and the family members. Stigma can cause individuals with an MHC and their families to become isolated and feel ashamed, or stigma can make individuals and family members engage in denial or a wish for things to appear normal, which may then discourage them from talking about their needs and seeking help. Family members living with a family member with an MHC frequently experience rejection, shame, and avoidance by others (Flood-Grady & Koenig Kellas, 2019; Shiraishi & Reilly, 2019).

Stigma and discrimination toward persons with an MHC can prevent care and treatment from reaching people with mental illnesses. For example, stigma toward a parent who has an MHC, or who is providing care to a child with an MHC, may prevent the parents from obtaining community support because of their fear that others may assume they are not a fit parent; they may not access care because of fears about losing custody of their child (Flood-Grady & Koenig Kellas, 2019). People with MHCs also may fear workplace reprisals if they seek mental health care through work-provided insurance.

Unfortunately, nurses and health care providers are not immune to demonstrating stigma toward individuals with MHCs and their families. For example, nurses providing care to a mother parenting a child with attention deficit-hyperactivity disorder (ADHD) may blame poor parenting for the child's behavioral challenges. In a qualitative study about stigma by association, spouses and parents reported being excluded from the treatment process despite having been the sole support of their family member with an MHC for years. They also reported feeling little to no support in coping with the burden of caregiving. Lack of information due to privacy regulations or confidentiality policies can be perceived as very stigmatizing by family members (van der Sanden et al., 2016).

There is cause to hope, however, because young people are decreasing stigma toward those with an MHC. For instance, there is a national trend for college students to seek treatment for mental health problems, and educational institutions are making efforts to help students identify and take advantage of these services (Daily, 2020).

Nursing Role in Reducing Stigma

Nurses can help decrease stigma in several ways. Words matter. The words and terms used by the general public to refer to people with mental disorders include: *crazy, nuts, mad, loony, one-fry-short-of-a-happy-meal, weirdo, psycho,* and *his elevator doesn't go all the way up,* to name a few. These expressions may resemble an attempt at humor to some people, but they have disrespectful intent. When a person asks, "Am I crazy?" and the nurse answers, "No, you have a mental disorder called schizophrenia," a small step is taken toward treating mental disorders equal to general medical disorders. When nurses discourage others from demeaning people with mental disorders, just as one would discourage racist, sexist, or homophobic speech, another step is taken in the direction toward what the culture and society will not tolerate (Burke et al., 2016).

Education of those working with those who have an MHC about specific disorders and their treatments can also help reduce or prevent behaviors or discrimination caused by stigma. Increased understanding about the symptoms and behaviors arising from an MHC promote the provision of optimal care. For instance, instead of blaming poor parenting, nurses working with a mother whose child has ADHD can focus on identifying those behaviors that are ADHD-related and work with the mother to develop targeted interventions that compensate for the executive function deficits and emotional dysregulation issues associated with this condition.

FAMILY MEMBERS OF INDIVIDUALS WITH AN MHC

The whole family may be affected by and involved in care of the member who has an MHC, or individual relationships and responsibilities may be more pronounced. For example, a spouse may be providing care to his or her partner. Parents may be providing care to young or adult children, or siblings may provide care for siblings. In some cases, the parent has the MHC, resulting in a child taking care of the parent. The "normal" relationships and dynamics within the family may be disrupted. Nurses need to pay attention to family dynamics and to the potential burdens faced by individual members and the family as a whole when a member has an MHC.

A systemic review of 39 studies conducted mostly in high-income countries found a high level of psychological problems (such as depression and anxiety) in family members, including parents, siblings, children, and grandchildren, of people with SMI. Difficulties in social relationships such as a higher divorce rate, fewer marriages, and a strained family environment were reported, as were financial issues related to the cost of treatment and inability to work. The children's level of functioning was also affected in terms of school performance, and they were often placed in special education and faced malnutrition (Fekadu et al., 2019).

This section focuses on family caregiving, the general burden of family caregiving, spousal caregiving, role changes within the family, children living with a parent or sibling who has an MHC, parenting a child who has an MHC, and the nursing role.

Family Caregiving

Family caregiving is a term used to describe family members or friends who provide unpaid care to chronically ill or functionally impaired persons. Family caregivers often take on their role because of a sense of responsibility and because of limited or no available resources or services. When a family member has an MHC, remaining members may feel marginalized and distanced from the care planning process. Common themes across international studies include family feelings of isolation, lack of information, lack of recognized role, and not feeling listened to or taken seriously by health care providers. Families also commonly report a belief that health care providers use the need for confidentiality as a way to avoid sharing important information about the identified client's condition and treatment (Eassom et al., 2014).

Disrupted Family Life Stages

Normative family life stages among family members are interrupted by the onset of a serious mental illness in a family member. For example, during the childbearing stage of the family life cycle, family tasks include adjusting to the new roles as parent(s). If the mother of the infant develops postpartum depression (PPD) or psychosis, this stage of development is disrupted, for example, because the mother may be hospitalized, and bonding with the infant is affected. PPD is associated with a number of detrimental outcomes for children and families, such as compromised parenting behaviors

including disengagement, impaired mother-infant interactions, and negative perceptions of the infant. Children of depressed mothers are at risk for mental health problems throughout their lives and are at further risk if the family lives in poverty (Newland & Parade, 2016). Other family members such as aunts, uncles, or grandparents of the infant may have to assume care of the infant for safety reasons even if the mother is not hospitalized.

Schizophrenia or bipolar illness often surfaces during late adolescence, just at the time when the task of the family is to help their adolescent prepare for adulthood as they go to college or join the workforce. DeTore et al. (2018) found that family burden was significantly higher in those families whose child was not working or in school. Social events, employment, and education were sacrificed due to the individual having schizophrenia. Both personal loss and stress may be central experiences of family members due to unwanted or unexpected changes in identity, future roles, routines, and aspirations as a result of the mental illness (Leith et al., 2018).

According to Family Life Cycle Theory, going to college is considered one of the distinct transitions to make as family members help their child launch. Mitchell and Abraham (2018) found that adolescents of a parent with a mental illness struggled more with the transition because they experienced more homesickness, depression, and anxiety than their peers who did not have a parent with an MHC.

Burden of Caregiving

Caregiver burden refers to the physical, psychological, emotional, social, and financial stressors that are associated with caregiving (Sharma et al., 2016). The age of the caregiver, educational level, and financial stress related to insufficient resources all affect caregiver burden. The mental health system in the United States has struggled to provide adequate support services for adults with an MHC, leaving family members to be the primary source of care. Parents usually provide this support for adult children with an SMI until they are no longer able to do so, at which point siblings have to take on this responsibility (Leith et al., 2018).

In their international quantitative study commonly known as C4C, Vermeulen et al. (2015) found that caregivers experience burdens in the following life domains: emotional (through the constant anxiety of caring), social (feeling isolated and lonely), physical (fear that the identified patient will relapse such that the caregiver's safety may be at risk and that the caregiving itself makes their own health worse), financial (worries about the financial situation of the person they care for), and finally the domain of relationship (fear that the person with the mental disorder will continue to be dependent on them in the future). Some of the caregivers studied felt that they were treated differently because of the mental illness of the person they cared for, which confirms that stigma extends beyond the identified patient to family members. On the other hand, the researchers also found that caregivers stated that they had become more understanding of others with problems and had discovered inner strength of their own. Finally, almost all the caregivers felt the need for additional support in their caregiving role. Some were able to use other family members for respite care, but only 6% to 8% had access to paid respite care.

Spousal Caregiving

Many family caregivers for those with MHCs are caring for a spouse or partner. Care is typically provided in the family home, and the most common tasks performed on a daily basis are providing companionship, providing emotional support during a crisis, and monitoring symptoms. Other aspects of care include providing or monitoring medications, paying bills, advocating for the person to receive help, arranging and coordinating services and appointments, assisting with personal grooming, taking more responsibility for child care and household chores, and going to appointments with the person who has an MHC (American Psychological Association, 2017). These tasks and aspects of care are common to anyone who has an MHC, regardless of whether the person is the spouse, child, sibling, and so on.

Spousal care providers may feel angry about the changes that they see in their spouse because of the onset, exacerbations, and remissions of the MHC. Spouses may find themselves blaming their spouse for having a character flaw rather than understanding the cause of and treatments for the MHC. Additional financial and parental responsibilities can also increase the stress and negatively affect the relationships between family members. A small qualitative study of female spousal caregivers of spouses with SMI in Iran found that they

experienced psychological distress in three categories: emotional detachment, emotional exhaustion, and loss of self (Rahmani et al., 2018). This is consistent among many studies reviewed by Sharma et al. (2016); after reviewing more than 100 studies worldwide, they also found inconclusive evidence regarding mental and physical strain experienced by the caregiver according to gender.

Family Role Changes

It is not unusual for family caregivers of persons with an MHC to change their relationships or roles within the family. For example, an adult younger brother may find it challenging to maintain his role as younger brother while also being caregiver and guardian to his older sister who has an SMI. Children may take on some parenting roles—such as providing personal and emotional care to a parent, engaging in household chores, providing care to brothers and sisters, administering medication to parents, or providing crisis support to a parent during an acute psychotic episode or self-harming (but not harming others). Thus, parents may maintain their role as parents, although there might be some interdependence between the child and parents. Being a child (under the age of 18 years) in the caregiver role to a parent can have a positive effect on the child's development, including improved family relationships, but it can also negatively affect the child's development and overall childhood experience. Källquist and Salzmann-Erikson (2019) found some adults suffered from relational issues because of the role reversal in the families, whereas Patrick et al. (2019) found that adult children had equally satisfying relationships as those in the general population.

Role changes may not be welcomed by the family. For instance, some family caregivers may feel obliged to provide care to their relative with an MHC. Family care providers often struggle with unexpected and unfamiliar expectations placed on them in their new roles. Legal and moral rights related to providing care to the family member with an MHC often cause conflict between the family caregiver and the health care providers. Frequently, health care providers neither appreciate nor understand the legal needs and moral rights of the family caregiver; rather, they focus on the legal and moral rights of the person with the MHC. For example, health care providers may pressure a parent or parents to take their adult child home with them because they believe that the person with the MHC will benefit by being cared for at home or because the person no longer meets the requirement for hospitalization and no other placement is available. However, the parents may not feel that they have the capacity to care for their adult child, or they may have made a decision not to attempt to provide care because of previous negative consequences to the family when the adult child has been at home. This difference in perspectives can cause barriers between health care providers and family caregivers. It is important to note that family caregivers and families in general want to be included and supported in the treatment and decision making about care for their family member. This reinforces the importance of including the family members to ensure an understanding of their needs as well as that of the family member with an MHC.

Children With a Family Member With an MHC

When an adult with an MHC accesses care, it is imperative that nurses ascertain whether there are children in the family, because research has shown that children living with a family member with an MHC are at increased risk for developing psychopathology, that is, developing emotional and behavioral problems including anxiety or personality disorders (Mental Health America, 2016). Adult children have reported dangerous and frightening situations when their parent was suffering from paranoia and had delusions that also included them. The parent may have been physically and verbally abusive. However, the most common experience was neglect (Källquist & Salzmann-Erikson, 2019).

Mental health care providers often overlook children who live with a family member with an MHC and do not ask about parental status (Christiansen et al., 2019). One recommendation to avoid omission of this important information is to change the hospital assessment forms to include a section that asks about children living in the home. Regardless, nurses should make it standard practice to ask the question.

Nurses should not only determine if there is a child in the family of a person with an MHC; they also need to understand how children perceive their role. Strained relationships between family members are not uncommon and can lead to a chaotic family life. Appropriate assessment and intervention are important to ameliorate any negative consequences for a child who is living with a person who has an MHC, regardless of whether that person is the child's parent or sibling or has another relationship with the child. At the same time, nurses should remember that, in spite of the associated risks, many of these children remain emotionally and mentally healthy.

Nurses need to be aware that children living with a family member with an MHC often believe they caused the MHC and may have feelings of guilt, anger, or anxiety (Mental Health America, 2016). In addition, the children may feel alone. Nurses must initiate a conversation with the children and not wait until they ask for help. It is important for nurses to tell the children that they did not cause the parent's illness or strange behavior nor are they responsible for taking care of the family member. Nurses should emphasize that there are health care professionals who will provide care to the family member. Providing age-appropriate information about the parent's MHC and treatment decreases the children's feelings of guilt and also decreases the children's negative feelings toward the MHC.

Developing a relationship with the children ameliorates the feelings of being isolated and alone. If there are several children of different ages in the living situation, the nurse must remember to provide teaching and answers to each child, appropriate to the child's developmental and cognitive ability. Children who are knowledgeable about a parent's illness are able to understand the parent's behaviors better in relation to the specific illness (Mental Health America, 2016). Children need thoughtful, developmentally appropriate information about their parent's illness and treatment. Children who are not given the whole story are left to make up their own explanations, which only adds to their emotional confusion and possible self-blame for parental symptoms. Support for family relationships and other networks must be part of the care that nurses provide to parents in any setting (Kouros et al., 2020). Support groups were found to help the children feel less alone and to understand that they were not at fault (Källquist & Salzmann-Erikson, 2019).

Although a primary role for a nurse who is providing care to an adult with an MHC is to identify the presence of children living in the family and to offer support and education to those children, the nurse also needs to perform a family-centered assessment of the children's needs (Tungpunkom et al., 2017), followed by referral to relevant services. Once needs are identified, nurses can develop a plan for assisting the child. For example, with parental consent and within the limits of confidentiality, nurses can contact a child's school to apprise teachers or administrators of the family situation affecting the child. Nurses can facilitate access to other professional services and family support, such as family and/or individual therapy. Therapy that teaches children and youth how to communicate easily and have fewer arguments with their parents may be beneficial because those factors have been shown to contribute to improved mental health among adolescents ages 11 to 15 years in a very large, cross-national study involving 43 countries and including 26,078 young Canadians (Freeman et al., 2011). In addition, it is important to provide services that can enhance a child's coping skills, because children with effective coping skills are less likely to have behavioral or emotional problems.

Although the majority of professional services for family members with an MHC are in the community, there are times when a family member may be hospitalized. Nurses need to remember to ask the hospitalized family member if there are children. Children whose family members are hospitalized want and need information about the hospitalized family member and appreciate having a nurse talk with them about visiting the psychiatric facility and having someone take a genuine interest in explaining what is happening to their family member. It is the responsibility of the nurse to provide age-appropriate information. Simple words and explanations can be used even with very young children and toddlers and may alleviate a lot of the child's anxiety.

Children Living With a Parent With an MHC

In addition to the more general areas noted previously, nurses also must recognize that specific issues may arise when a child is living with a parent with an MHC. Children growing up with a parent with an MHC may express anger toward this parent because their parent is not similar to other parents, and they may experience extreme sadness when they remember a time when the parent was healthy (Mental Health America, 2016). These children also frequently worry, often needlessly, that they will inherit and develop the MHC, but they will only share this concern with another person after the person has gained their trust. Circumstances such as maternal depression can have a negative impact on the child's normal development and on his or her likelihood of developing a mental health problem. Therefore, nurses need to pay particular attention to specific risks when the parent is the person with an MHC.

A study in the Netherlands examined parentification in adolescents in which the parent had an MHC. In a family systems framework, appropriate boundaries between parents and children are central to family functioning. When a parent has an MHC, parentification may result in unclear boundaries, which in turn may result in feelings of stress for the adolescent. From a developmental perspective, caring for a parent is a role reversal and often beyond the adolescent's capabilities. The researchers found that parentification can have negative consequences, but family intervention and psychoeducational support can facilitate coping skills (Van Loon et al., 2017).

Parents may experience a double burden because they need to manage their own illness and raise their children. Parents with an MHC often fear their children will inherit the illness, and this fear can be projected onto the children. Parents with an SMI sometimes cannot care for their children, which creates a great deal of pain and sorrow due to the separation for both the parent and child. They may have difficulty explaining their illness to their children, and they often experience the prejudice and stigma because they have a mental illness. The stigma may induce feelings that they are not a good parent, and they may avoid talking about it for fear of losing custody (Källquist & Salzmann-Erikson, 2019).

Risks to Normal Development

Several disorders, including depression, schizophrenia, and BD, not only affect an adult's ability to parent but also can have an impact on a child's growth and development. It is estimated that about 10% to 15% of women in the Unites States experience PPD (Guintivano et al., 2019). The impact of maternal depression on children from infancy to adolescence has been observed in clinic and community settings; maternal depression can have negative effects on a child. Problems with language development and intelligence (Lam-Cassettari & Kohlhoff, 2020), behavior, development of depressive symptoms, sleep patterns, physical health, parent-child relationship, and attachment have all been identified as possible results of parental depression (Claus et al., 2019). Sullivan et al. (2019) also examined socioeconomic status (SES) as a contextual risk factor in addition to parental depression. Findings highlighted that girls may be particularly vulnerable to high risk within the low SES context.

Parents with depression may communicate pessimism and sadness to their infants, and they may laugh less and demonstrate less affection, tenderness, and responsiveness. Decreased close and continuous contact with infants can have the most harmful effects for infants (Brockington et al., 2011). A child's mental health and social competence are predicted less by illness variables and categorical diagnosis than by multiple contextual risks (Brockington et al., 2011). The Australian Maternal Health Study found that psychoeducation for parents when the mother had been diagnosed with depression reduced depression relapse incidence in the mothers and reduced incidence of sleep disturbances in infants. The psychoeducation program included individual meetings with nurses about parental concerns, group meetings with other new parents, brief parenting education, information about normal infant sleeping and crying patterns, and follow-up calls to the primary caregivers when the baby was 4 and 12 weeks old (Brown et al., 2021).

Children benefit from consistency in parenting behavior. Similar to children of parents with depression, children of parents with BD are at increased risk for parenting disturbances related to the cyclical nature of the disorder. Women with BD are particularly vulnerable to relapse during the postpartum period. Inconsistent parenting behavior can be related to the parent's depression, manic/hypomanic or mixed state, chronicity of episodes, suicidality/suicide attempts, risky behavior associated with mania, problems with adherence to treatment, withdrawn and/or irritable behavior during a depressed mood, relapse in spite of treatment, and/or recovery time between episodes (Anke et al., 2019). Parenting difficulties

in themselves can be challenging stressors for any parent, but parents who have BD may experience exacerbation of the bipolar symptoms with increases in stress (Anke et al., 2019). Nurses can provide assistance to these parents by collaborating with the parent, child, family, and other health care providers to address the health needs determined by the family needs assessment.

Nurses, teachers, and family members may not recognize the concerns and issues that children who are living with a parent who has an MHC can face unless the child demonstrates a learning or behavior problem in school or a parent requests specific support for the child. Therefore, children of parents with an MHC should be routinely assessed for parent-child relational problems and possible developmental delays so that appropriate interventions can be implemented in a timely manner.

Risks of Developing an MHC

It has been estimated that 15% to 23% of children around the world have a parent with an MHC and that they are more likely than their peers to develop a mental health problem (Leijdesdorff et al., 2017). Children's development of depression may be influenced by genetic factors, environmental influences, marital or partner stress or violence, or even disruptions in parenting. Not only are children who live with a parent with an MHC at elevated risk for developing a mental health problem, including being developmentally delayed, but they are also at increased risk of being abused and neglected. Children of parents with an MHC should be routinely assessed for potential mental health concerns and, where warranted, appropriate interventions should be implemented. Accumulating evidence demonstrates the effect of early life stress and trauma on mental and physical health throughout the life span. The evidence indicates that increased investment in family economic resources and the health of young children, especially those with known risks, are the most effective strategies for helping children grow and achieve success in adulthood while reducing inequalities in health outcomes (National Academies of Sciences, Engineering, and Medicine, 2019).

Other Risks

Disruption of relationships within the family and increases in risky behaviors can be an issue, particularly for youth. They may struggle with the stigma associated with the MHC, and they may opt out of a relationship with the parent and instead use maladaptive coping mechanisms that can lead to risky behaviors or problems with the justice system. Nurses need to be cognizant of this possibility, make sure to assess teenagers for adaptive and maladaptive coping mechanisms, and then intervene as necessary.

Some children have parents with an MHC, such as schizophrenia, major depressive disorder (MDD), or BD, that is more likely than other MHCs to lead to hospitalization. These children often worry about what will happen to them if a parent is hospitalized.

Nurses also must remember to dispel the myth that parents with an MHC are unfit parents. Rather, nurses must emphasize that a parent with an MHC can be a very competent, effective, nurturing, and loving parent. Children and parents benefit from continuous assessment of the child's needs and ongoing professional support and treatment for the parents. Many effective psychotherapeutic and psychological interventions are available, including family therapies, mother and infant psychotherapies, and brief cognitive therapy appropriate to the age and stage of child development (Brockington et al., 2011). Nurses can provide support to parents who have an MHC by actively listening to the parents' concerns about parenting, providing realistic information about parenting skills, and assessing for the need for interventions to support the children.

Adult children who grew up living with a parent with an MHC may remember negative experiences caused by their parent's illness and the lack of information and support from mental health services. They may remember worrying about their parent's well-being, wondering if their parent was going to commit suicide, being fearful that the parent was not getting the care needed, and being anxious about coming home from school because they did not know how their parent was going to respond to them. These adult children may remember having to approach either the parent without the health condition or a health care provider to get information about their parent's condition rather than the health care provider offering this information to them (Källquist & Salzmann-Erikson, 2019). Children are not in a place to seek information; rather, nurses must offer and provide this information to

children so that they do not grow into adults with negative memories about their experience.

Children Living With a Sibling With an MHC

Prolonged mental health issues of one family member influence the whole family system, including siblings. Sibling relationships have a profound impact on the development of a child. The sibling relationship provides a connection for a child to learn how to interact with others, manage quarrels, handle rivalries, share secrets, and try on different roles (Kovacs et al., 2019). Siblings share a common genetic and social background, early life experiences, and a family cultural background that can last a lifetime. Brothers and sisters also share unique private information about their parents and families. The common bond that siblings experience can be a source of support and companionship for the sisters and brothers. But an MHC in one sibling can interfere negatively with sibling relationships. Siblings may experience a wide range of difficult emotions and experiences, such as anger, guilt, helplessness, social withdrawal, and loss of a relationship. Although siblings often experience the relationship with their brother or sister as stressful, they don't see cutting off the relationship as an option. Siblings who participate in caregiving may at the same time experience positive growth (Kovacs et al., 2019).

Liegghio (2017), as part of a larger study, found that young siblings had predominantly negative experiences. They struggled with understanding their sibling's MHC and experienced considerable family stress and overt family stigma resulting in stress, worry, and burden. The perceived their sibling with an MHC as having a character flaw and did not connect negative behavior to the MHC. Some siblings described being popular at school but would lose friends when it was discovered they had a sibling with an MHC (Liegghio, 2017). If the family members are not able to discuss the issues, this can lead to further shame or guilt. Unfortunately, these kinds of actions often lead to more silence and isolation for the unaffected sibling.

Sisters and brothers who have a sibling with an SMI, such as schizophrenia or BD, often struggle to understand what has happened to the affected sibling and the impact the condition has on their relationship with their affected sibling, as well as the entire family. For example, siblings who observe an affected sibling's first psychotic episode may be traumatized. Although the majority of those with an SMI are not violent, those who are violent tend to be so toward family members. Exposure to violence and fear of victimization by the family member with an SMI has a negative impact on the family system. Siblings of individuals with an SMI too often do not have their needs met. They often feel abandoned, invisible, or forgotten by parents (Sporer et al., 2019). Yet these siblings need more help; for example, they need health care providers to be available to answer their questions and to clarify their role in the future care of their sibling. When they get older, siblings may also have problems developing and keeping intimate relationships because they are fearful of passing on any genetic deficiencies to their own children.

Sibling participation in a support group specifically for siblings who have a brother or sister with an MHC has been shown to decrease the siblings' feelings of being alone, and it helps them gain information about their sibling's MHC and learn ways to support their affected sibling (Liegghio, 2017). Another study conducted by Sporer et al. (2019) found three themes that represented helpful strategies: gaining insight and knowledge, joining peer support groups, and identifying a silver lining. The silver lining may include family members having a greater sense of purpose, a sense of closeness with their families, greater empathy and compassion, resiliency, and assertiveness. However, Sporer et al. (2019) cautions that it would be insensitive for practitioners to suggest family members find a silver lining. Her research found that family members could be led indirectly to a more positive outlook by attending support groups.

Providing education to siblings can clarify misperceptions about the MHC and its treatment. Although it is important to address the needs of the brothers' and sisters' current experiences with their affected brother or sister, nurses must also be future-oriented and provide education and support to these siblings in preparation for becoming future primary-care providers for their sibling. Nurses also need to be aware of other ways in which the dynamic in the family might be problematic when one sibling has an MHC and the other does not. For example, parents may focus their time and energy on the sibling with the MHC, leaving the unaffected sibling feeling neglected and resentful

of the attention given to the sibling. It is important that the needs of healthy siblings are not ignored, no matter how unintentional the neglect by parents may be. Nurses can work with parents to help them shape how the unaffected sibling perceives the affected sibling and the MHC, as well as identify ways in which the parents can provide the needed attention to healthy siblings. Family assessment is critical, followed by appropriate psychoeducation, discussions about how parents might relate to the unaffected sibling, and referral to supports as needed.

Parenting Children With an MHC

Parents provide care to children with an MHC on a regular basis in what can often be a long-term, ongoing activity; they frequently are the caregivers for their adult child with an MHC. Parents often experience grief, isolation, and stigma when their child has an MHC or blame themselves for their child's MHC. They may face health care providers who are suspicious of parental involvement and do not allow parent participation in the care of the child, especially when the child is hospitalized. Often forgotten are grandparents who assume a caregiving role for their adult children who have an MHC and also have children.

Grief and chronic sorrow are common experiences that parents encounter after being told their child has an MHC. Wayment and Brookshire (2018) examined grief and distress in mothers who had a child with an autism spectrum disorder (ASD). They found that grief could persist for years when the mothers perceived their child's diagnosis as a loss and unjust. They worried their child would have difficulties and that their hopes for their child would not be realized. They also found that mothers who blamed themselves for the ASD diagnosis were more likely to report grief and distress.

Chronic grief can affect the parent's psychological well-being, health status, and the parent-child relationship. The grief can be prolonged because the parents may experience grief differently across the life course of their child's illness and as the child moves through different developmental stages. On the other hand, depending on the MHC, the child's development may be disrupted and impair his or her ability to move through the developmental phases, furthering the impact on the family's life cycle. Parents may experience grief for the loss of the child that they can no longer have or may even feel that they have a different child from the one they started with; parents grieve for their future losses, for what their child may not be able to accomplish (Wayment & Brookshire, 2018). Some parents may feel the need to provide regular care for their child well into adulthood, and thus they grieve not seeing their children grow up into independent individuals. They also may grieve losses in their own lives, such as not becoming empty nesters. Nurses need to recognize and validate the grief and sorrow that parents experience and provide interventions and referrals to resources that decrease their emotional distress and life disruption.

Some parents of children with an MHC experience isolation and stigma from family, friends, teachers, and school administrators. Many parents are forced to leave work to meet with teachers to address educational and/or behavioral concerns or health care providers. A mental health crisis may take them away from work longer. This may result in problems with their employers and potentially cause them to lose their job, thus adding further to the financial strain they may already be experiencing. Many parents of adult children with an SMI experience significant frustration as they try to navigate a health care system that they perceive as being full of obstacles.

Parent participation is particularly important for child and family treatment given the critical role that parents play in the child's life. Mental illness of a family member affects the entire family system, and the family context has a great influence on the child's development and behavior. However, parents face challenges to actively participating in treatment due to feeling blamed, judged, and not listened to by mental health providers (Haine-Schlagel & Walsh, 2015).

Many parents experience the hospitalization of their child with an MHC. Parents report that the admission process can be very difficult for them and that they often feel in crisis; they want nurses and other health care providers to understand these challenges. They typically need written and verbal information related to their child's care, such as an up-to-date handbook that tells them who to call for information about their child, what to expect during the hospitalization, hospital costs, what the child can or cannot do, what they should be doing about school, and a list of nearby inexpensive accommodations during the hospitalization, and they need easy access to the child and better access to care before, during, and after hospitalization. Parents welcome practical tips and timely, accurate, situation-specific information that is communicated to them in a clear and honest manner. In addition, parents strongly suggest that they be recommended to a parent support group and also be given a list of parents who have undergone a similar experience and are willing to talk with them. Many parents experience guilt and shame related to their child's hospitalization and find it helpful when nurses talk to them about their guilt and shame in a nonjudgmental manner.

Some parents whose child has an SMI and never achieves independence may need to assume the responsibility of caring for their grandchildren. Grandparents may experience divided loyalties: the toll of providing care to their grandchildren but also the rewards that come with raising them. In the United States in 2008, 5.7 million children, 8% of all children, lived with a grandparent. An MHC in the parent of the child was one of the 11 reasons why the grandparent was raising the child (Davey et al., 2016). Caring for grandchildren involves physical exertion and dedication over time. If the grandparent is also caring for an adult child with MHC, the physical and mental toll can be overwhelming. A particularly vulnerable time for the grandparent is when the grandchild approaches the age at which the child's mother or father began developing symptoms, which can be experienced much like the anniversary of the death of a loved one. Nurses should be aware of such dates and offer support to grandparents rather than waiting for the grandparents to request help.

Although grandparents often provide the daily care for their grandchildren, nurses must recognize that typically it is the child's parent who is recognized as the legal guardian. The grandparents may view the parent's influence as not beneficial to the child's well-being and so they may feel tempted to minimize visitations; however, many do try to sustain a relationship between the parent and child. Grandparent caretakers sometimes are put into adversarial positions with the parent and may even have to sue for custody of the child. The opioid crisis has resulted in adverse childhood experiences that often trigger a change in guardianship that can last for years. Grandparents must balance the needs of their adult child and their grandchildren. This creates stress for the grandparents because they need to shift their roles from grandparent to parent. For the grandchildren, the traumatic events resulting from their parent suffering from addiction often results in behavioral challenges, difficulties with socialization, anxiety, depression, and lower school performance (Davis et al., 2020). At the same time, grandparents may experience chronic grief for their children who are unable to care for their own children. They may feel a sense of guilt and blame themselves for making parenting mistakes that may have led to their current circumstances (Capous-Desyllas et al., 2020).

As children with a chronic MHC begin to transition from child/adolescent mental health care providers to adult mental health care providers, it is important to assist the parents and adolescent to avoid disrupting continuity of care (Broad et al., 2017). It is not unusual to have a child's eligibility for mental health care services change to different systems. The transition may put the adolescents at risk of disengaging from services. Their responses are influenced by concurrent life transitions and their preferences regarding autonomy and independence. A review of published and unpublished literature found that adolescents identified preparation, flexible and individualized transition planning, timing, and informational continuity as positive factors during transition (Broad et al., 2017). Even though the young adult is assumed and expected to be responsible for managing his or her own health care needs, it is not uncommon for these young adults to continue to depend on their parents' assistance for accessing their mental health care. Giving the parents ample time to prepare for this transition can help make it a smooth one without interrupting continuity of care.

Interventions that can lead to positive outcomes for family caregivers include support groups, various educational interventions, respite- and day-care services, and complementary interventions such as mindfulness and relaxation training. Recognizing when family caregivers need intervention(s) is an important role for nurses. Helping families connect with others who experience the same challenges combined with self-care education allows them to see that they are not alone. Nurses should be encouraged to connect family caregivers to the National Family Caregivers Association (NFCA) and the National Alliance on

Mental Illness (NAMI), both of which provide many resources for family caregivers, including information about treatment programs for their family member, benefits, legal matters, and several other support services. NAMI is the nation's leading voice on mental health advocacy and provides support and education that was not previously available to family members (Fitzpatrick, 2017).

SUMMARY OF NURSING CARE IN ASSISTING FAMILY CAREGIVERS

1. Include the family whenever possible because the family is an integral part in caring for those with an MHC; in general, family members want to be included and supported in the treatment and care decision making for their family member.
2. When an adult with an MHC accesses care, it should be standard practice that nurses ascertain whether there are children in the family. Nurses must recognize that specific issues may arise when a child is living with a parent with an MHC.
3. Ensure that hospital assessment forms include a section that asks about children living in the home.
4. Remember that many children of adults with an MHC remain emotionally and mentally healthy in spite of the associated risks.
5. Be aware that children living with a family member with an MHC often believe they caused the MHC and may feel alone and/or have feelings of guilt, anger, or anxiety.
6. Perform a family-centered assessment of the children's needs on a regular basis, followed by referral to relevant services, to avoid potential developmental delays. At the same time, dispel the myth that parents with an MHC are unfit parents. Emphasize that a parent with an MHC can be a very competent, effective, nurturing, and loving parent.
7. Develop a relationship with the child. Nurses must initiate a conversation with the child and not wait until a child asks for help.
8. Tell the child that she or he did not cause the parent's illness or strange behavior, nor is she or he responsible for taking care of the family member. Reinforce that the health

care team will provide care to the family member.

9. Provide age-appropriate information about the parent's MHC and treatment. Children who are knowledgeable about a parent's illness are able to understand the parent's behaviors better in relation to the specific illness.

10. Children who are not given the whole story are left to make up their own explanations, which only adds to their emotional confusion and possible self-blame for parental symptoms.

11. Support for family relationships and other networks must be part of the care that nurses provide to parents in any setting. Connect family caregivers to NAMI and/or NFCA.

12. Nurses can alleviate some of the concern and uncertainty by assisting families to develop a crisis intervention plan and inviting the entire family to participate.

13. Provide support to parents who have an MHC by actively listening to the parents' concerns about parenting, providing realistic information about parenting skills, and assessing for the need for interventions to support the children.

14. Nurses can work with parents of children with an MHC to help them shape how unaffected siblings perceive the affected sibling and the MHC, as well as identify ways in which the parents can provide the needed attention to healthy siblings.

FAMILIES OF INDIVIDUALS WITH A SPECIFIC MHC

Several MHCs warrant specific discussion, either because of the stigma associated with these disorders or the serious impact these disorders can have on family function and well-being. The following four disorders will be discussed:

- Schizophrenia
- Major depressive disorder (MDD)
- Bipolar disorder (BD)
- Attention deficit-hyperactivity disorder (ADHD)

This section will briefly describe each disorder, discuss the impact that these specific disorders can

have on families, and review implications for nursing practice. Note that substance use disorder is a common comorbidity with these conditions, so it too requires assessment and intervention. The Johnson family case study, which appears later in the chapter, discusses assessment and treatment for substance use disorder.

Schizophrenia, BD, and MDD should be considered potentially terminal illnesses for persons with these disorders due to the high suicide rate, which speaks to the devasting impact of these mental illnesses. An estimated 4.9% of people with schizophrenia die by suicide, with the highest risk in the early stages of the illness (NIMH, 2018).

Approximately two-thirds of people with MDD consider suicide, and about 10% to 15% of them complete suicide (Sadock et al., 2017). These high rates of attempted and completed suicides mean that nurses should consistently and diligently assess for suicidality/suicidal ideations in these populations. Several suicide screening tools are available on the internet, and the agencies where nurses work are required to have an identified validated suicide assessment screening tool available.

The Joint Commission's analysis of inpatient suicide methods suggests that additional prevention efforts should be targeted toward mitigating risks associated with suicide attempts and toward reducing the risk of suicide immediately following discharge (Williams et al., 2018). The Joint Commission (2019) has implemented seven new and revised elements of performance for accredited facilities that became effective on July 1, 2019. These performance elements were designed to improve the quality and safety of care for all those treated for an MHC and for those at risk for suicide. One requirement is to screen for suicidal ideation using a validated tool starting at age 12 (Joint Commission, 2019; Gottlieb, 2014).

Schizophrenia

Schizophrenia is a chronic condition of disturbed thought processes, perceptions, and affect that can lead to severe social and occupational dysfunction and sometimes hospitalization. International prevalence of schizophrenia among noninstitutionalized persons is 0.33% to 0.75% (NIMH, 2018). It is diagnosed most often when an individual experiences psychosis for the first time, usually in his or her late teens or early twenties. Schizophrenia is a severe disorder characterized by distorted thinking and perception and inappropriate emotions. The symptoms of schizophrenia tend to fall into three categories: psychotic, negative, and cognitive symptoms (NIMH, 2020).

Psychotic symptoms include altered perceptions, distorted thinking, and odd behaviors. People experiencing psychosis may have an altered sense of reality. Specifically, they typically experience auditory and/or visual hallucinations; delusions, which are firmly held beliefs that are not supported by facts but result instead from paranoid thinking and unusual thinking; or disorganized speech known as a thought disorder.

Negative symptoms include loss of motivation; loss of interest or enjoyment in daily activities; social withdrawal; and a flat affect, which affects engaging in everyday activities and normal functioning.

Cognitive symptoms vary from being subtle to pronounced, with problems in concentration and memory. There are often challenges in processing information in order to make decisions, which has an impact on judgment.

There is complete symptomatic and social recovery in about 30% of persons with schizophrenia; however, a person with schizophrenia may demonstrate disturbed behavior during some phases of the disorder, which can lead to unfavorable social consequences for the individual and family. Up to 80% of individuals with schizophrenia may have an MDD at some time in their lives, which is conjectured to be linked with the 20-fold increase in suicide compared to the general public (Sadock et al., 2017). Globally, schizophrenia decreases the person's life span by an average of 10 years (WHO, 2016), with the most frequent causes of premature death other than suicide being heart disease, liver disease, and diabetes (NIMH, 2018). People with schizophrenia also have a higher mortality rate from accidents and natural causes than does the general population (WHO, 2016).

Inpatient treatment for persons with an SMI such as schizophrenia is more likely to be limited to days rather than weeks or months. This approach means that treatment and symptom management tend to occur in the community. Some individuals with schizophrenia live with their families, but many do not. Some live on their own, others live with roommates or in a group setting, still others are homeless. Because they are adults who are considered competent when their condition is at least fairly well managed, it can be very challenging for families to help the person obtain the care he or she needs, especially if the person with schizophrenia is not managing well and is refusing care.

Whether or not the person with schizophrenia lives with the family, families need help understanding how to manage the situation. They need information about schizophrenia and guidance on how to cope with the symptoms. Individuals with schizophrenia and their family members benefit from family education and support, coordination of specialty care, and assertive community treatment (ACT). ACT is for those with schizophrenia who are at risk for multiple hospitalizations and homelessness. ACT is an evidence-based program that includes a multidisciplinary team, a medication prescriber, shared caseload among team members, high frequency of patient contact, low patient-to-staff ratios, and outreach to patients in the community (NIMH, 2020). Family members need to be aware of this program.

Psychological distress is a significant predictor of family functioning, and having a family member with schizophrenia is a major stressor for the family. Being informed and knowing what to look for can help family members recognize early signs of changes in the individual's symptoms and behaviors that may require professional involvement. If changes are addressed early, it is possible to avoid hospitalization and reduce family stress. For example, families need information about how to interact safely with a family member who may be having command hallucinations, especially if the hallucinations are commanding the individual to harm herself or others. Nurses need to inform family members that it is not appropriate to argue or disagree with the person who is actively hallucinating or having a delusion. Rather, family members should have a plan already in place to implement. If there are children in the household, the person's behavior may be frightening to them. Children should have a safe, prearranged place to go, such as a nearby neighbor, or they should have contact information to call a trusted person to come be with them. Nurses should engage in open discussions with family members about how to interact with their family member who may be hallucinating or having a delusional thought, preferably before the experience.

Families who have a family member with schizophrenia need nurses to understand the frustration and exhaustion they frequently experience; they also want to feel respected by health care providers. On the other hand, nurses need to remind family members to be patient with the affected family member. Family members may be aware of the positive symptoms (i.e., hallucinations and delusions) and negative symptoms (i.e., anergy, amotivation, apathy, avolition) of schizophrenia. Melton et al. (2020) found that families responded quickly to seek treatment when hallucinations and physical deterioration were present, but they found delusions confusing and were slower to respond. Families find negative symptoms very difficult to deal with, and the individual with these symptoms is often perceived as lazy and socially inept.

Most individuals with schizophrenia do not live with a family member, but when the person who has schizophrenia does live at home, the tasks that family caregivers typically provide on a daily basis are similar to those needed when anyone has an MHC: providing companionship, providing emotional support during a crisis, monitoring symptoms, assisting with personal grooming, and so on. The nature of this condition can make it difficult for families to provide the care they perceive the person needs, especially when the medications are not effective (or the person with schizophrenia has stopped taking them). Nurses need to provide assistance to these families in managing the individual's illness, including assistance with living arrangements, job placement, day-to-day activities, and medications. The family's coping ability and functioning are enhanced when appropriate social support systems are in place, and such supports can even buffer the family from the emotional distress that can occur when providing care to a family member with schizophrenia. Nurses need to remind families that there are limits to what they can do for their family member. Nurses should refer families to appropriate resources and support groups, including NAMI.

Medication adherence is a major part of treatment for managing the symptoms and behaviors of schizophrenia, but adherence is variable and frequently less than optimal. The side effects of medications can lead the person with schizophrenia to stop his or her medication, resulting in exacerbation of the condition. It is important to engage the individual and appropriate family members in administering medications and in monitoring the effects and effectiveness of the medications. Many of the medications have serious adverse effects. Neuroleptic malignant syndrome and extrapyramidal symptoms, including akathisia and tardive dyskinesia, which affect the muscles, are serious and life-threatening complications that can be caused by typical and atypical antipsychotic medications. The individual and appropriate family members need to know what to do and who to call should they observe a dangerous or life-threatening side effect, such as difficulty swallowing or breathing, and they should have emergency information readily available. In addition, interventions to prevent metabolic syndrome, such as eating healthy foods and participating in regular exercise, can help to maintain a healthy body and decrease the risk for developing this syndrome.

Hospitalization is not uncommon, partly because of nonadherence to medication regimens, and it is a stressful time for the individual and family. Family members often do not understand the use and purpose of physical restraints or seclusion, and they may need to be taught this information by nurses in a nonjudgmental and positive manner, making sure that they understand the temporary use of these safety measures. Related to issues of hospitalization is the topic of involuntary commitment. Nurses need to be familiar with their state or provincial involuntary commitment statutes and inform families about these laws so that families and individuals do not become overwhelmed or frustrated should involuntary commitment occur. Involuntary civil commitment means that an individual is admitted to a mental health unit against his or her will. The three main reasons for involuntary commitment are mental illness, substance use disorder, and developmental disability. Being dangerous to oneself, including being unable to provide for one's basic needs, or presenting a danger to others usually defines the typical commitment standard for mental illness. Most jurisdictions provide for a hearing, the right to counsel, and a periodic judicial review.

Family members of people with schizophrenia may be in the position of seeking involuntary commitment for their mentally ill family member, which can be a very stressful process. People with major mental illnesses often do not understand their disorders and disagree about receiving treatment even when they feel like acting out violently. Before police or emergency mental health intervention can be called in, the mentally ill person, under most state laws, must be already violent. Family members may see the situation escalating, but they may not receive help until treatment is no longer focused on the person's mental disorder but on the violence. Many people have been arrested and charged with crimes of violence during exacerbations of mental disorders (Robertson & Walter, 2014). Family members and caregivers are often significant members of the decision-making process to commit a person with schizophrenia and often find themselves in a position of role conflict, confusion, and misunderstanding (Arya, 2014).

Two final comments about schizophrenia are worthy of consideration for nurses. First, persons with schizophrenia should not be labeled or called "schizophrenics" but rather identified by their names to avoid further stigmatization. It is also more professional and respectful and less pejorative to identify the person by name and not by illness. Second, the number of children born to parents with schizophrenia has increased because of improved medications and deinstitutionalization; the fertility rate is close to that for the general population (Sadock et al., 2017). First-degree biological relatives of persons with schizophrenia have a greater than 10-fold risk for developing schizophrenia compared with the general population (Sadock et al., 2017). The aforementioned statements have teaching and education implications for nurses working with families who have a family member with schizophrenia.

MDD

MDD, also called major depression or clinical depression, is a medical condition that causes a persistent feeling of sadness and loss of interest; it affects how someone thinks, feels, and behaves, and it can lead to emotional and physical problems. More than 264 million people of all ages suffer from depression, making it a leading cause of disability worldwide (WHO, 2020a). People with MDD often have trouble doing normal day-to-day activities, and they may feel as if life is not worth living. A chronic illness that usually requires long-term treatment, MDD affects 4.7% of Canadians (Statistics Canada, 2020) and about 5% to 8% of Americans (NIMH, 2018).

Sadock et al. (2017) asserted that the life event most often associated with development of depression is the loss of a parent before a child is 11 years old, and the environmental stressor most associated with onset of a depressive episode is the loss of a spouse. The Patient Health Questionnaire-9 is one of the most validated tools (9-item depression scale) in mental health, used by nurses and other clinicians to screen for depression and for assessing treatment responses (University of Washington, 2021), which is in the public domain and available online. Adults with depression experience the following: anhedonia (the inability to experience pleasure from activities normally found to be enjoyable), anxiety (Sadock et al., 2017), decreased energy, feelings of guilt, and changes in appetite or sleep. Depression often coexists with physical medical conditions (NIMH, 2017). MDD interferes with social, occupational, and interpersonal functioning. Older adults may manifest depression with somatic symptoms. Unfortunately, many health care providers underdiagnose and undertreat older persons with depression because they assume that MDD is a natural part of aging—which it is not. At the same time, it is important for nurses to be aware of the multiple losses an older person may have experienced and her or his ability to cope with these losses and how much family support they have.

A holistic nursing assessment should include an assessment of contextual factors that may have led to the depressive symptoms. A Canadian study of university students found that depression, anxiety, and stress outcomes were significantly associated with a number of determinants grouped as family, interpersonal, social, socioeconomic, and political factors (Othman et al., 2019). This study reinforces the need for nurses to advocate beyond the support, education, and treatment needs of the individual and her or his family to address the social determinants of health.

MDD can jeopardize marriages and lead to marital discord. More than 50% of spouses report that they would not have married their spouse or had children had they known that their partner was going to develop a mood disorder (Sadock et al., 2017). Family therapy and couples therapy are important strategies to help families; they can be effective in improving the psychological well-being of the whole family.

Psychotherapy and psychopharmacology are common treatments for persons with depression.

Selective serotonin reuptake inhibitors (SSRIs) and serotonin-norepinephrine reuptake inhibitors (SNRIs) are two common types of drugs used to treat depression. Individuals who are prescribed these medications and their families need to be aware of a potentially life-threatening drug interaction—serotonin syndrome—that can occur if these drugs are inadvertently taken with other drugs or in case of overdose. Serotonin is a chemical produced by the body that allows nerve cells and the brain to function. Too much serotonin may cause mild symptoms such as shivering and diarrhea, but severe serotonin syndrome may lead to muscle rigidity, fever, and seizures, which can be fatal if not treated. Herbs, such as St. John's wort; stimulants, such as methylphenidate; and opioids, such as hydrocodone, can interact to produce serotonin syndrome. Families need to be educated about the signs and symptoms of serotonin syndrome and receive information on how to contact the health care provider or emergency support services. Nurses should be familiar with the classification of drugs that are prescribed to their clients, such as SSRIs, SNRIs, or norepinephrine-dopamine reuptake inhibitors (NDRIs), as well as the neurotransmitters and parts of the brain affected by these drugs. Drugs are used to treat symptoms and behaviors, not to treat diagnoses. There are numerous psychopharmacology textbooks, as well as many excellent online resources, available for nurses to learn more about these drugs.

Children and Depression

Depression is not always easily recognized in children because many everyday stresses, such as the birth of a sibling, can cause changes in a child's behavior. It is important to be able to tell the difference between typical behavior changes and those associated with more serious problems. Symptoms of depression in children often manifest as irritability and anger. It may be demonstrated by excessive clinging to parents or by phobias, and adolescents often exhibit poor academic performance, substance abuse, antisocial behavior, sexual promiscuity, or truancy, or they run away (Sadock et al., 2017). Other behaviors to pay special attention to include problems across a variety of settings, such as at school, at home, or with peers; withdrawal from social or other activities that used to be enjoyed; difficulty with concentration;

running away from home or talking about running away; suicidal ideation; change in sleep pattern; and comments that indicate hopelessness or low self-worth (Bhatia, 2018).

Children who live with a parent who has MDD are often aware of the parent's depression and are both emotionally affected and inappropriately involved in managing everyday life, such as taking over daily living or financial tasks that are normally completed by an adult. Even though children want to help their parent, they do not feel capable, which can often lead to feelings of guilt. Guilt is a feeling that children living with a depressed parent experience more often than other children. Some children worry that their depressed parent may attempt or complete suicide while they are away from home. Salo et al. (2020) found that the depressed parents were compromised in their ability to convey cognitive and affective empathy to their younger children.

It promotes children's health when the family as a whole learns about depression and learns how to talk more openly about it. It is important for nurses to help children understand that they did not cause the parent's depression and also to help the parents convey this message to their children. Children of depressed parents are at a higher risk for depression and anxiety (Maciejewski et al., 2018). Given this risk, nurses and other mental health providers need to integrate the promotion of child development services in the treatment of parents with depression. A study conducted in Finland (Niemelä et al., 2019) found that implementing the Let's Talk About Children Service Model (LT-SM), which is aimed at promoting child and family well-being and resilience and preventing child and family dysfunction, reduced referrals to child protective services. The community-based model uses integrated approaches to bring together health, social, and educational services in a coordinated effort to support children in their everyday life at home, school, and community environments (Mieli Mental Health Finland, n.d.). A key component of the program includes supporting parents and families to reduce barriers that impact development milestones and developing healthy coping skills for children.

A study in Greece by Maciejewski et al. (2018) found implementing both LT-SM and Family Talk Intervention (FTI) fostered family and child resilience by supporting parent-child relationships,

BOX 18-2
Let's Talk About Children Service Model (LT-SM)

LT-SM is a two- to three-session intervention intended to be offered to all psychiatric patients with dependent children. If there is a need for extra family support, a third meeting may be conducted. The premises of the program are that the routines, encounters, and interactions with children on an ordinary day are the foundation of child development, and parental mental health issues often compromise these daily routines of everyday life. The program also recognizes that children often need understanding and support in day care, at school, and in their social life with peers. Therefore, LT-SM also has a contextual, ecological element.

BOX 18-3
Family Talk Intervention (FTI)

FTI is designed for those treating parents with depression and/or anxiety. It includes six sessions with a family with one child, and the number of sessions increases with each additional child. Two parent sessions included individual and family history taking and psychoeducation regarding depression and resilience. Individual sessions with each child included the child's psychosocial status and family experiences. Parents discussed with the clinician how to respond to their children's questions, talk about depression, and cope effectively with potential family problems. In the family session, parents put mental illness into words and responded to their children's questions.

promoting protective factors in the family, and improving understanding of issues facing the family when a parent has an MHC and other family stress. These programs can be implemented by appropriately trained mental health professionals, including nurses. See Box 18-2 and Box 18-3 for a brief description of the LT-SM and FTI programs, respectively.

BD

BD affects about 2.8% of adult Americans, with nearly 83% of BD diagnoses classified as severe (NAMI, 2017), and worldwide the prevalence is around 0.4% (WHO, 2016). A large survey of 11 countries found that the overall lifetime prevalence of bipolar type 1 was 0.6% and of type 2 was 0.4% (Rowland & Marwaha, 2018). Bipolar I disorder, a subdiagnosis of BD that is characterized by one or more manic episodes, is more common in divorced and single persons than among married people (Sadock et al., 2017). BD is a recurring, treatable but incurable MHC that causes cycles of mania and depression. Episodes of mania or depression can last from 1 day to months, with euthymic (normal mood) periods between these mood shifts (NAMI, 2017). These dramatic shifts in mood can disrupt family function and cause damage to relationships; academic problems; financial problems caused by loss of jobs; and even legal problems, including confrontations with the police.

Family members can find it very difficult to interact with a family member who is demonstrating manic symptoms—euphoria, reduced need for sleep, excessive talking, irritability, overactivity, overconfidence, impaired concentration, increased pleasure-seeking or risk-taking behaviors, and elevated surges of energy. Children especially can become disturbed when living with a family member who is manic. The children's safety can be in jeopardy, and the children may feel afraid being near someone who is behaving irrationally. On the other hand, it can be equally disconcerting for families to live with or provide care to someone who is depressed and demonstrating hopelessness, extreme sadness, and loss of energy.

Families with a member who has BD are continually challenged by the fickleness and unpredictability that this MHC can cause. The family and the individual live with uncertainty, not knowing which mood to expect at any given time or when a change will occur. Parents of adult children with BD have more compromised mental and physical health and more difficulties in marriage and work life than comparison families. In addition, parents who already had an MHC before the onset of their child's BD are even more vulnerable to problems with mental health issues, psychological well-being, and work life than parents who do not have an existing MHC. Consequently, obtaining the history of MHC in parents and the immediate family is important to inform the nurse's interventions in promoting the well-being of each family member.

Family history of BD conveys a greater risk for BD disorders in general (Sadock et al., 2017). Nurses need to teach families about the genetic implications of this MHC and educate families on the signs and symptoms so that families can recognize them and initiate early professional treatment. BD is a difficult MHC to diagnose accurately, yet it is important that this MHC be differentiated from MDD, personality disorders, substance use, anxiety disorders, and schizophrenia (Sadock et al., 2017) because the treatments can be significantly different.

The average age of onset is 25, but BD can occur earlier during adolescence. Because adolescents can manifest symptoms of mania and depression differently from adults, they are often misdiagnosed as having antisocial personality disorder or schizophrenia rather than BD (Sadock et al., 2017). Adolescent symptoms of mania can include substance abuse, irritability that can lead to fights, academic problems, suicide attempts, obsessive-compulsive symptoms, somatic complaints, and antisocial behaviors. Misdiagnosis has tremendous implications in young people. Making differential diagnoses in adolescents is difficult, and it is important for nurses to advocate for additional assessments as new signs and symptoms emerge in adolescents so that they are treated appropriately and so that they can avoid unnecessary treatments and complications. It is crucial for nurses to consider the child's environment. Children who are being abused in the home, especially sexually, may exhibit behaviors that mimic an MHC. Child sexual abuse and other forms of maltreatment have been found to be significantly associated with a wide range of MHCs such as post-traumatic stress disorder (PTSD), panic disorder, substance abuse, schizophrenia, and antisocial personality disorder (Shrivastave et al., 2017). In these situations, the family needs treatment, even though the child is seen as the identified patient.

Caregivers who receive both psychoeducation and health promotion interventions have significantly less depression, improved health, and less subjective burden of care and role dysfunction. Not only might the caregivers receive benefit from these two interventions, but the family member with BD may demonstrate a decrease in mania and depression due in part to the improved health of the caregiver (Sampogna et al., 2018).

Caregivers of persons with BD often feel overlooked by health care providers, but they feel more supported if the mental health nurses collaborate with them, show understanding of the complexities associated with BD, and are nonjudgmental and noncritical of the family. Health care providers should recognize the uniqueness of the caregiver and the recipient of the care. It is also important to be honest with the family about the fact that BD is not curable and to maintain hope at the same time.

Although BD is treatable, the condition can cause significant social and economic stress for families. Educational interventions for family members living with a person with BD reduce stress for the family members, increase their understanding of the condition, and enhance their ability to remain socially functional. It is essential that nurses teach family members to observe for early signs of relapse into mania, such as provocative dressing, unrestrained buying sprees, hypersexuality, being more talkative than usual, or grandiosity; or signs of relapse into depression, such as increased sleeping, problems sleeping, problems with concentration, anhedonia, or recurrent thoughts of suicide (NIMH, 2020). It is important that family members monitor these changes in their family member who has BD and notify the appropriate health care provider when there are changes.

ADHD

The prevalence of ADHD around the world is 5.3% among children and at least 2.8% among adults (Speerforck, 2019). ADHD begins in childhood and is characterized by three core symptoms: attention deficit, impulsivity, and hyperactivity. Symptoms persist in about 60% of children into adulthood, resulting in detrimental impacts on social, financial, and professional functioning (Speerforck, 2019).

ADHD, behavior problems, anxiety, and depression are the most commonly diagnosed MHCs in children, with ADHD being the most prevalent in both the United States and Canada and with a higher incidence in boys. The general prevalence of ADHD in Canada is estimated to be between 5% to 9% for children and adolescents and 3% to 5% for adults (Canadian ADHD Resource Alliance [CADDRA], 2021). The prevalence in the United States is estimated at 9.4% of children aged 2 to 17 (CDC, 2020a). Boys (12.9%) are more often diagnosed with ADHD than girls (5.6%). The underrepresentation of girls may be attributed to underdiagnosis, however, because girls often present with the inattentive rather than hyperactive type of ADHD and are overlooked.

ADHD is one of the MHCs with the strongest genetic basis, according to epidemiological studies (Grimm et al., 2018), and so it is not uncommon to have more than one family member with ADHD, including one or both parents. Diagnosis is complex and requires collaborating with many key adults in the child's life, including teachers, parents, friends, and other community adults with whom the child may interact. Diagnosis in adults often follows a diagnosis for one of their children.

Children, adolescents, and adults with ADHD typically demonstrate diminished sustained concentration, increased levels of impulsivity, hyperactivity, and problems with social interactions. Other people may view them as lazy, stupid, reckless, or uncaring because of how the symptoms affect the person with ADHD. Some children, especially girls, may be inattentive rather than hyperactive, and the hyperactivity in adults is often internal rather than external. Young people who are diagnosed with ADHD often endure stigma from their peers, teachers, family, and society. Examples of stigma include teachers and peers thinking that a person with ADHD chooses to be inattentive in class or that the person with ADHD has a character flaw rather than an MHC. A study conducted by Metzger and Hamilton (2020) found that teachers are more likely to rate children with ADHD as performing below grade level regardless of their demonstrated ability on subject-specific tests.

Many young people struggle with the negative assumptions that others have toward them and that they have toward themselves. They often experience a lack of empathy and understanding from key adults in their lives. Young people with ADHD frequently feel that the diagnosis itself gives them a bad reputation, including thinking that others consider them stupid. Eccleston et al. (2019), in their review of the literature, found five overarching themes (see Table 18-3) that captured the life experiences of adolescents living with ADHD.

Parents and caregivers of children with ADHD experience a wide range of challenges. After examining and analyzing 80 publications, mostly from the United States, Corcoran et al. (2017) concluded that the major finding involved the parents' emotional burden of caring for a child with ADHD. Parents struggled with managing the hyperactive, impulsive, and inattentive behaviors, including forgetfulness, inability to listen and complete tasks, poor grades, tantrums, risk taking, and poor social relationships. Parents talked about the constant mess, chaos, and conflict in the home and finding it exhausting. Parents experienced a variety of intense and painful emotions as they attempted to manage family routines. Parents found disciplining children only worked in a limited way and took constant effort throughout the day. The challenges of parenting spilled into other areas of their lives, such as their physical and psychological health, marital relationship, and work.

What works best is a comprehensive, collaborative, and multimodal treatment approach that is individualized to meet the unique needs of the person with ADHD. The American Academy of Pediatrics (AAP) recommends that behavior therapy be the first mode of treatment for young children, and parent training has the most evidence for being effective. The Children and Adults with Attention-Deficit/Hyperactivity Disorder (CHADD) website has a wealth of resources, including information about a number of different programs for families to manage ADHD, some of which are offered through telehealth or online courses.

It is very beneficial for parents to learn about and use home management skills, such as eliminating screen time before bed to decrease sleep problems, supervising and providing homework to assist the child with staying organized and focused, and providing short movement breaks at regular intervals; it is also important that parents request appropriate neuropsychological and

Table 18-3	**Adolescent Experience of Living With ADHD**

1. Perspectives of the problem varied from being a physical condition; an academic disadvantage; part of their personality, behavior, and emotions; normal.

2. Societal pressures related to stigma and rejection, others' expectations, conflict and invalidation.

3. Sense of self (feeling different, needing acceptance, affected self-esteem, and maintained versus altered identity).

4. Feelings about medication (efficacy, burden, and weighing the costs and benefits).

5. Maturational shift from passive to active (shifting role of adolescent, scaffolding through support, and worry about the future).

Source: Eccleston et al., 2019.

psychoeducational evaluations for their child. These evaluations help to determine if the child might benefit from school-based supports, particularly if their child has academic difficulties, a learning disorder, or executive functioning difficulties. For example, in the United States, some children with ADHD qualify through a federal law, the Individuals with Disabilities Education Act (IDEA), to receive an individual education plan (IEP) that is unique to the child and supports the child's educational needs. Another plan, the 504 Plan, is provided by a civil rights law that protects children with ADHD from being discriminated against because of their MHC; therefore, some children who may not qualify for an IEP may receive additional educational support under the 504 Plan. IEPs are also common in Canada after appropriate assessment and evaluation.

Treatment for ADHD may include medications, psychotherapy such as behavioral therapy, psychoeducation including lifestyle changes, coaching, and other interventions to decrease the number and severity of stressors in the individual's and family's life. Family therapy helps to maintain and promote healthy family functioning. Family therapy is also indicated if the condition jeopardizes the marriage, for example, if a spouse whose partner has ADHD is considering leaving the marriage (Sadock et al., 2017). Family therapy is especially recommended if a child and a parent have ADHD because it may be difficult for a parent to recognize her or his own disorganization, inconsistent responses to the child's behaviors, and/or impulsivities and the impact they can have on the family.

Although AAP recommends that parents learn behavior management skills before medicating children under the age of 6, both medications and behavior therapy are recommended for children ages 6 and above (CDC, 2020a). Medications, in conjunction with other interventions, are often used to treat ADHD, but the decision to use these medications has to be based on the benefits of taking the medications versus the consequences of not taking them. The parent or adult needs to make these decisions without outside pressure from family or media who may be misinformed. Parents of children with ADHD often experience misgivings about administering a stimulant to their child based on feedback they get from their family, friends, or the media, even though

stimulants are the recommended treatment. Much of the information parents obtain about treating ADHD with medications is secondary and not evidence based.

Nurses have a responsibility to provide accurate information to parents so the parents can make a thoughtful and informed decision about whether or not to treat their child with medication. The child and adult who are prescribed a stimulant require regular checkups. Just as many clinical settings contact patients for follow-up visits, such as for diabetes management, these settings should likewise designate a nurse to be the point person to provide this service to persons with ADHD and their families. Nurses should educate families that medications neither cure ADHD nor necessarily eliminate the impulsive behaviors a child or adult may exhibit. Families should be aware of the advantages and disadvantages of taking medications several times during the day versus taking a long-acting stimulant.

ROLE OF THE FAMILY MENTAL HEALTH NURSE

In order to establish a collaborative relationship with the family, nurses must have a nonblaming and accepting attitude toward family members. Families value interactions with health care providers that demonstrate openness, cooperation, confirmation, and continuity. Family members increasingly have assumed the role of primary caregivers for mentally ill individuals, so it is more important than ever to include them as partners in the delivery of mental health care. Care delivery systems that involve family members acknowledge the effect mental disorders have on entire family systems. They seek to prevent the return or exacerbation of a disorder, and they alleviate pain and suffering experienced by family members. To fulfill these goals, Dixon et al. (2001) identified 15 evidence-based principles that continue to be relevant and can be incorporated into family nursing interventions for families of individuals with a mental illness (Box 18-4). This section briefly examines a few areas of focus for mental health nurses within care delivery systems: prevention of MHCs, psychoeducation, family recovery, crisis plans, and providing culturally sensitive care.

BOX 18-4

Evidence-Based Principles for Working With Families of Individuals With a Mental Illness

Following are evidence-based principles for health care providers who work with families that have an individual or individuals with mental illness:

- Coordinate care so that everyone involved is working toward the same treatment goals within a collaborative, supportive relationship.
- Attend to both the social and clinical needs of the primary patient.
- Provide optimal medication management.
- Listen to family's concerns and involve them in all elements of treatment.
- Examine family's expectations of treatment and expectations of the primary patient.
- Evaluate strengths and limitations of the family's ability to provide support.
- Aid in the resolution of family conflict.
- Explore feelings of loss for all parties.
- Provide pertinent information to patients and families at appropriate times.
- Develop a clear crisis plan.
- Help enhance family communication.
- Train families in problem-solving techniques.
- Promote expansion of the family's social support network.
- Be adaptable in meeting the family's needs.
- Provide easy access to another professional if current work with the family ceases.

Source: Adapted from Dixon, L., McFarlane, W., Lefley, H., Lucksted, A., Cohen, M., Falloon, I., . . . Sondheimer, D. (2001). Evidence-based practices for services to families of people with psychiatric disabilities. *Psychiatric Services, 52*(7), 903–910.

Prevention of MHCs

The most important role for the nurse in mental health care is to engage in professional activities that prevent MHCs. Toxic stress during childhood has the capacity physically to change a child's brain and be hardwired into the child's biology via genes in the DNA, according to epigenetics research (Sciaraffa et al., 2018). The CDC-Kaiser Permanente Adverse Childhood Experiences (ACE) Study was one of the first studies on the effects of childhood abuse, neglect, and household challenges on health and well-being later in life (CDC, 2021). According to the study, long-term exposure

to chronic severe stress and the absence of a supportive adult can profoundly affect the developing brain (CDC, 2021). Genetics influence brain development and exposure to significant stress can affect the way specific genes are expressed. There is a polymorphism (genetic variation within a population) in the 5-HTT gene that results in the occurrence of MDD only if the gene carrier experiences a major life stressor (Burke et al., 2016). Stress itself, such as physical, emotional, and sexual abuse; famine; and natural disasters, can also profoundly affect emotional, behavioral, cognitive, social, and physical functioning in children.

Secure attachments and ample nurturing not only allow for a positive environment for the brain to build neural connections to integrate the brain systems but also strengthen an infant's ability to cope with stress (Sciaraffa et al., 2018). When babies cry and their needs are taken care of, such as through food or attention and comfort, their neuronal pathways are strengthened, and they learn how to get their needs met both physically and emotionally. On the other hand, babies who are abused or neglected learn other lessons that can be damaging and may interfere with a child's ability to self-regulate. For instance, the child whose needs are not met and who endures repeated painful disappointments may abandon crying for help, resulting in problems with hyperarousal or dissociation. The Adverse Childhood Experiences (ACE) study reinforced these findings. The ACE study is addressed in more detail in Chapter 12 of this textbook.

Maltreatment at an early age may have enduring effects on the development and function of a child's brain. Child maltreatment can manifest internally, with depression, anxiety, or suicidality, or outwardly, with aggression, impulsiveness, hyperactivity, delinquency, or substance abuse. There is an association between maltreatment in childhood and a person being diagnosed with borderline personality disorder. Borderline personality disorder is characterized by seeing others and situations in black-and-white terms, having unstable relationships, having feelings of abandonment, exhibiting self-harm, having problems with anger, and escaping through substance abuse. The limbic system plays a key role in regulating emotion and memory of one's experiences. Research has shown that abuse in children can cause permanent damage to the neural structure and function of the brain. People with borderline personality disorder often have reduced integration between the left and right brain hemispheres, a smaller corpus callosum, and limbic electrical irritability (Hockenberry et al., 2017).

There is also some evidence that a mother smoking or drinking alcohol during pregnancy affects the growth of neural pathways, thereby increasing the risk of their children becoming smokers, whereas prenatal exposure to alcohol increased the risk of substance use disorder (O'Brien & Hill, 2014) and/or ADHD (Ware et al., 2014). Exposure to prenatal alcohol is associated with a variety of structural and functional brain changes (Sharma & Hill, 2017). Healthy lifestyle behaviors, including diet; exercise; stress reduction strategies; and nonconsumption of alcohol, cigarettes, and illegal substances, seem to play a role in reducing the risk of developing an MHC. Nurses should encourage and support healthy lifestyles, whether prenatally or for children, youth, or adults.

Nurses must advocate for good parenting and must offer parenting support in a nonjudgmental way. Nurses should be at the forefront of ensuring the prevention of childhood maltreatment. Early assessment and intervention are important to help prevent serious repercussions for children. Nurses can provide resources for caretakers of children so they learn the necessary skills to provide responsible care, support, and nurturing to their child. Nurses should be active in local, state, and national policies that affect child welfare.

Persons with SMI tend to have a 10- to 25-year lower life expectancy, compared with the general population, because of preventable diseases, especially cardiovascular disease, respiratory disease, infections, and suicide (Liu et al., 2017). These premature deaths can dramatically affect families because of the burden of physical care, financial costs, and role changes. Mental health nurses play a significant role in addressing the physical health care needs of persons with SMI; they must be able to assess and address the physical impact that the person's lifestyle (such as nutrition, exercise, and sleep), psychotropic medication adverse effects, and living environment can have on preventing cardiovascular, metabolic, and respiratory diseases among this population. However, multilevel interventions provide optimal prevention in order to take into consideration the social determinants of health such as public policies, socioeconomic status, environmental vulnerabilities, access to health care, housing, employment, and social support. It cannot be emphasized enough how intertwined these factors are at multiple levels, thus contributing to excess mortality. Addressing individual lifestyle is not enough (Liu et al., 2017).

Psychoeducation

A major role for a professional nurse working with families who have a member with an MHC is to provide psychoeducation. Psychoeducation includes teaching clients about the cause and treatments of the MHC while being attuned to each family member's unique needs. Family psychoeducation is an evidence-based therapeutic intervention that provides social support, education, and support for improved understanding and coping with an MHC, including SMI. Psychoeducation provides insight into the MHC and helps remove stigma, misunderstandings, and myths about mental illness (Singh et al., 2020).

The time commitment and emphasis on social support, education, and coping skills are what differ among the diverse psychoeducational models. Currently, these interventions may continue for months or years. Because psychoeducational programs are multifaceted and involve long-term relationships, they are typically delivered by teams of health care providers working together. Nurses' training and education make them well suited to participate in such interdisciplinary teams that emphasize client and family education, enhance coping skills, and develop supportive networks.

The educational element of these programs involves providing information to relatives regarding diagnoses, cause of mental illness, prognosis, and treatment. Skills training may include coping skills for family members and social skills training for the family member with the MHC. In addition, the entire family may work on developing communication skills so members can communicate more effectively with one another. Nurses can enhance social support for the family by actively including relatives as members of the treatment team and by helping to establish connections to other families with similar experiences. Through networking with one another, families can find support and share problem-solving strategies. A local chapter of NAMI is one support and advocacy organization that families may find helpful.

BOX 18-5
Family Intervention Strategies

- Coordinate information and treatment plans across settings and with multiple health care providers.
- Ensure that communication is bidirectional, from health care providers to families and from families to health care providers.
- Provide validation for commitment and work being done by all family members.
- Create ways for families to manage treatment plans that affect everyday routines.
- Identify realistic ways that the mentally ill family member can participate in and contribute to the family.
- Articulate an action plan to implement during times of crisis.
- Negotiate ways to manage specific problem behaviors.
- Connect with appropriate social resources (individual/group therapy, support groups, extended family, friends, religious organizations).
- Provide diagnostic and treatment-related family psychoeducation.
- Encourage self-care behaviors for all family members.
- Identify effective coping skills for individual family members.
- Advocate for policy changes that benefit individuals with MHCs and their family members.
- Challenge detrimental stereotypes and stigma of persons with an MHC.

Nurses can teach individuals and family members about no-cost relaxation techniques to reduce stress (e.g., breathing techniques and exercises, guided imagery, yoga, and progressive muscle relaxation) and provide pet and/or music therapy. Nurses have the skills to help families cope with feelings of anger and disappointment as they go through the grief process after learning about the MHC of one of their family members. It is important to realize that it may take time for families to accept the diagnosis and that the level of acceptance will vary between members of the family. A variety of family intervention strategies are outlined in Box 18-5.

Family Recovery

The recovery process of families who have a family member with an MHC (Spaniol & Nelson, 2015) involves four fluid phases that may not be the specific process for each individual: (1) shock, discovery, and denial; (2) recognition and acceptance; (3) coping; and (4) personal and political advocacy. Mental health nurses who are aware of these phases can provide specific interventions to these families in each of the phases.

Family members and relatives of persons with an MHC often experience challenging ethical dilemmas that affect the lives of everyone. For example, when should a family member make decisions on behalf of (1) oneself, (2) the person with the MHC, or (3) the entire family? It is often appropriate for a family member to encourage individual freedom and autonomy for the person with an MHC, but allowing this freedom can also have negative impacts on the family, such as not "making" a person take her psychiatric medication but then knowing that the possible emergence of psychosis will cause increased stress for all family members. Prioritizing among oneself, others in the family, and the person with the MHC can cause guilt for family members, such as deciding when to exclude a person with an MHC from a special family event. Mental health nurses can provide support to these families by listening nonjudgmentally and providing hope as families struggle to balance their lives with providing care to the person with an MHC.

There is strong evidence to support family-based interventions in the treatment of a patient with an MHC. Involving the family has been shown to improve symptoms among children with mood disorders (Young & Fristad, 2015) and when treating chronic and refractory MHCs, such as conduct disorder and substance abuse (Sharma & Sargent, 2015). A large Canadian study (Aldersey & Whitley, 2015) found that the family can be a positive influence on the recovery of the family. Family members being there for each other, such as listening, making telephone calls, and providing verbal encouragement, fostered family recovery. Practical support, such as providing financial assistance for housing and treatment, also facilitated family recovery. Families who provided motivation to recover assisted the recovery process.

Crisis Plans

Family members who provide care to relatives with a severe MHC experience a higher rate of violence than the general public. Yet these family caregivers frequently feel guilt, embarrassment, and hopelessness about experiencing violence from a family member. It is a topic that is difficult for family members to raise with health care providers and others. One major way to support families so they can manage violence is to include relatives as valuable sources of information (Kontio et al., 2017). For example, ask family members about how they have managed violence in the past and what signs and/or symptoms they have observed that indicate a family member's escalation of violence. Family members may feel guilty about having a family member involuntarily admitted to a hospital, especially if the police are involved.

Nurses are integral in assisting families to develop a crisis plan and putting it in place before the need for such a plan. It is more challenging to manage a crisis when families do not have a predetermined plan to follow. Nurses should suggest that families have the following information readily available:

- A list of health care providers, emergency professional contact names, and telephone numbers
- Suicide hotline telephone numbers
- Insurance information
- Details about the best route to the appropriate emergency department or health care facility, including specific directions to get to the sites
- Safe locations where children or other members of the family can go during escalation times

A psychiatric advance directive (PAD) is a legal document that allows a second party to act on behalf of the patient if he or she becomes acutely ill and unable to make decisions about treatment. The PAD has to be written when the person with an MHC is competent, and it details the patient's preferences for treatment (NAMI, n.d.a). Nurses can play a major role in helping the person with an MHC and their family plan ahead. Nurses should provide information for families to obtain support by participating in local support groups, such as through NAMI in the United States and CMHA in Canada.

Providing Culturally Competent Care

Nurses must remember that cultural norms and beliefs shape family members' perceptions of coping and managing care for relatives with an MHC. NAMI's informative website (NAMI, n.d.b) includes mental health fact sheets. Nurses are encouraged to review these fact sheets to become more informed. They will help them in practice and in decreasing myths and stereotypes about different ethnic groups.

NAMI also has fact sheets about depression among the following groups: veterans; lesbian, gay, bisexual, and transgender people; seniors; women; men; and children and adolescents. Misdiagnosis and undertreatment are not uncommon among some cultural groups; improved understanding about various cultural groups will enhance nursing practice. In addition, because psychiatric medications are a significant part of treating MHCs, it is important for nurses to know which populations may be fast metabolizers and which might be slow metabolizers in order to avoid overmedicating or undermedicating a specific individual. At the same time, it is important not to stereotype individuals or families based on their cultural identity but rather to use cultural identity as one aspect of the nursing assessment to consider when developing a nursing plan for the entire family.

Case Study: Johnson Family

This case study about the Johnson family demonstrates the assessment, diagnosis, outcome identification, planning, implementation, and evaluation for care of a family with a member who has been diagnosed with BD and substance use disorder.

Setting
Inpatient acute care hospital, cardiac intensive-care unit (ICU).

Nursing Goal
The family will identify a family-oriented community resource for people with family members with mental disorders or substance use disorders that they are willing to attend by the time the client is discharged. Tony is the member of the family

Case Study: Johnson Family—cont'd

who was hospitalized for mental health and substance abuse concerns. He was just diagnosed with BD and agreed to engage in a change conversation (Miller & Rollnick, 2013) in which he will list his own reasons for adhering to his mood-stabilizing medications and at least one strategy from his own life for making adherence possible or easier.

Family Members

- Steve: father (now married to Debbie), 49 years old, small-business owner
- Mary: mother (now married to Harold), 49 years old, server at a restaurant
- Debbie: stepmother, 54 years old, schoolteacher
- Harold: stepfather, 60 years old, successful building contractor
- Tony: identified patient, 23 years old, oldest child, son, unemployed, sleeping on couches of friends
- Susie: younger daughter, Tony's sister, 17 years old, overachiever and "perfect" child
- Thomas: Mary's father, 86 years old, wealthy businessman
- Emma: Mary's mother, 85 years old, substance use disorder

Johnson Family Story

Tony Johnson is a 23-year-old man who was admitted to the hospital through the emergency department in acute cardiac distress from an accidental methamphetamine overdose. He arrived at the emergency department by ambulance from his drug-free friend Doug's single-occupancy hotel room. Tony is currently homeless. For the past 2 weeks, he has been sleeping on Doug's floor.

When he was 12 years old, Tony was diagnosed with ADHD by his pediatrician, who was consulted about his disruptive behavior in school. He took methylphenidate (Ritalin) prescribed by the pediatrician, which made him feel "more quiet," in his words. When he was 13 years old and his sister was 7, his parents divorced. His father, Steve, left the home and started living with Debbie, whom he later married. Steve kept his children on his company health insurance. Tony felt responsible for the divorce because of all the arguments his parents had concerning how to manage his behavior and poor school performance. During the turmoil in their relationship, his parents did not take him back to the pediatrician nor to the recommended psychologist, but they continued to refill his prescription for methylphenidate. He continued to take it in high school. By this time, Tony stated that the medicine made him "feel energetic, like I didn't need as much sleep." When he was emotionally stable, Tony did well in school.

Tony had several episodes in high school during which he was unable to go to school. He felt angry and irritable yet tired; he was unable to concentrate mentally, had nightmares, and had difficulty with goal-oriented behavior (mealtime, personal hygiene, doing homework, and meeting friends, which he used to be able to do).

Tony started drinking alcohol at age 16. He stole his father's liquor, as well as money from his parents to buy beer illegally or alcohol from friends. During irritable episodes, he increased his drinking in an attempt to feel better. When he was arrested for driving under the influence of intoxicants at age 18, the court mandated an alcohol use disorder program that had a family counseling component. His father Steve was angry about the arrest and about how this might affect Steve's relationship with his new wife Debbie. Steve told Tony that if his behavior had a bad effect on Debbie, he would never speak to him again. Although his entire family was encouraged to participate in the program, only Tony's mother Mary, his sister Susie, and his grandfather Thomas (Mary's father) attended. His father, Steve, and stepmother, Debbie, accepted the family teaching literature but did not attend the group counseling sessions. The prescription for methylphenidate was stopped.

Tony stayed in the treatment program because of the legal requirement, but he did not believe that he had a problem with alcohol. He stated, "I can quit any time I want to." His sister wanted to protect him, so she minimized the impact of his illness when she described it in the group. His mother did not mention the stealing of money or liquor from the home. His grandfather said, "Boys will be boys. He's healthy and high-spirited. If he says he can control his drinking, he can."

Tony spent the next 2 years having episodes of either agitation or lack of energy and depression. He spent the night sleeping at the houses of various friends and occasionally at his mother's or later his stepfather's house. He used alcohol in an attempt to solve his problems and eventually started stealing prescription painkillers from his grandmother Emma. He also bought drugs from a dealer and continued to steal from his family, friends, and their families, and he burglarized one family's home while they were away. He stole credit cards and shoplifted at stores to pay for drugs and alcohol.

(continued)

Case Study: Johnson Family—cont'd

When his stepmother caught him stealing her jewelry, Tony promised to try rehabilitation again at a facility financed by his father's insurance; this program was a dual-diagnosis program, where he was diagnosed with BD and substance use disorder. He was prescribed new medications for mood stabilization. His parents and both stepparents, as well as his sister, participated in the family portion of the program. The family continued in the group portion of the program, even after Tony quit the program early.

Tony stopped taking his mood-stabilizing medications approximately 2 weeks ago, when his most recent binge use of methamphetamine started. Currently, his mental health care provider is withholding the mood-stabilizing medications until the methamphetamine is no longer affecting Tony's major systems.

Family Members

The admitting nurse and the social worker have gleaned familial information, described in the following paragraphs, from Steve, Mary, Debbie, and Harold. The Johnson family genogram is illustrated in Figure 18-1; the family ecomap is illustrated in Figure 18-2.

Steve is very concerned about his son's health and reminds him that the health care providers have said that his son will not survive another year if he continues to use methamphetamines. Steve recognizes his son's depression and anger and feels guilty that he did not notice sooner that Tony was depressed and "self-medicating" with alcohol and drugs. He blames himself for the divorce, which he believes precipitated Tony's alcohol and drug abuse. He also regrets working so much during Tony's early years and for ignoring Tony's alcohol use and stealing. Mary initiated the divorce when she discovered Steve was having affairs and using cocaine. Steve was diagnosed at the time of the divorce as having BD, with a manic episode that resulted in his hospitalization. He had also been drinking excessively for years and has alcohol use disorder. He has been clean and sober for 8 months, during which he has been regularly attending Alcoholics Anonymous. His BD is being managed by medications and is stable.

Mary, Tony's mother, became a stay-at-home mom when she gave birth to Tony. She resented that he was not a good student. She went back to work as a server in a restaurant shortly after Susie was born.

Susie has been under pressure all her life to "be good, not like Tony." Unlike Tony, she excels at school and is obedient to her parents and all authority figures. Despite all the comparisons to Tony, she loves her brother and wants to protect him. She does not tell her parents when she knows he breaks the family rules.

Debbie is a better limit-setter than Steve and is often more practical about recognizing and addressing Tony's needs. She is influential with both Steve and Mary in making decisions about Tony. There are no members in her extended family with substance use disorder.

Harold, Tony's stepfather, is 11 years older than Mary and in many ways is a father figure for his wife. He dotes on his 12-year-old son and largely ignores his stepson, Tony, and stepdaughter, Susie; he does brag about Susie's successes. He is a successful building contractor and is able to provide a luxurious life for his wife and son.

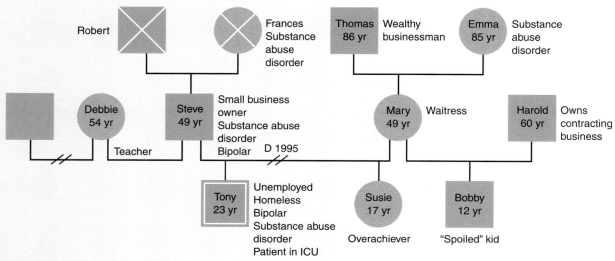

FIGURE 18-1 Johnson Family Genogram

Case Study: Johnson Family—cont'd

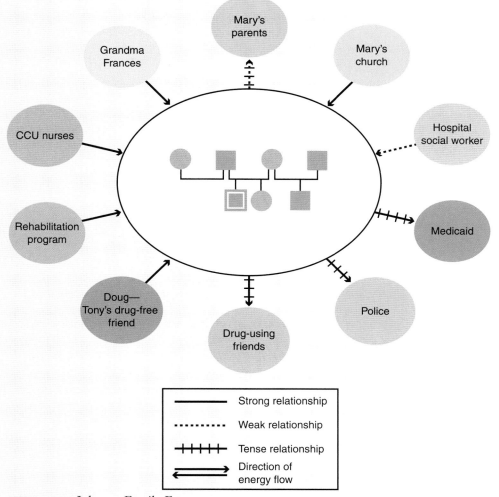

FIGURE 18-2 Johnson Family Ecomap

Susie, 17 years old, is bright and well behaved. Tony calls her the "perfect" child he never was. She is an honor student, talented in music and art, and well-liked by her fellow students and by adults. She worries about Tony and has always tried to please him.

Steve's mother, Frances, died 10 years ago of complications from a liver transplant. She had substance use disorder, which the family never admitted to anyone, even to themselves. Steve's father died when Tony was young. His parents owned a grocery store that they ran as a family.

Mary's parents, Thomas and Emma, live nearby. Thomas is a wealthy but distant businessman who believes that each person is a "master of his own destiny" and should just change behavior if it is a problem. Emma was a stay-at-home wife and mother; she has substance use disorder, mostly alcohol, but takes excessive prescription pain medications as well. Thomas is aware she drinks too much, but he protects her every way he can.

Discharge Plans

Tony will be discharged in 3 days, with the discharge diagnosis of acute methamphetamine poisoning resolved.

(continued)

Case Study: Johnson Family—cont'd

Family Systems Theory in Relation to the Johnson Family

The health event that the Johnson family is managing will be viewed through the lens of a nurse who used Family Systems Theory as the foundational approach to working with this family. A more detailed discussion of Family Systems Theory can be found in Chapter 5.

Concept 1—All Parts of the System Are Interconnected

In the Johnson case, all members of the family are affected by Tony's dual *DSM-5* diagnoses of substance abuse disorder and BD, and his dramatic overdoses and near-death experiences. His father feels enormous guilt and is afraid to confront and set limits with his son for fear of sending him to his death. Steve is humiliated that his son knows that he himself misused drugs. He is much more concerned about the stigma of drug use than that of alcohol use. There were times when Tony was growing up that his father drank alcohol with him. Now, Steve is trying to understand what role BD plays in the problems that both Tony and he have. Tony's mother, Mary, believes that she can help Tony change his self-destructive behavior. Tony's stepmother is more realistic because she is not as emotionally attached to Tony, but she worries about the effects of Steve's drug use, and she fears a relapse of Steve's own bipolar symptoms.

Concept 2—The Whole Is More Than the Sum of Its Parts

In the Johnson family case study, the complexity of the blended family increases the interconnectedness and interdependence of the family members. It is not just parents and children or grandparents and parents; instead, it is a complex system involving different permutations of the family relationships that can deteriorate over time as the stress of Tony's illness takes its toll on the entire system.

Concept 3—All Systems Have Some Form of Boundary or Border Between the System and Its Environment

In the Johnson family, the normal boundaries of self and others, and of family and outsiders, are dysfunctional. Spousal boundaries are violated by infidelity; parent-child boundaries are violated by theft. When Steve drank alcohol with his son Tony, parent-child boundaries were violated. Some of the boundaries are closed by distant, aloof parents and spouses.

Concept 4—Systems Can Be Further Organized Into Subsystems

The Johnson family has many subsystems: parent, parent-stepparent, parent-child, grandparent-parent, sibling, grandparent, and in-law. Each of these subsystems can be mobilized to help with the goals defined for the family. Specifically, the mother-father-stepmother-son subsystem will probably prove most influential in discharge planning.

Family Impact

In the Johnson family, objective impact includes the financial costs of treatment, physical strain and damage, effects on the health of other family members, and disruption in the daily lives of many of the family members. The subjective impact is the enormous guilt and fear felt by the family members; the damage to Tony's mental and social health; the disruption felt by other children in the family; the strain placed on the marriages; and the disrupted family routines, such as regular mealtimes and leisure time.

Social Support and Stigma

The Johnson family has been moderately successful in previous generations at hiding the substance abuse and dysfunction. Although more acceptable now than in previous generations, some social stigma is attached to divorce, remarriage, substance use disorder, and mental illness—all of which affect the Johnson family. Methamphetamine use carries a large social stigma today. Family and health care providers need information that is evidence-based to increase the understanding of the immense physical, mental, and social impact that this combination of problems has on the family. Providing family members with accurate information about the disorder and the treatments and medications can improve family functioning.

Coping and Resiliency

The Johnson family would benefit from an intervention designed to enhance their success with dealing with Tony's and others' behaviors, and with feelings of worry and concern. Most mental health care providers would suggest that they attend 12-step meetings for families affected by substance use, such as Alcoholics Anonymous and Al-Anon, and that they have family

Case Study: Johnson Family—cont'd

counseling with Tony. All subsystems need help learning more effective coping strategies, from those who remain aloof from the problems to those who become overly enmeshed in the lives of other family members.

Assistance From Mental Health Care Providers

The Johnson family needs referral to a treatment facility that focuses on the dual-diagnosis approach to treatment for the identified client and family members. In addition, the extended family needs counseling concerning the impact of these disorders and the maladaptive coping styles being used. Tony needs treatment for both his substance use disorder and his BD at the same time. These disorders are intertwined and respond poorly when treated in isolation.

Family psychoeducation for the Johnson family would include education about substance use and BDs; coping skills for Tony and the family members, especially in dealing with grief and anger; and effective communication skills to express feelings constructively. Tony would also receive medication teaching about his mood stabilizer.

Mental Health Care Nursing From a Family Systems Perspective

This section will identify the needs of each member of the Johnson family and address the family as a whole by looking at the family from the perspective of Family Systems Theory.

Assessment

The nurse and a social worker conduct the assessment of the Johnson family with Tony, Steve, Mary, and Debbie. It includes the following:

- *Perception of and understanding of the illness:* The Johnson family has some experience with substance abuse and BD. The diagnosis of BD is newer, and they have a poorer understanding of it alone and combined with substance use. The nurse assesses whether the knowledge is accurate and current.
- *The primary complaint, symptoms, or concerns:* The Johnson family believes that Tony's illness is the family's "problem." In reality, the dysfunctional family dynamics are more central needs. Since this crisis has arisen, the family's biggest concern is Tony's safety. They now fear that Tony will either end up dead or in prison.
- *Physical, developmental, cognitive, mental, and emotional health status:* The Johnson family is in a great deal of emotional pain and is in a crisis state at this time. The family's stress level is at an all-time high.
- *Health history:* The Johnson family has a history of mental health problems but appears to be physically healthy otherwise.
- *Treatment history:* Tony has a history of unsuccessful treatment attempts, with brief periods of abstinence from alcohol and drugs, and minimal treatment for his BD. Tony takes mood-stabilizing medication intermittently but has not had a long-term relationship with a psychiatrist since he was 17.
- *Family, social, cultural, racial, ethnic, and community systems:* The Johnson family systems have been described and are reflected in the ecomap of the family (see Figure 18-2). Mary is involved with church activities. Tony is in contact with friends from high school in addition to his friends who use drugs.
- *Activities of daily living and health habits:* These activities are seriously disrupted for Steve, Debbie, Mary, and Susie. The stress, worry, and concern they have for Tony, and the time and energy they are using to help Tony find a place to live and get into treatment, are affecting their own abilities to spend time focusing on their own health and well-being.
- *Substance use:* The Johnson family has alcohol, cocaine, and methamphetamine abuse in its history.
- *Coping mechanisms used:* Although some healthy mechanisms are used by the Johnson family, the family members also use rationalization, projection, denial, and substance use as ways of coping. Susie is coping by making everyone else happy. She is compliant with the demands of everyone else and may not be making the personal growth during adolescence that she needs to move into a healthy adulthood.
- *Spiritual and religious beliefs or values:* The Johnson family members state that they are Christians, but the only family members to attend services or admit to spiritual practices are Steve, Susie, and Mary. Steve uses meditation to maintain focus in his life but has been unable to do so for many months because of his increased time spent on attempting to keep track of Tony.
- *Economic, legal, or other environmental factors that affect health:* Steve's finances have been strained by Tony's illness. Harold and Mary refuse to accept any of the monetary burden of his care, saying that "he needs to take care of himself," but they remain emotionally involved.

(continued)

Case Study: Johnson Family—cont'd

- *Health-promoting strengths:* Tony and his father, and Tony and his grandfather remain involved with each other, and they hope that Tony can become more independent which can be mobilized to promote healthy family behaviors and communication.
- *Complementary therapies used:* Tony's friends have recommended acupuncture for his substance use disorder, but he has not been clean long enough to try it. Debbie is trying meditation to ease the stress and is trying to get Steve to join a yoga group with her.
- *Family conflicts:* Numerous unresolved family conflicts continue in the Johnson family.
- *Familial roles and responsibilities:* In the Johnson family, Mary alternates between being overprotective and being harsh and critical with her children. Steve is an enabler and unable to set appropriate limits. Susie is pseudomature in her relationship with Tony.
- *The person's ability to remain safe:* Without long-term treatment and medication management, Tony is at great risk for harm.

Treatment Goals

- In the short term, the goals are for the family to identify a family-oriented community resource for people with family members with mental disorder or substance use disorder that they are willing to attend by the time Tony is discharged. The nurse wants Tony to engage in a change conversation (Miller & Rollnick, 2013) in which he lists his own reasons to adhere to his mood-stabilizing medications and at least one strategy from his own life for making adherence possible and easier.
- The longer-term treatment goals for the Johnson family are to admit Tony into a short-term residential treatment facility and to find a long-term treatment program for families with a member with dual diagnoses. The family desires social support from others with similar experiences, education regarding Tony's ongoing treatment options, and skills training that will help them communicate better with one another and teach them to manage the impact of these disorders on the family in between these intermittent crises.

Diagnosis

Tony's dual diagnosis of BD with substance use disorder helps determine the best treatment approach for Tony as an individual. His dual disorder probably began when he was an adolescent. Tony describes the feelings of depression and hopelessness preceding his misuse of drugs.

Family Diagnoses

Most experts advocate for the inclusion of the family in treatment of a family member diagnosed with a mental illness. In addition to the plan of care that staff nurses have established to address Tony's individual nursing diagnoses, family diagnoses for the Johnson family include the following:

- Compromised family coping related to situational crisis, as evidenced by Tony's overdose and hospitalization, the family's disruption in their daily activities, and the increased need for support.
- Dysfunctional family process related to drug abuse, as evidenced by familial conflict and ineffective problem solving.
- Ineffective family therapeutic regimen management related to decisional conflict (discharge decision), economic difficulty, and excessive demands on the family, as evidenced by verbalization of the desire to manage Tony's treatment and prevent the negative sequelae of his methamphetamine abuse and untreated BD.

Outcome Identification

For Tony and the rest of the Johnson family, treatment attempts have failed to date, and it appears that Tony will need to aim for abstinence and control of his mental illness to survive. The desired outcomes for the Johnson family include, but are not limited to, Tony's recovery from his methamphetamine substance use disorder and control of his BD. Outcomes for the whole family include identifying familial support systems in the community, exploring financial options to pay for Tony's treatment, making a family decision regarding the best treatment option available for Tony, facilitating Tony's acceptance into a residential treatment facility, expressing anger appropriately, discussing openly substance abuse and other open family secrets, setting limits on inappropriate and enabling behavior, and honoring individual and family boundaries and needs.

Case Study: Johnson Family—cont'd

Planning

For the Johnson family, an integrated program in the community is most appropriate, but such programs are not easy to find and are often quite expensive. Discharge planning for the Johnson family includes the following: the family will be given information about appropriate referrals for residential care, the family (and Tony) will seek out and accept an appropriate referral, and Tony will be discharged to the referral facility. The family will also be given referrals to the Meth Family and Friends Support Group as well as NAMI. The family will also be referred for counseling to a therapist or counselor who is available through Steve's insurance plan so family members may work on their communication and coping skills, develop more appropriate boundaries with one another, and address some of their own needs.

Implementation

Tony and his family accepted a referral to a Volunteers of America drug-free facility and treatment program in which family members participate on a regular basis. This program is free to Tony as long as he continues to work at the facility. He was willing to accept this placement, and it did not burden Steve economically.

Evaluation

Follow-up is necessary to determine the effectiveness of the referral in assisting the family to function more appropriately, helping Tony to be drug free, and providing treatment for Tony's BD.

Benefits of Involving Family

In the Johnson family, Tony is reaching out for help from his family. He has been unsuccessful in receiving and accepting treatment on his own, and he needs the resources of his family (insurance and finances) to get the treatment he needs. The family needs him to be healthy to improve its self-image and its own successful functioning.

Barriers to Involving Family

Many of the barriers to involving the Johnson family are a result of the family dynamics that the family exhibits. The family has a pattern of blaming Tony for family problems and then rescuing him during periods of crisis, and it has difficulty setting appropriate limits and insisting that Tony take responsibility for his actions. The family members tend to become overly involved during some periods and to remain aloof at others, resulting in inconsistent participation. They are in need of long-term partnership with a treatment team. Tony's lack of commitment to treatment hinders any type of healthy long-term relationship being established with his family. In addition, Steve may experience a sense of guilt that Tony may have inherited the BD from him, and he may need counseling to express some of these feelings. The stress of Tony's illness and recent crisis may exacerbate Steve's own disorder.

You are the nurse caring for Tony in the ICU on the day of his discharge. Thus, your ability to influence is limited.

Questions for reflection on the nursing care of the Johnson family:

1. Discuss your feelings in response to the case study.
2. What approach would you take in caring for Tony? How might an understanding of Family Systems Theory and SBN guide your nursing practice in working with Tony?
3. What are your priority discharge instructions?

Case Study: Anderson Family

The following brief case study illustrates how a school nurse's interaction with a student led to psychoeducation and support for members of the entire family. The Anderson family consists of a grandmother and the two older children she is raising. See Figure 18-3 for the family genogram.

Karen, age 14, has an older brother, Tom, who is 21 and still lives at home. Tom was diagnosed with paranoid schizophrenia when he was 17. Their grandmother, Ellen, is raising Karen and Tom because both of their parents were killed in a motor vehicle accident 5 years ago. Ellen is 67 and is a retired schoolteacher with a limited income. Karen seldom brings friends to the house because she does not want to be embarrassed by her brother. Tom has been acting paranoid and frequently mumbles sentences

(continued)

Case Study: Anderson Family—cont'd

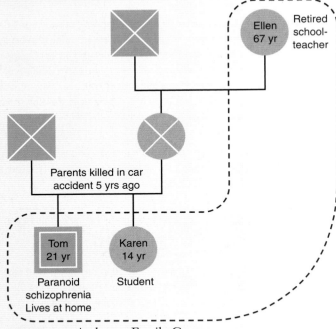

FIGURE 18-3 Anderson Family Genogram

under his breath that don't make any sense to Karen. Karen is aware that the psychiatric mental health nurse practitioner (PMHNP) is in the process of regulating his psychiatric medications, but she thinks that things will just never get better. Karen is afraid that she's going to develop the same traits as her brother when she gets older and worries that her grandmother won't be able to take care of both of them. Karen's grandmother takes Tom to his psychiatric medication appointments and also to individual therapy and is preoccupied with the thought that she is going to have to take care of Tom for the rest of her life—she loves Tom, but she had been looking forward to living independently and doing things with her friends.

The school nurse was aware of Karen's living situation and asked Karen to come and see her after school. The nurse did a brief assessment (see Figure 18-4 for the family ecomap) and was able to help Karen voice her fears and concerns about her brother's disorder. She spent some time teaching Karen about schizophrenia and treatments. Karen felt relieved to be able to talk to someone and learn more information that helped her understand why her brother did and said things that did not make sense to her. The nurse was aware of a local NAMI chapter that had a separate parent and sibling support group for families who had a family member with schizophrenia. Karen went to a meeting reluctantly, but she was relieved to hear the stories from other kids her age and was surprised to learn that they had similar experiences. Karen's grandmother hesitatingly went to a support group—she had driven Karen to the NAMI meeting and sat in the car, but she eventually decided to attend a meeting herself. Karen and her grandmother began to talk more openly about their worries and concerns.

Tom's psychiatric-mental health nurse practitioner (PMHNP) learned from Tom that his sister and grandmother were attending NAMI support groups. The PMHNP asked Tom if it would be okay if Karen and his grandmother could come to one of his appointments, and he agreed. The PMHNP spent time explaining the purpose and adverse effects of the medications Tom was taking and encouraged Karen and Ellen to contact her if they noticed changes in his behavior that might suggest his symptoms were increasing or he was experiencing a side effect from the medications.

As Tom became stabilized on his medication, he began to be more involved in communicating with his sister and grandmother. Eventually, Karen became more comfortable bringing her friends to the house. Ellen was able to learn more about community training programs that Tom could attend during the day to learn a skill that could eventually lead to a job. The job-training program was part of a community grant and so did not add a financial burden to Ellen. Ellen was now able to do more

Case Study: Anderson Family—cont'd

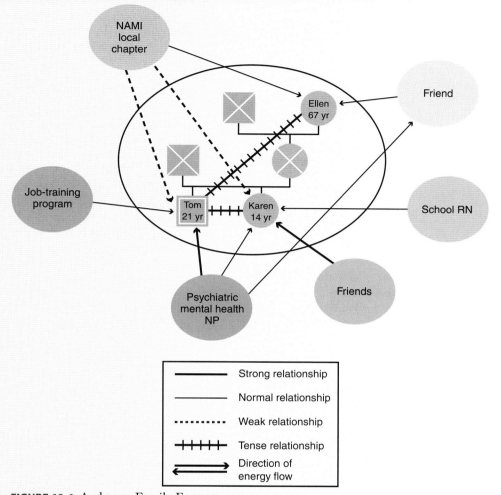

Strong relationship
Normal relationship
Weak relationship
Tense relationship
Direction of energy flow

FIGURE 18-4 Anderson Family Ecomap

things during the day with her friends. Psychoeducation decreased not only the family stress as a unit but also Karen and Ellen's stress. The school nurse was instrumental in providing psychoeducation, which led Karen and Ellen to peer-led support groups.
   Questions for reflection on the nursing care of the Anderson family:

1. You are the school nurse at Karen's school. The case study stated that the nurse was aware of Karen's living situation. Is that enough to warrant asking her to come see you?
2. What behavior(s) might Karen exhibit that would alert you to conduct an assessment?
3. What are some risk factors that you might be concerned about related to complicated grief?
4. As a nurse, what do you need to be aware of when working with families who have a family member suffering from schizophrenia?

SUMMARY

Nurses play an important role not only by helping families manage their lives when a member of the family has an MHC, but also by preventing MHCs from occurring. Providing mental health nursing care may be challenging because of the stigmas associated with MHCs, but it is also a privilege. The nurse-family relationship is very important in effecting positive outcomes: Nurses can reduce stigmas; correct myths about MHCs; offer family-centered interventions that promote family health, including referrals to appropriate resources; and provide nursing approaches that change a potentially negative experience into a positive one. The following points highlight critical concepts that are addressed in this chapter:

- A family-focused approach to providing mental health care to families—that is, viewing the family as a unit—includes supporting families in their natural caregiving roles and thus in ways that encourage family collaboration and choice in treatment decisions.

- There are improved outcomes for the person with an MHC if the health care provider collaborates with her or his family when providing treatment to the individual.
- Physical and/or mental comorbidities are frequently present when someone has an MHC.
- Common needs for families living with a family member with an MHC are support, information, skills and training, advocacy, and referral sources.
- Families value interactions with health care providers that demonstrate openness, cooperation, confirmation, and continuity.
- Nurses must have an attitude toward family members that is perceived as nonblaming and accepting in order to establish a collaborative relationship with the family.
- There are many effective psychotherapeutic and psychological interventions available, including family therapies, mother and infant psychotherapies, and brief cognitive therapy appropriate to the age of the child and his or her stage of child development.

chapter 19

Families and Population Health

Annette Bailey, PhD, RN

Jacqueline F. Webb, DNP, FNP-BC, RN

Kimberly Dupree Jones, PhD, FNP, FAAN

Critical Concepts

- Population health refers to the well-being of defined groups of individuals and differences in health between population groups.
- Care of families and communities requires a transition from an individual-focused to a community- and population-focused perspective.
- Community and public health nurses care for diverse families in a variety of settings.
- Community and public health nurses view families as subunits of the community or as clients in the context of the community.
- Community and public health nurses aim to meet the holistic needs of families and communities while prioritizing health needs.
- Healthy families contribute to healthy communities.
- Community and public health nursing is grounded in social justice and culturally safe, ethical practice.
- Community and public health nurses consider health inequalities from intersecting social, political, economic, and environmental factors that affect the health and well-being of families and communities.
- Using a combination of health promotion strategies and principles, community and public health nurses work to address health inequities that produce differential health outcomes among families and communities and improve the health of populations.
- Family interventions in the community are targeted toward primary, secondary, and tertiary prevention. The nurse-family relationship is central in interventions at all three levels of prevention.
- Community and public health nursing are evidence based and policy driven.
- Interventions for families are planned, implemented, and evaluated from a health promotion perspective.
- Community and public health nurses understand that population health status is relevant to the distribution of health resources and opportunities across defined groups and communities.
- Community and public health nurses are advocates for programs, policies, and research that improve population health outcomes.

A definition of *health* provided by the World Health Organization (WHO) (2021c), which has not changed since 1948, suggests that "health is a state of complete physical, mental, and social well-being and not merely the absence of disease or infirmity" (para. 1). This definition implies that achieving health is much more than treating diseases. Health is not just physical; it is also emotional and social. Community and public health nurses understand that creating a balance in the various dimensions of people's lives—culture, society, economic, politics, and the physical environment—is crucial in helping them to cultivate health (WHO, 2021c). Community and public health nurses recognize that people interact in communities and societies and that these interactions affect their health in profound ways. Therefore, disease patterns are not simply a result of unhealthy behavior but are the most obvious and extreme manifestation of unfavorable interactions between human beings and their environments. The interactions produce significant health inequities between different groups and communities in society, with social injustice at the root of these differences. Guided by an understanding that population health is predictive of the cumulative impact of social inequality based on race, gender, and social class, community and public health nurses work to modify social factors that impinge on the physical, mental, and social well-being of different groups (McGibbon & Lukeman, 2019). This more holistic understanding of nursing practice demands that we engage communities and populations in envisioning what health means to them. But how do community and public health nurses transform this understanding of health into health promotion for families?

A broad definition of *family* guides community and public health nurses toward inclusiveness in working with and understanding complex family systems. Family, for purposes of this chapter, comprises two or more individuals who depend on one another for emotional, physical, and economic support. The members of the family are self-defined. Along with this broad definition of *family*, community and public health nurses utilize two prevalent schools of thought. One view sees the family as the unit of care and the community as context. The other view focuses on the community as client with the family as context. The commonality between these views is that family, and thus family health, is indistinguishably linked to community health. Healthy communities are comprised of healthy families. Hence, families as units of relationship are important components of communities, and undoubtedly they are heavily affected by their community's state of health. The word *community* means more than just a geographical space; it includes population groups and individuals who share similar interests, needs, and outcomes, regardless of geographical location or setting (Goodman et al., 2014). Most people are members of multiple types of communities based on their social norms, personal priorities, interests, and cultures. Community and public health nurses understand the effects that communities can have on individuals and families, and they recognize that a community's health is reflected in the health experiences of its members and their families (Canadian Public Health Association, 2021). Therefore, health promotion actions should be concurrent and encompassing for both contexts. Identifying family needs and developing a plan of care for families cannot be done in isolation from the broader context of their surroundings and experiences. When working with families, nurses need to consider environmental, psychological, and behavioral health issues, as well as those of a more physiological nature.

Key considerations for the role of nurses are tackling social injustice that cause health inequities and addressing social determinants of health (SDOHs) affecting the well-being of families. Doing so recognizes that family health problems have roots in economic, political, and social structures. SDOHs have a significant impact on all aspects of health (Braveman & Gottlieb, 2014; Heiman & Artiga, 2015). WHO (2021b) defines SDOHs as the conditions in which individuals are born, grow, live, work, and age. The WHO definition of SDOHs goes on to state that these conditions are shaped by the distribution of money, power, and resources globally, nationally, and locally. SDOHs create disparities in experiences with health issues such as cancer, diabetes, HIV/AIDS, mental health, smoking, obesity, drug use, suicide, and homicide (Singh et al., 2017). In short, SDOHs constitute much of the individual's and family's contextual roots.

It is important for nurses to understand the impact that SDOHs have on the families they work with in order to assess their circumstances. Issues of violence, homelessness, unemployment, unclean physical environments, unsupportive relationships, and poor access to needed resources (e.g., food, shelter) are a few indications of risks in a community. These issues are inextricably linked to the health of families. Promoting and sustaining health for families means helping them tap into their personal strength, access social and economic resources, and cope with stressors (Canadian Public Health Association, 2021). Community and public health nurses use health promotion strategies, such as facilitating access to resources, to improve the health of families. A more detailed discussion of SDOHs comes later in this chapter.

Community and public health nursing emphasize the social, political, and economic aspects of health to help individuals, families, and communities gain a higher degree of harmony within the mind, body, and soul. A community or public health nurse who visits a new mother in her home and realizes that a bed used for the newborn baby is infested with bedbugs cannot simply focus on the physical health of the mom and baby. In the same way, for example, it is necessary to focus on the ways that broader social contexts and political decisions create and exacerbate homelessness. Paying attention to the lack of resources caused by poverty becomes an essential aspect of the nurse's role in promoting health for families. In fact, the degree to which nurses can contribute positively to the well-being of vulnerable families in communities depends on their convictions and commitments to modify these factors as well as on society's support and recognition of the importance of their work.

This chapter offers a description of population health that encompasses nursing care of families delivered in the context of community and public health. It begins with a definition of *population health* and *community and public health nursing*, and follows with a discussion of concepts and principles that guide the work of nurses, the roles they enact in working with families and communities, and the various settings where they work. This discussion is organized around a visual representation of community health nursing. The chapter ends with a discussion of current trends in community and public health nursing.

WHAT IS POPULATION HEALTH? WHAT IS COMMUNITY AND PUBLIC HEALTH NURSING?

Population health signifies a shift in the focus of health care delivery. At first, the term *population health* seemed to be used more frequently in Canada than in the United States; however, the approach seems to have emerged from a focus on the SDOHs (Glauberman et al., 2020; Kindig & Stoddart, 2003). One definition of population health refers to "the health outcomes of a group of individuals, including the distribution of such outcomes within the group" and is distinguished from the more common term *public health*, which consists of a set of activities carried out by organizations with official health functions for the public (Glauberman et al., 2020, p. 60). Population health interventions are designed to promote health and prevent disease among an aggregate, or a subgroup, of the population, and those served may have certain characteristics or conditions in common (Minnesota Department of Health, 2019). Examples of population health interventions include (1) implementing a COVID-19 or influenza vaccine clinic in a residential community serving older adults, (2) performing an outreach intervention to raise awareness on the effects of hypertension on Black men, and (3) organizing a helmet safety campaign for youth in the community. Table 19-1 includes roles that nurses may serve in population health.

According to the Canadian Public Health Association (2021), community and public health nursing involves a synthesis of nursing theory and public health science that focuses on population health promotion and primary health care with the intention of maintaining and promoting health, preventing illnesses and injuries, and developing communities. The American Public Health Association (2021) defines *public health nursing* in a similar way: as the practice of promoting and protecting the health of populations using knowledge from nursing, social, and public health sciences. The key characteristics of public health nursing practice include:

- A focus on the health needs of the public, addressing inequities
- Assessment of community and population health using a comprehensive, systematic approach

Table 19-1	Roles That Nurses Serve in Population Health

- Vaccine coordinator, county health department
- Community diabetes educator
- Care management nurse
- Population health nurse educator
- Grant coordinator, population health focus
- Researcher, population health
- Family nurse practitioner, primary care
- School nurse
- Correctional nurse
- Oncology nurse navigator
- Advanced practice nurse, gerontology
- Coordinator of care across disciplines
- Telehealth chronic illness care nurse (e.g., congestive heart failure)
- In-home skilled care nurse for medically fragile children
- Coordinator specialty telephone triage care

- Attention to multiple determinants of health
- An emphasis on primary prevention
- Application of interventions at all levels—individuals, families, communities, and the systems that have an impact on their health (American Public Health Association, 2021).

For organizations guiding professional nursing curricula in the United States, the recommendations are consistent and focus on competencies and skills needed for community and public health nurses currently and in the future. The definitions communicate the critical role of community and public health nurses in fostering care for families beyond a clinical perspective. In their work, community and public health nurses rely on various concepts and principles to promote health for individuals, families, communities, and populations. Drawing from various health promotion frameworks and set standards of practice, they enact principles in various settings, with modifications based on families' and communities' needs. This is done through a process of collaboration and empowerment with families, with the goal of improving the health of individuals and families and enabling them to express aspirations and develop their capacity to lead a fulfilling life. Nurses are aware of the role they have in recognizing social injustices and advocating for equity for all people

through policy development and capacity building within the community. This work may include developing strategies for improved engagement with families, adopting partnership models for all work with families and communities, and challenging institutional and social structures that foster injustice, health inequities, and social oppression (McGibbon & Lukeman, 2019). The model in Figure 19-1 helps to contextualize community and public health nursing.

HEALTH PROMOTION FRAMEWORKS, STANDARDS, AND PRINCIPLES

Health promotion and disease prevention are foundational to community and public health nurses' work. Interventions for families are planned, implemented, and evaluated from a health promotion perspective. From this perspective, nurses help to reduce health inequities by engaging families in processes that promote their control over their own health. This work includes developing families' skills, increasing their participation in their care process, and improving their access to resources. To prevent illness and injuries, nurses employ health education to help families modify lifestyles and behaviors (e.g., healthy eating, wearing bicycle helmets and seat belts, tobacco use prevention, and physical activity). For families to modify their behaviors, nurses know that they must address specific barriers beyond their control, such as poverty, racism, discrimination, and trauma. Rather than blaming families for their situations, community and public health nurses shift their thinking and focus on population health, which is concerned with changing the social, economic, political, and environmental conditions that affect families' health choices and outcomes.

The nurse can intervene in public policy at the community, organizational, and/or the individual level to help improve outcomes for individuals and families. For the most sustainable outcomes, nurses rely on the socioenvironmental/socioecological approach pictured in Figure 19-1 to guide their actions in addressing factors that impede families' choices to improve their health. The socioenvironmental/socioecological model is based on systems theory and is grounded in an understanding that vulnerability in health results from

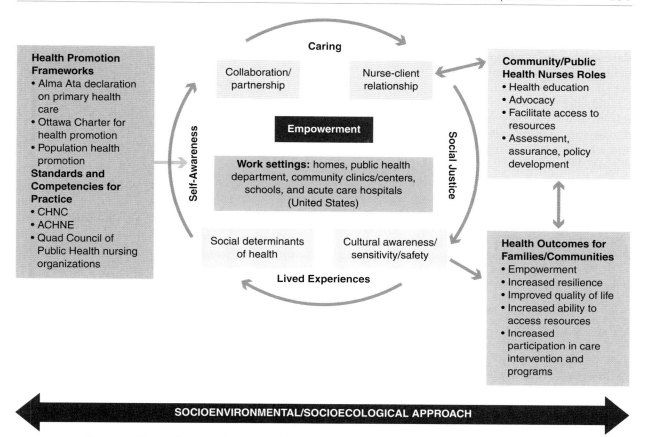

FIGURE 19-1 Contextualizing Community and Public Health Nursing

the interrelationships and intersections between personal and environmental factors (Kuran et al., 2020). Focusing on these environmental factors, including SDOHs (U.S. Department of Health and Human Services, 2021b), shifts the blame from the family to the conditions in which they live and the choices that they do or do not have.

The health of vulnerable families in various settings in society (e.g., families experiencing homelessness, refugees, victims of intimate partner violence, racialized families, and families in poverty) is affected negatively by many factors that intersect and are compounded for prolonged and devastating health impacts. An understanding of the factors that negatively affect family health and the strategies to modify these factors is a priority for the role of community and public health nurses. The use of health promotion strategies is crucial to helping nurses to fulfill this priority. For example, Hill (2020) explores a socioecological framework to address maternal obesity prevention,

highlighting that maternal obesity is a complex interplay between individual, interpersonal, community, and societal factors and not simply a matter of lifestyle change. Using the socioecological model, nurses are able to identify and address influences at the individual level (e.g., culture, lack of personal breastfeeding skills), interpersonal level (e.g., lack of support from family and friends, lack of encouragement from health care providers), community/environmental level (e.g., neighborhood stress, lack of community breastfeeding accommodations, workplaces, and hospitals), and organizational level (e.g., public health organizations, pediatric groups, and the formula industry). Community and public health nurses can target these influences using various health promotion strategies. From the perspective of maternal obesity, nurses can work at the individual level to address cultural-specific barriers and needs and build mothers' capacity for behavior change. At the interpersonal level, nurses can provide education and facilitate access to support services to address key influences to address in turn maternal obesity and support mothers' efforts. At the community/environment level, community and public health nurses can get involved in advocacy activities such as organizing community activities to influence public- or private-sector support for resources for mothers. At the organizational level, nurses can employ advocacy, coalition building, and lobbying to demand policy action in maternal obesity (Hill, 2020).

Health Promotion Frameworks

Whether working with individuals, families, or a community, nurses use key health promotion frameworks to guide their work: (1) the Alma Ata Declaration on Primary Health Care, (2) the Ottawa Charter for Health Promotion, and (3) the Population Health Promotion Model. Although various health promotion documents exist, these three frameworks remain central to health promotion interventions with families and communities. We discuss each framework next.

Alma Ata Declaration on Primary Health Care

The Alma Ata Declaration on Primary Health Care (WHO, 1978) laid the foundation for subsequent health promotion frameworks. It proposed five interconnected primary health care principles: health promotion, accessibility, public participation, appropriate technology, and intersectoral collaboration. The principles are based on access to health and health care, equity, and empowerment. Because families' SDOHs influence how they access resources, manage chronic conditions, and engage in healthy behaviors, addressing SDOHs for families by integrating primary health care principles is an integral component of nurses' work. For example, community and public health nurses who work with families to increase access to needed resources that are cost- or distance-prohibitive are practicing the primary health care principle of accessibility.

Ottawa Charter for Health Promotion

The Ottawa Charter for Health Promotion of 1986 (WHO, 2021a) proposed five overarching strategies: develop personal skills, create supportive environments, build healthy public policy, strengthen community action, and reorient health services. The strategies are intended to enable families and communities to increase control over and improve their health. Using these strategies, nurses work with families to address their physical, mental, and social needs, and help them attain prerequisites of health, such as shelter, food, sustainable resources, social justice, and equity. For example, to allow newcomers to acquire and sustain needed resources, nurses may facilitate personal skill development in résumé writing, job seeking, and interviews for them to acquire employment.

Population Health Promotion Model

The Population Health Promotion Model (Hamilton & Bhatti, 1996) draws on two decades of health promotion knowledge to guide practical actions. Key assumptions of this model include the recognition of determinants of health, the use of knowledge gained from research and practice, collaboration with families about the most appropriate actions to care for them, and building relationships with families based on mutual respect and caring rather than on professional power. In addition to incorporating these assumptions into their work, nurses applying this model are able to focus on the concerns of at-risk groups, such as youth and women in at-risk families.

Interventions to modify these issues are targeted at a broad social, political, and economic level, and the interventions are tailored to meet the needs of groups at the community and family level. For example, the model can be applied to the care of a family with a child suffering from obesity. Knowing there are societal, system, community, family, and individual factors involved, nurses can target assessment and interventions to the unique needs of the child and family (Public Agency of Canada, 2014), for example:

- *Socioeconomic issues:* Are there concerns with food insecurity?
- *Social support:* Are there social support and time for play or friend groups?
- *Community:* Are there opportunities for support in the community?
- *Education:* What are the child's experiences at school? Are there opportunities for collaboration with teachers or counselors?
- *Environment:* Does the family have access to safe exercise outdoors?
- *Supportive environment:* Would the family benefit from education about supportive communication and engaging activities?

- *Biology, physical assessment:* Are there familial or genetic predispositions?
- *Personal health:* How are the child and family members feeling? Do they regularly seek or have access to health care?
- *Personal coping skills:* Would the family benefit from teaching about coping skills?
- *Child development:* When was the child's last checkup? Are there developmental concerns?

Health Promotion Standards of Practice

To be effective in their roles, community and public health nurses integrate a broad range of competencies and interrelated standards of practice in their work. The Community Health Nurses of Canada (CHNC) is a national organization for registered nurses to support and advance practice and to improve the health of Canadians. The organization represents community health nurses and advocates for their role as community health nurses; advocates for healthy public policy to address SDOHs; and promotes a publicly funded, universal system for public health (CHNC, 2019). Community health nurses also work within the Canadian Community Health Nursing Professional Practice Model, which is guided by seven standards:

- Health promotion, prevention, and health protection
- Health maintenance
- Restoration and palliation
- Professional relationships
- Capacity building
- Access and equity
- Professional responsibility and accountability (CHNC, 2019)

In addition, "Core Competencies for Public Health in Canada" (Government of Canada, 2019) provides a baseline for nurses to fulfill effective public health functions. The competencies guide community and public health nurses in delivering acceptable, safe, and ethical care in an effort to protect, preserve, and promote the health of families. Areas of focus include public health sciences, assessment and analysis, policy and program planning, partnerships and collaboration, diversity, communication, and leadership (Government of Canada, 2019).

Standards and competencies are also an integral part of U.S. community and public health nursing practice. In the United States, community and public health nursing practice at the generalist and advanced or specialist level is competency based, and it is divided into three tiers of practice: the public health nursing generalist, the public health nursing specialist or manager, and the public health nursing organization leader or administrator (Council of Public Health Nursing Organizations, 2021). Partnering with communities, populations, and organizations is essential for public health practice at all levels and is a primary principle of public health nursing practice (Quad Council Coalition Competency Review Task Force, 2018). In addition, the American Association of Colleges of Nursing (AACN), developed a supplement to "The Essentials of Baccalaureate Education for Professional Practice in Nursing" (AACN, 2013) that includes recommended baccalaureate competencies and curricular guidelines for public health nursing that inform course offerings in nursing programs that are preparing community and public health nurses for now and the future. Clearly, the role of the community and public health nurse has been evolving through collaboration and partnership (relational skill building, including cultural sensitivity), and through the evaluation of outcomes (understanding data collection and analysis).

Public health nursing competencies include analytic and assessment skills, policy development and program planning skills, communication skills, cultural competency skills, community dimensions of practice (using an ecological perspective), public health sciences skills, financial planning and management skills, and leadership and systems thinking skills (Quad Council Coalition Competency Review Task Force, 2018).

Principles in the Process of Community and Public Health Nurses' Work

Underlying the role of the community and public health nurse in any context is a focus on maintenance and promotion of health and prevention of illnesses and injuries. These concepts and principles include, but are not limited to, SDOHs; cultural awareness, sensitivity, and safety; collaboration and partnership; nurse-client relationship; and empowerment. These principles are rooted in the values of caring, social justice, self-awareness, and honoring of families' and communities' lived experiences.

SDOHs

One of the most important concepts that influence community and public health nurses' thinking and action when they are working with families and communities include the SDOHs, which were discussed in Chapter 7. These SDOHs, or conditions necessary for living, can include factors such as education, poverty, unemployment, climate change, social support and status, racism, housing, childhood development, planetary sustainability, and access to health and social services (Divakaran, 2016; Goodman, 2014). These and other determinants shape peoples' vulnerability, put them at risk for illnesses, and influence their social status and the level of respect they receive in society. For example, vulnerability to homelessness is shaped by complex and connected determinants of health, such as issues including mental health challenges, substance abuse, precarious immigration status, and domestic and sexual abuse, which are intricately tied to poverty that requires global legislative changes (Mackie, 2015). Social injustice occurs when the health outcomes of individuals, groups, or communities are disproportionately affected because of differences in access and exposure to opportunities (e.g., education, employment). For example, the COVID-19 pandemic revealed significant demarcations in global health inequities because of social and racial inequalities. Across several countries, the spread of COVID-19 was more severe among vulnerable populations due to poverty, barriers to accessing service, low socioeconomic status, immigration status, and living in densely populated and disadvantaged neighborhoods. These conditions, also associated with increased comorbidity among already socially vulnerable groups, put them at greater risks of disease burden (Ivers & Walton, 2020; Shadmi et al., 2020). People of color have disproportionately grappled with the mental health impacts of COVID-19 resulting from job loss, financial insecurity, grief from the death of loved ones, and social isolation. Structural racism and other structural factors such as racist policing, racial bias, and medical mistreatment intersect to reinforce the mental health impacts of COVID-19 specifically on Blacks in the United States (Egede & Walker, 2020). Laurencin

and Walker (2020) referred to this intersecting impact of structural racism and COVID-19 as a pandemic on a pandemic for Black people.

The influence of health equity on disease patterns and process is so profound, and it is critical that community and public health nurses recognize and address SDOHs and social injustice as the root of many health problems faced by families and communities. For instance, community and public health nurses in Toronto, Ontario, working in the Investing in Families Program (Table 19-2), provide resources, mental health care, and other support to sole-parent families with children between the ages of 6 and 18 years who are receiving social assistance. For families in this program, determinants of health can be many and interrelated. Thus, community and public health nurses target prioritized health needs while trying to meet the holistic needs of families. Key determinants of health needs assessed by nurses include emotional, economic, employment, educational, housing, and mental health needs.

Cultural Awareness, Cultural Safety, and Antiracism

Community and public health nurses often find themselves working with culturally diverse communities. Within this diversity are differences in health between groups of people, with worst health outcomes seen among groups with more intense and continuous inequities in key SDOHs. This difference in health outcome is referred to as health disparities. Health disparities are predominantly a result of unequal distribution of resources and opportunities between groups that is moderated by race, gender, and social class. Social injustice is at the root of health differences between groups in our society (McGibbon & Lukeman, 2019; U.S. Department of Health and Human Services, 2021b). Although the Institute of Medicine (IOM, 2003) *Unequal Treatment* report came out in 2003, recent studies are still finding unequal treatment, even when access is improved. For example, Shaw and Santry (2015) conducted a retrospective study of more than 49,000 patients who depended on ventilators at 185 academic medical centers in the United States. Early tracheostomy for these patients is associated with increased survival. Yet patients who were women, Black, Hispanic, and/or on Medicaid were all found to be less likely to receive early tracheostomy. Similarly,

Table 19-2   **Examples of Community and Public Health Nursing**

NAME OF PROGRAM	PROGRAM DESCRIPTION	ROLE OF THE COMMUNITY AND PUBLIC HEALTH NURSES	SPECIFIC EXAMPLE OF PROGRAMMING	INTERPROFESSIONAL PROGRAM COLLABORATION
Healthy Baby Healthy Children	To enable all children to attain and sustain optimal health and developmental potential in the areas of • Positive parenting • Breastfeeding • Healthy family dynamics • Healthy eating, healthy weights, and physical activity • Growth and development	Assessments Referrals and recommendations Service coordination Supportive counseling Health promotion Health teaching Advocacy	Supports families with children from birth to the age of 4 years Assesses growth and development, mother-child attachment Links and refers to various community agencies	Family home visitors Registered dietitians Nutrition promotion consultants Community nutrition educators High-risk consultants Health promotion consultants Mental health nurse consultants Infant hearing screeners Family support worker/social workers Speech-language pathologist Program evaluators
Mental Health Promotion	To promote mental health in Toronto's diverse communities through competent clinical and consultative practice along with education, both internally to Toronto Public Health (TPH) programs and externally to relevant community agencies	The mental health nurse consultant provides consultation to a variety of internal and external programs Education and training	Using a narrative approach, the mental health promotion team focuses on suicide prevention, violence prevention, and mental health promotion	Examples of internal consultations: • Healthy communities • Chronic disease prevention • Healthy families • Communicable disease control • Healthy environments Examples of external consultations: • Children's aid society • Parks, forestry, and recreation • Shelter, support, and housing • Toronto social services • Toronto community housing cooperation
Investing in Families	To improve the economic, health, and social status of select families receiving social assistance in Toronto Overall goal of investing in family public health nursing service is to meet the health needs of select, vulnerable families receiving social assistance in Toronto • To promote healthy lifestyles • To increase personal resilience • To improve physical and mental health • To enhance social and community supports • To improve the family's circumstances through greater access to employment training and supports	Assessments Referrals and recommendations Service coordination Supportive counseling Health promotion Health teaching Advocacy	Supports families with children from 6 to 18 years old Receives referrals from Toronto social services Conducts detailed assessments Uses a strengths-based approach assessing the positive assets of the client	Toronto social services caseworker Public health nurse Health promotion consultant Mental health nurse consultant Recreationist

(continued)

Table 19-2	Examples of Community and Public Health Nursing—cont'd			
NAME OF PROGRAM	**PROGRAM DESCRIPTION**	**ROLE OF THE COMMUNITY AND PUBLIC HEALTH NURSES**	**SPECIFIC EXAMPLE OF PROGRAMMING**	**INTERPROFESSIONAL PROGRAM COLLABORATION**
School Health	• To enhance the physical, mental, social, and spiritual well-being of all the members of the school community • To strengthen the capacity of school communities to achieve optimal health • To enhance resilience in all school-age children and youth in the city of Toronto	Develop working relationships with all members of the school community to promote healthy schools Work with school communities to increase their capacity to identify health issues, develop and implement a plan of action, evaluate, and build on their successes Participate in existing health committees and advocate for the establishment of new school health committees Engage students and parents in healthy school initiatives Identify and consult with school communities on emerging health issues and trends Link between schools and TPH services and programs Partner with community organizations that support healthy schools	Liaison public nurse establishes a healthy school committee that assesses the needs of the school in a comprehensive manner The work of the school health committee includes • Creating a shared vision for a healthy school • Assessing strengths and needs of the school community • Prioritizing the issues • Developing a plan • Implementing the plan • Monitoring and evaluating the plan • Celebrating success	School administration School boards Teachers Students Parent council Internal programs in TPH Community agencies

Tignanelli et al. (2020) looked at racial disparity in mortality rates among Black and White males treated for high-grade splenic injuries across different hospitals. They found that Black males had significantly higher mortality rates than White males with similar splenic injuries. Factors contributing to this disparity include racial disparities in resource allocations, socioeconomic status, residential segregation, quality of hospital care, and access to high-quality providers and services. Race-based health care barriers are not only relevant to the U.S. health care system but also in Canada, where quality health care and social service access for Indigenous and racialized people are marked by historic and ongoing systems of oppression and multilevel racism (Wylie & McConkey, 2019). The role of nurses is to advocate for the equitable opportunity for Indigenous and underrepresented people to access high-quality health care that is grounded in the principles of cultural safety. Rectifying these inequalities is not as simple as the nurse developing cultural competencies because each individual, family, and community has variations in values and practices based on its unique experiences (Harrison et al., 2019). That is, underrepresented populations and diverse communities are heterogeneous. There are wide variations within groups as well as between them.

It is important for nurses working with diverse populations to reflect deliberately on cultural similarities and differences and on principles of diversity, equity, and social justice in the context of ethical nursing practice. From this understanding, nurses can situate their roles and accountability to nurse-client relationships in order to take actions that reduce barriers and improve equity in health care. Because community and public health nurses work with people of diverse cultural and racial backgrounds in various settings, it is crucial for them to engage in continuous reflective practice that explores their assumptions, values, and beliefs, as well as strategies for structurally competent nursing care for the groups and families they serve. This critical reflection can lead to sensitive and empowering client-centered care.

Many families that community and public health nurses care for may not speak English in their homes, or they may have other cultural differences that challenge the provision of culturally safe care. Increasing the numbers of bilingual, bicultural, underrepresented health care providers is identified as one of the solutions aimed at improving health disparities and as a way for institutions and organizations providing care to demonstrate their commitment to diversity, equity, and inclusion.

Promoting diversity in the health care workforce has many benefits. It is shown that when providers share a similar ethnic or racial background with their patients, the result is higher patient satisfaction and higher-quality health outcomes (Noone et al., 2016). Illness states are becoming increasingly complex due to the intersecting and complicating impacts of cultural and social factors. Racism, especially, has an impact on all dimensions of health, making this a crucial area of consideration in nursing care. Because peoples' unique lived experiences with racism and racial trauma affects their illness experiences, health care providers who are mindful of professional ethics, empathy, and culturally sensitive care in their engagements with diverse patients can help to facilitate positive health outcomes.

Added to this context are refugee families, who may have survived war, disaster, and devastating trauma such as torture, rape, and/or watching family members or others die. Often, refugee families are enduring post-traumatic stress disorder, depression, or both, which may intensify the life challenges they face. In understanding a family's context, nurses need to be aware of not only how to satisfy language deficits but also how to understand both their own and the family's cultural background and perspectives and how these influence the caring process. With this understanding, nurses can ensure that care is provided with heightened personal and professional awareness.

To facilitate culturally safe care for families, community and public health nurses working with diverse populations recognize that self-awareness and continuous self-reflection are as much nursing skills as they are tools for health promotion. Originally developed in New Zealand, cultural safety goes beyond cultural sensitivity and competence to address the attitudes of health care providers, with an emphasis on discrimination, power imbalance, and the effects of colonization (Horrill et al., 2018). Culturally safe care involves the nurse's reflection and self-awareness of his or her attitudes and beliefs related to culture, ethnicity, age, gender, political and religious beliefs, and sexual orientation with regard to the background of the individual (Doutrich et al., 2012). This approach shifts the focus from the nurse's expertise to the expertise of the community, which defines whether the care has been safe or not (Brascoupé & Waters, 2009; Doutrich et al., 2014). Culturally safe care is provided to all within their cultural norms and values and in a manner that garners their trust and promotes their empowerment. For example, in promoting health for Indigenous families hurt by colonization processes, community and public health nurses would invite the families to partner with them. This process helps to build their capacity, facilitate trust, and acknowledge their right to self-determination in an effort to promote equal access to health care (Brascoupé & Waters, 2009; Richmond & Cook, 2016). Patient safety is at risk when health care interactions lack open communication and empowerment. More specifically, patients and families may feel unsafe if they are unable to use interpreters, if their family cannot be involved, or if they are experiencing socioeconomic barriers (Chauhan, 2020). Nurses have the opportunity to promote culturally safe care that is sensitive to cultural differences by staying aware of their own cultural biases and values and being open to culturally safe practices as defined by the clients.

Collaboration and Partnership

Community and public health nurses are usually members of teams promoting health and well-being for families and communities. They work in collaboration with other key members of a community and/or family team. Effective collaborative relationships can improve the experience and the outcome for all involved. Nurses' participation in collaboration depends on the type and purpose for which the collaboration was formed. For example, nurses working on a school health team collaborate with various stakeholders—teachers, parents, school board members, government officials, and others—to promote health in schools. On such teams, nurses may share specialized public health knowledge, share needed resources, interface with external partners, advocate, and/or contribute to decision-making processes. The essence of these collaborations is to share knowledge and power among key stakeholders to produce solutions that no one partner could achieve independently. Collaborations are ways in which nurses honor families and community members' lived experience. The lived experiences, knowledge, and expertise that other members bring to the team represent an important piece of the puzzle toward better health outcomes for families and communities. For example, from a public health perspective, management of the COVID-19 pandemic requires the urgent collaboration of different professional teams locally, regionally, and nationally. Given public health nurses' critical decision-making skills and their relationship with families and communities, many were diverted from their usual roles to assist in a diverse range of activities with other decision makers in various jurisdictions. Their roles in contact tracing, advocacy, education, and supporting families were complementary to team efforts to control and manage the spread of COVID-19 (Edmonds et al., 2020).

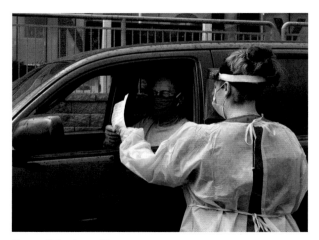

Source: © istock.com/Hoptocopter

Interprofessional collaboration refers to a collaborative partnership between two or more health professionals or human services providers who work to promote and protect the health of individuals, families, and communities (Minnesota Department of Health, 2019). Collaboration involves a high level of commitment, coordination, and cooperation toward a mutual goal.

When multiple providers and patients communicate and consider each other's perspectives, they can better address several factors that affect the health of individuals, families, and communities (Sullivan et al., 2015). One example of interprofessional collaboration can be found in the family health teams of Ontario, Canada. These primary-care teams feature different professionals working in collaboration with each other and the families. These teams address the shortage of family physicians in Ontario, increase access to and quality of care, and decrease the number of individuals visiting the emergency department for minor issues. Rather than going to see a family physician, residents of Ontario are able to receive primary-care services from an entire team of health care providers in the community. A family health team might include a physician, registered nurse, nurse practitioner, pharmacist, social worker, and dietitian. Instead of being referred elsewhere, patients of the family health team are able to acquire services from this team, which collaborates on the provision of their care. As another example, the Investing in Families Program involves collaboration between various divisions across the city of Toronto—parks, forestry and recreation, social services, children's services, and public health. At any point, public health nurses can collaborate with any of these partners in the provision of care for families in the program.

Supporting families in their journey toward healthy change within their lives requires the development of collaborative partnerships between nurses and individuals, families, and communities (CHNC, 2021). Because of the complex nature of SDOHs, community and public health nurses find themselves engaging in interdisciplinary teamwork. These interdisciplinary teams feature collaboration between individuals from a broad variety of disciplines, such as business, nutrition, sociology, economics, education, human services, government, and health sciences. The collaborative relationships and partnerships with other professionals, disciplines, clients, families, and communities are critical to addressing the complexities of health care.

Nurse-Client Relationship With Families and Communities

Community and public health nurses caring for families in the community rely on the nurse-client relationship as the foundation of their care (Minnesota Department of Health, 2019). The relationship allows the nurses to maximize client involvement; recognize strengths and available resources; and ultimately facilitate empowerment at the individual, family, and community level. The nurse-client relationship relies on the development of trust. For example, the early phase of

home visitation programs is based on the development of trust through helping clients identify problems, engaging in mutual problem solving, making decisions about necessary health services, and adopting health-promoting behaviors. This trust-building phase is crucial to the success of a program such as this because longer-term home visitation programs seem to be more effective than shorter-term ones. For some clients with traumatic pasts, however, developing trust and maintaining it over time are challenges (Dmytryshyn et al., 2015). In addition to developing trust, the nurse-client relationship is established for the nurse and the clients and families to work as partners toward accomplishing a mutual goal in health. As partners, the expertise of all is valuable to an interactive and therapeutic process.

The nurse-client relationship is key to the success of intervention programs. In a study of relationship building between public health nurses and single mothers living on public assistance, Porr (2013) found that this interactional strategy was a key practice standard for public health nurses and was instrumental in improving SDOHs in this population. Components of relationship building included engaging in a positive manner as well as offering verbal commendations.

In spite of budgetary barriers, relational practice continues to be intensely necessary for holistic, family-oriented care (Spadoni et al., 2015). Nurses working in the Healthy Baby Healthy Children (HBHC) program (see Table 19-2), for instance, are trained in implementing principles of home visitation, which includes establishing therapeutic relationships with families.

In an early but still relevant example of relational practice, Doutrich et al. (2012) paired students enrolled in a community health nursing course with local public health nurses in their clinical rotations. The students reported that they learned to value relationship building with community clients as critical to practice. They described this relationship as the key to "finding the door," getting through it, and establishing a trust relationship with clients. Other important skills these students identified included becoming aware of their own biases, getting the client's story, and not blaming or judging the client. This ability to remain nonjudgmental usually occurred when the students were truly engaged with families and understood each family's context. For example, if issues such as poverty, discrimination, and racism are not explored as underlying factors in Indigenous people's overrepresentation in homelessness in Canadian and other societies (Patrick, 2014), we are likely to approach these families with bias and blame, hence sabotaging opportunities to establish therapeutic working relationships.

Empowerment

Empowerment can be viewed as a nurse-facilitated, strengths-based process in which nurses and families work actively to share knowledge that promotes families' capacity to find and sustain solutions for improved health outcomes as well as advance health equity and well-being for communities (Torres et al., 2014). Although nurses can facilitate empowerment, they cannot "give" it. Empowerment is a process as well as an outcome. Although hierarchical relationships still characterize the power dynamics within many provider-client relationships in health care, it should be the goal of all nurses to facilitate empowerment within their community and public health practice.

Facilitating healthy change can be difficult because of the complex and fluctuating nature of the family in its unique environment, and it requires considerable skill in various empowerment strategies. Nurses must have the skills to build trusting, nonjudgmental relationships that allow and encourage families to tell their stories so they can jointly uncover the family's needs. In addition, community and public health nurses must have skills that facilitate empowering families to make decisions about their health (CHNC, 2021). For example, nurses can adopt the role of mediator or coach rather than director or decision maker. Nurses using a family-centered approach can collaborate with families to solve problems and build on their strengths, and to utilize each other and the resources that they have available to them.

Emphasizing individual and family responsibility can support self-management of chronic conditions, which moves beyond educating individuals to helping them identify challenges and solve problems related to their illness (Grady & Gough, 2014). Families that have barriers to participating actively in processes that empower them and support their independence may need an advocate. Community family nurses can speak out as advocates for the issues that affect individuals and families they care for. For years, Toronto street nurse Cathy Crowe has used political advocacy and activism to bring attention to the social injustice surrounding access to housing. Recognizing that issues such as homelessness occur at the intersection of power, politics, and families' personal lives, Crowe has used political activism to question unjust political decisions and inactions as a moral obligation to promote equity and access (Falk-Rafael & Bradley, 2014). She has strategically galvanized the use of print, social media, documentaries, and the involvement of key stakeholders at the community and governmental levels. By doing so, nurses such as Crowe uncover the policy and environmental factors that affect families while also providing support for the individual, family, community, and population as they begin to advocate for themselves. These actions are important in transforming families and communities from a state of powerlessness to recognition of their own strengths.

SETTINGS WHERE COMMUNITY AND PUBLIC HEALTH NURSES WORK

Community and public health nurses care for families in a variety of settings, such as the following:

- The home
- Community settings such as schools, clinics, adult day-care or retirement centers, and correctional facilities
- The streets or an alternative environment for families experiencing homelessness
- Temporary housing such as shelters or transitional or recovery programs
- Community-wide programs outside a traditional "place"

Although diversity exists in settings and families specific to sociodemographics (i.e., race, ethnicity, age, gender, sexual orientation, socioeconomic status, and family type), geographical location, attitudes, values, and subjective well-being, nurses use health promotion principles to act as go-betweens for people and their interactions with their environments in order to prevent illnesses and promote health (Kemppainen et al., 2013). Knowing what strategies to use with different families requires an understanding of their diverse needs.

This section covers three common settings where community and public health nurses work: family homes, community-based care settings, and public health departments.

Family Homes

Community and public health nurses working with families make home visits to assess family health status, needs, and the family's environment in order to develop specific interventions and identify available resources. For example, community and public health nurses conduct visits with clients, usually in a client's home, after a baby is born. They visit the home to determine safety, nutrition status, emotional needs, and relationship support needs. They then provide education, counseling, and referral as needed. Nurses help new mothers set goals for making healthy lifestyle choices and fostering personal growth. In some cases, nurses meet with families and their infants to conduct genetic counseling and inform them about the different tests that are possible. In other situations, nurses work with older adults in their homes to help them remain in their homes through case management, home care, and telehealth services. Assessment of the social, emotional, and physical development of families across the age span is a key role of the nurses in home visitation programs. Nurses assess the physical environment of the home, including safety hazards, such as availability of smoke detectors and fire extinguishers; any dangerous equipment; and the adequacy of running water and indoor plumbing.

In the HBHC program, for example, nurses promote the health of mothers and children in their homes. The HBHC program is a free public health initiative implemented in Ontario, Canada, to foster social, emotional, and physical health for vulnerable children. Families with anticipated poor birth outcomes, children who are failing to thrive, family stress, little social support, and low income are often referred to the program. In this program, public health nurses and family home visitors work together to assess families' situations (breastfeeding; nutrition; literacy; and social development, such as mother-child bonding), help them to access services and supports, and facilitate skill development of parents (Ontario Ministry of Children and Youth Services [OMCYS], 2020). Community nurses working with the Victorian Order of Nurses (VON) (2021) for Canada provide home-care services to families recovering from an illness. These nurses conduct assessments, provide personal support, and provide referrals to community services.

Research has demonstrated the effectiveness of home visitation programs in the United States as well. The seminal work of David Olds (2002) in the development and evaluation of the Nurse-Family Partnership program illustrates the effectiveness of family-centered care and community and public health nursing home visitation. Nurses visited low-income, unmarried mothers and their children. The families with home visitation had significantly improved health outcomes. The home visitation was found to contribute to reductions in the following: number of the mothers' subsequent pregnancies, use of welfare, child abuse and neglect, and criminal behaviors for up to 15 years after the first child's birth. At this early stage, there was little research about the effectiveness of this and other home visitation programs by nurses. However, a recent systematic review of home visiting in the United States from 2005 to 2015 found that nursing home and visitation intervention programs by nurses provided an effective route to empower people at risk for health disparities to avoid injury, maintain health, and prevent and manage chronic disease (Abbott & Elliott, 2016).

Community-Based Care Settings

Community and public health nurses also practice in community-based care settings. Community-based care settings, found in both rural and urban communities in the United States, offer the public access to a wide array of nursing services in a single setting. Community-based programs typically provide services that are not available elsewhere and are likely to focus on the needs of underserved populations. Within these settings, nurses focus on promoting health and preventing disease; they offer health screening, education, and well-child care. In addition, such settings may offer secondary and tertiary prevention services, such as management of acute and chronic health conditions, and mental health counseling.

The model for these settings is usually multidisciplinary and strives to provide affordable, accessible, acceptable care that serves to empower individuals across the life span to meet their own health care goals. The focus on social justice in many of these settings is realized by attempts to reach out to marginalized populations and to provide comprehensive, quality, nonjudgmental health care. In keeping with the community-as-mindset concept, community-based care settings may be either physical places or they may be embedded in more traditional health care settings. Some community-based care settings provide educational experiences for nursing students and students from other disciplines, making these settings a place where nursing practice, theory, and research can blend in a model that serves those who need health care the most. With the national focus on interprofessional education, nurse-led interprofessional collaborative practice teams have been integrated into many nurse-led community-based programs. These programs are often affiliated with or attached to schools of nursing and offer practice and research opportunities for faculty members as well as students (Pilon et al., 2015).

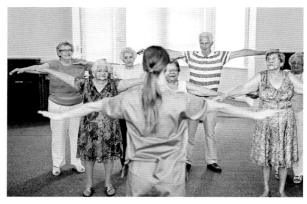

Source: © istock.com/Cecilie_Arcurs

The Ontario Early Years Centers (OEYCs) is a similar model in Canada. OEYCs are government-funded, early learning drop-in programs for parents, caregivers, and children that are located in communities across the province of Ontario. Community and public health nurses and other early childhood experts from the community, including primary care providers and pre-school educators, assist parents and caregivers to get the help they need to promote health, long-term learning, and positive behavior among children within the first 6 years of their lives. Parents, caregivers, and children participate actively in educational activities together, whereas public health nurses provide guidance and support for new parenting skills

and links to other services in the community, such as prenatal nutrition programs (OMCYS, 2020).

Public Health Departments

Probably the most widely known and accepted model for community-based services for families is the county and state departments of health. The role of governmental health departments at all levels (local, state, national) is to address public health care functions, including assessment, policy development, and assurance (Towne & Chaudry, 2017). Public health departments serve the needs of individuals and families across the life span in both health department and home-based models and, more recently, in acute-care settings in the United States. These programs include services to vulnerable groups, such as pregnant and childbearing families (Women, Infants, and Children [WIC] programs), children with special health care needs, individuals at risk for or diagnosed with infectious diseases, and those with chronic conditions. Recent health care reform and budget-reduction measures have resulted in reduced direct-care clinical service provision in most local health departments (Beck & Boulton, 2016). Still, public health nurses represent the largest group of public health practitioners working in U.S. local and state health departments, in spite of administrative and educational barriers to their practice. Regardless of the type of health department, public health nurses provide essential population health services such as diagnosis and treatment, epidemiology, health promotion, disease surveillance, community health assessment, and policy development (Centers for Disease Control and Prevention [CDC], 2020a).

Chronic pain is the number one reason patients seek care, as well as the number one cause of disability, addiction, and opioid dependency, leading to more deaths than motor vehicle accidents (CDC, 2020b; Jones et al., 2013). Chronic pain is also the number one driver of health care costs, exceeding the costs of cancer, heart disease, and diabetes combined.

Chronic pain is now known to be a disease rather than a symptom, a finding supported by nurse researchers (Clauw et al., 2018, 2019). Pain is termed chronic when it exceeds the time expected to heal an acute injury. Chronic pain may arise without an inciting event (Raja et al., 2020). In addition to pain assessment and management, nurses are expected to address the personal impact of chronic pain in terms of suffering, loss of function, disability, depression, addiction, and other comorbidities and consequences (Toye et al., 2017). However, when the authors of this chapter reviewed the literature about chronic pain management by nurses in the community, it was determined that many studies focused on pain assessment tools, with less instruction on pain management and what community resources are available to help families.

Related to chronic pain management in the United States and Canada is the increasing problem of opioid addiction and overdose. In July 2016, the Comprehensive Addiction and Recovery Act (CARA) was signed into law. It contains multiple initiatives to help address the current opioid crisis (Roberts et al., 2016). Before the national focus, local agencies had attempted a variety of preventative interventions, including the use of naloxone in the community, needle exchange programs, and takeback medication programs. Community and public health nurses and nursing students have often been involved in these injury prevention programs. One such academic-practice collaboration was described as "service learning for injury prevention" and involved a multiyear public health nursing clinical practicum with students involved with community stakeholders engaged in multiple interventions (Alexander et al., 2014, p. 175).

Rather than blaming individuals and families for their situations regarding chronic pain and opioid dependence and addiction, it is important that community and public health nurses think upstream to consider how social, political, economic, and environmental conditions affect families' health choices and outcomes. Indeed, journalist Sam Quinones's (2016) best-selling book, *Dreamland*, details the role of multiple stakeholders beyond the patient and family that have created the opioid crisis: the pharmaceutical industry, drug wholesalers and other suppliers, pill-mill prescribers, and well-intended prescribers who followed the best science in the 1990s through early 2000s regarding the need to assess and treat nonmalignant pain (e.g., pain as the fifth vital sign) (Kutlutürkan & Urvaylıoğlu 2019; Tompkins et al., 2017). In sum, chronic pain is common and costly, and its treatment sequelae are complex. An individualized nurse-patient relationship is important in comprehensive assessment and management of pain.

Elder abuse is emerging as an area of major concern nationally and internationally, and is called out as such in Healthy People 2020 (U.S. Department of Health and Human Services, 2020). Public health nurses are often on the front lines in detecting such abuse in a variety of settings. In a study of elder maltreatment in assisted-living facilities, public health nurses played key roles in abuse detection as well as policy and education development and delivery (Phillips & Ziminski, 2012). Nurses also must be aware of the omission of needed support and attention as a type of abuse. Nurses need to know how to report elder abuse in their communities and be willing to take quick action to prevent further abuse. In many U.S. states, nurses are mandatory reporters of elder abuse. For example, in the states of Oregon and Washington, nurses must report abuse of older adults who experience physical harm, financial exploitation, verbal or emotional abuse, lack of basic care, involuntary seclusion, wrongful restraint, unwanted sexual contact, or abandonment by the caregiver. Each state has an individual policy for reporting to protective services. More information about reporting elder abuse in the United States can be found at the National Clearinghouse on Abuse in Later Life (NCALL) (2021) website.

In the United States, 85% of providers have seen an increase of families experiencing homelessness in recent years (Bassuk Center, 2015). Despite this growing social problem, most research about homelessness focuses on individuals, often men. In an attempt to understand the families experiencing homelessness and to respond appropriately, Slesnick et al. (2012) interviewed mothers experiencing homelessness and their caseworkers to assess alignment between needs and available services. Persistent lack of social support was a key theme. Understanding how public health nurses can assist with the process of rehousing while supporting family agency and self-efficacy can lead to a rich new role for public health nurses. The researchers suggested that services address practical supports but also be trauma-informed, help build self-esteem, repair and rebuild family relationships, and develop healthy communities (Slesnick et al., 2012).

Engaging nurses and nursing students in caring for families experiencing homelessness, a growing segment of our population, is challenging, and creativity is warranted. Breen and Robinson (2016) found that that participation in a service-learning clinical rotation with families experiencing homelessness increased Registered Nurse to Bachelor of Science Degree in Nursing (RN to BSN) students' awareness of the circumstances for people who have socioeconomic disadvantages, causing them to question their previously held assumptions and make practice changes. Similarly, Rasmor et al. (2014) found that nurse practitioner students who completed an experience working with vulnerable families in free clinics increased their interest in working with these populations after graduation. With decreasing funding for targeted services for vulnerable populations such as families experiencing homelessness, nurses need to engage in providing care where the families can access it.

ROLES OF COMMUNITY AND PUBLIC HEALTH NURSES WORKING WITH FAMILIES AND COMMUNITIES

In their capacities, community and public health nurses play several roles. These include, but are not limited to, health education, advocacy, facilitation of access to health resources, assessment, assurance, policy development, referrals, building capacity, and consultation. Table 19-2 describes some of the diverse roles assumed by these nurses. In this section, we discuss community and public health nursing roles in health education, facilitation of resources, assessment, assurance, and policy development.

Health Education

Health education is essential to the promotion of health and the prevention of disease in families. Using information gained through family health appraisals and assessments, community health nurses reinforce health-promoting behaviors and provide health information and teaching in identified at-risk areas. The CDC lists five major determinants of health: (1) health care access and quality, (2) education access and quality, (3) social and community context, (4) economic stability, and (5) neighborhood and built environment (CDC, 2021a). Community and public health nurses have a role in facilitating high-level wellness for their

clients by advocating for positive changes in health determinants, including health behaviors, social environment and characteristics, physical environment and ecology, and health services.

Community health nurses use a variety of strategies to modify behaviors, characteristics, or care limitations identified in the health appraisal. Teaching and health information can be used to discuss immunizations, nutrition, rest, exercise, use of seat belts, and abuse of harmful substances such as alcohol and drugs. Community health nurses may refer families to programs and resources that assist in their lifestyle modifications (e.g., smoking cessation classes, exercise programs).

Health teaching, based on appraisal of the physical environment, might also include information on child safety and prevention of falls for older adults. Other teaching might focus on psychological or social environmental problems, such as family communications or dealing with peer pressure. In some situations, community health nurses promote a healthy and safe environment by meeting with the school board to provide evidence about playground hazards or poor food-handling practices.

Facilitate Access to Resources

A major health promotion strategy is to ensure access to health promotion and prevention services, including immunizations, family planning, prenatal care, well-child care, nutrition, exercise classes, and dental hygiene. These services may be provided directly by community health nurses, or community health nurses may facilitate access to these services through referrals, case management, discharge planning, advocacy, coordination, and collaboration.

Nurses must consider access to resources within a context of what choices families realistically have. For example, eating healthy meals requires that healthy foods be available in locations that families can access easily and without expensive transportation. Also, accessing health providers and facilities requires that, in the United States, families have some type of health insurance or other means to pay. The Affordable Care Act's (ACA's) major coverage provisions went into effect in January 2014 and have led to significant coverage gains. In the second half of 2019, 35.7 million persons of all ages (11.0%) were uninsured—significantly higher than the first 6 months of 2019 (30.7 million, 9.5%) (National Center for Health Statistics, 2020). There has been movement toward patient-, client-, and family-centered care, and toward upstream thinking and preventative care. Although there are still some Americans without insurance, the change in coverage since the implementation of ACA is significant. In addition to providing (and mandating) coverage, ACA did not allow health insurance companies to deny individuals health insurance based on preexisting conditions. The Kaiser Family Foundation found in a recent study that 52 million Americans (or 27%) have a preexisting condition "that would likely make them uninsurable if they applied for health coverage under medical underwriting practices that existed in most states before insurance regulation change" (Kaiser Family Foundation, 2016, para. 1).

Facilitating access to resources for families who are deprived because of race, social class, and gender requires understanding of how social injustice operates on a social level to cause such depravity. Paul Farmer is a physician and author best known for his medical work in Haiti and worldwide with tuberculosis and AIDS. He wrote about structural violence in his book, *Pathologies of Power: Health, Human Rights and the New War on the Poor* (Farmer, 2003). Structural violence refers to historical, economic, and political roots of generational oppression. It is about unequal treatment, racism, classism, and discrimination. We see these factors dominating the experiences of gun violence victims and survivors. These structural inequities work to perpetuate the disproportional occurrence and impact of gun violence among Blacks, while shaping their experience with gun violence trauma and access to service and supports (Bailey et al., 2013, 2015). These same factors are intimately involved as predictors and facilitators in diverse homeless populations' experience (Paul et al., 2019). Whether homelessness or structural violence, several social issues are rooted in systematized, unequal access to resources. Working toward social justice requires a partnership between families and professionals. The community and public health nurses' responses to the structural violence perpetuated by policy, the myth of meritocracy (that anyone who is hard-working and deserving can succeed), and our biases make it an ethical obligation to engage in deep relational practice with the families we serve.

Assessment, Assurance, and Policy Development

Community and public health nurses are engaged in the core public health functions of assessment, assurance, and policy development. These core functions include assessing and monitoring the health of communities and populations at risk to identify health problems and priorities, ensuring that all populations have access to appropriate and cost-effective care (assurance), and formulating policies designed to solve identified local and national health problems and priorities. Assessment is facilitated by the trust that public health nurses have earned from their clients, agencies, and private providers—trust that provides ready access to populations that are otherwise difficult to access and engage in health care. In addition, these nurses are deeply informed about current and emerging health issues through their daily contact with high-risk and vulnerable populations. This trust and knowledge provide the foundation for ways that nurses can work with communities (populations) and families and individuals. Table 19-3 lists the different assessment approaches nurses can use in the community, based on the focus of the health care.

Assurance activities are the direct, individual-focused services that public health nurses provide. Although the current shift in emphasis is toward assessment and policy development, critical assurance activities remain for the public health nurse. Assurance activities at the community, family, and individual levels are outlined in Table 19-4.

In 1988, IOM compiled a report called *The Future of Public Health*, which led to the Current Core Functions of Public Health (e.g., assessment, policy development, assurance) and the 10 Essential Services of Public Health in the United States. These core functions and essential services remain the guiding framework for U.S. public health (CDC, 2020a). Over time and in some areas, this framework changed the focus of public health from delivering primary health care or providing safety-net services to individuals to a more population, upstream, data-driven, policy-focused health care system. See Table 19-5 to review ways that policy comes about relative to public health. Although many local health departments still provide some level of health care to individuals or families, this movement toward the core functions has meant

Table 19-3 **Comparison of Assessment Approaches**		
COMMUNITY	**FAMILY**	**INDIVIDUAL**
Analyze data on and needs of specific populations or geographical area. Identify and interact with key community leaders, both formally and informally. Identify target populations that may be at risk. These populations may include families living in high-density, low-income areas, preschool children, primary and secondary school children, and older adults. Participate in data collection on a target population. Conduct surveys or observe targeted populations, such as preschools, jails, and detention centers, to gain a better understanding of needs.	Evaluate a specific family's strengths and areas of concern. This involves a comprehensive assessment of the physical, social, and mental health needs of the family. Evaluate the family's living environment, looking specifically at support, relationships, and other factors that might have a significant impact on family health outcomes. Assess the larger environment in which the family lives (their block or specific community) for safety, access, and other related issues.	Identify individuals within the family in need of services. Evaluate the functional capacity of the individual through the use of specific assessment measures, including physical, social, and mental health screening tools. Develop a nursing diagnosis for the individual that describes a problem or potential problem, causative factors, and contributing factors. Develop a nursing care plan for the individual.

Table 19-4 **Assurance Activities in Community, Family, and Individual Care**		
COMMUNITY	**FAMILY**	**INDIVIDUAL**
Provide service to target populations, such as child-care centers, preschools, worksites, underrepresented communities, jails, juvenile detention facilities, and homeless shelters. Interventions may include health screening, education, health promotion, and injury prevention programs. Improve quality assurance activities with various health care providers in the community. Examples include education on new immunization policies, educational programs for communicable disease control, assistance in developing effective approaches, and support techniques for high-risk populations. Maintain safe levels of communicable disease surveillance and outbreak control. Participate in research or demonstration projects. Provide expert public health consultation in the community. Ensure that standards of care are met within the community (assurance).	Provide services to a cluster of families within a geographical setting. Services may be provided in a variety of settings, including homes, child-care centers, preschools, and schools. Services may include physical assessment, health education and counseling, and health and developmental screening. Provide care in a nursing clinic to a specific group of families in a geographical location.	Provide nursing services based on standards of nursing practice to individuals across the age continuum. These services may encompass a variety of programs, including, specifically, First Steps and Children With Special Health Care Needs, and more generally, child abuse prevention, immunizations, well-child care, and HIV/AIDS programs. Assess and support the individual's progress toward meeting outcome goals. Consult with other health care providers and team members regarding the individual's plan of care. Prioritize individual's needs on an ongoing basis. Participate on quality assurance teams to measure the quality of care provided.

changes in what it means to be a public health nurse or provider. For example, the growing number of new cases of pertussis in the United States requires us to consider all health as public health. Most serious morbidity and mortality from pertussis occurs in infants who are too young to mount an immune response to active vaccines, so community and public health nurses are actively working in acute-care and long-term care facilities to vaccinate all adults to provide herd immunity that shields our youngest and most vulnerable family members.

Coalitions of community partners that include academic-practice partnerships, traditional public health services, councils for people who are homeless, peer mentors, and regional acute- and ambulatory-care systems are joining together in some areas. Coalitions involve groups of individuals, including public health workers, researchers, clinicians, researchers, educators, and citizens, to promote the health of the public and reduce health inequities (CDC, 2021b). Their purposes in these coalitions are to use data to influence the provision

Table 19-5 **Activities That Influence Policy Development**		
COMMUNITY	**FAMILY**	**INDIVIDUAL**
Provide leadership in convening and facilitating community groups to evaluate health concerns and develop a plan to address the concerns. Recommend specific training and programs to meet identified health needs. Raise awareness of key policymakers about health regulations, budget decisions, and other factors that may negatively affect the health of communities. Recommend programs to target populations such as child-care centers, retirement centers, jails, juvenile detention facilities, homeless shelters, worksites, and underrepresented communities. Act as an advocate for the community and individuals who are not willing or able to speak to policymakers about issues and programs of concern. Work with business and industry to develop employee health programs.	Recommend new or increased services to families based on identified needs. Recommend programs to meet specific families' needs within a geographical area. Facilitate networking with families with similar needs or issues. Guide policymakers on specific issues that affect clusters of families. Request additional data and analyze information to identify trends in a group or cluster of families. Identify key families in a community who may either oppose or support specific policies or programs, and develop appropriate and effective intervention strategies to use with these families.	Recommend or assist in the development of standards for individual client care. Recommend or adopt risk classification systems to assist with prioritizing individual client care. Participate in establishing criteria for opening, closing, or referring individual cases. Participate in the development of job descriptions to establish roles for various team members who will provide service to individuals.

of coordinated efforts to address services and to influence policies aimed toward "making living better—for everyone" (Healthy Living Collaborative of Southwest Washington [HLCSW], 2021, para. 1). Current priorities for HLCSW include bringing communities and organizations together to identify and remove barriers to health and equity, build a workforce of skilled community health workers, remove barriers to school attendance, and shape public policy.

TRENDS IN PUBLIC HEALTH

Community and public health nursing positions in the United States, rather than growing with population and health care needs, have declined significantly in the past two decades (Young et al., 2014). The factors contributing to this trend include an aging nursing workforce, challenges with funding in the public health system, and a shortage of sites for clinical training (Young et al., 2014). Similar to nurses in many contexts, community and public health nurses with positions in public health are being asked to do more with less. Responding to workforce and economic constraints, some public health services have switched to a focus on the core functions and community and neighborhood interventions. Skills in connecting planning to

SDOHs, understanding the multiple perspectives of all stakeholders, and being able to translate (almost in a multilingual way) the contextual realities of clients are among the skills required. Community and public health nurses today must become comfortable with geographical information system (GIS) (Box 19-1) mapping and epidemiology, and they should know and be able to connect with the communities these representations depict. It is important that nurses be willing to engage in political actions to address issues not easily ameliorated at the individual level. Thus, establishing proactive policies should be an important health

BOX 19-1
Geographical Information Systems (GISs)

A GIS visually displays, analyzes, and manipulates spatial data to locate geographical areas, potential hazards, water sources, and other important information. This digital technology helps the user to understand trends and issues of concern by rendering data visually, in the forms of maps, charts, histograms, and a variety of reports. Having access to this type of detailed data in a visual format allows community and public health nurses to intervene more quickly and accurately to enhance public health and safety.

goal for public health and community nurses to facilitate improved health for vulnerable families and groups.

Nurse Practitioner Roles in Community and Public Health Nursing

In April 2013, the National Organization of Nurse Practitioner Faculties (NONPF) released the following six nurse practitioner population-foci competencies: Family/Across the Lifespan, Neonatal, Acute Care Pediatric, Primary Care Pediatric, Psychiatric–Mental Health, and Women's Health/Gender Related. NONPF incorporated population health into nursing education programs for nurse practitioners and into its accreditation for these programs, with the intent that all nurse practitioners be educated and competent in population health.

One example of a program employing nurse practitioners in population health takes place in Oregon. Oregon has a comprehensive network of child abuse assessment and intervention centers designed to minimize trauma to child abuse victims by coordinating the local community's response to reports of suspected child abuse. This community-based, interprofessional, child maltreatment intervention model offers population-focused nurse practitioners the opportunity to prevent, recognize early, and treat families that have experienced dysfunction and/or child maltreatment in order to prevent some of the negative life impacts of these early experiences. Services include interviews of suspected victims of child abuse, medical evaluations, mental health treatment and/or referrals, provision or coordination of other victim services, and individual- and community-specific needs. This important work grew, in part, out of findings from the Adverse Childhood Experiences study (Felitti et al., 1998). The study revealed the following: (1) more than half of study participants had experienced at least one of the adverse experiences studied (psychological, physical, or sexual abuse; violence against mother;

or living with household members who were substance abusers, mentally ill or suicidal, or ever imprisoned); (2) persons who had experienced four or more categories of childhood exposure, compared with those who had experienced none, had a 4- to 12-fold increased health risk for alcoholism, drug abuse, depression, and suicide; (3) persons who had experienced four or more categories of childhood exposure had a two- to fourfold increase in smoking, poor self-rated health, greater than 50 sexual intercourse partners, and sexually transmitted infection; and (4) persons who had experienced four or more categories of childhood exposure had a 1.4- to 1.6-fold increase in physical inactivity and severe obesity (Felitti et al., 1998). Findings from this foundational study have been replicated in more recent work (Gilbert et al., 2015).

Several very creative and successful community programs integrate knowledge about adverse childhood experiences and resilience. For example, the Walla Walla Valley's Children's Resilience Initiative in Washington State grew out of an understanding of adverse childhood experiences (ACEs) and their consequences. The initiative is a learning community whose goal is to build a toolbox of resilience-based strategies to confront the challenges of life. This is a community-wide project that exists outside a traditional nursing "space." Quality care for families in the community can be enhanced when rigid understandings of place and/or position of nursing care are rethought and made more flexible to match family and community needs.

Population-focused nurse practitioners often fill positions in inpatient and outpatient settings that focus on the care of groups of clients with particular chronic illnesses, such as diabetes or heart disease. These nurse practitioners provide primary care to these clients and offer individual and group health education and other health promotion activities. Their interest and expertise in a particular health condition lend themselves well to advocating for necessary resources for their population of interest and to becoming active in health policy change on behalf of their clients.

Case Study: Davis Family

Three weeks ago, two senior nursing students, who were participating in their community and population health clinical as members of an outreach team at a homeless outreach program, were asked by one of the case managers on the team to do an assessment of a client named John Davis at his apartment. John had been refusing help from his case manager and denied offers to connect him with medical care. The students completed a physical assessment to the best of their abilities and observed the following: urine, feces, and blood-stained clothing; more than two instances of bilateral pitting edema of the lower extremities; diminished bilateral lung sounds in all quadrants; numerous open sores on John's neck and upper extremities; disorientation to time; overgrown toenails that embedded themselves into the bottoms of his toes; muscle wasting; and extreme generalized weakness. It was clear to them that the client's safety was in jeopardy, and they made the decision to call emergency medical services for transport to the hospital. Their decision was fully supported by the case manager and outreach team. The homeless outreach program does not provide any health services, nor does it employ any health care providers. Nursing students do community and population health clinical rotations at this site every semester.

Following his transport to the hospital, John was admitted for a 3-week stay to address concerns associated with his mental illness, addiction to drugs and alcohol, severe dehydration, open skin sores, and extreme weakness. John is a 57-year-old male who had been estranged from his family and chronically homeless for many years until recently, when he was placed in a Housing First apartment in a small town 10 miles from the hospital. Housing First is a program that prioritizes permanent housing as a basic necessity, like access to food, that must be met in order for individuals to be successful addressing other issues such as unemployment or addiction issues ((National Alliance to End Homelessness, 2016).

John resembles an 80-year-old man, has a long list of problem health issues, and uses drugs and alcohol to self-medicate for an underlying chronic mental illness (see the Davis family's genogram in Figure 19-2 and the ecomap in Figure 19-3).

A day after his discharge from the hospital and return to his Housing First apartment, John was sent for treatment to the emergency room of the local hospital. His symptoms included severe shortness of breath, weakness, confusion, and chest pain. He was immediately readmitted to the hospital with a unilateral pneumothorax.

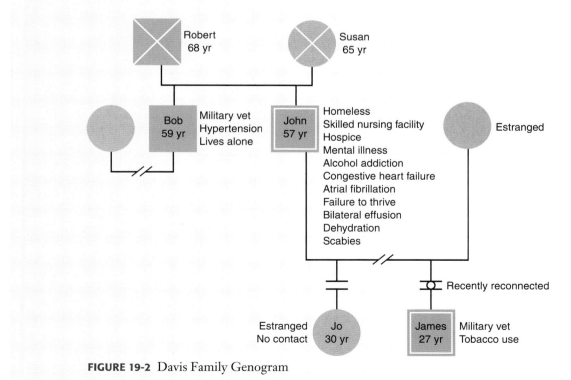

FIGURE 19-2 Davis Family Genogram

(continued)

Case Study: Davis Family—cont'd

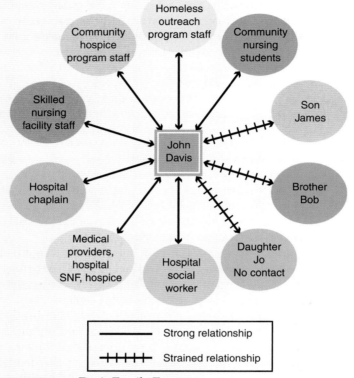

FIGURE 19-3 Davis Family Ecomap

The senior nursing students who worked with John visited him at the hospital. They noticed a drastic decline in his neuro/ mental status from the day before and were concerned that he was unable to feed himself or get to the bathroom. When they discussed these issues with the primary nurse, she mentioned that he would likely show progressive decline because of his compromised respiratory status. She also said that the social worker was in the process of contacting his family, per his request, and assisting him in the process of filling out an advance directive.

During the next week, the primary nurse and social worker began to make arrangements for John to be transferred to a skilled nursing facility upon discharge from the hospital. Because he continued to decline, they realized that his current needs for support and caregiving would exceed what could be provided at the homeless outreach program. The outreach team was involved with the discharge plan and agreed that John was no longer capable of caring for himself independently.

During the week that he was in the hospital, John had several visits with family members who had agreed to visit him. His son and his brother both visited, and the family was supported by members of the homeless outreach program and the hospital staff, including the nurses, social worker, and chaplain. With John's consent, his family was involved in the discussions about his declining condition and transfer to the skilled nursing facility. On the day of his discharge from the hospital, the nurse also placed a call to the local hospice program that would admit him to the hospice program once he got settled in the skilled nursing facility. In the referral to the hospice program, John's diagnosis list was updated to include the following: congestive heart failure, atrial fibrillation, bilateral pleural effusion, failure to thrive, dehydration, scabies, and a sacral pressure ulcer. He was now dependent on oxygen, confined to a wheelchair and hospital bed, and required 24-hour skilled care.

When John arrived in the skilled nursing facility, he became combative and began refusing assistance. He also refused to wear his oxygen or take his medication for comfort, which caused increased hypoxia, pain, and confusion. It is important to remember that John had multiple mental health issues, making his acceptance of any help very difficult. In addition, his confusion from what

Case Study: Davis Family—cont'd

appeared to be oxygen deprivation increased the risk that he could become combative. Meanwhile, John exhibited signs of air hunger: tripod position, respiratory rate of 36, and agitation. The care team and family set up his room and called to schedule the hospice admission sooner rather than later. His son and his brother took turns staying with him and provided much of the care that he needed, including medication administration of comfort medications when he would take them. He was no longer eating or drinking and declined quickly.

Outcome

John died in the skilled nursing facility 3 days after his transfer from the hospital. His son and his brother were at his bedside providing loving support and care.

Questions for reflection on the nursing care of the Davis family:

1. Reflect on the care that John received leading up to his death. Discuss the strengths and challenges.
2. Describe the settings, or care environments, where John's care was delivered.
3. What concepts and principles for care were utilized by the nurse and the health care team?
4. What were the roles provided by the nurse?

SUMMARY

Community and public health nurses forge strong nurse-client partnerships as they maneuver through the maze of interventions and resources in providing family-centered nursing. They are concerned with the health of families and the ways in which family health influences the health of communities.

- Nurses foster interconnectedness among families in the community.
- The settings in which community and public health nurses work with families vary and include, but are not limited to, public and private health agencies, schools, and occupational sites.
- Population health and community and public health nursing roles vary according to whether the nurse is focusing on the family as the unit of care in the context of the community, focusing on the health of the community with families being a subunit, or focusing on an aggregate of the population.

- Community and public health nurses aim to meet the holistic needs of families and communities while targeting prioritized health needs.
- Rather than blaming families for their situations, community and public health nurses consider how social, political, economic, and environmental conditions affect families' health choices and outcomes.
- Family interventions in the community are targeted toward primary, secondary, and tertiary prevention. The nurse-family relationship is central in interventions at all three levels of prevention.
- Interventions for families are planned, implemented, and evaluated from a health promotion perspective.
- Using a combination of relational collaboration and health promotion strategies and principles, community and public health nurses strive to partner with families to assist with all levels of healthy change.

NCLEX®-Style Questions

1. The nurse prepares to assess a family, which includes several members with chronic health problems. Which definition of assessment does the nurse use when meeting with this family?

1. The use of an instrument to quantify a particular family attribute.
2. The use of a tool to collect family information within 15 minutes.
3. The collection of subjective and objective data that begins on first contact with the family.
4. The process of assigning numbers or symbols to variables to assist nurses in measuring family member characteristics.

2. The nurse plans to use a family genogram during a family assessment. What assessment information does this tool provide?

1. Tension between family members.
2. Multigenerational patterns and health conditions.
3. Communication patterns among family members.
4. Relationships between family members and the community.

3. The nurse meets with a family to complete a genogram. The nurse understands that there should be a minimum of how many generations represented on the genogram?

1. One.
2. Two.
3. Three.
4. Four.

4. The nurse begins to assess a family. Based on the nurse's initial assessment of the family,

which of the following best describes the family story?

1. The analysis of outcomes.
2. The gathering of data from a variety of sources to see the whole picture of the family experience.
3. The process of establishing intervention plans.
4. The clustering of data into meaningful groups and identifying pertinent relationships between variables.

5. A nurse is working with a family and has completed an ecomap. The nurse understands that an ecomap assists in the assessment of a family in which of the following ways? **Select all that apply.**

1. Pinpoints health conditions.
2. Analyzes multigenerational patterns.
3. Highlights tension among family members.
4. Includes pets and non-blood-related family members.
5. Identifies the relationship between family members and the community.

6. The nurse is working with a family and learns that the family members are moving and will no longer be able to meet with the nurse for continuing care. What should the nurse do as this relationship is terminated? **Select all that apply.**

1. Write a therapeutic letter.
2. Schedule a summary meeting.
3. Ask the physician to write a letter.
4. Encourage the family members to keep in touch.
5. Refer the family members to resources in the new community.

7. The nurse plans to use the Family Assessment and Intervention Model when working with a family. Which of the following demonstrate(s) the purpose of this model? **Select all that apply.**

1. Health promotion.
2. Family change strategies.
3. Restoration of family stability and family functioning.
4. Family reaction and instability at lines of defense and resistance.
5. Large amount of information that may not relate to the family problem.

8. A nursing instructor is discussing the determinants of health with a group of community health nursing students. The nursing instructor asks the students to identify examples of determinants of health that may affect family health. Which of the following is an example of an environmental determinant of health?

1. The family's ability to access libraries and theaters.
2. The availability of low-cost housing or apartments.
3. The presence of a coal-fired, electricity-generating plant in the community.
4. The student-to-teacher ratio at the local elementary school.

9. A nurse has volunteered to provide a community talk at the local library on disasters. Which of the following in the nurse's talk would be an example of the mitigation phase of the disaster management cycle?

1. Advocating to state officials to provide funds for rebuilding an earthquake-proof water system.
2. Eliminating sources of standing water in yards to reduce mosquito-breeding sites.
3. Recommending families practice an escape plan if a wildland fire threatened their community.
4. Setting up temporary food distribution centers at the local high school.

10. A community health nurse is completing an environmental assessment and reports that each summer, migrant workers are hired to help with harvesting fruit trees, which are frequently sprayed with pesticides to minimize crop damage. The nurse reports inadequate availability of protective clothing and washing stations for the migrant workers. The owners of the orchards indicate that it is too expensive to provide these resources for the short harvest season. Based on this information, the nurse understands that this is an example of which of the following?

1. Environmental health literacy.
2. Environmental injustice.
3. Environmental justice.
4. Environmental policy.

11. The nurse reviews assessment data before creating a family plan of care. Which definition of family health promotion should the nurse keep in mind when selecting interventions for the family?

1. Having resources to pay for medical bills.
2. Living in a location where health resources are readily available.
3. Planning for retirement and achieving a quality and dignified death.
4. Improving or maintaining the physical, social, emotional, and spiritual well-being of the family.

12. The nurse is assessing the rituals that a family follows. Which definition of a family ritual should the nurse use when identifying these activities?

1. Process of family members learning to do things together.
2. Repetitive pattern of formal behavior around a specific event that is repeated.
3. Process of getting the family members back together after a conflict.
4. Action that the family takes to keep the family heritage and history.

13. A health care system is planning to implement telehealth in all facilities. Which outcome should the nurse expect when this approach to care is fully implemented?

1. Reduced incidences of chronic disease development.
2. Improved health care access, quality, and efficiency.

3. Decreased time for diagnosing health problems.
4. Elimination of the need for face-to-face interactions with care providers.

14. Which factor(s) should the nurse identify as influencing the promotion of a family's health? **Select all that apply.**

    1. Being a role model.
    2. Teaching self-care behavior.
    3. Supporting family member(s) during illness.
    4. Focusing primarily on younger family members.
    5. Providing care for family members across the life course.

15. Family empowerment is a process, outcome, and intervention. On what should the nurse focus when assisting a family to become more empowered? **Select all that apply.**

    1. Providing information.
    2. Problem solving for the family.
    3. Encouraging family participation in goal setting.
    4. Providing encouragement and support.
    5. Using strategies to increase family strength.

16. During a health assessment, a middle-aged male who identifies as gay asks the nurse not to document his sexual preference because his primary health care provider is not aware. What should this request indicate to the nurse?

    1. Fear of not receiving required care.
    2. Fear of having to pay more for care.
    3. Fear of not having anyone to help as aging occurs.
    4. Fear that family members will be discriminated against.

17. The nurse manager suggests that the nursing staff include an assessment of mental health for all clients who are members of the LGBTQ+ community. Why is the manager most likely making this suggestion? **Select all that apply.**

    1. The higher risk of substance abuse within this community.
    2. The greater risk for depression within this community.

3. The high level of social stigma and discrimination that this community often experiences.
4. A preexisting bias against this community.
5. The fact that suicide is a leading cause of death within this community.

18. The nurse is aware of several children adopted into same-sex families that are scheduled to participate in the community preschool program. What can the nurse do to facilitate the acceptance of these children's family structure into the preschool learning environment? **Select all that apply.**

    1. Ensure that teaching materials demonstrate diverse family structures.
    2. Provide toys, books, and games that emphasize traditional gender roles.
    3. Select materials that show both genders performing a variety of roles.
    4. Instruct the preschool staff members on ways to reduce the stigma of these children.
    5. Encourage these children to play with toys that are opposite from their parents' gender.

19. A community health nurse who works with COPD patients wants to help lower the rate of prevalence. The nurse can implement which of the following interventions as effective methods to lower prevalence of chronic illnesses like COPD?

    1. Develop a quit plan with each patient who smokes.
    2. Advocate for policy-based strategies to prevent or discourage smoking, such as implementing a higher excise tax on cigarettes and creating workplace programs.
    3. Educate children on how encourage their parents to stop smoking.
    4. Advocate for exercise workplace programs for employees.

20. The nurse is caring for a patient with progressing dementia. During a family meeting to discuss how the family members can best support each other, the nurse

implements which important intervention to help the family cope?

1. Identify one family member who will drive the patient to the next provider appointment.
2. Discuss meal planning and where food should be bought.
3. Discuss redistribution of family roles to help ease role strain, and discuss how relationships might change throughout the process of providing care and the changing health needs of their family member.
4. Bring comfort food to the meeting to help the family feel better when discussing difficult topics.

21. A patient with Parkinson's disease is in the clinic for a follow-up visit. The primary caregiver, who is the patient's eldest daughter, has accompanied the patient. During the visit, the nurse makes sure to assess which of the following?

1. The caregiver's understanding of the condition and the type of care needed, and the ability of the caregiver to identify problem-solving strategies when issues arise.
2. Whether the caregiver slept well last night and was able to eat breakfast this morning.
3. If there is anyone else that could provide care because having a family member provide care often does not work out well.
4. The size of the family, because small families have a difficult time with caregiving.

22. The nurse is attempting to empower a patient and his or her family members to feel control in order to provide self-management of the family member's chronic disease. The nurse implements which of the following strategies?

1. Gives specific directions of when and how care should be provided.
2. Gives the patient a list of all the patient's health care providers and encourages the patient to contact each one so care can be coordinated.

3. Explains the need to be rigid in care routines.
4. Provides education to build confidence and skills of the patient and the family members.

23. Nurses know routines are beneficial for coping with chronic illness, particularly during times of change, crisis, and illness events. To promote routines, the nurse implements which of the following with the patient and family with a new chronic illness diagnosis?

1. Map out the routine the patient and family members should follow every day.
2. Identify only one or two realistic important family traditions to try to incorporate into the new routines.
3. Identify important daily routines with activities of daily living (ADLs) and care needs and important family traditions or celebrations in order to collaborate on realistic goal setting.
4. Create goals for the patient and share them with the family members, along with the routines they should be following.

24. The family members of a client with a terminal illness hesitate to agree to palliative care because they do not want to give up on a possible cure. How should the nurse respond while also including a principle of palliative care?

1. "Most people don't realize that palliative care means there is no cure."
2. "There will not be another opportunity if palliative care is refused now."
3. "The client can continue to receive treatment intended to cure the disease."
4. "Palliative care and curative treatments cannot be provided at the same time."

25. The family members of a client receiving palliative care for a terminal illness hesitate to call for the nurse because all staff members seem to be too busy to address the client's needs. Which action should the

nurse take to improve the connection with the family?

1. Vary the number and type of caregivers who respond to the client's needs.
2. Enter the room and stand or sit at the bedside to talk with the client and family members.
3. Provide the family with reading material that explains the role of palliative care.
4. Attend to infusions and environmental issues while talking with the client and family.

26. The spouse of a client nearing death is concerned because the client's breathing is "so noisy." Which statement by the nurse would be appropriate when referring to the client's respiratory status?

   1. "The noise is due to pneumonia."
   2. "The noise is due to respiratory congestion."
   3. "The noise is referred to as the death rattle."
   4. "The noise is due to fluid in the lungs."

27. The family members of a client nearing the end of life ask if they can leave to get dinner. Which client observation causes the nurse to suggest that the family wait a while longer before leaving the client?

   1. Cheyne-Stokes respiration pattern.
   2. Apneic periods of 15 to 30 seconds.
   3. Shallow respirations at 30 per minute.
   4. Use of neck and shoulder muscles to breathe.

28. A client assigned to a student nurse for care dies shortly after the student completes morning care. What should the nurse do to support the student at this time?

   1. Suggest that the student leave the clinical area.
   2. Encourage the student to participate in postmortem care.
   3. Talk with the student about the experience and answer any questions.
   4. Assign the student to another client for the remainder of the clinical day.

29. An interprofessional team meeting is scheduled to discuss the care needs for a client with a terminal illness. What should the nurse expect when participating in this meeting? **Select all that apply.**

   1. Control is centralized.
   2. Client goals direct care.
   3. The focus is on problem solving.
   4. The client's family can be in attendance.
   5. Decisions are made by the team leader.

30. The nurse providing palliative care to a client with a terminal illness is experiencing moral distress. Which situation(s) most likely caused the nurse to experience this emotional response? **Select all that apply.**

   1. The nurse continues to provide chemotherapy to the client upon the family's request.
   2. The nurse is unable to relieve dyspnea because of a fear of overmedicating the client.
   3. The team members decide to withhold routine fluids unless the client is thirsty.
   4. Another health care provider suggested that another course of treatment might "do the trick."
   5. The adult children of the client want everything possible done, but the client is exhausted and wants it to end.

31. The nurse notes that a client who returned from war is having difficulty remembering recent events and is unable to perform simple self-care tasks. Which part of the client's physiology is responsible for these behaviors?

   1. Amygdala.
   2. Hippocampus.
   3. Adrenal glands.
   4. Prefrontal cortex.

32. A nurse is reassigned to assist with triaging victims of a train derailment in the emergency department. The next day, the nurse returns to providing care in the intensive-care unit and is assigned the victims. If this pattern continues, which

health problem is the nurse prone to developing?

1. Apathy.
2. Depression.
3. Poor self-esteem.
4. Secondary traumatization.

33. A client with PTSD arrives for a follow-up clinic appointment. The nurse should confirm that the client is continuing to follow which of the following interventions?

1. Drinks 2 to 3 liters of fluid per day.
2. Measures blood pressure every week.
3. Adheres to an 1,800 calorie/day eating plan.
4. Attends cognitive-behavioral therapy sessions.

34. The nurse plans care for a client recovering from a gunshot wound received during the robbery of a convenience store. Which intervention(s) does the nurse select to promote trauma-informed care for this client? **Select all that apply.**

1. Coaches the client in calming skills.
2. Builds positive social support.
3. Suggests returning to the scene of the event.
4. Reminds the client that the injuries were not life-threatening.
5. Encourages connectiveness between family members.

35. The nurse suspects that an adult client experienced domestic violence as a child. Which observation(s) cause the nurse to come to this conclusion? **Select all that apply.**

1. Several arrests for armed robbery.
2. Meets with friends once a week to play poker.
3. Red-flagged for suicide precautions when incarcerated.
4. Repeatedly admitted to a rehabilitation facility for heroin use.
5. Worked for a company for 2 years and then sought new employment.

36. The nurse suspects that a family has closed boundaries. Why will this family not be amenable to nursing interventions?

1. They are unstable.
2. They do not have children.
3. They do not interact with each other.
4. They reject influences from the outside environment.

37. The nurse is planning care for a family with a new baby. Which reason should the nurse identify as a risk for conflict between the nurse and the client during this time?

1. Acute illness occurring in the new mother.
2. Agreement between the father or partner and the mother.
3. Agreement between grandparents and the nurse.
4. Different advice from family members versus the nurse.

38. The nurse plans to discuss an expectant client's decision regarding infant feeding. What is important for the nurse to do when considering feeding management for this family?

1. Inform the client that she should breastfeed.
2. Assist the parents to form a nurturing relationship surrounding the feeding of the infant.
3. Encourage bottle-feeding because this will guarantee proper nutrition for the infant.
4. Encourage the father or partner to leave the feeding decision up to the mother.

39. The nurse plans care to address the communication pattern within a family with a new infant. What intervention should the nurse select for this family?

1. Encourage talking when the baby is sleeping.
2. Hold the baby while talking with each other.
3. Teach the family members how to recognize and respond to the baby's cues.
4. Keep voice tone low when discussing a difficult situation.

40. The female partner of a family is upset because the spouse will not talk about the inability to conceive. Which response should the nurse make to this client?

   1. "Talking about the problem can increase your spouse's anxiety about it."
   2. "Men deny the amount of emotional distress they experience."
   3. "Most men do not share their feelings."
   4. "Men only want to talk to other men and won't do that unless they know someone else has the same problem."

41. The nurse suspects that a new mother is at risk for poor attachment with her newborn. What could be a reason (or the reasons) for poor attachment? **Select all that apply.**

   1. Family stress.
   2. Poor self-image.
   3. Family violence.
   4. Low self-esteem.
   5. Maternal depression.

42. What information does the family health nurse use to determine the most appropriate health promotion activities in a family with young children?

   1. The children's health practices.
   2. The parents' and grandparents' health beliefs.
   3. The patterns of daily routines and family rituals.
   4. The patterns of disease and illness reorganization task management.

43. During a home visit, the nurse learns that a family is experiencing a situational transition. Which event most likely occurred in this family?

   1. The parents filed for divorce.
   2. A child was diagnosed with cystic fibrosis.
   3. The oldest daughter was accepted into college.
   4. A grandparent retired from a full-time job.

44. The nurse learns that the parents of a family are rarely at home and are not involved in the children's activities or interests. Which type of parenting style is represented by this family?

   1. Permissive.
   2. Uninvolved.
   3. Authoritative.
   4. Authoritarian.

45. The nurse prepares health promotion information for a family with a toddler. Which intervention does the nurse recommend to the parents?

   1. Place the child on its back to sleep.
   2. Provide headgear when the child plays outside.
   3. Place medications in a locked cabinet.
   4. Instruct about the dangers of drinking and driving.

46. The nurse is preparing to assess a family with small children. Why should the nurse focus on the family transition points during this assessment? **Select all that apply.**

   1. At transition points, the family has a large amount of time to plan.
   2. The family has to spend a great deal of money at transition points.
   3. At transition points, families are most likely to reorganize and change.
   4. Individuals within the family are at greatest risk for illness at transition points.
   5. Individuals within the family are most likely to change roles and related tasks at transition points.

47. The nurse prepares an educational seminar about families for a community health fair. What should the nurse explain as the overall major function(s) or task(s) of parents? **Select all that apply.**

   1. To help children learn to read.
   2. To provide food, shelter, and clothing.
   3. To socialize children into schools and the community.
   4. To encourage children to leave the home after college.
   5. To assist children in developing spiritual beliefs to guide daily tasks.

48. Which action(s) does the nurse take to promote well-being in a family with children? **Select all that apply.**

    1. Communicate with the family.
    2. Reinforce the use of discipline.
    3. Understand the family's routines.
    4. Encourage modeling positive behavior.
    5. Support development of parenting skills.

49. What are some behaviors nurses can model to embrace a family-centered care model in acute- and critical-care settings? **Select all that apply.**

    1. The nurse calls the family at home to communicate a change in a patient's condition.
    2. The nurse provides the family with explanations in understandable terms.
    3. The nurse spares the family any news about the patient's prognosis.
    4. The nurse keeps the family from having to assist with patient care.
    5. The nurse develops a trusting connection with family members and the patient.

50. How can hospital policies support family-centered care models?

    1. Banning cell phone use in the hospital.
    2. Asking families to leave during nurse bedside report.
    3. Providing clean, quiet waiting rooms with privacy and computer access.
    4. Limiting visitation hours to protect patients.

51. How can nurses improve communication with families and patients in the hospital setting?

    1. Use whiteboards effectively in patient rooms.
    2. Prevent families from visiting during rounds so they are not confused by jargon.
    3. Avoid going to waiting rooms to share information with families because of confidentiality.
    4. Allow the physician to share pertinent information so there is no confusion.

52. When the family has reached a decision to withdraw life-sustaining therapies (LSTs) in the hospital, what nursing action prepare and support the family?

    1. Informing family members that they should not touch the body.
    2. Telling the family that nursing care is now completed for the patient.
    3. Preparing the family members for when death appears imminent.
    4. Telling the family members that everyone must be present at the bedside during withdrawal of therapies.

53. As a nurse caring for a patient at high risk for dying, what can be done to improve advance care planning?

    1. Provide accurate, understandable information.
    2. Ask the provider if she or he is educated in advance care planning.
    3. Leave an advance directive form with the patient to fill out on admission to the unit.
    4. Tell the patient you will get an expert to talk to her or him about advance directives.

54. Which approach describes a growing trend in the care of individuals with a mental health condition?

    1. Use of family members as caregivers.
    2. Implementation of wraparound services in all communities.
    3. Practice of multigenerational assessments in all settings.
    4. Decreased use of psychotropic medications in the treatment.

55. The nurse learns that a client with a mental health condition has an 8-year-old child. What action should the nurse take?

    1. Arrange for another family member to care for the child.
    2. Complete a family-centered assessment of the child's needs.
    3. Discuss placing the client in a treatment center to protect the child.
    4. Identify medication that might help the child to be more helpful to the client.

56. The nurse provides care to a client with dementia. Which of the following

statements by the nurse is most appropriate when assisting this client with mealtime?

1. "Let me help you, honey."
2. "How can I help you, Mrs. Smith?"
3. "Oh my! You made a messy!"
4. "Let me feed you so you don't dirty your clothes."

57. A child with ADHD is prescribed a stimulant. What information regarding this medication should the nurse include when instructing the family? **Select all that apply.**

1. The stimulant can lead to slow bone growth.
2. A long-acting form of the stimulant is available.
3. Regular health checkups are required.
4. This medication will cure the disorder.
5. Impulsive behaviors will be eliminated.

58. The health care provider suggests that a family participate in psychoeducation. What should the nurse instruct the family to expect when participating in this type of instruction? **Select all that apply.**

1. Social support.
2. Family education.
3. Home-care support.
4. Training in coping skills.
5. Behavioral therapy techniques.

59. A family is concerned because one family member with schizophrenia frequently has violent outbursts. The nurse is working with the family to create a crisis plan. Which statement by the family would require further education?

1. "We need to identify a safe location."
2. "We need to know what dose of a sedative to give."
3. "We need to have insurance information easily available."
4. "We need to include suicide hotline telephone numbers."

60. A spouse plans to provide care at home to a client with a mental health condition. Which common task(s) should the nurse instruct the spouse to expect to perform when providing care? **Select all that apply.**

1. Providing companionship.
2. Offering emotional support.
3. Performing behavioral therapy.
4. Monitoring symptoms.
5. Attending group therapy.

61. The nurse learns that a family is providing care to a client with bipolar disorder. Which action by the nurse would not be appropriate when offering support to the family?

1. Not being critical when working with the family.
2. Not being judgmental when working with the family.
3. Assuring the family that cures are available.
4. Providing honest information.

62. The nurse prepares material to share during a community health fair. Which definition of *community* should the nurse keep in mind while preparing this material?

1. A group of vulnerable people.
2. A group of people with the same illness.
3. A group of people with similar characteristics.
4. A group of people living in the same environment.

63. The nurse prepares health promotion activities for a family. Which statement best describes the nurse's purpose for planning activities for this family?

1. To teach the family to resolve conflicts.
2. To improve or maintain the well-being of family members.
3. To help the family identify strengths and trust personal decisions.
4. To protect family members from diseases and their outcomes.

64. The nurse provides care to people within an urban community. What should be established in order for interventions to be successful?

1. The nurse-client relationship.
2. Payment for services provided.
3. Times when the nurse is available.
4. Frequency of visits to the families.

65. A family is having difficulty with health promotion activities. Which barrier(s) should the nurse realize is hindering this family's success if the family members are dealing with behavior modification? **Select all that apply**.

   1. Stress
   2. Conflict.
   3. Disinterest.
   4. Lack of time.
   5. Lack of money.

66. Which action(s) should the nurse take to reduce health inequities within a community? **Select all that apply.**

   1. Develop families' skills.
   2. Improve access to resources.
   3. Increase the use of home-care services.
   4. Reduce the cost for health care services.
   5. Increase participation in family care processes.

67. The nurse plans to visit families within a community. What should the nurse focus on when meeting with these families to reduce the risk for health disparities? **Select all that apply.**

   1. Ways to avoid injuries.
   2. Actions to maintain health.
   3. Strategies to manage chronic disease.
   4. Reasons to receive required immunizations.
   5. Approaches to adhere to prescribed eating plans.

Index

References followed by the letter "f" are for figures, "t" are for tables, and "b" are for boxes.